BMJ

clinical evidence concise

The international source of the best available evidence for effective health care

Editorial Office
BMJ Publishing Group, BMA House, Tavistock Square, London, WC1H 9JR, United Kingdom. Tel: +44 (0)20 7387 4499 • Fax: +44 (0)20 7383 6242 • www.bmjpg.com

Subscription prices for *BMJ Clinical Evidence*
BMJ Clinical Evidence Concise is published six monthly (June/December) by the BMJ Publishing Group. The annual subscription rates (for December, Issue 16 and June, Issue 17) are:

Print format
Personal: £107 • €158 • US$198
Institutional: £225 • €333 • US$416
Student/nurse: £53 • €78 • US$98

Online format
Personal: £129 • €191 • US$239
Student/nurse: £65 • €96 • US$120

Institutional subscriptions are for print editions only. Institutions may purchase online site licenses separately. For information on site licenses, and special combined rates if you wish to purchase print and online formats together, please visit the subscription pages of our website www.clinicalevidence.com or email us at CEsubscriptions@bmjgroup.com (UK and ROW) or clinevid@pmds.com (Americas). You may also telephone us or fax us on the following numbers:
UK and ROW Tel: +44 (0)20 7383 6270 • Fax: +44 (0)20 7383 6402
Americas Tel: +1 800 373 2897/240 646 7000 • Fax: +1 240 646 7005

Bulk subscriptions for societies and organisations
The Publishers offer discounts for any society or organisation buying bulk quantities for their members/specific groups. Please contact us at CEfeedback@bmjgroup.com.

Institutional site license
The Publishers offer institutions the opportunity to purchase online access to clinicalevidence.com. To discuss your institutional needs further please contact us at consortiasales@bmjgroup.com.

Rights and permission to reproduce
For information on translation rights, please contact Caroline Gomm at cgomm@bmjgroup.com.
To request permission to reprint all or part of any contribution in *BMJ Clinical Evidence* please contact Michelle Patten at mpatten@bmjgroup.com.

British Library Cataloguing in Publication Data. A catalogue record for this book is available from the British Library. ISSN 1475-9225, ISBN 1-905545-12-6.

Legal Disclaimer
The information contained in this publication, is intended for healthcare professionals. Categories presented in *BMJ Clinical Evidence* indicate a judgement about the strength of the evidence available to our authors prior to publication and the relative importance of benefits and harms.

We rely on our authors to confirm the accuracy of the information presented, and to describe generally accepted practices, and therefore we as the publisher, and our editors, cannot warrant its accuracy. Readers should be aware that professionals in the field may have different opinions. Because of this fact and also because of regular advances in medical research, we strongly recommend that readers independently verify specified treatments and drugs, including manufacturers' guidance. Also, the categories do not indicate whether a particular treatment is generally appropriate or whether it is suitable for a particular individual. Ultimately it is the readers' responsibility to make their own professional judgements, so to appropriately advise and treat their patients.

Description or reference to a product or publication does not imply endorsement of that product or publication, unless it is owned by the BMJ Publishing Group Limited.

To the fullest extent permitted by law, BMJ Publishing Group Limited and its editors, are not responsible for any losses, injury or damage caused to any person or property, (including under contract, by negligence, products liability or otherwise), whether they be direct or indirect, special, incidental or consequential, resulting from the application of the information in this publication.

Printed in Italy by Legoprint S.P.A.

Designed by Pete Wilder, The Designers Collective, London, UK.

Team and Advisors

Acknowledgements

The BMJ Publishing Group thanks the following people and organisations for their advice and support: The Cochrane Collaboration, and especially Iain Chalmers, Mike Clarke, Phil Alderson, and Carol Lefebvre; Tom Mann, Ron Stamp, Ben Toth, Veronica Fraser, and Nick Rosen; the British National Formulary, and especially Dinesh Mehta, Eric Connor, and John Martin; Martindale: The Complete Drug Reference, and especially Sean Sweetman; the Health Information Research Unit at McMaster University, and especially Brian Haynes and Ann McKibbon; the United Health Foundation (UHF), and especially Reed Tuckson and Yvette Krantz; Bazian Ltd, and especially Anna Donald and Vivek Muthu; previous staff who have contributed to this issue and the clinicians, epidemiologists, and members of patient groups who have acted as contributors, advisors, and peer reviewers.

The BMJ Publishing Group values the ongoing support it has received from the global medical community for *BMJ Clinical Evidence*. In addition to others, we wish to acknowledge the efforts of the UHF, who have provided educational funding to support wide dissemination to health professionals in the USA. We are grateful to the clinicians and patients who have taken part in focus groups, which are crucial to the development of *BMJ Clinical Evidence*. Finally, we would like to acknowledge the readers who have taken the time to send us their comments and suggestions.

Contents

BMJ Clinical Evidence is available in other non-English language editions. The Spanish translation (published in collaboration with the Iberoamerican Cochrane Centre and Legis) now comes in both formats: concise and online.[4] The full text is available in Russian[5] (seven broad speciality editions). The concise edition is also available in German[6], Hungarian[7] and Portuguese.[8] Finally, *BMJ Clinical Evidence* continues to be available free online to people in developing countries as part of the HINARI initiative spearheaded by the World Health Organization and the BMJ Publishing Group. Details of those countries that qualify are available from the *BMJ Clinical Evidence* website (www.clinicalevidence.com).

FEEDBACK

We encourage and appreciate all feedback via our website. You can contact us at CEfeedback@bmjgroup.com or use the 'Contact Us' button on every page. Alternatively, you can send a response for publication by clicking on the button on the left hand side of every webpage marked 'Your response'. Responses are screened before publication and may not be posted if they do not meet the requirements described in the guidance provided to potential correspondents. Users who do not have access to email or the website can contact the Editor of *BMJ Clinical Evidence*, Dr Charles Young, on +44 (0)20 7383 6257. We are particularly interested to know the clinical question that led you to consult *BMJ Clinical Evidence* and the extent to which this was answered. If you have comments on any of our content, or think that important evidence might have been missed, or have suggestion for new topics or questions please let us know.

Readers who would like to contribute either as authors or peer reviewers are also invited to send a letter and a brief CV or résumé to mpatten@bmjgroup.com.

REFERENCES

1. Kawamoto K, Houlihan CA, Balas EA, et al. Improving clinical practice using clinical decision support systems: a systematic review of trials to identify features critical to success. *BMJ*, doi:10.1136/bmj.38398.500764.8F (published 14 March 2005); accessed 22 March 2006.
2. 'User's Guides to the Medical Literature', The Evidence-Based Medicine Working Group. Edited by Guyatt G, Rennie D, AMA Press 2002.
3. *Clinical Evidence Conciso: La fonte delle migliori prove de efficacia per la pratica clinica*. Milan, Italy: Centro Cochrane Italiano/Editore Italiano/Editore Zadig, 2003.
4. *Evidencia Clinica*. Barcelona, Spain/Bogotá, Colombia: Asociacón Colaboración Cochrane Iberoamerican/Legis, 2004.
5. *Dokazatel'naya meditsina*. Moscow, Russia: Media Sphera Publishing Group, 2003.
6. *Kompendium evidenzbasierte Medizin*. Bern, Switzerland Verlag Hans Huber, 2004.
7. *Clinical Evidence Concise*. Budapest, Hungary: Medition Kiadó Kft, 2005.
8. *Evidência Clinica – Conciso*. Porto Alegre, Brazil: Artmed Editora SA, 2005.

and to read and respond. All 'responses' are screened before publication on the website. This service is very similar to the BMJ's successful **'Rapid Responses'** service and we have adopted the same publication policy for the responses that we receive.

To submit your comments, go to **'Your Responses'** in the left hand menu within each review, and follow the instructions. Examples received since the service opened include suggestions for research questions not yet covered within *BMJ Clinical Evidence*, and comments on how the research evidence relates to clinical practice. We hope that this will become a valued and well-used feature as the number of responses grows.

USER GROUPS AND WORKSHOPS

We have a well-established international advisory board for *BMJ Clinical Evidence* and its sister product *BestTreatments*. The aims of the board are to act as a sounding board to consider the direction of our products, to bring forward new ideas to meet our user and customer needs, and to extend the skill mix and expertise of people involved in creating our products. We have also set up a number of user groups. These are groups of nurses, general practitioners, junior doctors and patients that meet to allow us to market test our products and new ideas. Finally we are providing a series of educational workshops in evidence based medicine for clinicians in the UK. The aim of all these initiatives is to make sure we meet the needs of practicing clinicians and patients by continually interacting with these groups, by actively soliciting discussion and through feedback.

GOING BEYOND THE EVIDENCE

As a result of consistent feedback from clinicians about the need for *BMJ Clinical Evidence* to provide some interpretation of the evidence, we have changed our editorial policy of simply reporting the research for a given clinical situation, and highlighting gaps in current knowledge.

We now encourage our authors to provide some clinical interpretation of the evidence they are describing. This can be found in many topics and interventions under the heading **'Clinical Guide'** within the **'Comments'** section for interventions, on the website (www.clinical evidence.com). We are in the process of revising guidance to authors in order to develop this explanatory material further.

To support our policy of seeking to explain and contextualise evidence, within this Issue we are also pleased to include an article written by Stacey Sheridan, Assistant Professor of Medicine, University of North Carolina, USA, examining different approaches to primary prevention of ischaemic heart disease. This can be found adjacent to the Cardiovascular risk tables in Appendix 1.

ADDING 'DIAGNOSIS' TO *BMJ CLINICAL EVIDENCE*

We have undertaken preliminary work to include material on diagnosis within *BMJ Clinical Evidence*. In pursuit of this we have been fortunate to have the input of a range of experts in this field, including Paul Dieppe, Tonya Fancher and Richard Kravitz. Simultaneously, the Cochrane Collaboration is also planning the construction of a database of diagnostic research and systematic reviews which would further our potential coverage of evidence based diagnosis.

Already, we are incorporating diagnostic content within the background section of *BMJ Clinical Evidence* topics and are keen to ensure that this is as useful to healthcare professionals and patient users as possible. We would particularly value suggestions on how this material could be improved to increase its utility. This might include suggestions on preferred terminology, or whether approaches based on clinical presentations, symptoms and their differential diagnosis, or test interpretation would be most valuable.

INTERNATIONAL REACH

BMJ Clinical Evidence has an international circulation, reaching more than a million clinicians worldwide in six languages. In the USA, 500 000 clinicians will receive copies of the concise edition thanks to the United Health Foundation. In the UK, the National Health Services in Scotland and Wales fund the provision of free online access to a total of over 660 000 clinical staff. Additionally, the BMJ Publishing Group will distribute 40 000 copies of the concise edition to clinical staff in England. The BMA sends the concise edition to 10 500 UK medical students once a year. The governments of Norway and New Zealand now provide everyone in their countries with free online access, and thanks to the Italian Ministry of Health and the work of the Italian Cochrane Centre, 300 000 doctors in Italy receive a copy of the concise edition in Italian.[3]

Figure 1 illustrates the percentage of treatments falling into each category. Dividing treatments into categories is never easy. It always involves a degree of subjective judgement and is sometimes controversial. Why do we do it? Because users tell us it is helpful, but in the knowledge that clinical decisions must always be informed by more than simply the evidence,[2] and in particular informed by individual circumstances and patient's preferences. However, as Figure 1 shows, the research community still has a large task ahead. Even this assessment underestimates the extent of what is 'unknown' since within many of the treatments categorised as beneficial or potentially harmful, this may reflect only one comparison. So, for example, treatment A might be 'likely to be beneficial' because of proven benefit in comparison with placebo, but whether it is better or worse than treatment B may be unproven.

We are continuing to make use of what is 'unknown' in *BMJ Clinical Evidence* by feeding back to the UK NHS Health Technology Assessment Programme (HTA) with a view to help inform the commissioning of primary research. Every six months we evaluate *BMJ Clinical Evidence* interventions categorised as 'unknown effectiveness' and submit those fitting the appropriate criteria to the HTA via their website http://www.ncchta.org/.

OTHER PARTNERSHIPS

LINKS WITH THE JAMES LIND ALLIANCE

The James Lind Alliance has been established to build a coalition of organisations representing patients and clinicians, collaborating to confront important uncertainties about the effects of treatments. It aims to establish partnerships between patients and clinicians to identify and prioritise current uncertainties and to ensure that the future research agenda is informed by the priorities of these front line groups.

One important product of the James Lind Alliance will be the free access Database of Uncertainties about the Effectiveness of Treatments (DUET). The alliance will attempt to gather from both the public and healthcare professionals clinical questions for which there do not appear to be satisfactory evidence based answers at present. So far the conditions of particular interest include schizophrenia, asthma and epilepsy. Both we and the James Lind Alliance are keen to receive suggestions from any reader of *BMJ Clinical Evidence*, either via the usual *BMJ Clinical Evidence* feedback (CEfeedback@bmjgroup.com) or the 'Your Responses' facility, or directly to Charles Young on cyoung@bmjgroup.com. We will be pleased to pass on any suggested questions to the James Lind Alliance.

LINKS TO DRUG PRESCRIBING INFORMATION AND GUIDELINES

We are keen to support the drive to implement evidence based decision making in clinical practice. We are aware that one of the barriers to evidence based clinical decision making is the lack of a single resource for all the information needed during a clinical decision making process. Difficulties in accessing relevant information about therapeutic drugs can arise when the evidence about the clinical effects of therapeutic drugs is provided in one resource and practical prescribing information is provided by a different resource.

BMJ Clinical Evidence is the international source of the best available evidence, whereas the British National Formulary (BNF) provides practical information for UK healthcare professionals on selection and clinical use of medicines. UK-based healthcare professionals using the *BMJ Clinical Evidence* website will have noticed that we now link our content to the relevant sections of the BNF. These links are regularly updated to reflect changes in content of both *BMJ Clinical Evidence* and BNF. We are interested in exploring the possibilities of expanding this function to other countries and providing electronic links between *BMJ Clinical Evidence* content and location-specific drug-prescribing information.

BMJ Clinical Evidence also provides Drug Safety Alerts to warn clinicians about important adverse effects of therapeutic drugs. In addition we provide links to guidelines from around the world for practical information relating to our systematic reviews.

DEVELOPMENTS

'YOUR RESPONSES'

The *BMJ Clinical Evidence* website now has a **'Your Responses'** facility that appears in every systematic review and for every intervention. Users are encouraged to both post comments

Welcome to Issue 16

Welcome to Issue 16 of *BMJ Clinical Evidence*, the international source of the best available evidence on the effects of common clinical interventions. *BMJ Clinical Evidence* summarises the current state of knowledge and uncertainty about interventions used for prevention and treatment of important clinical conditions. To achieve this, we systematically search and appraise the world literature to provide rigorous systematic reviews of evidence on the benefits and harms of clinical interventions. Our aim is to support clinical decision making.

EVIDENCE BASED PRACTICE AT THE POINT OF CARE

Evidence based medicine (EBM) is well into its second decade, and yet worldwide the challenges of bringing EBM into clinical practice are a constant cause for debate.

In a systematic review published in the *BMJ*, Kawamoto, Houlihan, Balas and Lobach identified four features that, where present, improved the likelihood of clinical decision support systems improving practice:

- automatic provision of decision support as part of clinician workflow
- provision of recommendations rather than just assessments
- provision of decision support at the time and location of decision making
- and computer based decision support[1]

Of 32 systems possessing all four features, 30 (94%) significantly improved clinical practice. This review provides a guide to where evidence based resources should be positioning themselves in the future. We are very pleased that not only has *BMJ Clinical Evidence* been successfully integrated into clinical record systems, but we have also undertaken experimental work in which our content underpins different decision support applications.

HOW MUCH DO WE KNOW?

So what can *BMJ Clinical Evidence* tell us about the state of our current knowledge? In *BMJ Clinical Evidence* we try to summarise the evidence in order to support an effectiveness category:

- Beneficial
- Likely to be beneficial
- Trade off between benefits and harms
- Unlikely to be beneficial
- Likely to be ineffective or harmful
- Unknown effectiveness

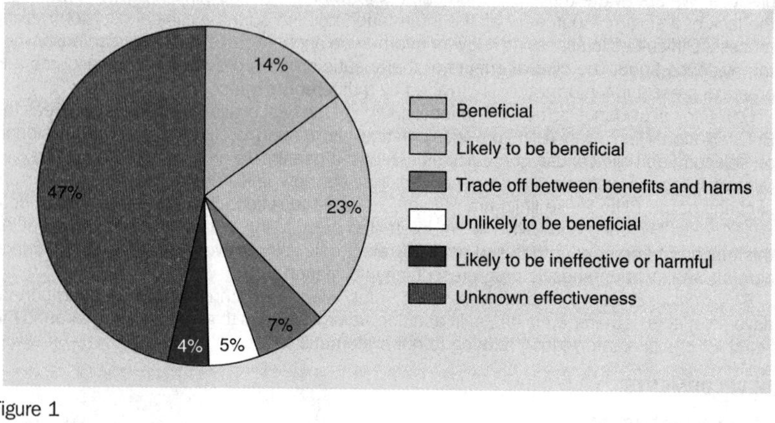

Figure 1

A guide to BMJ Clinical Evidence Concise

SUMMARY PAGE

BMJ Clinical Evidence Concise contains the summary information from the most recent version of each section of the *BMJ Clinical Evidence* website (www.clinicalevidence.com). It contains evidence relating to thousands of therapeutic or preventive interventions, derived from original research studies, and presents it in around 800 pages. For each condition, interventions are categorised according to whether they have been found to be effective or not. The full evidence detail behind these summaries, including clinical questions, figures, tables, and appendices, are featured online at www.clinicalevidence.com, along with quantified, referenced, and up to date information about each condition.

Making summaries involves discarding detail, and users of *BMJ Clinical Evidence Concise* need to be aware of the limitations of the evidence presented. It is not possible to make global statements that are both useful and apply to every patient or clinical context that occurs in practice. For example, when stating that we found evidence that a drug is beneficial, we mean that there is evidence that the drug has been shown to deliver more benefits than harms when assessed in at least one group of people, using at least one outcome at a particular point in time. It does not mean that the drug will be effective in all people given that treatment or that other outcomes will be improved, or even that the same outcome will be improved at a different time after the treatment.

MEASURE OF TREATMENT EFFECTS

The dilemma is how to present summaries that are useful but not misleading. We have experimented with providing statements with no numerical information at all, with NNTs only, with a batch of absolute and relative risks, or with just the odds ratio. Each measure has its advantages and disadvantages, and not all are available from the included studies. Quantitative results may be misleading in the absence of discussion of their precision, reliability, and applicability. In *BMJ Clinical Evidence Concise*, we present non-numerical information only. Detailed quantitative results are presented online, where we are able to discuss their interpretation in more detail. Your suggestions on improvements are welcome.

USING *BMJ CLINICAL EVIDENCE* ONLINE

BMJ Clinical Evidence Concise is intended to be used as a first point of call when trying to decide what the options for treatment might be. A detailed exploration of the evidence will require looking up the detail on *BMJ Clinical Evidence* online (www.clinicalevidence.com). The electronic versions link, whenever possible, to abstracts of the original research in PubMed or published online versions. In this way, *BMJ Clinical Evidence* is also designed to act as a pointer, connecting the clinician rapidly to the relevant original evidence.

INDEX PAGE

Each systematic review online contains a page which lists interventions and describes whether they have been found to be effective or not. Key Points provide a summary of the evidence and background information in the review. The full evidence detail supporting the categorisation, consisting of the question, a summary statement, benefits, harms, and a comment can be accessed by a hyperlink from the categorisation table or from the Key Points page. We would value your feedback on the presentation of interventions in future issues.

CATEGORISATION

We have developed these categories of effectiveness from one of the Cochrane Collaboration's first and most popular products, *A guide to effective care in pregnancy and childbirth*.[1] The categories are explained in the table below.

TABLE Categorisation of treatment effects in *BMJ Clinical Evidence*

Beneficial	Interventions for which effectiveness has been demonstrated by clear evidence from RCTs, or the best alternative source of information, and for which expectation of harms is small compared with the benefits.
Likely to be beneficial	Interventions for which effectiveness is less well established than for those listed under 'beneficial'.
Trade off between benefits and harms	Interventions for which clinicians and patients should weigh up the beneficial and harmful effects according to individual circumstances and priorities.
Unknown effectiveness	Interventions for which there are currently insufficient data or data of inadequate quality.
Unlikely to be beneficial	Interventions for which lack of effectiveness is less well established than for those listed under 'likely to be ineffective or harmful'.
Likely to be ineffective or harmful	Interventions for which ineffectiveness or harmfulness has been demonstrated by clear evidence.

Fitting interventions into these categories is not always straightforward. For one thing, the categories represent a mix of several hierarchies: the size of benefit (or harm), the strength of evidence (RCT or observational data), and the degree of certainty around the finding (represented by the confidence interval). Another problem is that much of the evidence most relevant to clinical decisions relates to comparisons between different interventions rather than to comparison with placebo or no intervention. Where necessary, we have indicated the comparisons. A third problem is that interventions may have been tested, or found to be effective, in only one group of people, such as those at high risk of an outcome. Again, we have indicated this where possible. But perhaps most difficult of all has been trying to maintain consistency across different systematic reviews. We continue to work on refining the criteria for putting interventions under each category.

Interventions that cannot be tested in an RCT for ethical or practical reasons are sometimes included in the categorisation table and are identified with an asterisk.

NEGATIVE FINDINGS

A surprisingly hard aspect to get right is the reporting of negative findings. Saying that there is no good evidence that a treatment works is not, of course, the same as saying that the treatment doesn't work. In trying to get this right, we may have erred too much on the side of caution; when in doubt, instead of saying, for example, that "the review found no difference", we say that "the review found no evidence of a difference". We recognise that, to get this right, we need a better handle on the power of individual systematic reviews and trials to demonstrate statistically significant differences between groups, and better information on what constitutes clinically important differences in the major outcomes for each intervention. In the meantime, we hope that the text makes a clear distinction between lack of benefit and lack of evidence of benefit.

OUTCOMES

BMJ Clinical Evidence focuses on outcomes that matter to patients, meaning those that patients themselves are aware of, such as symptom severity, quality of life, survival, disability, walking distance, and live birth rate. We are less interested in proxy outcomes such as blood lipid concentrations, blood pressure, or ovulation rates. Each systematic review includes a list of the main patient oriented outcomes, and where possible describes how these are measured. We have for the moment decided not to address the vexed question of what constitutes a clinically important change in an outcome, but we would welcome suggestions on how to do this.

EFFECTS, NOT EFFECTIVENESS

A key aim of *BMJ Clinical Evidence* is to emphasise the important trade offs between advantages and disadvantages of different treatment options. We therefore talk about the effects of interventions, both positive and negative, rather than the effectiveness, and for each question or intervention option we present data on benefits and harms under separate headings.

HARMS

Information about harms is often more difficult to synthesise than information about benefits.[2] Most controlled trials are designed to investigate benefits. Many either fail to document harms, or present the information in a form that is difficult to analyse or interpret. When drugs are licensed they may have been used clinically in only a few thousand people; the absence of documented harms is not strong evidence that harms will not be discovered in the years after licensing.

BMJ Clinical Evidence recognises that the evidence about harms is often weaker than that about benefits. In an attempt to correct for this bias, *BMJ Clinical Evidence* has lowered the threshold for evidence to be included in the harms section. Much of the evidence for harms comes from observational studies ranging from prospective controlled cohort studies to case reports, and these are included when the harm is serious or when there is good corroborating evidence that the harm can be attributed to the treatment.

AN INTERNATIONAL APPROACH

BMJ Clinical Evidence takes an international approach to the evidence. This means including drugs that are not licensed in some countries. It also means keeping in mind the practicalities of treating people in poorer countries, by covering some interventions even if they have been superseded (for example, single drug treatment for HIV infection as opposed to three drug treatment).

REFERENCES

Full references to the individual studies cited in *BMJ Clinical Evidence Concise* are available online. References cited in the definition, incidence/prevalence, aetiology/risk factors, and prognosis sections are listed in the text but are available as hyperlinks from the equivalent section online.

SYSTEMATIC REVIEW GLOSSARY

Reviews may contain glossary listings; these are available in full online and can be accessed from the hyperlinks within the review.

TABLES AND FIGURES

The presence of figures and tables online are flagged up in a similar way to the glossary with the use of Ⓕ for figures and Ⓣ for tables.

FEEDBACK

The design of *BMJ Clinical Evidence Concise* will change progressively over the next few years. We will perform evaluation studies ourselves to measure the relevance of the material to the questions being asked in practice, the ease of use, and to check that the message extracted from the summary corresponds closely with that intended. If you have any comments, suggestions, or detect any errors, please let us know at CEfeedback@bmjgroup.com.

For more information on any of our products or processes, please visit our website at www.clinicalevidence.com.

REFERENCES

1. Enkin M, Keirse M, Renfrew M, et al. *A guide to effective care in pregnancy and childbirth*. Oxford: Oxford University Press, 1998.
2. Derry S, Loke YK, Aronson JK. Incomplete evidence: the inadequacy of databases in tracing published adverse drug reactions in clinical trials. BMC Medical Research Methodology 2001;1:7. http://www.biomedcentral.com/1471-2288/1/7 (last accessed 13 October 2003).
3. Smith R. Beyond conflict of interest. BMJ 1998;317:219–292.

Hodgkin's lymphoma

Search date May 2005

Evangelos Terpos and Amin Rahemtulla

What are the effects of single regimen chemotherapy treatments for first presentation stage 1 or 2 non-bulky disease?

BENEFICIAL

ABVD (as effective as combined regimens with radiotherapy but with fewer adverse effects) *New*

One RCT found no significant difference between ABVD alone and radiotherapy in progression free or overall survival at 5 years in those with favourable prognostic factors. Two RCTs found no significant difference in overall survival between ABVD alone and ABVD plus extended field radiotherapy at 5 years but found different results for progression free survival. One RCT found that ABVD reduced permanent azoospermia compared with MOPP. One prospective cohort study found that ABVD was associated with pulmonary toxicity, commonly producing cough and dyspnoea during treatment, and rarely death. Despite a lack of direct comparisons, ABVD is generally preferred to MOPP due to its lower toxicity and similar effectiveness.

TRADE OFF BETWEEN BENEFITS AND HARMS

MOPP *New*

One RCT found no significant difference between MOPP chemotherapy (6 cycles) and radiotherapy alone in disease free or overall survival at a median follow up of 7.5 years. It also found that MOPP chemotherapy increased hospital admissions, episodes of febrile neutropenia, documented infections, and blood transfusions compared with radiotherapy alone. One RCT found that MOPP chemotherapy increased permanent azoospermia compared with ABVD chemotherapy. Despite a lack of direct comparisons, ABVD is generally preferred to MOPP due to its lower toxicity and similar effectiveness.

What are the effects of combined chemotherapy and radiotherapy treatments compared with radiotherapy alone for first presentation stage 1 or 2 non-bulky disease?

TRADE OFF BETWEEN BENEFITS AND HARMS

MOPP plus radiotherapy *New*

One systematic review found that MOPP plus radiotherapy increased relapse free survival and decreased mortality from refractory disease at 10 years compared with radiotherapy alone in people with early stage Hodgkin's lymphoma. There was no significant difference between treatments in overall survival. One additional RCT found similar results but another found no significant difference between treatments in 10 year relapse free survival or overall survival. Common adverse effects with MOPP plus radiotherapy included paresthesias and anaemia. Despite a lack of direct comparisons, ABVD is generally preferred to MOPP due to its lower toxicity and similar effectiveness.

Hodgkin's lymphoma

UNLIKELY TO BE BENEFICIAL

VBM plus radiotherapy *New*

One small RCT found no significant difference between VBM plus radiotherapy and radiotherapy alone in disease free or overall survival at 5 years.

What are the effects of combined chemotherapy and radiotherapy treatments compared with the same chemotherapy agent alone for first presentation stage 1 or 2 non-bulky disease?

BENEFICIAL

ABVD plus radiotherapy* *New*

Two RCTs found no significant difference in overall survival between ABVD alone and ABVD plus extended field radiotherapy in overall survival at 60 months. One of them also found no significant difference in complete remission and progression free survival but the other RCT found that ABVD plus radiotherapy reduced progression free survival at 5 years compared with ABVD (6 cycles). Despite the lack of robust RCT evidence, two to four cycles of ABVD in combination with 20–30 Gy involved field radiotherapy is considered the international gold standard for early stage Hodgkin's lymphoma.

UNLIKELY TO BE BENEFICIAL

CVPP plus radiotherapy *New*

One RCT found no significant difference between CVPP plus radiotherapy and CVPP alone (6 cycles) at 7 years in people with a favourable prognosis. Subgroup analysis found that combination therapy increased disease free but not overall survival in people with an unfavourable prognosis.

What are the effects of specific combined chemotherapy and radiotherapy treatments versus each other in stage 1 or 2 non-bulky disease?

BENEFICIAL

ABVD plus radiotherapy (improved progression free survival compared with MOPP plus radiotherapy and less gonadal toxicity) *New*

One RCT found that ABVD plus radiotherapy increased 6 year progression free survival but not overall survival compared with MOPP plus radiotherapy. It also found that ABVD plus radiotherapy increased the proportion of people with a normal spermogram at 1 year compared with MOPP plus radiotherapy. Two to four cycles of ABVD is considered the international gold standard for early stage Hodgkin's disease in combination with 20–30 Gy involved field radiotherapy.

UNLIKELY TO BE BENEFICIAL

EBPV plus radiotherapy (reduced failure free survival compared with MOPP-ABV plus radiotherapy) *New*

One RCT found that EBVP plus radiotherapy reduced failure free but not overall survival compared with MOPP-ABV plus radiotherapy.

What are the effects of different radiotherapy treatment strategies in stage 1 or 2 non-bulky disease?

BENEFICIAL

Involved field radiotherapy (as effective as extended field radiotherapy with less adverse effects) *New*

Five RCTs found no significant difference in overall survival between involved field and extended field radiotherapy between 4 and 25 years. Involved field radiotherapy also reduced the proportion of people with radiotherapy related complications, the most common of which were pulmonary.

UNKNOWN EFFECTIVENESS

Increased dose regimens *New*

Two RCTs provided insufficient evidence to assess the effectiveness of different dose regimens in the treatment of early stage Hodgkin's disease.

What are the effects of single regimen chemotherapy treatments for first presentation stage 2 bulky disease, stage 3, or stage 4 disease?

BENEFICIAL

ABVD *New*

One RCT found that both ABVD and ABVD plus MOPP increased complete remission post treatment and disease free survival compared with MOPP but there was no significant difference in overall survival at 5 years. One RCT found no significant difference between ABVD and MOPP plus ABV in complete remission post treatment, disease free survival, and overall survival at 5 years. One RCT found that ABVD increased complete remission, and failure free survival at 3 years but not overall survival compared with Stanford V. One RCT found that both MEC and ABVD increased complete remission and failure free survival at 3 years, but not overall survival compared with Stanford V. Expert consensus is that ABVD presently demonstrates the best combination of efficacy and toxicity and should be considered the gold standard of care for advanced stage Hodgkin's lymphoma (with or without consolidative radiotherapy).

TRADE OFF BETWEEN BENEFITS AND HARMS

MOPP *New*

One RCT found that MOPP decreased complete remission post treatment and disease free survival compared with ABVD but there was no significant difference in overall survival at 5 years. Three RCTs found that MOPP reduced complete clearance post treatment and disease free survival but not overall survival compared with ABVD plus MOPP. RCTs found that MOPP increased adverse effects such as life threatening leukaemia and permanent azoospermia compared with ABVD.

Hodgkin's lymphoma

What are the effects of dose intensified chemotherapy treatments for first presentation stage 2 bulky disease, stage 3, or stage 4 disease?

TRADE OFF BETWEEN BENEFITS AND HARMS

Escalating dose BEACOPP (more effective than COPP-ABVD but increased adverse effects) New

One RCT found that escalating dose BEACOPP increased freedom from treatment failure and overall survival at 5 years compared with COPP-ABVD and fixed dose BEACOPP. It also found that escalating dose BEACOPP increased the proportion of men with sterility, haematological adverse effects, and acute myeloid dysplastic syndrome compared with COPP-ABVD and BEACOPP.

UNKNOWN EFFECTIVENESS

ChlVPP-EVA (more effective than VAPEC-B) New

One RCT found that ChlVPP-EVA increased freedom from progression, event free survival, and overall survival at 5 years compared with VAPEC-B. More RCTs are required to asses the effectiveness and safety of ChlVPP-EVA and VAPEC-B compared with standard treatments in Hodgkin's disease.

What are the effects of combined chemotherapy plus radiotherapy treatments compared with chemotherapy alone for first presentation stage 2 bulky disease, stage 3, or stage 4 disease?

UNLIKELY TO BE BENEFICIAL

ABVPP plus radiotherapy New

One RCT found that ABVPP plus radiotherapy reduced overall survival at 5 years compared with ABVPP alone, after induction with ABVPP.

COPP-ABVD plus radiotherapy New

One RCT found no significant difference between COPP plus ABVD compared with radiotherapy alone in the proportion of people who relapsed at 8 weeks, after induction with COPP plus ABVD.

MOPP-ABV plus radiotherapy New

Two RCTs found no significant difference between MOPP-ABV plus radiotherapy and MOPP-ABV alone in disease free or overall survival at 5 years, after induction with MOPP-ABV.

MOPP plus radiotherapy New

A systematic review found no significant difference between MOPP plus radiotherapy and MOPP alone in overall survival at 10 years, after induction with MOPP.

*Categorisation based on consensus.

DEFINITION Hodgkin's lymphoma, also known as Hodgkin's disease, is a malignancy of the lymph nodes and lymphatic system. The majority of people present with an enlarged but otherwise asymptomatic lump, most often in the lower neck or supraclavicular region. Mediastinal masses are frequent and are revealed after routine chest X rays. Approximately one fourth of people present systemic symptoms at diagnosis, such as unexplained fever, profuse sweating, fatigue, itchy skin, and unexplained weight loss. Hepatosplenomegaly, anaemia, lymphocytopenia, and eosinophilia are also non-specific manifestations of the disease. Hodgkin's lymphoma is categorised according to appearance under the microscope (histology) and extent of disease (stage). **Histology:** Diagnosis is based on the recognition of Reed-Stenberg cells and/or Hodgkin cells in an appropriate cellular background in tissue sections from a lymph node or another organ, such as the bone marrow, lung, or bone. Fine needle aspiration biopsy is not adequate for diagnosis of Hodgkin's lymphoma; an open biopsy is always required.[1] Reed-Stenberg cells are typically multinucleated giant cells, which, in 98% of cases, are thought to be derived from the germinal centre of peripheral B cells.[2,3] The WHO classification is based on histological subtype (see table 1Ⓣ). The distribution of histological subtypes varies between age groups, with young adults reportedly showing a greater proportion of nodular sclerosis compared with older adults.[4] Nodular lymphocyte predominant (LP) Hodgkin's lymphoma is a rare subtype which usually has a more indolent natural history, and is often treated differently.[5] This subtype has been excluded in the trials of this review. **Stage:** There are several different staging classification systems for Hodgkin's lymphoma. Computerised tomography scanning is the major method of staging both intra-thoracic and intra-abdominal disease, while bone marrow trephine biopsy is used for the detection of marrow infiltration by malignant cells. Magnetic resonance imaging (MRI) scanning and fluorodeoxyglucose positron emission tomography (FDG-PET) scanning may also have a role in Hodgkin's lymphoma staging, mainly by revealing disease in sites difficult to be discovered by computerised tomography imaging. Classification systems include the Ann Arbor classification (see table 2Ⓣ)[6] and the Cotswolds (see table 3Ⓣ). Staging methods have changed substantially over the last 20 years. Staging laparotomy with splenectomy is no longer routine practice due to a number of possible complications (including post-splenectomy sepsis, small bowel obstruction, and even mortality), delay to the start of treatment, similar survival rates between people with or without a staging laparotomy, and the introduction of combined modality treatment for all stages.[7-9] **Population:** For the purposes of this review, we considered adults with a first presentation of Hodgkin's lymphoma. We considered treatments separately in two groups of people: stage I or II non-bulky disease, and II (bulky), III, or IV disease; most studies used the Ann-Arbor classification system.

INCIDENCE/ PREVALENCE The annual incidence of Hodgkin's lymphoma is about 3/100 000 in the UK, without any very large variations in incidence or in nature between countries or population groups.[10] However, the age distribution of Hodgkin's lymphoma differs across geographical areas as well as ethnic groups. In the developed world, there is a bimodal age distribution with peaks at 15–34 years and over 60 years with nodular sclerosis being the most common subtype.[11] Early stage nodular sclerosis Hodgkin's lymphoma is the most common form in children living in developed countries, but advanced mixed cellularity and lymphocyte rich subtypes are seen most commonly in developing countries.[12,13] In children in Europe and the USA, incidence in men is double that of incidence in women, but in adolescents there is an equal distribution between sexes.[14] The incidence rate of Hodgkin's lymphoma in general increases with the level of economic development.[15]

AETIOLOGY/ RISK FACTORS The exact cause of Hodgkin's lymphoma remains unclear. However, it is well accepted that Hodgkin's lymphoma is a heterogeneous condition that most probably consists of more than one aetiological entity. The Epstein Barr virus has been implicated in the development of Hodgkin's lymphoma, but this association varies with age, with positivity being most prominent in children and the elderly. Epstein Barr virus positivity is high in childhood Hodgkin's lymphoma worldwide, but low in adolescents in developed countries with nodular sclerosis Hodgkin's lymphoma. Histological subtype, age, sex, socioeconomic status,

Hodgkin's lymphoma

and ethnic background have all been shown to influence the association between the Epstein Barr virus and Hodgkin's lymphoma.[16] Although the pathogenesis of Hodgkin's disease is not yet fully understood, the nature of the Hodgkin/Reed-Stenberg (H/RS) cell has been recognised. The H/RS cell is derived from a B lymphocyte with clonal rearrangements in the V, D, and J segments of the IgH chain locus. Regulation of Fas mediated apoptosis, and the nuclear factor-kappa B pathway seem to be strongly implicated in the pathogenesis of Hodgkin's lymphoma.[2]

PROGNOSIS **Overall survival:** The outcome in both localised and advanced Hodgkin's lymphoma has improved greatly over the last 20 years. The disease is now considered curable in the majority of cases. Even if first line treatment fails, the person may be cured later. Therefore, the doctors confront the dilemma of whether it is better to use more intensive therapy initially to cure the maximum number of people possible or whether it is better to use less aggressive therapy initially and rely on more intensive salvage therapy in a greater proportion of people. The overall survival differs in terms of disease extent. People with localised disease (stage I/II) have a 6 year overall survival of more than 90% even in poor risk groups. People with advanced disease (stage III/IV) have a 5 year overall survival of almost 85%.[17] **Relapse:** The event free survival at 4 years is near 99% for people with localised disease and almost 80% in people with advanced disease.[17] **Prognostic indicators:** Despite an enormous effort to define clinically relevant and generally acceptable prognostic factors, stage and systemic B cell symptoms are still the two major determinants for stratifying people with Hodgkin's lymphoma. Bulky disease (> 10 cm nodal mass) has recently emerged as a third prognostic factor that meets general acceptance. In the USA, most centres treat people according to the traditional classifications of early stages (I–IIA or B) and advanced stages (III–IVA or B; I–IIB with bulky disease), which is the classification used for the purposes of this review. Additional prognostic factors often used in adults are shown in table 4 ❶. The International Prognostic Score (IPS) has been used by several study groups that are currently tailoring treatment strategies at first diagnosis depending on the risk for treatment failure (IPS 0–2 and 3–7), but stratifying people on the basis of the IPS is still an experimental approach (see table 4 ❶).[18] Another group looked at prognostic factors specifically for children and young adults with Hodgkin's disease treated with combined modality treatment. They analysed 328 people aged 2–20 years old (48% were aged > 14 years) and multivariate analysis identified five pretreatment factors that correlated with inferior disease free survival: male sex; stage IIB, IIIB, or IV disease; bulky mediastinal disease; white blood count of more than 13.5×10^9 /L; and haemoglobin less than 11.0 g/dL. In the study, age was not a significant prognostic factor (≤ 14 years compared with > 14 years old). Using this prognostic score, people with Hodgkin's lymphoma could be stratified into four groups with significantly different 5 year disease free survivals. Response to initial chemotherapy was also shown to be a predictor of outcome.[19] Other paediatric studies found nodular sclerosis histology and B symptoms also correlated with inferior outcome.[20,21]

Please refer to clinicalevidence.com for full text and references.

Myeloma (multiple)

Search date November 2004

Ambuj Kumar and Benjamin Djulbegovic

What are the effects of treatment in people with asymptomatic early stage multiple myeloma (stage I)?

UNLIKELY TO BE BENEFICIAL

Early chemotherapy plus corticosteroids in stage I disease (no benefit over deferred treatment)

One systematic review of three small RCTs found that early chemotherapy plus corticosteroids in people with early stage multiple myeloma reduced disease progression compared with deferred treatment. However, it found no significant difference between early and deferred treatment in response rate or survival. The RCTs included in the review are likely to have been underpowered to detect clinically important differences in survival.

What are the effects of first line treatments in people with advanced stage multiple myeloma (stages II and III)?

BENEFICIAL

Adding prednisolone to single agent chemotherapy (increased survival compared with melphalan alone)

One RCT found that adding prednisolone to melphalan increased survival compared with melphalan alone. Another RCT found that in people with favourable prognostic features adding prednisolone to melphalan increased median survival compared with melphalan. However, it found that in people with poor prognostic features adding prednisolone to melphalan reduced median survival and increased severe and fatal infections compared with melphalan alone, although the significance of these findings was unclear. One RCT found no significant difference in survival between melphalan plus prednisolone and cyclophosphamide.

Combination chemotherapy (increased survival compared with melphalan)

One RCT found that combination chemotherapy (adriamycin plus carmustine plus cyclophosphamide plus melphalan) increased survival compared with melphalan.

Combination chemotherapy plus corticosteroids (similar survival with different regimens, no survival benefit compared with melphalan plus prednisolone or cyclophosphamide)

One RCT found that adding increased dose cyclophosphamide and prednisolone to a regimen of vincristine plus carmustine plus melphalan plus cyclophosphamide plus prednisolone did not improve overall response or survival. One RCT found that adding ranimustine to a regimen of cyclophosphamide plus vincristine plus melphalan plus prednisolone did not improve response or survival. One RCT found no significant difference between cyclophosphamide and combination chemotherapy (cyclophosphamide plus melphalan plus prednisolone plus lomustine). One systematic review and two subsequent RCTs found no significant difference in survival between melphalan plus prednisolone and combination chemotherapy plus prednisolone.

Myeloma (multiple)

High dose chemotherapy plus stem cell rescue (increased survival compared with conventional dose chemotherapy)

Two RCTs, which randomised participants at diagnosis, found that high dose chemotherapy plus stem cell rescue increased progression free survival and overall survival compared with conventional dose chemotherapy. One RCT, which randomised participants only if they responded to initial chemotherapy, found that high dose chemotherapy plus stem cell rescue increased complete remission rate compared with conventional dose chemotherapy. It found no significant difference in progression free survival and similar overall survival between groups. Two further RCTs were published in abstract form only, so we could not assess study quality fully.

High dose melphalan conditioning regimen before autologous stem cell transplantation (increased overall survival compared with melphalan plus total body irradiation)

One RCT found limited evidence that high dose melphalan alone (200 mg/m^2) increased overall survival, but not event free survival compared with high dose melphalan (140 mg/m^2) plus total body irradiation (8 Gy). Melphalan plus total body irradiation increased severe mucositis and the duration of neutropenia compared with melphalan alone. There was also a trend towards increased treatment related mortality with melphalan plus total body irradiation.

Intermediate dose chemotherapy plus stem cell rescue (increased survival compared with conventional dose chemotherapy)

One RCT found that in people aged 50–70 years old, intermediate dose melphalan plus stem cell rescue improved response rate, event free survival, and overall survival compared with conventional dose chemotherapy. One RCT found that intermediate dose chemotherapy plus myeloablative therapy plus autologous stem cell rescue increased complete remission compared with intermediate dose chemotherapy alone, but it found no significant difference in survival.

Relative effectiveness of different single agent chemotherapy plus corticosteroid regimens (similar survival with bendamustine plus prednisolone, melphalan plus prednisolone, or melphalan plus dexamethasone)

One RCT found that bendamustine plus prednisolone increased complete response and progression free survival compared with melphalan plus prednisolone. Median overall survival was similar in both groups. One RCT found no significant difference in survival between melphalan plus prednisolone and melphalan plus dexamethasone.

Relative effectiveness of different single agent chemotherapy regimens (similar survival with melphalan, cyclophosphamide, lomustine, and carmustine)

Two RCTs found no significant difference between cyclophosphamide and melphalan in survival. One RCT provided limited evidence that melphalan increased overall response but not survival compared with lomustine or carmustine.

Single agent chemotherapy (more effective than placebo)

We found no systematic review comparing chemotherapy versus placebo solely in people with multiple myeloma who had not received previous treatment, although we found two RCTs in people who had received previous treatment. There is consensus that chemotherapy is beneficial for the treatment of multiple myeloma.

LIKELY TO BE BENEFICIAL

Autologous stem cell transplant (increased survival compared with allogeneic transplant)

We found no systematic review, RCTs, or prospective cohort studies. Two retrospective comparative case matched analyses found that syngeneic transplantation in multiple myeloma increased survival compared with autologous transplant if a twin donor was available. If a twin donor was not available, autologous stem cell transplantation increased survival compared with allogeneic bone marrow transplant. Treatment related toxicity was higher with allogeneic bone marrow transplant than with autologous stem cell transplantation. These are best available data to date.

Peripheral blood stem cells (similar survival, reduces duration of neutropenia and thrombocytopenia compared with bone marrow stem cells)

One RCT found no significant difference between autologous peripheral blood stem cells and bone marrow transplant in response, event free survival, or overall survival. However, it found that peripheral blood stem cell transplant reduced the duration of neutropenia and thrombocytopenia compared with bone marrow transplant.

Syngeneic transplantation (increased survival compared with autologous transplant if a twin donor was available)

We found no systematic review, RCTs, or prospective cohort studies. Two retrospective comparative case matched analyses found that syngeneic transplantation in multiple myeloma increased survival compared with autologous transplant if a twin donor was available.

Timing of autologous stem cell transplant (increased event free survival compared with late transplantation)

One RCT found that early autologous stem cell transplantation increased event free survival compared with late autologous stem cell transplantation. It found no significant difference in overall survival.

TRADE OFF BETWEEN BENEFITS AND HARMS

Interferon

One systematic review and two subsequent RCTs found that adding interferon to chemotherapy in induction or maintenance phase increased response and progression free survival, although they found no significant difference in overall survival. The review and RCTs found that interferon increased toxicity.

Optimum priming regimen

One RCT found that stem cell factor plus filgrastim plus cyclophosphamide enhanced yield of CD34+ after a single leukapheresis compared with filgrastim plus cyclophosphamide. It also found that stem cell factor plus filgrastim plus cyclophosphamide increased treatment related adverse events. One RCT found that filgrastim alone reduced the time taken to collect peripheral blood progenitor cells compared with filgrastim plus cyclophosphamide, and filgrastim plus cyclophosphamide increased admission to hospital, fever, and pneumonia/sepsis compared with filgrastim alone.

Myeloma (multiple)

UNKNOWN EFFECTIVENESS

Bortezomib

We found no systematic review or RCTs of bortezomib as first line treatment for multiple myeloma.

Double versus single autologous transplant

One RCT found that in people who have received high dose chemotherapy, double autologous stem cell transplant increased event free and overall survival at 7 years compared with single autologous stem cell transplant.

Non-myeloablative allogeneic stem cell transplant (reduced intensity conditioning, mini-transplant)

One non-randomised study with historical control found no significant difference in overall survival between non-myeloablative transplant and conventional allogeneic bone marrow transplant, but low treatment related mortality with mini-transplants. These are best available data to date.

Thalidomide and thalidomide derivatives

We found no systematic review or RCTs of thalidomide or its derivatives, published as a full paper, for the first line treatment of advanced stage multiple myeloma.

UNLIKELY TO BE BENEFICIAL

Purging of autologous stem cells

One RCT found that purging autologous stem cells reduced myeloma cell contamination in peripheral blood cell collection. However, it found no significant difference in survival between selected and unselected cell autograft.

LIKELY TO BE INEFFECTIVE OR HARMFUL

Allogeneic stem cell transplant (increased treatment related mortality compared with autologous transplant)

We found no systematic review, RCTs, or prospective cohort studies. Two retrospective comparative case-matched analyses found that autologous stem cell transplantation increased survival compared with allogeneic bone marrow transplant. Treatment related toxicity was higher with allogeneic bone marrow transplant. These are best available data to date.

What are the effect of salvage treatments in people with advanced stage multiple myeloma (stages II and III)?

BENEFICIAL

Bortezomib

We found one RCT of bortezomib for salvage treatment of advanced multiple myeloma. It found that bortezomib increased response rate, time to progression, and overall survival compared with dexamethasone.

UNLIKELY TO BE BENEFICIAL

Salvage therapy regimens

Eleven RCTs found no significant difference in response and survival between different salvage therapy regimens.

What are the effect of treatments (supportive therapy) in people with advanced stage multiple myeloma (stages II and III)?

BENEFICIAL

Bisphosphonates

One systematic review found that bisphosphonates, particularly pamidronate and clodronate, reduced skeletal fractures and pain compared with placebo or no therapy. One RCT in people with multiple myeloma or breast carcinoma found no difference between zoledronic acid and pamidronate.

LIKELY TO BE BENEFICIAL

Epoetin alpha

One systematic review found that epoetin alpha improved anaemia compared with placebo or no therapy.

TRADE OFF BETWEEN BENEFITS AND HARMS

Infection prophylaxis

One systematic review found that trimethoprim–sulphamethoxazole and immunoglobulin reduced infections, although they may increase toxicity.

UNKNOWN EFFECTIVENESS

Plasmapheresis

Two small RCTs found that plasmapheresis improved renal function in people with multiple myeloma.

DEFINITION Multiple myeloma is characterised by neoplastic proliferation of plasma cells, mainly contained within the bone marrow. It is a debilitating malignancy that is part of a spectrum of diseases ranging from monoclonal gammopathy of unknown significance (MGUS) to plasma cell leukaemia.[1] Multiple myeloma can present outside the bone marrow as solitary plasmacytoma or extramedullary plasmacytoma; however, this chapter does not currently deal with these forms. The most common symptoms of multiple myeloma are those relating to anaemia, renal dysfunction, infections, or bone lesions. Multiple myeloma is most common in people over the age of 40 years. A diagnosis of symptomatic myeloma requires the presence of monoclonal protein (M-protein) in serum, urine, or both; bone marrow clonal plasma cells (> 10%) or plasmacytoma; and related organ or tissue impairment (ROTI) (see table 1)Ⓣ. Ninety-seven per cent of people with multiple myeloma have a presence of M-protein in serum, urine, or both. A diagnosis of asymptomatic myeloma (also known as smouldering myeloma) requires the presence of M-protein in serum of 30 g/L or more, bone marrow clonal plasma cells of 10% or more, or both, and no ROTI or symptoms. The most common differential diagnoses of symptomatic multiple myeloma are MGUS and asymptomatic (smouldering) multiple myeloma (see table 2)Ⓣ.[2,3] Other less common differential diagnoses include non-secretory myeloma, solitary and extramedullary plasmacytoma, plasma cell leukaemia, primary systemic amyloidosis, and Waldenstorm's macroglobulinaemia and other non-Hodgkin's lymphoma. Durie and Salmon proposed the initial clinical staging system for

Myeloma (multiple)

multiple myeloma in 1975.[4] People with Durie Salmon stage I disease are usually asymptomatic (see table 3)🅣. In addition to the World Health Organization classification,[5] a new international staging system for multiple myeloma was recently proposed, based on clinical and laboratory data from 10 750 people with previously untreated symptomatic myeloma (see table 4)🅣.[6]

INCIDENCE/ PREVALENCE Multiple myeloma is the most common primary cancer of the bones in adults, representing about 1% of all cancers diagnosed in the US in 2004 and 14% of all haematological malignancies.[7] The annual incidence of multiple myeloma in the US is three or four cases per 100 000 population[8] and prevalence is 43 cases per 100 000.[9] In the UK, multiple myeloma accounts for 1% of all new cases of cancer diagnosed each year.[10] In 2001, the incidence of multiple myeloma in the UK was 6.1 cases per 100 000 population.[10]

AETIOLOGY/ RISK FACTORS The exact aetiology of multiple myeloma remains unclear.[1] Genetic and environmental factors have been associated with the occurrence of multiple myeloma. However, evidence linking the genetic or environmental factors has not been substantiated.[1]

PROGNOSIS Currently, no cure is available for multiple myeloma. The recently proposed new international staging system for multiple myeloma found median survival to be 29–62 months, based on clinical and laboratory data from 10 750 people with previously untreated symptomatic myeloma (see table 4)🅣.[6]

Please refer to clinicalevidence.com for full text and references.

Non-Hodgkin's lymphoma (diffuse large B cell lymphoma)

Search date April 2006

Ellen R Copson and J. Paul Kerr

What are the effects of first line treatments for aggressive non-Hodgkin's lymphoma (diffuse large B cell lymphoma)?

BENEFICIAL

CHOP 21 (no alternative regimen [MACOP-B, m-BACOD, ProMACE-CytaBOM, PACEBOM] shown to be superior)

CHOP 21 is the standard treatment for aggressive non-Hodgkin's lymphoma (not including Burkitt's lymphoma), and placebo controlled trials or no treatment would be considered unethical. Six RCTs identified by two systematic reviews found that MACOP-B, m-BACOD, ProMACE-CytaBOM, and PACEBOM were not consistently superior to CHOP 21 in terms of overall survival. Toxicity was generally similar with these different regimens. Two RCTs comparing CHOP 21 versus CHOEP found a superior complete response rate and 5 year event free survival with CHOEP but with increased toxicity. Two RCTs (one in people with low risk, localised lymphoma and the other in people with poor prognosis, aggressive lymphoma) found no difference in complete response rates between CHOP plus radiotherapy and ACVBP; however, they found that ACVBP increased 5 year event free survival and overall survival, but increased treatment related deaths and other adverse effects. For data on CHOP 21 in combination with radiotherapy or rituximab, or for data comparing CHOP 21 versus CHOP 14, see separate options.

CHOP 21 plus radiotherapy (increases disease free survival compared with CHOP 21 alone)

One RCT identified by a systematic review found that short schedule CHOP 21 (3 cycles) plus radiotherapy improved 5 year progression free survival and overall survival compared with longer schedule CHOP 21 (8 cycles) alone in people with early stage disease. Longer schedule CHOP 21 alone increased the risk of congestive heart failure compared with short schedule CHOP 21 plus radiotherapy, and slightly increased the risk of myelosuppression, although this increase did not reach significance. One subsequent RCT in people with early stage disease found that low dose radiotherapy in people who had achieved complete response with longer schedule CHOP 21 (8 cycles) improved disease free survival at 6 years compared with longer schedule CHOP 21 alone, but found no significant difference between treatments in overall survival at 6 years. One RCT found that application of adjuvant radiotherapy to sites of nodal bulky disease in people with advanced (stage IV) diffuse large B cell lymphoma who had achieved a complete response after initial chemotherapy was associated with significantly greater 5 year event free survival and overall survival compared with patients treated with chemotherapy alone. Another RCT found significantly improved progression free and overall survival in patients with high or intermediate risk diffuse large B cell lymphoma with residual disease after chemotherapy who received involved field radiotherapy compared with those who received no radiotherapy.

CHOP 21 plus rituximab (increases survival compared with CHOP 21 alone)

One RCT found that, in people aged 60–80 years with stage II–IV disease, CHOP 21 plus rituximab increased response rate, and reduced events (progression, ▶

relapse, or need for second line treatment) and death compared with CHOP 21 alone at 5 years. A subsequent RCT found that CHOP 21 plus rituximab increased 3 year event free survival and overall survival compared with CHOP 21 in patients aged 18–60 with stage II–IV disease.

LIKELY TO BE BENEFICIAL

CHOP 14

We found one RCT comparing CHOP 21 versus CHOP 14 in people aged 18–60 years with good prognosis aggressive lymphoma, and a second RCT comparing CHOP 21 versus CHOP 14 in people aged 61–75 years with aggressive lymphoma. The RCT in younger people found no significant difference between CHOP 14 and CHOP 21 in complete response rates or 5 year event free survival. However, overall 5 year survival was higher with CHOP 14. The RCT in older people found that CHOP 14 improved complete response rate, 5 year event free survival, and overall survival compared with CHOP 21. Toxicity was similar with CHOP 14 and CHOP 21 in both studies.

What are the effects of treatments for relapsed aggressive non-Hodgkin's lymphoma (diffuse large B cell lymphoma)?

LIKELY TO BE BENEFICIAL

Conventional dose salvage chemotherapy (consensus that treatment should be given but relative benefits of different regimens unclear)*

We found no RCTs comparing different conventional dose salvage chemotherapy regimens (PACEBOM, ESHAP, RICE, IVAC) in people with relapsed aggressive non-Hodgkin's lymphoma. The consensus is that people with relapsed disease should be treated with salvage chemotherapy. One systematic review identified 22 phase II trials of various conventional dose salvage chemotherapy regimens. All regimens reported similar response rates and no single superior regimen could be identified.

High dose chemotherapy plus autologous transplant stem cell support (increases survival compared with conventional dose chemotherapy in people with chemosensitive disease)

Two systematic reviews identified one RCT comparing high dose chemotherapy plus autologous bone marrow transplantation versus conventional dose chemotherapy in people with a chemotherapy sensitive relapse of aggressive non-Hodgkin's lymphoma. It found that high dose chemotherapy plus autologous bone marrow transplantation improved 5 year event free survival and overall survival compared with conventional chemotherapy. We found no RCTs in people with chemotherapy resistant disease.

*Based on consensus.

UNKNOWN EFFECTIVENESS

Allongeneic stem cell support

We found no systematic review or RCTs.

DEFINITION Non-Hodgkin's lymphoma (NHL) consists of a complex group of cancers arising mainly from B lymphocytes (85% of cases) and occasionally from T lymphocytes. NHL usually develops in lymph nodes (nodal lymphoma) but can arise in other tissues almost anywhere in the body (extranodal lymphoma). NHL is categorised according to its appearance under the microscope (histology) and the extent of the disease (stage). **Histology:** Since 1966, four major different methods of classifying NHLs according to their histological appearance have been published (see tables 1T, 2T, 3T, and 4T). At present, the World Health Organization (WHO)[1] system is accepted as the gold standard of classification. The WHO system is based on the underlying principles of the REAL classification system.[2] Historically, NHLs have been divided into slow growing "low grade" lymphomas and fast growing "aggressive" lymphomas. This chapter deals only with the most common aggressive NHL — diffuse B cell lymphoma (WHO classification [see table 1]T). Interpretation of older studies is complicated by the fact that histological methods have changed and there is no direct correlation between lymphoma types in the WHO and other classification systems. Attempts to generalise results must therefore be treated with caution. We have, however, included some older studies referring to alternative classification methods if they included people with the following types of aggressive lymphomas, which overlap substantially with the WHO classification of interest: Working Formulation classification — primarily intermediate grades (grades E–H [see table 2]T);[3] Kiel classification — centroblastic, immunoblastic, and anaplastic (see table 3)T;[4] and Rappaport classification — diffuse histiocytic, diffuse lymphocytic, poorly differentiated, and diffuse mixed (lymphocytic and histiocytic [see table 4]T).[5] **Stage:** NHL has traditionally been staged according to extent of disease spread using the Ann Arbor system (see table 5)T.[6] The term "early disease" is used to describe disease that falls within Ann Arbor stage I or II, whereas "advanced disease" refers to Ann Arbor stage III or IV disease. However, all people with bulky disease, usually defined as having a disease site larger than 10 cm in diameter, are treated as having advanced disease, regardless of their Ann Arbor staging. **Relapsed disease:** Relapsed disease refers to the recurrence of active disease in a person who has previously achieved a complete response to initial treatment for NHL. Most studies of treatments in relapsed disease require a minimum duration of complete response of 1 month before relapse.

INCIDENCE/ PREVALENCE It is the sixth most common cancer in the UK; 9443 new cases were diagnosed in the UK in 2002 and it caused 4418 UK deaths in 2003. Incidence rates show distinct geographical variation, with age standardised incidence rates ranging from 17 per 100 000 in Northern America to 4 per 100 000 in south-central Asia. NHL occurs more commonly in males than in females, and the age standardised UK incidence increased by 10.3% between 1993 and 2002.[7]

AETIOLOGY/ RISK FACTORS The aetiology of most NHLs is unknown. Incidence is higher in individuals who are immunosuppressed (congenital or acquired). Other risk factors include viral infection (human T cell leukaemia virus type-1, Epstein–Barr virus, human immunodeficiency virus), bacterial infection (e.g. *Helicobacter pylori*), previous treatment with phenytoin or antineoplastic drugs, and exposure to pesticides or organic solvents.[8]

PROGNOSIS **Overall survival:** Untreated aggressive NHLs would generally result in death in a matter of months. High-grade lymphomas, particularly diffuse large B cell lymphomas and Burkitt's lymphomas, have a high cure rate with both initial and salvage chemotherapy.[9] The 5 year relative age standardised survival for people diagnosed with and treated for NHL between 2000 and 2001 was 55% for men and 56% for women.[7] **Relapse:** About 50% of people with NHL will be cured by initial treatment. Of the rest, about 30% will fail to respond to initial treatment (so called "chemotherapy refractory disease") and about 20–30% will relapse. Most relapses occur within 2 years of completion of initial treatment. Up to 50% of these have chemotherapy sensitive disease; the remainder tend to have chemotherapy resistant disease. **Prognostic indicators:** Prognosis depends on histological type, stage, age, performance status, and lactate dehydrogenase levels. Prognosis varies substantially within each Ann Arbor stage, and further information regarding prognosis can be obtained from applying the

Non-Hodgkin's lymphoma (diffuse large B cell lymphoma)

International Prognostic Index (IPI).[8] The IPI model stratifies prognosis according to the presence or absence of five risk factors: age (< 60 years *v* > 60 years), serum lactate dehydrogenase (normal *v* elevated), performance status (0 or 1 *v* 2–4), Ann Arbor stage (I or II *v* III or IV), and number of extranodal sites involved (0 or 1 *v* 2–4). People with two or more high risk factors have a less than 50% chance of relapse free and overall survival at 5 years. IPI staging is currently the most important system used to define disease stage and treatment options. However, most studies identified by our search predate the IPI staging system.

Please refer to clinicalevidence.com for full text and references.

Sickle cell disease

Search date August 2005

Martin M Meremikwu

What are the effects of interventions to prevent sickle cell crisis and other acute complications in people with sickle cell disease?

BENEFICIAL

Penicillin prophylaxis in children under 5 years of age

One systematic review found that penicillin prophylaxis in children younger than 5 years reduced invasive pneumococcal infections compared with no penicillin or placebo, irrespective of pneumococcal vaccination status.

LIKELY TO BE BENEFICIAL

Hydroxyurea

One RCT in adults identified by a systematic review found that hydroxyurea reduced the incidence of painful crisis, acute chest syndrome, and the need for blood transfusion over a mean of 21 months compared with placebo. It found no significant difference in stroke, hepatic sequestration, and mortality between hydroxyurea and placebo, but it may have lacked power. Another RCT in children identified by a systematic review found that hydroxyurea reduced the duration of hospital stay compared with placebo. Fewer people taking hydroxyurea than taking placebo had these outcomes. Hydroxyurea has been associated with neutropenia, hair loss, skin rash, and gastrointestinal disturbances. We found no RCTs assessing the long term effects of hydroxyurea.

Malaria chemoprophylaxis

Falciparum malaria is believed to precipitate sickle cell crisis and to increase the risk of death in children with sickle cell anaemia; therefore, regular chemoprophylaxis with antimalarial drugs is advocated by consensus. However, one quasi-randomised trial identified by a systematic review and one additional RCT provided insufficient evidence to assess routine malaria chemoprophylaxis in people with sickle cell disease.

Piracetam

One RCT identified by a systematic review found that piracetam reduced the incidence of sickle cell crisis in children compared with placebo.

Zinc sulphate

One RCT identified by a systematic review found that zinc sulphate reduced the incidence of sickle cell crisis compared with placebo.

UNKNOWN EFFECTIVENESS

Avoidance of cold environment

We found no RCTs or observational studies of sufficient quality evaluating avoiding exposure to cold environment to prevent sickle cell crisis and other life threatening complications of sickle cell disease.

Limiting physical exercise

We found no RCTs or observational studies of sufficient quality evaluating limiting exercise to prevent sickle cell crisis and other life threatening complications of sickle cell disease.

▶

Sickle cell disease

Penicillin prophylaxis in children over 5 years of age

One RCT in children who had received prophylactic penicillin for at least 2 years and polysaccharide pneumococcal vaccine found no significant difference between continuing penicillin beyond 5 years of age and placebo in either pneumococcal infections.

Pneumococcal vaccines

One RCT found no significant difference in the incidence of pneumococcal infection between polysaccharide pneumococcal vaccination and control. Three RCTs did not evaluate the clinical benefits of pneumococcal conjugate vaccines. RCTs found that both polysaccharide pneumococcal and pneumococcal conjugate vaccines caused no severe adverse events, but were associated with mild fever, local pain, and swelling.

What are the effects of interventions to treat pain in people with sickle cell crisis?

LIKELY TO BE BENEFICIAL

Patient controlled analgesia

Two small RCTs in adults with sickle cell crisis found no significant difference in pain between patient controlled analgesia using either meperidine or morphine and intermittent parenteral treatment using either meperidine or morphine. The incidence of adverse effects was also similar in both regimens.

TRADE OFF BETWEEN BENEFITS AND HARMS

Controlled release oral morphine given after an initial intravenous bolus dose of morphine versus repeated doses of intravenous morphine

We found no RCTs comparing morphine versus placebo in people with sickle cell crisis. One RCT in children with painful crisis found that, after an intravenous loading dose of morphine at onset of treatment, controlled release oral morphine was as effective as intravenous morphine for reducing pain. However, oral morphine may be associated with an increased risk of acute chest syndrome compared with intravenous morphine.

Corticosteroid as adjunct to narcotic analgesics

One RCT found that adding high dose intravenous methylprednisolone to intravenous morphine reduced the duration of inpatient analgesia compared with placebo in people with acute severe sickle cell crisis. It found no significant difference between adding methylprednisolone and placebo in the proportion of people readmitted to hospital for recurrent pain within 2 weeks of stopping treatment, although more people taking methylprednisolone were readmitted. Another RCT found that adding dexamethasone to intravenous morphine reduced the number of doses and duration of intravenous analgesia compared with placebo in people with acute sickle cell chest syndrome. Some of the known adverse effects of corticosteroids are increased risk of infections, weight gain, hypertension, poor glucose metabolism, cataracts, and poor growth in children.

UNKNOWN EFFECTIVENESS

Acupuncture

We found no RCTs of acupuncture in people with sickle cell crisis.

Aspirin

We found no RCTs of aspirin in people with sickle cell crisis.

Codeine

We found no RCTs of codeine in people with sickle cell crisis.

Diflunisal

One RCT in adults with vaso-occlusive sickle cell crisis found no significant difference between adding diflunisal to intramuscular meperidine compared with adding placebo, in pain or in dose of meperidine administered, but it is likely to have been underpowered to detect a clinically important difference.

Hydration

We found no RCTs on the effects of routinely giving extra fluids to treat people with sickle cell crisis.

Ibuprofen

We found no RCTs of ibuprofen in people with sickle cell crisis.

Ketorolac

Four small RCTs provided insufficient evidence to assess ketorolac in people with vaso-occlusive sickle cell crisis.

Oxygen

One RCT in children provided insufficient evidence to assess oxygen treatment in people with sickle cell crisis.

Paracetamol

We found no RCTs of paracetamol (acetaminophen) in people with sickle cell crisis.

DEFINITION **Sickle cell disease** refers to a group of disorders caused by inheritance of a pair of abnormal haemoglobin genes, including the sickle cell gene. It is characterised by chronic haemolytic anaemia, dactylitis, and acute episodic clinical events called "crises".[1] Vaso-occlusive (painful) crises are the most common and occur when abnormal red cells clog small vessels, causing tissue ischaemia. The others are hyper-haemolytic crisis (excessive haemolysis), acute chest syndrome, sequestration crisis, and aplastic crisis. A common variant of sickle cell disease, also characterised by haemolytic anaemia, occurs in people with one sickle and one thalassaemia gene. **Sickle cell trait** occurs in people with one sickle gene and one normal gene. People with sickle cell trait do not have any clinical manifestation of illness. This chapter covers people with sickle cell disease with or without thalassaemia.

INCIDENCE/ PREVALENCE Sickle cell disease is most common among people living in or originating from sub-Saharan Africa.[2] The disorder also affects people of Mediterranean, Caribbean, Middle Eastern, and Asian origin. The sickle cell gene is most common in areas where malaria is endemic: sickle cell trait affects about 10–30% of Africa's tropical populations.[3] Sickle cell disease affects an estimated 1–2% (120 000) of newborns in Africa annually. About 178 babies (0.28/1000 conceptions) are affected by sickle cell disease in England annually.[4] About 60 000 people in the USA[4] and 10 000 in the UK suffer from the disease.[5]

AETIOLOGY/ RISK FACTORS Sickle cell disease is inherited as an autosomal recessive disorder. For a baby to be affected, both parents must have the sickle cell gene. In parents with sickle cell trait, the risk of having an affected baby is one in four for each

Sickle cell disease

pregnancy. Painful (vaso-occlusive) crisis is the most common feature of the disease, and these episodes start in infancy and early childhood.[6] Factors that precipitate or modulate the occurrence of sickle cell crisis are not fully understood, but infections, hypoxia, dehydration, acidosis, stress (such as major surgery or childbirth), and cold are believed to play some role. In tropical Africa, malaria is the most common cause of anaemic and vaso-occlusive crisis.[3] High levels of fetal haemoglobin are known to ameliorate the severity and incidence of sickle cell crisis and other complications of the disease.

PROGNOSIS People affected by sickle cell disease are predisposed to bacterial infections, especially to those caused by encapsulated organisms such as *Pneumococcus*, *Haemophilus influenzae*, *Meningococcus*, and *Salmonella* species. Severe bacterial infections such as pneumonia, meningitis, and septicaemia are common causes of morbidity and mortality, especially among young children.[7] About 10% of children with sickle cell anaemia may develop a stroke, and more than 50% of these may suffer recurrent strokes.[8] Abnormal features of cerebral blood vessels shown by transcranial Doppler scan predict a high risk of stroke in children with sickle cell disease.[9] Frequent episodes of crisis, infections, and organ damage reduce the quality of life of people with sickle cell disease. A high rate of vaso-occlusive (painful) crisis is an index of clinical severity that correlates with early death. Life expectancy remains low, especially in communities with poor access to health services. In some parts of Africa, about 50% of children with sickle cell disease die before their first birthday.[3] The average life expectancy with sickle cell disease in the USA for men is about 42 years and for women is about 48 years.[10] Frequent blood transfusions could increase the risk of immune reactions and infections, such as HIV and hepatitis B or C viruses, and Chagas' disease. The need for repeated blood transfusions in people with sickle cell disease predisposes them to the risk of iron overload.[11]

Please refer to clinicalevidence.com for full text and references.

Acute myocardial infarction

Search date August 2004

Nicholas Danchin and Eric Durand

Which treatments improve outcomes in acute myocardial infarction?

BENEFICIAL

Angiotensin converting enzyme inhibitors

One systematic review in people treated within 14 days of acute myocardial infarction found that angiotensin converting enzyme inhibitors reduce mortality after 6 weeks compared with placebo. However, a non-systematic review found that angiotensin converting enzyme inhibitors increase persistent hypotension and renal dysfunction at 6 weeks compared with placebo.

Aspirin

One systematic review in people with acute myocardial infarction found that aspirin reduced mortality, reinfarction, and stroke at 1 month compared with placebo.

Beta-blockers

Two systematic reviews and one subsequent RCT found that beta-blockers reduced mortality compared with no beta-blockers. One RCT in people receiving thrombolytic treatment found that immediate treatment with metoprolol reduced rates of reinfarction and chest pain at 6 days compared with delayed treatment, but had no significant effect on mortality at 6 days or at 1 year.

Primary percutaneous transluminal coronary angioplasty versus thrombolysis (performed in specialist centres)

One systematic review found that primary percutaneous transluminal coronary angioplasty reduced a combined outcome of death, non-fatal reinfarction, and stroke compared with thrombolysis.

Thrombolysis

One non-systematic review of large RCTs in people with acute myocardial infarction and ST segment elevation or bundle branch block on their initial electrocardiogram found that prompt thrombolytic treatment (within 6 hours and perhaps up to 12 hours and longer after the onset of symptoms) reduced mortality compared with placebo. RCTs comparing different types of thrombolytic agents with each other found no significant difference in mortality. One non-systematic review found that thrombolytic treatment increased the risk of stroke or major bleeding compared with control. The review also found that intracranial haemorrhage was more common in people of advanced age and low body weight, those with hypertension on admission, and those given tissue plasminogen activator rather than another thrombolytic agent. One non-systematic review found conflicting results for intracerebral haemorrhage with bolus treatment compared with infusion of thrombolytic agents. One systematic review found that thrombolysis was less effective at reducing a combined outcome of death, non-fatal reinfarction, and stroke compared with primary percutaneous transluminal coronary angioplasty.

Acute myocardial infarction

LIKELY TO BE BENEFICIAL

Adding low molecular weight heparin (enoxaparin) to thrombolytics (reduces acute myocardial infarction rates)

One RCT found that adding enoxaparin (a low molecular weight heparin) to streptokinase reduced further acute myocardial infarction rates compared with adding placebo in people with early evidence of a developing infarction. One systematic review identified five RCTs comparing enoxaparin (a low molecular weight heparin) plus thrombolytic treatment versus unfractionated heparin plus thrombolytic treatment. Two of the RCTs identified by the review found that enoxaparin plus thrombolytics reduced further acute myocardial infarction rates compared with unfractionated heparin plus thrombolytics, whereas three RCTs found no significant difference between treatments. The review found no significant difference in mortality between enoxaparin and unfractionated heparin when added to thrombolytic treatment and no significant difference between added enoxaparin and added unfractionated heparin in the risk of intracranial or other major bleeding.

Nitrates (in the absence of thrombolysis)

One systematic review of the trials conducted in the prethrombolytic era found that nitrates reduced mortality in people with acute myocardial infarction compared with placebo.

TRADE OFF BETWEEN BENEFITS AND HARMS

Glycoprotein IIb/IIIa inhibitors

Two large RCTs found that combined treatment with half dose thrombolysis plus abciximab did not reduce mortality at 1 month in people with acute myocardial infarction compared with full dose thrombolysis, but one RCT found limited evidence that the combined treatment reduced non-fatal cardiovascular events. However, the RCTs found that combined treatment with abciximab increased bleeding complications, particularly extracranial haemorrhage. One meta-analysis of four RCTs with abciximab and one additional RCT in people treated with primary angioplasty found a reduction in the combined end point of death, reinfarction, and target vessel revascularisation at 30 days and 6 months compared with control, but found no significant reduction in death alone. The meta-analysis found an increased risk of major bleeding with abciximab compared with control. Two additional RCTs comparing early versus late administration of tirofiban in people undergoing primary coronary angioplasty found no significant difference in survival or morbidity outcomes between groups.

UNLIKELY TO BE BENEFICIAL

Adding unfractionated heparin to thrombolytics

Two RCTs found no significant difference in mortality or further acute myocardial infarction rates between unfractionated heparin plus thrombolytics and thrombolytics alone. One systematic review identified five RCTs comparing enoxaparin (a low molecular weight heparin) plus thrombolytic treatment versus unfractionated heparin plus thrombolytic treatment. Two of the RCTs identified by the review found that enoxaparin plus thrombolytics reduced further acute myocardial infarction rates compared with unfractionated heparin plus thrombolytics, whereas three RCTs found no significant difference between treatments. The review found no significant difference in mortality between enoxaparin and unfractionated heparin when added to thrombolytic treatment. The systematic review found no significant difference between added enoxaparin and added unfractionated heparin in the risk of intracranial or other major bleeding.

Nitrates (in addition to thrombolysis)

Two RCTs in people with acute myocardial infarction (after thrombolysis was introduced) found no significant difference in mortality between nitrates and placebo.

LIKELY TO BE INEFFECTIVE OR HARMFUL

Calcium channel blockers

We found evidence that neither dihydropyridines nor verapamil reduce mortality compared with placebo. One RCT found limited evidence that, in people with left ventricular dysfunction, nifedipine given in the first few days after acute myocardial infarction may increase mortality compared with placebo.

Which treatments improve outcomes for cardiogenic shock after acute myocardial infarction?

BENEFICIAL

Early invasive cardiac revascularisation

One large RCT found that early invasive cardiac revascularisation reduced mortality after 6 and 12 months compared with medical treatment alone in people with cardiogenic shock within 48 hours of acute myocardial infarction. A second, smaller RCT found similar results, although the difference was not significant.

UNKNOWN EFFECTIVENESS

Early cardiac surgery

We found no RCTs evaluating early surgical intervention for ventricular septal rupture, free wall rupture, or mitral valve regurgitation complicated by cardiogenic shock after acute myocardial infarction.

Intra-aortic balloon counterpulsation

An RCT presented only in abstract form found limited evidence of no significant difference in mortality at 6 months between intra-aortic balloon counterpulsation plus thrombolysis and thrombolysis alone in people with cardiogenic shock.

Positive inotropes

We found no RCTs comparing inotropes versus placebo.

Pulmonary artery catheterisation

We found no RCTs comparing pulmonary artery catheterisation versus no catheterisation.

Thrombolysis

Subgroup analysis of one RCT found no significant difference in mortality after 21 days between thrombolysis and no thrombolysis in people with cardiogenic shock.

Vasodilators

We found no RCTs comparing vasodilators versus placebo.

Ventricular assistance devices and cardiac transplantation

We found no RCTs evaluating either ventricular assistance devices or cardiac transplantation.

Acute myocardial infarction

DEFINITION **Acute myocardial infarction (AMI):** The sudden occlusion of a coronary artery leading to myocardial cell death. **Cardiogenic shock:** Defined clinically as a poor cardiac output plus evidence of tissue hypoxia that is not improved by correcting reduced intravascular volume.[1] When a pulmonary artery catheter is used, cardiogenic shock may be defined as a cardiac index below 2.2 L/minute/m^2 despite an elevated pulmonary capillary wedge pressure (≥ 15 mm Hg).[1-3]

INCIDENCE/ PREVALENCE **AMI:** Acute myocardial infarction is one of the most common causes of mortality worldwide. In 1990, ischaemic heart disease was the world's leading cause of death, accounting for about 6.3 million deaths. The age standardised incidence varies among and within countries.[4] Each year, about 900 000 people in the USA experience AMI, about 225 000 of whom die. About half of these people die within 1 hour of symptoms and before reaching a hospital emergency room.[5] Event rates increase with age for both sexes and are higher in men than in women and in poorer than richer people at all ages. The incidence of death from AMI has fallen in many Western countries over the past 20 years. **Cardiogenic shock:** Cardiogenic shock occurs in about 7% of people admitted to hospital with AMI.[6] Of these, about half have established cardiogenic shock at the time of admission to hospital, and most of the others develop it during the first 24–48 hours after their admission.[7]

AETIOLOGY/ RISK FACTORS **AMI:** Identified major risk factors for cardiovascular disease include increasing age, male sex, raised low density lipoprotein cholesterol, reduced high density lipoprotein cholesterol, raised blood pressure, smoking, diabetes, family history of cardiovascular disease, obesity, and sedentary lifestyle. For many of these risk factors, observational studies show a continuous gradient of increasing risk of cardiovascular disease with increasing levels of the risk factor, with no obvious threshold level. The immediate mechanism of AMI is rupture or erosion of an atheromatous plaque causing thrombosis and occlusion of coronary arteries and myocardial cell death. Factors that may convert a stable plaque into an unstable plaque (the "active plaque") have yet to be fully elucidated. Shear stresses, inflammation, and autoimmunity have been proposed. The changing rates of coronary heart disease in different populations are only partly explained by changes in the standard risk factors for ischaemic heart disease (particularly a fall in blood pressure and smoking). **Cardiogenic shock:** Cardiogenic shock after AMI usually follows a reduction in functional ventricular myocardium, and is caused by left ventricular infarction (79% of people with cardiogenic shock) more often than by right ventricular infarction (3% of people with cardiogenic shock).[8] Cardiogenic shock after AMI may also be caused by cardiac structural defects, such as mitral valve regurgitation due to papillary muscle dysfunction (7% of people with cardiogenic shock), ventricular septal rupture (4% of people with cardiogenic shock), or cardiac tamponade after free cardiac wall rupture (1% of people with cardiogenic shock). Major risk factors for cardiogenic shock after AMI are previous myocardial infarction, diabetes mellitus, advanced age, hypotension, tachycardia or bradycardia, congestive heart failure with Killip class II–III, and low left ventricular ejection fraction (ejection fraction < 35%).[7,8]

PROGNOSIS **AMI:** May lead to a host of mechanical and cardiac electrical complications, including death, ventricular dysfunction, congestive heart failure, fatal and non-fatal arrhythmias, valvular dysfunction, myocardial rupture, and cardiogenic shock. **Cardiogenic shock:** Mortality rates for people in hospital with cardiogenic shock after AMI vary between 50–80%.[2,3,6,7] Most deaths occur within 48 hours of the onset of shock (see figure 1) Ⓕ.[9] People surviving until discharge from hospital have a reasonable long term prognosis (88% survival at 1 year).[10]

Please refer to clinicalevidence.com for full text and references.

Angina (stable)

Search date December 2004

Laurence O'Toole

What are the effects of long term single drug treatment for stable angina?

LIKELY TO BE BENEFICIAL

Beta Blockers*

One small RCT identified by a systematic review found no significant difference between a beta blocker (propranolol) and placebo in angina frequency or exercise duration after 6 months. However, this trial may have lacked power to detect a clinically important difference between groups. There is consensus that beta blockers are effective for treating the symptoms of stable angina. RCTs found no significant difference between beta blockers and calcium channel blockers in the frequency of angina attacks, exercise duration, mortality, or non-fatal cardiovascular events at 6 months to 3 years. However, these RCTs may have lacked power to detect clinically important differences between groups. One RCT also found no significant difference between beta blockers and calcium channel blockers in quality of life. We did not find any systematic reviews or RCTs that compared longer use of beta blockers with long acting nitrates or potassium channel openers.

Calcium channel blockers*

One small RCT identified by a systematic review found no significant difference between bepridil and placebo in the frequency of angina attacks. It found that bepridil increased exercise duration compared with placebo at 6 months. There is consensus that calcium channel blockers are effective for treating the symptoms of stable angina. RCTs identified by the review found no significant difference between calcium channel blockers and beta blockers in the frequency of angina attacks, exercise duration, mortality, or non-fatal cardiovascular events at between 6 months and 3 years. However, these RCTs may have lacked power to detect clinically important differences between groups. One RCT also found no significant difference between calcium channel blockers and beta blockers in quality of life. One RCT found no significant difference between amlodipine and isosorbide mononitrate in the frequency of angina attacks or in quality of life. It found that amlodipine increased exercise duration compared with isosorbide mononitrate at 6 months. The RCT found that peripheral oedema was more common with amlodipine than with isosorbide mononitrate, whereas headache was more common with isosorbide mononitrate. We found no systematic review or RCTs that compared long term calcium channel blockers with potassium channel openers.

Nitrates*

We found no RCTs comparing long term single drug treatment with nitrates versus placebo for stable angina. However, there is consensus that nitrates are effective for treating the symptoms of stable angina. One RCT found no significant difference between amlodipine and isosorbide mononitrate in the frequency of angina attacks or in quality of life. It found that amlodipine increased exercise duration compared with isosorbide mononitrate at 6 months. The RCT found that peripheral oedema was more common with amlodipine than with isosorbide mononitrate, whereas headache was more common with isosorbide mononitrate.

Angina (stable)

Potassium channel openers*

We found no RCTs on the effects of long term single drug treatment with potassium channel openers for stable angina. However, there is consensus that potassium channel openers are effective for treating the symptoms of stable angina.

*Based on consensus.

DEFINITION Angina pectoris, often simply known as angina, is a clinical syndrome characterised by discomfort in the chest, shoulder, back, arm, or jaw.[1] Angina is usually caused by coronary artery atherosclerotic disease. Rarer causes include valvular heart disease, hypertrophic cardiomyopathy, uncontrolled hypertension, or vasospasm or endothelial dysfunction not related to atherosclerosis. The differential diagnosis of angina includes non-cardiac conditions affecting the chest wall, oesophagus, and lungs. Angina may be classified as stable or unstable. **Stable angina** is defined as regular or predictable angina symptoms that have been occurring for over 2 months. Symptoms are transient and are typically provoked by exertion, and alleviated by rest or nitroglycerin. Other precipitants include cold weather, eating, or emotional distress. This chapter deals specifically with long term treatment of stable angina caused by coronary artery atherosclerotic disease, and therefore, only includes RCTs with a follow up of more than 6 months. **Unstable angina** is diagnosed if there is a rapid decline in exercise capacity or if there are episodes of pain at rest. This is usually associated with atherosclerotic plaque instability and, as myocardial infarction and death may ensue, should be treated as a medical emergency, usually requiring hospital admission (see chapter on unstable angina).

INCIDENCE/ PREVALENCE The prevalence of stable angina remains unclear.[1,2] Epidemiological studies in the UK estimate that 6–16% of men and 3–10% of women aged 65–74 years have experienced angina.[3-5] Annually, about 1% of the population visit their general practitioner with symptoms of angina[4] and 23 000 people with new anginal symptoms present to their general practitioner each year in the UK.[6] These studies did not distinguish between stable and unstable angina.[3-6]

AETIOLOGY/ RISK FACTORS Stable angina resulting from coronary artery disease is characterised by focal atherosclerotic plaques in the intimal layer of the epicardial coronary artery. The plaques encroach on the coronary lumen and may limit blood flow to the myocardium, especially during periods of increased myocardial oxygen demand. The major risk factors that lead to the development of stable angina are similar to those that predispose to coronary heart disease. These risk factors include increasing age, male sex, overweight, hypertension, elevated serum cholesterol level, smoking, and relative physical inactivity.[7]

PROGNOSIS Stable angina is a marker of underlying coronary heart disease, which accounts for 1 in 4 deaths in the UK.[8] People with angina are 2–5 times more likely to develop other manifestations of coronary heart disease than people who do not have angina.[7,9] One population based study (7100 men aged 51–59 years at entry) found that people with angina had higher mortality than people with no history of coronary artery disease at baseline (16 year survival rate: 53% with angina *v* 72% without coronary artery disease *v* 34% with a history of myocardial infarction).[10] Clinical trials in people with stable angina have tended to recruit participants who were not felt to be in need of coronary revascularisation and in these people prognosis is better, with an annual mortality of 1–2% and annual rate of non-fatal myocardial infarction of 2–3%.[11-14] Features that indicate a poorer prognosis include: more severe symptoms, male sex,[15] abnormal resting electrocardiogram[16] (present in about 50% of people with angina[17]), previous myocardial infarction,[10,18] left ventricular dysfunction,[19] easily provoked or widespread coronary ischaemia on stress testing (present in about one third of people referred to hospital with stable angina), and significant stenosis of all three major coronary arteries or the left main coronary artery.[6,19] In addition, the standard coronary risk factors continue to exert a detrimental and additive effect on prognosis in people with stable angina.[9,20,21] Control of these risk factors is dealt with in the *Clinical Evidence* chapter on secondary prevention of ischaemic cardiac events.

Please refer to clinicalevidence.com for full text and references.

Angina (unstable)

Search date March 2004

Madhu Natarajan

What are the effects of antiplatelet treatments?

BENEFICIAL

Aspirin

One systematic review found that antiplatelet treatment, mostly medium dose aspirin 75–325 mg/day, reduced the risk of death, myocardial infarction, and stroke compared with placebo in people with unstable angina. The evidence suggested no added cardiovascular benefit, and possible added harm, from doses of aspirin over 325 mg daily.

LIKELY TO BE BENEFICIAL

Clopidogrel/ticlopidine

Two RCTs found that adding clopidogrel to aspirin or ticlopidine to conventional treatment reduced mortality and myocardial infarction compared with aspirin alone or conventional treatment alone. One of the RCTs found that adding clopidogrel to aspirin increased major bleeding, but not haemorrhagic strokes, compared with aspirin alone after 6–9 months. Ticlopidine may cause reversible neutropenia. These drugs may be an alternative in people who are intolerant of or allergic to aspirin.

Intravenous glycoprotein IIb/IIIa inhibitors

One systematic review found that intravenous glycoprotein IIb/IIIa inhibitors reduced death or myocardial infarction at up to 6 months compared with placebo, but increased major bleeding complications. Longer term follow up of one of the RCTs included in the review found no significant difference between abciximab and placebo in mortality at 1 year.

LIKELY TO BE INEFFECTIVE OR HARMFUL

Oral glycoprotein IIb/IIIa inhibitors

One RCT identified by a systematic review found that the oral glycoprotein IIb/IIIa inhibitor sibrafiban did not significantly reduce the combined outcome of death, myocardial infarction, or recurrent ischaemia compared with aspirin at 90 days. However, the review found that oral glycoprotein IIb/IIIa inhibitors with or without aspirin increased bleeding compared with aspirin alone.

What are the effects of antithrombin treatments?

LIKELY TO BE BENEFICIAL

Direct thrombin inhibitors

One systematic review found that treatment with direct thrombin inhibitors for 7 days reduced death and myocardial infarction compared with heparin after 30 days.

Low molecular weight heparin

One systematic review in people taking aspirin found that adding low molecular weight heparin reduced death and myocardial infarction, and did not significantly increase bleeding complications in the first 7 days after unstable angina compared with adding placebo or no treatment. However, it found that longer ▶

term treatment with low molecular weight heparin (up to 90 days) did not significantly reduce death or myocardial infarction after 90 days compared with placebo. One systematic review found that low molecular weight heparin reduced myocardial infarction but not mortality, recurrent angina, or major bleeding compared with unfractionated heparin.

Unfractionated heparin

One systematic review found that adding unfractionated heparin to aspirin for 7 days in people with unstable angina reduced death or myocardial infarction at 1 week. However, a second review found no significant effect on death or myocardial infarction after 12 weeks. One systematic review found that unfractionated heparin was less effective than low molecular weight heparin at reducing myocardial infarction, but found no significant difference between treatments in mortality, recurrent angina or major bleeding.

UNLIKELY TO BE BENEFICIAL

Warfarin

Five RCTs found no significant effect of adding warfarin to usual treatment (usually aspirin) for recurrent angina, myocardial infarction, or death at up to 1 year. One of the RCTs found that warfarin was associated with an increase in major bleeding compared with usual treatment alone.

What are the effects of anti-ischaemic treatments?

UNKNOWN EFFECTIVENESS

Beta-blockers (for myocardial infarction or death)

We found insufficient evidence on the effects of beta-blockers on mortality or myocardial infarction, although one RCT suggested that beta-blockers may reduce the frequency and severity of chest pain.

Nitrates (for myocardial infarction or death)

We found insufficient evidence on the effects of nitrates on mortality or myocardial infarction, although RCTs suggested that nitrates may reduce the frequency and severity of chest pain.

UNLIKELY TO BE BENEFICIAL

Calcium channel blockers

One systematic review found no significant difference between calcium channel blockers and either placebo or standard treatment in mortality or myocardial infarction. Observational studies suggest that short acting dihydropyridine calcium channel blockers may increase mortality.

What are the effects of invasive treatments?

UNKNOWN EFFECTIVENESS

Routine early cardiac catheterisation and revascularisation

We found five RCTs that reported on different composite outcomes at different time points. Two RCTs found that early invasive treatment reduced death and other cardiac events or hospital readmission compared with conservative treatment at 4–6 months. However, three RCTs found no significant difference in death or other cardiac events between early invasive treatment and conservative treatment at 12 or more months.

Angina (unstable)

DEFINITION Unstable angina is distinguished from stable angina, acute myocardial infarction, and non-cardiac pain by the pattern of symptoms (characteristic pain present at rest or on lower levels of activity), the severity of symptoms (recently increasing intensity, frequency, or duration), and the absence of persistent ST segment elevation on a resting electrocardiogram. Unstable angina includes a variety of different clinical patterns: angina at rest of up to 1 week of duration; angina increasing in severity to moderate or severe pain; non-Q wave myocardial infarction; and post-myocardial infarction angina continuing for longer than 24 hours. Unstable angina and non-ST segment elevation myocardial infarction (non-STEMI) are clinically overlapping entities in terms of diagnosis and treatment strategies. Unstable angina, broadly defined as new or persistent chest pain, becomes classified as non-STEMI if in addition to chest pain there is elevation of cardiac enzymes, such as troponin, or persistent ST depression on electrocardiogram. Many trials include people with either unstable angina or non-STEMI. We have included RCTs in a mixed population of people with unstable angina or non-STEMI, as well as RCTs solely in people with unstable angina.

INCIDENCE/ PREVALENCE In industrialised countries, the annual incidence of unstable angina is about 6/10 000 people in the general population.

AETIOLOGY/ RISK FACTORS Risk factors are the same as for other manifestations of ischaemic heart disease: older age, previous atheromatous cardiovascular disease, diabetes mellitus, smoking cigarettes, hypertension, hypercholesterolaemia, male sex, and a family history of ischaemic heart disease (see Appendix 1). Unstable angina can also occur in association with other disorders of the circulation, including heart valve disease, arrhythmia, and cardiomyopathy.

PROGNOSIS In people with unstable angina taking aspirin, the incidence of serious adverse outcomes (such as death, acute myocardial infarction, or refractory angina requiring emergency revascularisation) is 5–10% within the first 7 days and about 15% at 30 days. Between 5% and 14% of people with unstable angina die in the year after diagnosis, with about half of these deaths occurring within 4 weeks of diagnosis. No single factor identifies people at higher risk of an adverse event. Risk factors include severity of presentation (e.g. duration of pain, speed of progression, evidence of heart failure), medical history (e.g. previous unstable angina, acute myocardial infarction, left ventricular dysfunction), other clinical parameters (e.g. age, diabetes), electrocardiogram changes (e.g. severity of ST segment depression, deep T wave inversion, transient ST segment elevation), biochemical parameters (e.g. troponin concentration), and change in clinical status (e.g. recurrent chest pain, silent ischaemia, haemodynamic instability).

Please refer to clinicalevidence.com for full text and references.

Atrial fibrillation (recent onset)

Search date October 2005

Gregory Y H Lip

What are the effects of interventions to prevent embolism in people with recent onset atrial fibrillation who are haemodynamically stable?

UNKNOWN EFFECTIVENESS

Antithrombotic treatment before cardioversion

We found no systematic review or RCTs on use of aspirin, heparin, or warfarin as thromboprophylaxis before attempted cardioversion in acute atrial fibrillation.

What are the effects of interventions for conversion to sinus rhythm in people with recent onset atrial fibrillation who are haemodynamically stable?

TRADE OFF BETWEEN BENEFITS AND HARMS

Flecainide

Five RCTs found that oral or intravenous flecainide increased the proportion of people who reverted to sinus rhythm within 1–24 hours compared with placebo. Flecainide was associated with serious adverse events, such as severe hypotension and torsades de pointes. Two RCTs found that oral flecainide increased the proportion of people who reverted to sinus rhythm within 8 hours compared with intravenous amiodarone. We found insufficient evidence to draw any conclusions about comparisons between intravenous flecainide and intravenous amiodarone, and between flecainide and quinidine. Three RCTs found no consistent evidence of a difference in rates of conversion to sinus rhythm between flecainide and propafenone. Flecainide and propafenone are not used in people with known or suspected ischaemic heart disease because they may cause arrhythmias.

Propafenone

One systematic review and subsequent RCTs found that propafenone increased the proportion of people converting to sinus rhythm within 1–24 hours compared with placebo in people with acute or chronic atrial fibrillation. Two RCTs found a faster rate of conversion to sinus rhythm with propafenone, but no significant difference between amiodarone and propafenone after 12 hours. One RCT found that propafenone increased conversion to sinus rhythm after 8 hours compared with amiodarone. One RCT found no significant difference between conversion to sinus rhythm between amiodarone and propafenone at 1 hour. One RCT found no significant difference in conversion to sinus rhythm between propafenone and digoxin at 1 hour. Three RCTs found insufficient evidence to compare rates of conversion to sinus rhythm between propafenone and flecainide. Propafenone and flecainide are not used in people with known or suspected ischaemic heart disease because they may cause arrhythmias.

UNKNOWN EFFECTIVENESS

Amiodarone

We found insufficient evidence from five RCTs about the effects of amiodarone as a single agent compared with placebo for conversion to sinus rhythm in ▶

people with acute atrial fibrillation who are haemodynamically stable. Four small RCTs found no significant difference in rate of conversion to sinus rhythm at 24–48 hours for amiodarone compared with digoxin, although the studies may have lacked power to exclude clinically important differences. One RCT found that amiodarone increased the rate of cardioversion compared with verapamil at 3 hours. Two RCTs found a faster rate of conversion to sinus rhythm with propafenone, but no significant difference between amiodarone and propafenone after 12 hours. One RCT found that propafenone increased conversion to sinus rhythm after 8 hours compared with amiodarone. One RCT found no significant difference between conversion to sinus rhythm between amiodarone and propafenone at 1 hour. Two RCTs found that intravenous amiodarone reduced the proportion of people who reverted to sinus rhythm within 8 hours compared with oral flecainide. We found insufficient evidence to draw any conclusions about comparisons between intravenous amiodarone and intravenous flecainide. We found no RCTs comparing amiodarone with direct current cardioversion.

Direct current cardioversion

We found no systematic review or RCTs of direct current cardioversion in acute atrial fibrillation in people who are haemodynamically stable.

Quinidine

We found no systematic review or RCTs that compared quinidine versus placebo. One small RCT in people with onset of atrial fibrillation within the last 48 hours found that quinidine plus digoxin increased the proportion of people converting to sinus rhythm within 12 hours compared with sotalol. We found insufficient evidence to draw any conclusions about comparisons between quinidine and flecainide.

Sotalol

We found no systematic review or RCTs comparing sotalol versus placebo. One small RCT in people with onset of atrial fibrillation of less than 48 hours found that quinidine plus digoxin increased the proportion of people who converted to sinus rhythm within 12 hours compared with sotalol.

UNLIKELY TO BE BENEFICIAL

Digoxin

We found no placebo controlled RCTs limited to people with acute atrial fibrillation. Four RCTs in people with atrial fibrillation of up to 7 days' duration found no significant difference between digoxin and placebo in conversion to sinus rhythm. The evidence suggests that digoxin is no better than placebo for restoring sinus rhythm in people with recent onset atrial fibrillation. The peak action of digoxin is delayed for up to 6–12 hours. Four small RCTs found no significant difference between digoxin and amiodarone in conversion to sinus rhythm at 24–48 hours, although these trials may have lacked power to detect clinically important differences. One RCT found no significant difference in conversion to sinus rhythm between digoxin and propafenone at 1 hour.

Verapamil

We found no placebo controlled RCTs limited to people with acute atrial fibrillation. One small crossover RCT in people with atrial fibrillation or atrial flutter for 2 hours to 2 years found no significant difference in the rate of cardioversion between verapamil and placebo. One RCT found that verapamil reduced the rate of cardioversion compared with amiodarone at 3 hours.

What are the effects of interventions to control heart rate in people with recent onset atrial fibrillation who are haemodynamically stable?

LIKELY TO BE BENEFICIAL

Digoxin

We found no placebo controlled RCTs limited to people with acute atrial fibrillation. Two RCTs found that intravenous digoxin reduced ventricular rate compared with placebo at 30 minutes or 2 hours in people with atrial fibrillation of up to 7 days' duration. One RCT found that, compared with intravenous digoxin, intravenous diltiazem reduced heart rate within 5 minutes in people with acute atrial fibrillation and atrial flutter.

Diltiazem

One RCT in people with atrial fibrillation (of unspecified duration) or atrial flutter found that intravenous diltiazem reduced heart rate in people within 15 minutes compared with placebo. One RCT found that in people with acute atrial fibrillation or atrial flutter, intravenous diltiazem reduced heart rate within 5 minutes compared with intravenous digoxin. One RCT found no significant difference between intravenous verapamil and intravenous diltiazem in rate control or measures of systolic function in people with acute atrial fibrillation or atrial flutter, but verapamil caused hypotension in some people.

Timolol

We found no placebo controlled RCTs limited to people with acute atrial fibrillation. One small RCT in people with atrial fibrillation (of unspecified duration) found that intravenous timolol (a beta-blocker) reduced ventricular rate within 20 minutes compared with placebo.

Verapamil

Two RCTs found that intravenous verapamil reduced heart rate at 10 or 30 minutes compared with placebo in people with atrial fibrillation or atrial flutter. One RCT in people with atrial fibrillation or acute atrial flutter found no significant difference between intravenous verapamil and intravenous diltiazem in rate control or measures of systolic function, but verapamil caused hypotension in some people.

UNKNOWN EFFECTIVENESS

Amiodarone

We found no systematic review or RCTs on the effects of amiodarone to control heart rate in people with acute atrial fibrillation who are haemodynamically stable.

Sotalol

We found no systematic review or RCTs on the effects of sotalol to control heart rate in people with acute atrial fibrillation who are haemodynamically stable.

DEFINITION **Acute atrial fibrillation** is rapid, irregular, and chaotic atrial activity of less than 48 hours' duration. It includes both the first symptomatic onset of chronic or persistent atrial fibrillation and episodes of paroxysmal atrial fibrillation. It is sometimes difficult to distinguish new onset atrial fibrillation from long standing atrial fibrillation that was previously undiagnosed. Atrial fibrillation within 72 hours of onset is sometimes called recent onset atrial fibrillation. By contrast, chronic atrial fibrillation is more sustained and can be

Atrial fibrillation (recent onset)

described as paroxysmal (with spontaneous termination and sinus rhythm between recurrences), persistent, or permanent atrial fibrillation. This review deals only with people with acute atrial fibrillation who are haemodynamically stable. The consensus is that people who are not haemodynamically stable should be treated with immediate direct current cardioversion. We have excluded studies in people with atrial fibrillation arising during or soon after cardiac surgery.

INCIDENCE/ PREVALENCE We found limited evidence of the incidence or prevalence of acute atrial fibrillation. Extrapolation from the Framingham study suggests an incidence in men of 3/1000 person years at age 55 years, rising to 38/1000 person years at 94 years.[1] In women, the incidence was 2/1000 person years at age 55 years and 32.5/1000 person years at 94 years. The prevalence of atrial fibrillation ranged from 0.5% for people aged 50–59 years to 9% in people aged 80–89 years. Among acute emergency medical admissions in the UK, 3–6% had atrial fibrillation, and about 40% were newly diagnosed.[2,3] Among acute hospital admissions in New Zealand, 10% (95% CI 9% to 12%) had documented atrial fibrillation.[4]

AETIOLOGY/ RISK FACTORS Common precipitants of acute atrial fibrillation are acute myocardial infarction and the acute effects of alcohol. Age increases the risk of developing acute atrial fibrillation. Men are more likely to develop atrial fibrillation than are women (38 years' follow up from the Framingham Study, RR after adjustment for age and known predisposing conditions 1.5).[5] Atrial fibrillation can occur in association with underlying disease (both cardiac and non-cardiac) or can arise in the absence of any other condition. Epidemiological surveys found that risk factors for the development of acute atrial fibrillation include ischaemic heart disease, hypertension, heart failure, valve disease, diabetes, alcohol abuse, thyroid disorders, and disorders of the lung and pleura.[1] In a British survey of acute hospital admissions of people with atrial fibrillation, a history of ischaemic heart disease was present in 33%, heart failure in 24%, hypertension in 26%, and rheumatic heart disease in 7%.[3] In some populations, the acute effects of alcohol explain a large proportion of the incidence of acute atrial fibrillation. Paroxysms of atrial fibrillation are more common in athletes.[6]

PROGNOSIS **Spontaneous reversion:** Observational studies and placebo arms of RCTs found that more than 50% of people with acute atrial fibrillation revert spontaneously within 24–48 hours, especially if atrial fibrillation is associated with an identifiable precipitant such as alcohol or myocardial infarction. **Progression to chronic atrial fibrillation:** We found no evidence about the proportion of people with acute atrial fibrillation who develop more chronic forms of atrial fibrillation (e.g. paroxysmal, persistent, or permanent atrial fibrillation). **Mortality:** We found little evidence about the effects on mortality of acute atrial fibrillation where no underlying cause is found. Acute atrial fibrillation during myocardial infarction is an independent predictor of both short term and long term mortality.[7] **Heart failure:** Onset of atrial fibrillation reduces cardiac output by 10–20%, irrespective of the underlying ventricular rate,[8,9] and can contribute to heart failure. People with acute atrial fibrillation who present with heart failure have worse prognoses. **Stroke:** Acute atrial fibrillation is associated with a risk of imminent stroke.[10-13] One case series used transoesophageal echocardiography in people who had developed acute atrial fibrillation within the preceding 48 hours; 15% had atrial thrombi.[14] An ischaemic stroke associated with atrial fibrillation is more likely to be fatal, have a recurrence, and leave a serious functional deficit among survivors than a stroke not associated with atrial fibrillation.[15]

Please refer to clinicalevidence.com for full text and references.

Heart failure

Search date February 2006

Robert McKelvie

What are the effects of non-drug treatments for heart failure?

BENEFICIAL

Multidisciplinary interventions

Three systematic reviews found that multidisciplinary programmes reduced all cause mortality, all cause hospitalisations, and heart failure hospitalisations compared with conventional care.

LIKELY TO BE BENEFICIAL

Exercise

Two systematic reviews found that exercise training reduced death rates compared with usual care, but the reduction was not statistically significant in one review. Two systematic reviews found that exercise training improved exercise performance compared with usual care.

What are the effects of drug and invasive treatments for heart failure?

BENEFICIAL

Angiotensin converting enzyme inhibitors

Systematic reviews and RCTs found that angiotensin converting enzyme inhibitors reduced ischaemic events, mortality, and hospital admission for heart failure compared with placebo. Relative benefits were similar in different groups of people, but absolute benefits were greater in people with severe heart failure. For a report on studies comparing angiotensin converting enzyme inhibitors versus angiotensin II receptor blockers, and the effects of combined angiotensin converting enzyme inhibitors and angiotensin II receptor blockers, see the section on angiotensin II receptor blockers.

Angiotensin II receptor blockers

One systematic review found that angiotensin II receptor blockers reduced mortality and admission for heart failure compared with placebo in people with New York Heart Association functional class II–IV heart failure, and were an effective alternative in people who were intolerant to angiotensin converting enzyme inhibitors. One systematic review found no significant difference between angiotensin II receptor blockers and angiotensin converting enzyme inhibitors in all cause mortality or hospital admission. One systematic review found that angiotensin II receptor blockers plus angiotensin converting enzyme inhibitors reduced cardiovascular mortality and admission for heart failure compared with angiotensin converting enzyme inhibitors alone. Effects on all cause mortality remained uncertain.

Beta-blockers

Systematic reviews found strong evidence that adding a beta-blocker to an angiotensin converting enzyme inhibitor decreased mortality and hospital admission in symptomatic people with heart failure of any severity. One systematic review found similar results for all cause mortality and heart failure hospitalisation for beta-blockers with or without angiotensin converting enzyme ▶

inhibitors or angiotensin II receptor blockers. One RCT found that bisoprolol may be as effective as enalapril to initiate treatment for heart failure. One systematic review found that beta-blockers significantly reduced all cause mortality in the elderly. Limited evidence from a subgroup analysis of one RCT found no significant effect on mortality in black people.

Digoxin (improves morbidity in people already receiving diuretics and angiotensin converting enzyme inhibitors)

One systematic review found that digoxin reduced hospitalisations and clinical deterioration compared with placebo in people in sinus rhythm but found no significant difference between digoxin and placebo for mortality.

Implantable cardiac defibrillators in people at high risk of arrhythmia

One systematic review found that implantable cardiac defibrillators reduced mortality in people with heart failure who have experienced a near fatal ventricular arrhythmia or are at high risk of sudden death. A second systematic review found that implantable cardiac defibrillators reduced mortality in people with heart failure due to non-ischaemic cardiomyopathy.

LIKELY TO BE BENEFICIAL

Cardiac resynchronisation therapy

One systematic review and one subsequent RCT found that cardiac resynchronisation therapy improved functional capacity, reduced heart failure hospitalisation, and reduced all cause mortality compared with standard care.

Eplerenone (in people with myocardial infarction complicated by left ventricular dysfunction and heart failure already on medical treatment)

One large RCT in people with recent myocardial infarction complicated by left ventricular dysfunction and clinical heart failure already on medical treatment (which could include angiotensin converting enzyme inhibitors, angiotensin II receptor blockers, diuretics, beta-blockers, or coronary reperfusion therapy) found that adding eplerenone (an aldosterone receptor antagonist) reduced mortality compared with adding placebo.

Spironolactone in people with severe heart failure

One large RCT in people with severe heart failure taking diuretics, angiotensin converting enzyme inhibitors, and digoxin found that adding spironolactone reduced mortality after 2 years compared with adding placebo.

UNKNOWN EFFECTIVENESS

Amiodarone

Systematic reviews found weak evidence that amiodarone may reduce mortality compared with placebo. However, we were unable to draw firm conclusions about the effects of amiodarone in people with heart failure.

Anticoagulation

A preliminary report from one RCT found no significant difference between warfarin and no antithrombotic treatment or between warfarin and aspirin in the combined outcome of death, myocardial infarction, and stroke after 27 months. However, the RCT may have lacked power to detect a clinically important difference. The effects of antiplatelet treatment in combination with angiotensin converting enzyme inhibitors require further research.

Antiplatelet agents

A preliminary report from one RCT found no significant difference between aspirin and no antithrombotic treatment or between aspirin and warfarin in the combined outcome of death, myocardial infarction, and stroke after 27 months. However, the RCT may have lacked power to detect a clinically important difference. The effects of antiplatelet treatment in combination with angiotensin converting enzyme inhibitors require further research.

LIKELY TO BE INEFFECTIVE OR HARMFUL

Calcium channel blockers

One systematic review found no significant difference in mortality between second generation dihydropyridine calcium channel blockers and placebo. RCTs comparing other calcium channel blockers versus placebo also found no evidence of benefit. Calcium channel blockers have been found to exacerbate symptoms of heart failure or increase mortality after myocardial infarction in people who also have pulmonary congestion or left ventricular dysfunction.

Non-amiodarone antiarrhythmic drugs

Evidence extrapolated from one systematic review in people treated after a myocardial infarction suggested that other antiarrhythmic drugs (apart from beta-blockers) may be associated with increased mortality in people with heart failure.

Positive inotropes (other than digoxin)

RCTs in people with heart failure found that positive inotropic drugs other than digoxin (ibopamine, milrinone, and vesnarinone) increased mortality over 6–11 months compared with placebo. One systematic review in people with heart failure found that intravenous adrenergic inotropes non-significantly increased mortality compared with placebo or control, and found insufficient evidence about effects on symptoms. Another systematic review found that phosphodiesterase III inhibitors also increased mortality. It suggested that their use may not be safe.

What are the effects of angiotensin converting enzyme inhibitors in people at high risk of heart failure?

BENEFICIAL

Angiotensin converting enzyme inhibitors in people with asymptomatic left ventricular dysfunction or other risk factors

RCTs in people with asymptomatic left ventricular systolic dysfunction found that angiotensin converting enzyme inhibitors delayed the onset of symptomatic heart failure, reduced cardiovascular events, and improved long term survival compared with placebo.

What are the effects of treatments for diastolic heart failure?

LIKELY TO BE BENEFICIAL

Angiotensin II receptor blockers

One RCT found that candesartan, an angiotensin II receptor blocker, reduced the combined outcome of cardiovascular death or hospital admission for heart failure compared with placebo, although the difference was not significant. It found no significant difference in cardiovascular death between the two groups, but found that candesartan reduced hospital admission compared with placebo.

UNKNOWN EFFECTIVENESS

Other treatments

We found no RCTs examining effects of other treatments in people with diastolic heart failure.

DEFINITION Heart failure occurs when abnormality of cardiac function causes failure of the heart to pump blood at a rate sufficient for metabolic requirements under normal filling pressure. It is characterised clinically by breathlessness, effort intolerance, fluid retention, and poor survival. Fluid retention and the congestion related to this can often be relieved with diuretic therapy. However, generally diuretic therapy should not be used alone and, if required, it should be combined with the pharmacological therapies outlined in this chapter. Heart failure can be caused by systolic or diastolic dysfunction and is associated with neurohormonal changes.[1] Left ventricular systolic dysfunction (LVSD) is defined as a left ventricular ejection fraction below 0.40. It may be symptomatic or asymptomatic. Defining and diagnosing diastolic heart failure can be difficult. Recently proposed criteria include: (1) clinical evidence of heart failure; (2) normal or mildly abnormal left ventricular systolic function; and (3) evidence of abnormal left ventricular relaxation, filling, diastolic distensibility, or diastolic stiffness.[2] However, assessment of some of these criteria is not standardised.

INCIDENCE/ PREVALENCE Both the incidence and prevalence of heart failure increase with age. Studies of heart failure in the USA and Europe found that under 65 years of age, the annual incidence is 1/1000 for men and 0.4/1000 for women. Over 65 years of age, the annual incidence is 11/1000 for men and 5/1000 for women. Under 65 years of age, the prevalence of heart failure is 1/1000 for men and 1/1000 for women; over age 65 years the prevalence is 40/1000 for men and 30/1000 for women.[3] The prevalence of asymptomatic LVSD is 3% in the general population.[4-6] The mean age of people with asymptomatic LVSD is lower than that for symptomatic individuals. Both heart failure and asymptomatic LVSD are more common in men.[4-6] The prevalence of diastolic heart failure in the community is unknown. The prevalence of heart failure with preserved systolic function in people in hospital with clinical heart failure varies from 13–74%.[7,8] Fewer than 15% of people with heart failure under 65 years of age have normal systolic function, whereas the prevalence is about 40% in people over 65 years of age.[7]

AETIOLOGY/ RISK FACTORS Coronary artery disease is the most common cause of heart failure.[3] Other common causes include hypertension and idiopathic dilated congestive cardiomyopathy. After adjustment for hypertension, the presence of left ventricular hypertrophy remains a risk factor for the development of heart failure. Other risk factors include cigarette smoking, hyperlipidaemia, and diabetes mellitus.[4] The common causes of left ventricular diastolic dysfunction are coronary artery disease and systemic hypertension. Other causes are hypertrophic cardiomyopathy, restrictive or infiltrative cardiomyopathies, and valvular heart disease.[8]

PROGNOSIS The prognosis of heart failure is poor, with 5 year mortality ranging from 26–75%.[3] Up to 16% of people are readmitted with heart failure within 6 months of first admission. In the USA, heart failure is the leading cause of hospital admission among people over 65 years of age.[3] In people with heart failure, a new myocardial infarction increases the risk of death (RR 7.8, 95% CI 6.9 to 8.8). About a third of all deaths in people with heart failure are preceded by a major ischaemic event.[9] Sudden death, mainly caused by ventricular arrhythmia, is responsible for 25–50% of all deaths, and is the most common cause of death in people with heart failure.[10] The presence of asymptomatic

LVSD increases an individual's risk of having a cardiovascular event. One large prevention trial found that the risk of heart failure, admission for heart failure, and death increased linearly as ejection fraction fell (for each 5% reduction in ejection fraction: RR for mortality 1.20, 95% CI 1.13 to 1.29; RR for hospital admission 1.28, 95% CI 1.18 to 1.38; RR for heart failure 1.20, 95% CI 1.13 to 1.26).[11] The annual mortality for people with diastolic heart failure varies in observational studies (1.3–17.5%).[7] Reasons for this variation include age, the presence of coronary artery disease, and variation in the partition value used to define abnormal ventricular systolic function. The annual mortality for left ventricular diastolic dysfunction is lower than that found in people with systolic dysfunction.[11]

Please refer to clinicalevidence.com for full text and references.

Peripheral arterial disease

Search date December 2005

Kevin Cassar and Paul Bachoo

What are the effects of treatments for people with chronic peripheral arterial disease?

BENEFICIAL

Antiplatelet agents

Systematic reviews found that antiplatelet agents (aspirin, clopidogrel, aspirin plus dipyridamole, or ticlopidine) reduced major cardiovascular events over an average of about 2 years compared with control treatment. Systematic reviews also found that antiplatelet agents (aspirin and ticlopidine) reduced the risk of arterial occlusion and revascularisation procedures compared with placebo or no treatment. The balance of benefits and harms is in favour of treatment for most people with symptomatic peripheral arterial disease, because as a group they are at much greater risk of cardiovascular events. One systematic review in people undergoing peripheral endovascular intervention found no significant difference between low dose aspirin plus dipyridamole and placebo in restenosis or reocclusion at 6 months.

Exercise

Systematic reviews and subsequent RCTs in people with chronic stable claudication found that regular exercise at least three times weekly for between 3 and 6 months improved total walking distance and maximal exercise time after 3–12 months compared with no exercise. One RCT found that vitamin E plus regular exercise increased walking duration compared with placebo at 6 months. One RCT found that a "stop smoking and keep walking" intervention increased the maximal walking distance compared with usual care at 12 months.

LIKELY TO BE BENEFICIAL

HMG-CoA reductase inhibitors (statins)

Three RCTs including people with peripheral arterial disease found that statins (simvastatin, atorvastatin, and pravastatin) reduced cardiovascular events (including non-fatal myocardial infarction, coronary death, total coronary events, and fatal and non-fatal stroke) compared with placebo. However, people with peripheral arterial disease formed only a small proportion (5–13%) of all people included in these RCTs. One RCT found that simvastatin increased time to onset of claudication compared with placebo at 12 months. One RCT found that simvastatin increased pain free walking distance and total walking distance compared with placebo at 6 months. One RCT found that atorvastatin increased pain free walking time compared with placebo at 12 months.

Percutaneous transluminal angioplasty (transient benefit only)

Two small RCTs identified by a systematic review, in people with mild to moderate intermittent claudication, found limited evidence that percutaneous angioplasty improved walking distance after 6 months compared with no angioplasty but found no significant difference after 2 or 6 years. Two small RCTs identified by a systematic review and four additional RCTs in people with stenosis between the femoral and popliteal arteries or between the aorta and iliac arteries found no significant difference between angioplasty alone and angioplasty plus stent placement in patency rates, occlusion rates, or clinical improvement. The RCTs may have lacked power to detect a clinically important ▶

effect. One RCT found no significant difference between percutaneous transluminal angioplasty plus lovastatin and percutaneous transluminal angioplasty alone in restenosis rates at 12 months. One systematic review found, in people with chronic progressive peripheral arterial disease, that percutaneous transluminal angioplasty was less effective in improving patency compared with surgery after 12–24 months but found no significant difference after 4 years. The review found no difference in mortality after 12–24 months.

Smoking cessation*

RCTs of advice to stop smoking would be considered unethical. The consensus view is that smoking cessation improves symptoms in people with intermittent claudication. One systematic review of observational studies found inconclusive results of stopping smoking, both in terms of increasing absolute claudication distance and reducing the risk of symptom progression, compared with people who continue to smoke.

*Based on observational evidence and consensus.

TRADE OFF BETWEEN BENEFITS AND HARMS

Cilostazol

One non-systematic meta-analysis and one additional RCT found that cilostazol improved claudication distance at 12–24 weeks compared with placebo. However, adverse effects of cilostazol were common in the RCTs, and included headache, diarrhoea, and palpitations. One RCT found limited evidence that cilostazol increased initial and absolute claudication distance compared with pentoxifylline.

UNKNOWN EFFECTIVENESS

Bypass surgery (compared with percutaneous transluminal angioplasty)

One systematic review found that surgery in people with chronic progressive peripheral arterial disease improved primary patency after 12–24 months compared with percutaneous transluminal angioplasty, but it found no significant difference after 4 years. The review found no significant difference in mortality after 12–24 months. Although the consensus view is that bypass surgery is the most effective treatment for people with debilitating symptomatic peripheral arterial disease, we found inadequate evidence from RCTs reporting long term clinical outcomes to confirm this view.

Pentoxifylline

One systematic review and one subsequent RCT found insufficient evidence to compare pentoxifylline versus placebo. One RCT found limited evidence that pentoxifylline was less effective at improving initial and absolute claudication distance compared with cilostazol after 24 weeks.

DEFINITION Peripheral arterial disease arises when there is significant narrowing of arteries distal to the arch of the aorta. Narrowing can arise from atheroma, arteritis, local thrombus formation, or embolisation from the heart or more central arteries. This topic includes treatment options for people with symptoms of reduced blood flow to the leg that are likely to arise from atheroma. These symptoms range from calf pain on exercise (intermittent claudication) to rest pain, skin ulceration, or symptoms of ischaemic necrosis (gangrene) in people with critical limb ischaemia.

INCIDENCE/ PREVALENCE Peripheral arterial disease is more common in people aged over 50 years than in younger people, and it is more common in men than in women. The prevalence of peripheral arterial disease of the legs (assessed by non-invasive

Peripheral arterial disease

tests) is about 13.9–16.9% in men and 11.4–20.5% in women over 55 years of age.[1,2] The overall annual incidence of intermittent claudication is 4.1–12.9/1000 in men and 3.3–8.2/1000 in women.[3]

AETIOLOGY/ RISK FACTORS Factors associated with the development of peripheral arterial disease include age, gender, cigarette smoking, diabetes mellitus, hypertension, hyperlipidaemia, obesity, and physical inactivity. The strongest associations are with smoking (RR 2.0–4.0) and diabetes (RR 2.0–3.0).[4] Acute limb ischaemia may result from thrombosis arising within a peripheral artery or from embolic occlusion.

PROGNOSIS The symptoms of intermittent claudication can resolve spontaneously, remain stable over many years, or progress rapidly to critical limb ischaemia. About 15% of people with intermittent claudication eventually develop critical limb ischaemia, which endangers the viability of the limb. The annual incidence of critical limb ischaemia in Denmark and Italy in 1990 was 0.25–0.45/1000 people.[5,6] Coronary heart disease is the major cause of death in people with peripheral arterial disease of the legs. Over 5 years, about 20% of people with intermittent claudication have a non-fatal cardiovascular event (myocardial infarction or stroke).[7] The mortality rate of people with peripheral arterial disease is two to three times higher than that of age and sex matched controls. Overall mortality after the diagnosis of peripheral arterial disease is about 30% after 5 years and 70% after 15 years.[7]

Please refer to clinicalevidence.com for full text and references.

Primary prevention: dyslipidaemia

Search date March 2006

Michael Pignone

What are the effects of pharmacological cholesterol lowering interventions in people at low risk (< 0.6% annual coronary heart disease risk)?

UNKNOWN EFFECTIVENESS

Fibrates

We found no RCTs examining the effects of fibrates in people at low risk of coronary heart disease events.

Niacin

We found no RCTs examining the effects of niacin for lowering cholesterol in people at low risk of coronary heart disease events.

Resins

We found no RCTs examining the effects of resins in people at low risk of coronary heart disease events.

Statins

We found no RCTs examining the effects of statins in people at low risk of coronary heart disease events.

What are the effects of pharmacological cholesterol lowering interventions in people at medium risk (0.6–1.4% annual coronary heart disease risk)?

BENEFICIAL

Fibrates

One large RCT in men found that gemfibrozil reduced coronary heart disease events, but not overall mortality, over 5 years compared with placebo.

LIKELY TO BE BENEFICIAL

Resins

One RCT in men found that cholestyramine reduced the combined outcome of non-fatal myocardial infarction and coronary heart disease death compared with placebo at 7 years, although the difference did not reach significance.

Statins

One large RCT in people (mainly men) at medium risk of coronary heart disease (CHD) events found that lovastatin reduced cardiovascular events after 5 years compared with placebo. The RCT found no significant difference between statins and placebo for all cause mortality, but it may have been underpowered to detect a clinically important difference in this outcome. Another RCT found no significant difference between pravastatin and usual care for all cause mortality or a combined outcome of nonfatal myocardial infarction or CHD death after a mean follow up of 4.8 years among men and women at medium risk. However, about 30% of people in the usual care group started lipid lowering drugs during the study, thus diluting the treatment effect.

Primary prevention: dyslipidaemia

UNKNOWN EFFECTIVENESS

Niacin

We found no RCTs examining niacin for lowering cholesterol in people at medium risk of coronary heart disease events.

What are the effects of pharmacological cholesterol lowering interventions in people at high risk (≥ 1.5% annual coronary heart disease risk)?

BENEFICIAL

Statins

Three RCTs provided mixed evidence that statins reduced coronary heart disease (CHD) events in predominantly male populations at high risk for future CHD events with a wide range of initial lipid levels. We found evidence that the magnitude of the benefit with statin treatment is related to an individual's baseline risk of CHD events and to the degree of cholesterol lowering, rather than to the initial cholesterol concentration. One systematic review and meta-regression analysis of all of the major primary and secondary prevention statin RCTs found that mortality benefits of statins outweigh risks in people with a 10 year CHD risk of more than 13%.

UNKNOWN EFFECTIVENESS

Fibrates

We found no RCTs examining effects of fibrates in people at high risk of coronary heart disease events.

Niacin

We found no RCTs examining effects of niacin in people at high risk of coronary heart disease events.

Resins

We found no RCTs examining effects of resins in people at high risk of coronary heart disease events.

What are the effects of reduced or modified fat diet?

LIKELY TO BE BENEFICIAL

Reduced or modified fat diet

One systematic review of people in all risk groups found limited evidence that reduced or modified fat diet reduced primary cardiovascular events compared with usual diet, but it found no significant difference in mortality. One small RCT with an extended follow up found that a diet low in saturated fat reduced mortality at year 24 in middle aged men with combined hyperlipidaemia compared with control. A second large RCT found that a low total fat diet had no effect on total cardiovascular disease in postmenopausal women compared with usual diet.

DEFINITION Dyslipidaemia, defined as elevated total or low density lipoprotein (LDL) cholesterol levels or low levels of high density lipoprotein (HDL) cholesterol, is an important risk factor for coronary heart disease (CHD) and stroke (cerebrovascular disease). This chapter examines the evidence for treatment of

dyslipidaemia for primary prevention of CHD. Primary prevention in this context is defined as long term management of people at increased risk but with no clinically overt evidence of cardiovascular disease, such as acute myocardial infarction, angina, stroke, and peripheral vascular disease, and who have not undergone revascularisation. Most adults at increased risk of cardiovascular disease have no symptoms or obvious signs, but they may be identified by assessment of their risk factors (see aetiology/risk factors below). We have divided people with no known cardiovascular disease into three groups: low risk (< 0.6% annual CHD risk), medium risk (0.6–1.4% annual CHD risk), and high risk (≥1.5% annual CHD risk). Prevention of cerebrovascular events is discussed in detail elsewhere in *BMJ Clinical Evidence* (see chapter on stroke prevention). In the USA the preferred method to calculate cardiovascular disease risk would be to use the Framingham risk equations, the best validated method from a US population (see Appendix 1).[1]

INCIDENCE/ PREVALENCE Dyslipidaemia, defined as elevated total or LDL cholesterol, or low HDL cholesterol, is common. Data from the US NHANES survey conducted in 1999–2000 found that 25% of adults had total cholesterol greater than 6.2 mmol/L or were taking a lipid lowering medication.[2] According to the World Health Report 1999, ischaemic heart disease was the leading single cause of death in the world, the leading single cause of death in high income countries, and second only to lower respiratory tract infections in low and middle income countries.[3] In 1998 it was still the leading cause of death, with nearly 7.4 million estimated deaths a year in member states of the World Health Organization and causing the eighth highest burden of disease in the low and middle income countries (30.7 million disability adjusted life years).[3]

AETIOLOGY/ RISK FACTORS Major risk factors for ischaemic vascular disease include increased age, male sex, raised LDL cholesterol, reduced HDL cholesterol, raised blood pressure, smoking, diabetes, family history of cardiovascular disease, obesity, and sedentary lifestyle. For many of these risk factors, including elevated LDL cholesterol, observational studies show a continuous gradient of increasing risk of cardiovascular disease with increasing levels of the risk factor, with no obvious threshold level. Although by definition event rates are higher in high risk people, most ischaemic vascular events that occur in the population are in people with intermediate levels of absolute risk because there are many more of them than there are people at high risk (see Appendix 1).[4]

PROGNOSIS One Scottish study found that about half of people who suffer an acute myocardial infarction die within 28 days, and two thirds of acute myocardial infarctions occur before the person reaches hospital.[5] People with known cardiovascular disease are at high risk for future ischaemic heart disease events (see chapter on secondary prevention of ischaemic cardiac events) as are people with diabetes (see chapter on prevention of cardiovascular disease in diabetes). For people without known cardiovascular disease, the absolute risk of ischaemic vascular events is generally lower but varies widely. Estimates of absolute risk can be based on simple risk equations or tables (see Appendix 1).[6,7] Such information may be helpful in making treatment decisions.

Please refer to clinicalevidence.com for full text and references.

Primary prevention of hypertension

Search date December 2003

Stacey Sheridan and Michael Pignone

What are the effects of treating hypertension with single drug therapy?

BENEFICIAL

Antihypertensive drugs versus placebo

Systematic reviews found that antihypertensive drug treatment decreased the risk of fatal and non-fatal stroke, cardiac events, and total mortality in people with essential hypertension compared with placebo.

What are the effects of different antihypertensive drugs for people with hypertension?

UNKNOWN EFFECTIVENESS

Antihypertensive drugs versus each other

Systematic reviews and large subsequent RCTs found no significant difference in the ability of different antihypertensive agents to reduce total mortality, cardiovascular mortality, and myocardial infarction. Compared with other antihypertensive drugs, however, ACE inhibitors and alpha-blockers were less effective in reducing rates of stroke and combined cardiovascular events; ACE inhibitors, calcium channel blockers and alpha-blockers were less effective in reducing heart failure; and calcium channel blockers were more effective in reducing stroke.

What are the effects of dietary modification for people with hypertension?

LIKELY TO BE BENEFICIAL

Fish oil supplementation

We found no systematic review or RCTs examining the effects of fish oil on morbidity or mortality in people with hypertension. One systematic review found that fish oil supplementation in large doses of 3 g daily modestly lowered blood pressure compared with placebo in people with hypertension.

Low salt diet

One systematic review found that too few RCTs assessed the effects of salt restriction on cardiovascular morbidity and mortality to draw conclusions. Systematic reviews found that dietary intervention to reduce salt intake modestly reduced blood pressure compared with usual diet in people with hypertension.

Potassium supplementation

We found no systematic review or RCTs examining the effects of potassium supplementation on morbidity or mortality in people with hypertension. One systematic review and one subsequent RCT found that daily potassium supplementation of about 60 mmol (approximately the amount contained in 5 bananas) reduced blood pressure by small amounts compared with placebo or no supplements.

UNKNOWN EFFECTIVENESS

Calcium supplementation

We found no systematic review or RCTs examining the effects of calcium supplementation on morbidity or mortality in people with hypertension. One systematic review in people both with and without hypertension found that calcium supplementation may reduce systolic blood pressure by small amounts compared with placebo or no supplements.

Magnesium supplementation

We found no systematic review or RCTs examining the effects of magnesium supplementation on morbidity or mortality in people with hypertension. One systematic review found no significant difference in blood pressure between magnesium supplementation and placebo in people with hypertension.

DEFINITION Hypertension, a clinically important elevation in blood pressure, is usually defined in adults as a diastolic blood pressure of 90 mm Hg or higher or a systolic blood pressure of 140 mm Hg or higher.[1,2] The World Health Organization defines grade 1 hypertension as office blood pressures ranging from 140–159 mm Hg systolic or 90–99 mm Hg diastolic, grade 2 hypertension as pressures of 160–179 mm Hg systolic or 100–109 mm Hg diastolic, and grade 3 hypertension as pressures equal to or greater than 180 mm Hg systolic and 110 mm Hg diastolic.[1] It is usually recommended that clinicians diagnose hypertension only after obtaining two or more elevated blood pressure readings at each of two or more separate visits over a period of one or more weeks.[2] This recommendation follows the pattern of blood pressure measurement in the RCTs of antihypertensive therapy and represents a compromise between reliable detection of elevated blood pressure and clinical practicality. This review focuses on the effects and treatment of essential hypertension, namely the elevation of systolic and diastolic blood pressures (in isolation or combination) with no secondary underlying cause.

INCIDENCE/ PREVALENCE Coronary heart disease is a major cause of morbidity and mortality throughout the world.[3] It is a leading cause of disability and rising health care costs, and it is responsible for 13% of deaths worldwide. Most of this burden of heart disease can be linked to several "traditional" risk factors, including age, sex, increasing blood pressure, increasing cholesterol, smoking, diabetes, and left ventricular hypertrophy.[4] Of these, hypertension is most common, affecting 20% of the world adult population.[5] The relative risk of adverse events associated with hypertension is continuous and graded.[6] The absolute risk of adverse outcomes from hypertension depends on the presence of other cardiovascular risk factors, including smoking, diabetes, and abnormal blood lipid levels, as well as the degree of blood pressure elevation.[7] Even modest elevations in blood pressure in young adulthood are associated with increased risk of cardiovascular events in middle age.[8]

AETIOLOGY/ RISK FACTORS Identified risk factors for hypertension include age, sex, race/ethnicity, genetic predisposition, diet, physical inactivity, obesity, and psychological and social characteristics.[9]

PROGNOSIS People with hypertension have a two to four times increased risk of stroke, myocardial infarction, heart failure, and peripheral vascular disease than those without hypertension.[6] Additionally, they have an increased risk of end stage renal disease, retinopathy, and aortic aneurysm.[10-12] The absolute risk of adverse outcomes from hypertension depends on other cardiovascular risk factors and the degree of blood pressure elevation (see incidence/prevalence section).[7]

Please refer to clinicalevidence.com for full text and references.

Secondary prevention of ischaemic cardiac events

Search date July 2004

Apoor Gami

What are the effects of antithrombotic treatment?

BENEFICIAL

Aspirin

Two systematic reviews found that aspirin reduced the risk of serious vascular events and reduced all cause mortality compared with placebo. One of the reviews found that doses of 75–325 mg daily were as effective as higher doses (500–1500 mg).

Oral anticoagulants in the absence of antiplatelet treatment

One systematic review found that moderate or high intensity oral anticoagulation reduced the risk of cardiovascular events in people with coronary artery disease but substantially increased the risks of haemorrhage compared with placebo or aspirin.

Thienopyridines

Two systematic reviews and two RCTs found that thienopyridines were more effective than aspirin for reducing the risk of further cardiovascular events.

LIKELY TO BE BENEFICIAL

Combinations of antiplatelets

One RCT found that clopidogrel reduced serious cardiovascular events in people already taking aspirin compared with aspirin alone. One systematic review and one RCT found that adding oral glycoprotein IIb/IIIa inhibitor to aspirin increased mortality and serious bleeding compared with aspirin alone.

LIKELY TO BE INEFFECTIVE OR HARMFUL

Oral anticoagulants in addition to antiplatelet treatment

One systematic review found that when added to aspirin, moderate or high intensity oral anticoagulation reduced the risk of serious cardiovascular events compared with aspirin alone but increased the risk of major haemorrhage. One RCT found that adding fixed, low dose warfarin to aspirin had no effect on cardiovascular outcomes compared with aspirin alone. Another RCT found that fixed dose ximelagatran reduced serious cardiovascular events compared with aspirin alone. We found no RCTs comparing oral anticoagulants plus aspirin versus any other drugs.

Oral glycoprotein IIb/IIIa receptor inhibitors

One systematic review found that oral glycoprotein IIb/IIIa receptor inhibitors (in people not taking aspirin) increased mortality, myocardial infarction, and haemorrhage compared with aspirin alone. We found no comparisons between oral glycoprotein IIb/IIIa receptor inhibitors and placebo or anticoagulants.

What are the effects of other drug treatments?

BENEFICIAL

Amiodarone

Two systematic reviews found that amiodarone (a class III antiarrhythmic agent) significantly reduced the risk of all cause and cardiac mortality compared with placebo in people with recent myocardial infarction and high risk of death from cardiac arrhythmia (including left ventricular dysfunction).

Angiotensin converting enzyme inhibitors (in people with and without left ventricular dysfunction)

Two large RCTs found that angiotensin converting enzyme inhibitors reduced the risk of serious cardiac events in people at high risk of cardiovascular events (but with normal ventricular function and without heart failure). Two systematic reviews found that angiotensin converting enzyme inhibitors reduced mortality in people with recent myocardial infarction or left ventricular dysfunction, one finding a smaller benefit in women, but equal benefit in people with and without diabetes and in black and white people.

Angiotensin II receptor blockers

One RCT found a reduction in cardiovascular events and a death with use of low dose angiotensin II receptor blockers compared with usual care in people with coronary artery disease, most of whom were not taking angiotensin converting enzyme inhibitors.

Beta–blockers

Systematic reviews have found strong evidence that beta–blockers reduce the risk of all cause mortality, coronary mortality, recurrent non-fatal myocardial infarction, and sudden death in people after myocardial infarction. One systematic review found no differences in effect between men and women. Another systematic review found that beta–blockers reduced risk of death from heart failure compared with placebo in people with left ventricular dysfunction and that relative benefit was similar in people with and without diabetes. Relative efficacy of different types of beta–blockers is not clear.

UNKNOWN EFFECTIVENESS

Angiotensin II receptor blockers added to angiotensin converting enzyme inhibitors

We found no systematic review or RCTs comparing angiotensin II blockers plus angiotensin converting enzyme inhibitors versus placebo. Two RCTs found conflicting evidence about the effects on mortality and morbidity of adding angiotensin II receptor blockers to treatment for people already taking angiotensin converting enzyme inhibitors versus angiotensin converting enzyme inhibitors alone, though one of these RCTs may have lacked power to detect a clinically important effect.

LIKELY TO BE INEFFECTIVE OR HARMFUL

Calcium channel blockers

One systematic review found no significant difference in mortality between calcium channel blockers and placebo in people after myocardial infarction or with chronic coronary heart disease. However, subgroup analysis by drug type found that diltiazem and verapamil reduced rates of refractory angina in people

Secondary prevention of ischaemic cardiac events

without heart failure after myocardial infarction. The review found non-significantly higher mortality with dihydropyridines compared with placebo.

Class I antiarrhythmic agents (quinidine, procainamide, disopyramide, encainide, flecainide, and moracizine)

One systematic review found that class I antiarrhythmic agents after myocardial infarction increased the risk of cardiovascular mortality and sudden death compared with placebo. One RCT found that in people with myocardial infarction and symptomatic ventricular arrhythmia, class I antiarrhythmic drugs increased risk of cardiac arrest or death compared with placebo.

Hormone replacement therapy

Two RCTs found no significant difference between combined oestrogen and progestin and placebo in cardiac events among postmenopausal women with coronary artery disease. A third RCT found no significant difference between oestrogen and placebo on mortality in women after myocardial infarction. A fourth RCT found that in men with pre-existing coronary heart disease, high dose oestrogen increased the risk of cardiac events compared with placebo. Hormone replacement therapy led to higher rates of venous thromboembolism, gall bladder disease, and vaginal bleeding in women.

Sotalol

One RCT found that, in people with myocardial infarction and left ventricular dysfunction, sotalol increased mortality compared with placebo.

What are the effects of cholesterol reduction?

BENEFICIAL

Non-specific cholesterol reduction

One systematic review and one RCT found that multiple lipid lowering treatments in people with coronary heart disease substantially reduced overall mortality, cardiovascular mortality, and non-fatal cardiovascular events compared with not lowering cholesterol.

Statins

One systematic review and subsequent RCTs found that, compared with control, statins reduced the risk of mortality and cardiac events in people at high risk of cardiovascular events or with evidence of prior disease. Two RCTs found that intensive statin treatment was more effective than moderate statin treatment in reducing mortality and cardiac events. One RCT found that pravastatin reduced the risk of cardiac outcomes in men, but not in women. Another RCT found that simvastatin was associated with similar relative risk reductions in women and the elderly compared with that in younger men. Pravastatin was shown by one RCT to be effective in reducing cardiovascular events in the elderly.

LIKELY TO BE BENEFICIAL

Fibrates

One RCT found that gemfibrozil reduced the risk of cardiac mortality and cardiac events in people with coronary heart disease compared with placebo. Three RCTs found different results regarding the effect of clofibrate on cardiac or all cause mortality in men with a history of myocardial infarction. A large RCT found no significant difference between bezafibrate and placebo in all cause mortality or cardiac events in people with myocardial infarction or stable angina and a low density lipoprotein level less than 4.7 mmol/L (180mg/dl). A smaller RCT found that bezafibrate reduced cardiac events (mortality, reinfarction, revascularisation, or a combination of these) compared with placebo in men with a history of myocardial infarction and elevated serum cholesterol.

What are the effects of blood pressure reduction?

BENEFICIAL

Blood pressure reduction

One systematic review found that the magnitude of cardiovascular risk reduction in people with coronary artery disease correlated directly with the magnitude of blood pressure reduction and there was little evidence for significant differences of treatment effect for different drugs classes.

What are the effects of non-drug treatments?

BENEFICIAL

Cardiac rehabilitation (including exercise)

One systematic review found that, compared with usual care, cardiac rehabilitation reduced mortality and cardiac events in people with coronary heart disease. Adverse events during or after exercise were rare.

LIKELY TO BE BENEFICIAL

Mediterranean diet

One RCT found that advising people with coronary heart disease to eat a Mediterranean diet (more fruit and vegetables, bread, pasta, potatoes, olive oil, and rapeseed margarine) had a substantial survival benefit over a Western diet.

Psychosocial treatment

One systematic review and two subsequent RCTs provided limited evidence that psychological treatment improved symptoms and reduced the risk of serious cardiac events compared with usual care in people with coronary artery disease.

Smoking cessation

We found no RCTs of the effects of smoking cessation on cardiovascular events in people with coronary heart disease. Observational studies have found that smoking cessation significantly reduced the risk of myocardial infarction and death in people with coronary heart disease.

UNKNOWN EFFECTIVENESS

Advice to eat less fat

We found no strong evidence from RCTs on the effect on secondary ischaemic cardiac events of advising people to eat a low fat diet.

Advice to eat more fibre

There was no evidence from one RCT included in a systematic review that high fibre diets had any effect on cardiac or all cause mortality.

Secondary prevention of ischaemic cardiac events

Fish oil consumption (from oily fish or capsules)

Three RCTs, one included in a systematic review, found conflicting evidence that advice to people with coronary heart disease to eat more fish (particularly oily fish) or to take fish oil capsules reduced cardiac events. One RCT found that use of fish oil capsules reduced mortality at 3.5 years.

UNLIKELY TO BE BENEFICIAL

Antioxidant vitamin combinations

Three RCTs included in a systematic review found no benefit of antioxidant combinations on cardiovascular events or cardiac mortality.

Multivitamins

One RCT included in a systematic review found a reduction in cardiac events with multivitamins but no effect on cardiac mortality.

Vitamin C

We found no RCTs examining the effects of vitamin C on risk of cardiovascular events or death.

LIKELY TO BE INEFFECTIVE OR HARMFUL

Beta-carotene

One RCT from a systematic review found no effect of beta carotene on cardiovascular events or death in people with mild angina. It found that in people with previous myocardial infarction beta carotene increased cardiac mortality.

Vitamin E

Two systematic reviews found inconclusive evidence about the benefits of vitamin E, two RCTs finding that high doses increased cardiac and all cause mortality.

What are the effects of revascularisation procedures?

BENEFICIAL

Coronary artery bypass grafting versus medical treatment alone

One systematic review and one subsequent RCT found that coronary artery bypass grafting reduced revascularisations and angina after 1 year and reduced cardiac and all cause mortality up to 10 years after surgery compared with medical treatment. People with left ventricular dysfunction had a larger absolute reduction in mortality than people with normal ventricular function, though relative benefits were similar. A significant survival benefit was observed in people with left main stem or three vessel disease, but not in people with single or double vessel disease.

Intracoronary stents (versus percutaneous coronary transluminal angioplasty alone)

One systematic review found no significant difference between routine stenting and standard percutaneous angioplasty in mortality rates, risk of myocardial infarction or risk of future coronary artery bypass grafting. However it found that stenting reduced rates of restenosis and future percutaneous transluminal angioplasty. One subsequent RCT found that stents increased event free survival but not mortality after 5 years compared with percutaneous transluminal angioplasty. One systematic review found that stenting significantly reduced cardiac events, restenosis, and revascularisation compared with percutaneous transluminal angioplasty in small (< 3 mm) coronary arteries. However, a subsequent RCT found similar rates of restenosis and cardiac events following either treatment in small coronary arteries. One RCT found that stents reduced cardiac events after 6 months compared with percutaneous transluminal angioplasty in saphenous vein graft lesions in people with prior coronary artery bypass grafting. Three RCTs found that stents reduced restenosis and improved angina in people with total occlusions. There is conflicting evidence from two RCTs about effects of stents compared with percutaneous transluminal angioplasty in people with stenosis after initial percutaneous transluminal angioplasty on further restenosis and cardiac events.

LIKELY TO BE BENEFICIAL

Coronary artery bypass grafting (versus percutaneous transluminal angioplasty with or without stenting for multivessel disease)

One systematic review found no significant difference in mortality or myocardial infarction between percutaneous transluminal angioplasty (with or without stenting) and coronary artery bypass grafting after 3 years. However, percutaneous transluminal angioplasty (with or without stenting) led to a higher rate of repeat revascularisation and recurrent angina. The review lacked power to detect less than a 20–30% relative difference in mortality.

Coronary percutaneous transluminal angioplasty versus medical treatment

One systematic review found no significant difference between coronary percutaneous transluminal angioplasty and medical treatment in survival. However, percutaneous transluminal angioplasty improved physical functioning and general health and vitality after 1 year and reduced angina severity in those with severe or moderate angina compared with medical treatment alone. The review found an increase in subsequent coronary artery bypass grafting with percutaneous transluminal angioplasty. One RCT in elderly people found that percutaneous transluminal angioplasty reduced anginal symptoms and adverse cardiac events, but not mortality or non-fatal myocardial infarction.

DEFINITION Secondary prevention in this context is the long term treatment to prevent recurrent cardiac morbidity and mortality and to improve quality of life in people who either had a prior acute myocardial infarction or are at high risk of ischaemic cardiac events for other reasons, such as severe coronary artery stenoses, angina, or prior coronary surgical procedures.

INCIDENCE/ PREVALENCE Coronary artery disease is the leading cause of mortality in developed countries and is becoming a major cause of morbidity and mortality in developing countries. There are international, regional, and temporal differences in incidence, prevalence, and death rates. In the USA, the prevalence of coronary artery disease is over 6%, and the annual incidence is over 0.33%.[1]

AETIOLOGY/ RISK FACTORS Most ischaemic cardiac events are associated with atheromatous plaques that can lead to acute obstruction of coronary arteries. Coronary artery disease is more likely in people who are older or have risk factors, such as smoking, hypertension, high cholesterol, and diabetes mellitus.

PROGNOSIS Within 1 year of having a first myocardial infarction, 25% of men and 38% of women will die. Within 6 years of having a first myocardial infarction, 18% of men and 35% of women will have another myocardial infarction, 22% of men and 46% of women will have heart failure, and 7% of men and 6% of women will have sudden death.[1]

Please refer to clinicalevidence.com for full text and references.

Stroke management

Search date January 2005

Elizabeth Warburton

What are the effects of specialised care in people with acute stroke?

BENEFICIAL

Specialised care (specialist stroke rehabilitation)

One systematic review found that specialist stroke rehabilitation reduced death or dependency after a median follow up of 1 year compared with conventional (less specialised) care. Prospective observational data suggest that these findings may be reproducible in routine clinical settings. A second systematic review of one RCT provided insufficient evidence to compare care based on in-hospital care pathways versus standard care. One small subsequent pilot study found that intensive monitoring reduced mortality at 3 months compared with standard care. It found no significant difference between intensive monitoring and usual stroke unit care in rates of poor outcome at 3 months but may not have been large enough to detect clinically important differences in function.

What are the effects of medical treatment in people with acute ischaemic stroke?

BENEFICIAL

Aspirin

One systematic review in people with ischaemic stroke confirmed by computerised tomography scan found that aspirin taken within 48 hours of stroke onset reduced death or dependency at 6 months and increased the proportion of people making a complete recovery compared with placebo. Another systematic review found no significant difference between aspirin and systemic anticoagulants (unfractionated and low molecular weight heparin) taken within 48 hours of stroke onset in death or dependency at 3–6 months and found that the risk of symptomatic intracranial haemorrhage or extracranial haemorrhage was lower with aspirin than systemic anticoagulants.

TRADE OFF BETWEEN BENEFITS AND HARMS

Systemic anticoagulation (unfractionated heparin, low molecular weight heparin, heparinoids, oral anticoagulants, or specific thrombin inhibitors)

Two systematic reviews comparing systemic anticoagulants (unfractionated heparin, low molecular weight heparin, heparinoids, oral anticoagulants, or specific thrombin inhibitors) versus control (placebo or no treatment) or versus aspirin found no significant difference in death or dependency after 3–6 months. Both reviews found that systemic anticoagulation reduced the risk of symptomatic deep venous thrombosis in people with ischaemic stroke compared with control (placebo or no treatment) or aspirin. However, systemic anticoagulants increased the risk of intracranial haemorrhage or extracranial haemorrhage.

Thrombolysis (increased overall mortality and fatal haemorrhages but reduced dependency in survivors; beneficial effects on dependency do not extend to streptokinase)

One systematic review in people with confirmed ischaemic stroke found that thrombolysis reduced the risk of the composite outcome of death or dependency after 1–6 months compared with placebo. However, thrombolysis increased the risk of death from intracranial haemorrhage measured in the first 7–10 days and risk of death after 1–6 months. The excess in mortality was offset by fewer people being alive but dependent 6 months after stroke onset, and the net effect was a reduction in people who were either dead or dependent. Systematic reviews that pooled results for specific thrombolytic agents found that benefits and harms of recombinant tissue plasminogen activator were similar to the overall results. However, streptokinase increased mortality compared with placebo, and this harm was not offset by reduced dependency in survivors. Results of the reviews may not extrapolate to people with the most mild or most severe strokes.

UNLIKELY TO BE BENEFICIAL

Neuroprotective agents (calcium channel antagonists, citicoline, gamma-aminobutyric acid agonists, glycine antagonists, lubeluzole, magnesium, N-methyl-D-aspartate antagonists, tirilazad)

RCTs found no evidence that calcium channel antagonists, citicoline, lubeluzole, gamma-aminobutyric acid agonists, tirilazad, glycine antagonists, magnesium, antineutrophil inhibitory factor, or N-methyl-D-aspartate antagonists improved clinical outcomes compared with placebo. One systematic review found that lubeluzole increased the risk of having Q-T prolongation to more than 450 ms on electrocardiography compared with placebo.

LIKELY TO BE INEFFECTIVE OR HARMFUL

Acute reduction in blood pressure

One systematic review in people with acute stroke provided insufficient evidence to assess the effects of lowering blood pressure compared with placebo on clinical outcomes. However, other studies found conflicting results. Two RCTs suggested that people treated with antihypertensive agents may have a worse clinical outcome and increased mortality.

What are the effects of surgical treatment for intracerebral haematomas?

UNKNOWN EFFECTIVENESS

Evacuation

We found that the balance between benefits and harms has not been clearly established for the evacuation of supratentorial haematomas. We found no evidence from RCTs on the role of evacuation or ventricular shunting in people with infratentorial haematoma whose consciousness level is declining.

DEFINITION Stroke is characterised by rapidly developing clinical symptoms and signs of focal, and at times global, loss of cerebral function lasting more than 24 hours or leading to death, with no apparent cause other than that of vascular origin.[1] Ischaemic stroke is stroke caused by vascular insufficiency (such as cerebrovascular thromboembolism) rather than haemorrhage.

Stroke management

INCIDENCE/ PREVALENCE Stroke is the third most common cause of death in most developed countries.[2] It is a worldwide problem; about 4.5 million people die from stroke each year. Stroke can occur at any age, but half of all strokes occur in people over 70 years old.[3]

AETIOLOGY/ RISK FACTORS About 80% of all acute strokes are ischaemic, usually resulting from thrombotic or embolic occlusion of a cerebral artery.[4] The remainder are caused either by intracerebral or subarachnoid haemorrhage.

PROGNOSIS About 10% of all people with acute ischaemic strokes will die within 30 days of stroke onset.[5] Of those who survive the acute event, about 50% will experience some level of disability after 6 months.[6]

Please refer to clinicalevidence.com for full text and references.

Stroke prevention

Search date September 2005

Gregory Y H Lip, Peter Rothwell, and Cathie Sudlow

What are the effects of preventive interventions in people with previous stroke or transient ischaemic attack?

BENEFICIAL

Antiplatelet treatment

One systematic review found that prolonged antiplatelet treatment reduced the risk of serious vascular events, including stroke, in people with previous stroke or transient ischaemic attack compared with placebo or no antiplatelet treatment.

Blood pressure reduction

One systematic review found that blood pressure lowering treatment reduced stroke, myocardial infarction, and major vascular events (stroke, myocardial infarction, or vascular death) compared with placebo or no treatment in people with a prior stroke or transient ischaemic attack, whether or not they were hypertensive and irrespective of the type of qualifying cerebrovascular event (ischaemic or haemorrhagic).

Carotid endarterectomy in people with moderately severe (50–69%) symptomatic carotid artery stenosis

Evidence from a pooled analysis of individual patient data from three RCTs in people with symptomatic carotid artery stenosis found that carotid endarterectomy reduced stroke and death in people with 50–69% carotid stenosis compared with no endarterectomy.

Carotid endarterectomy in people with severe (> 70%) symptomatic carotid artery stenosis

Evidence from a pooled analysis of individual patient data from three RCTs in people with symptomatic carotid artery stenosis found that carotid endarterectomy reduced stroke and death compared with no endarterectomy in people with more than 70% carotid stenosis, although no benefit was found in people with near occlusion. Benefit in symptomatic people with more than 70% stenosis was greater than in people with lower grade stenosis.

Cholesterol reduction

We found no systematic reviews comparing statins or non-statin cholesterol lowering treatments versus placebo that reported results separately for people with previous stroke or transient ischaemic attack. One systematic review found that statins reduced major vascular events, including stroke, compared with placebo or no treatment in various different types of people, including those with prior ischaemic stroke or transient ischaemic attack, irrespective of baseline cholesterol or of the presence or absence of coronary artery disease. One systematic review and three additional RCTs in broader populations found that non-statin cholesterol lowering drug treatments did not reduce stroke compared with placebo or no treatment.

Stroke prevention

LIKELY TO BE BENEFICIAL

Carotid endarterectomy in people with asymptomatic but severe carotid artery stenosis

One systematic review and one subsequent RCT found that carotid endarterectomy reduced perioperative stroke, death, and subsequent ipsilateral stroke in people with asymptomatic but severe stenosis compared with medical treatment. However, because the risk of stroke without surgery in asymptomatic people is relatively low, the benefit from surgery is small.

UNKNOWN EFFECTIVENESS

Alternative antiplatelet regimens to aspirin (no evidence that any regimen is more or less effective than aspirin alone)

Two systematic reviews and one subsequent RCT in people at high risk of vascular events found no good evidence that thienopyridines (ticlopidine or clopidogrel) were superior to aspirin for long term prevention of serious vascular events (stroke, myocardial infarction, or vascular death), but found that clopidogrel was a safe and effective alternative to aspirin. One systematic review in people at high risk of vascular events found that dipyridamole plus aspirin reduced non-fatal stroke compared with aspirin alone, but found no significant difference between treatments in serious vascular events (stroke, myocardial infarction, or vascular death). One systematic review and two subsequent RCTs in people at high risk of stroke found no significant difference between triflusal and aspirin in serious vascular events.

Carotid and vertebral percutaneous transluminal angioplasty

RCTs provided insufficient evidence about the effects of carotid and vertebral percutaneous transluminal angioplasty, or stenting compared with medical treatment or carotid endarterectomy in people with a recent carotid or vertebral territory transient ischaemic attack, or non-disabling ischaemic stroke who have severe stenosis of the ipsilateral carotid or vertebral artery.

Different blood pressure lowering regimens (no evidence that any regimen is more or less effective than any other)

We found no RCTs or systematic reviews that compared different blood pressure lowering regimens exclusively in people with a prior stroke or transient ischaemic attack. One systematic review found no significant difference between thiazide diuretics and beta-blockers in death, stroke, coronary artery disease, or total cardiovascular events. A second systematic review found that calcium channel blockers reduced stroke compared with angiotensin converting enzyme inhibitors, but the decrease was of borderline significance. It also found that diuretics or beta-blockers reduced stroke compared with angiotensin converting enzyme inhibitors, but the decrease was of borderline significance.

UNLIKELY TO BE BENEFICIAL

Carotid endarterectomy in people with moderate (30–49%) symptomatic carotid artery stenosis

Evidence from a pooled analysis of individual patient data from three RCTs in people with symptomatic carotid artery stenosis found that carotid endarterectomy was of no benefit in people with 30–49% stenosis compared with no endarterectomy.

Carotid endarterectomy in people with symptomatic near occlusion of the carotid artery

Three RCTs found no evidence that carotid endarterectomy increased the risk of stroke or death owing to surgery in symptomatic people with near occlusion of the ipsilateral carotid artery.

High dose versus low dose aspirin (no additional benefit but may increase harms)

One systematic review and one subsequent RCT in people at high risk of vascular events found that low dose aspirin (75–150 mg/day) was as effective as higher doses for preventing serious vascular events (stroke, myocardial infarction, or vascular death). It also found no significant difference in serious vascular events between doses of 75 mg or more and doses lower than 75 mg. However, the comparison lacked power to detect a clinically important difference. Systematic reviews found no evidence of an association between aspirin dose and risk of intracranial, major extracranial, or gastrointestinal haemorrhage. RCTs found that high dose aspirin (500–1500 mg/day) increased the risk of upper gastrointestinal upset compared with medium dose aspirin (75–325 mg/day).

LIKELY TO BE INEFFECTIVE OR HARMFUL

Anticoagulation in people in sinus rhythm

Systematic reviews found no significant difference between oral anticoagulation and placebo or antiplatelet treatment for preventing recurrent stroke after presumed ischaemic stroke in people in normal sinus rhythm. Anticoagulants increased the risk of fatal intracranial and extracranial haemorrhage compared with placebo or no treatment. High intensity anticoagulation increased the risk of intracranial or major bleeding compared with antiplatelet treatment.

Carotid endarterectomy in people with less than 30% symptomatic carotid artery stenosis

In a pooled analysis of individual patient data from three RCTs of carotid endartectomy for symptomatic carotid artery stenosis, carotid endarterectomy increased the risk of stroke or operative death in people with less than 30% carotid stenosis compared with no endarterectomy.

What are the effects of preventive anticoagulant and antiplatelet treatments in people with atrial fibrillation and previous stroke or transient ischaemic attack?

BENEFICIAL

Oral anticoagulants

One systematic review found that adjusted dose warfarin reduced the risk of stroke compared with control in people with previous stroke or transient ischaemic attack. The best time to begin anticoagulation after an ischaemic stroke is unclear. The review provided insufficient evidence to compare warfarin versus aspirin.

Stroke prevention

UNKNOWN EFFECTIVENESS

Aspirin

One RCT found no significant difference between aspirin and placebo in stroke or death in people with previous stroke or transient ischaemic attack. One systematic review provided insufficient evidence to compare aspirin versus warfarin.

What are the effects of preventive anticoagulant and antiplatelet treatment in people with atrial fibrillation and without previous stroke or transient ischaemic attack?

LIKELY TO BE BENEFICIAL

Aspirin in people with contraindications to anticoagulants

One systematic review found that aspirin reduced the risk of stroke compared with placebo. However, another review found no significant difference. One systematic review found that aspirin reduced stroke and major vascular events in people with non-valvular atrial fibrillation at a similar level to the effect found in other people at high risk (by approximately 25%). Aspirin is used in people with atrial fibrillation and when contraindications exist for anticoagulants, but the thromboprophylactic effect of aspirin may be on the associated vascular comorbidities rather than on the atrial fibrillation.

Oral anticoagulation

One systematic review found that warfarin reduced fatal and non-fatal ischaemic stroke compared with placebo in people at high risk of stroke, provided that there was a low risk of bleeding and careful monitoring. One overview in people less than 65 years old found no significant difference in the annual stroke rate between warfarin and placebo in people at low risk of stroke. Two systematic reviews found that warfarin reduced the risk of stroke compared with aspirin in people at high risk of stroke. One systematic review found no significant difference in stroke between warfarin and the anticoagulant ximelagatran. Ximelagatran has been voluntarily withdrawn worldwide due to a potential increased risk of liver damage.

DEFINITION Prevention in this context is the long term management of people with previous stroke or transient ischaemic attack, and of people at high risk of stroke for other reasons such as atrial fibrillation. **Stroke:** See definition under stroke management. **Transient ischaemic attack:** This is similar to a mild ischaemic stroke, except that symptoms last for less than 24 hours.[1]

INCIDENCE/ PREVALENCE See incidence/prevalence under stroke management.

AETIOLOGY/ RISK FACTORS See aetiology under stroke management. Risk factors for stroke include previous stroke or transient ischaemic attack, increasing age, hypertension, diabetes, cigarette smoking, and emboli associated with atrial fibrillation, artificial heart valves, or myocardial infarction. The relationship with cholesterol is less clear. Overviews of prospective studies of healthy middle aged people found no association between total cholesterol and overall stroke risk.[2-4] However, two of the overviews found that increased cholesterol increased the risk of ischaemic stroke but reduced the risk of haemorrhagic stroke.[3,4]

PROGNOSIS People with a history of stroke or transient ischaemic attack are at high risk of all vascular events, such as myocardial infarction, but are at particular risk of subsequent stroke (about 10% in the first year and about 5% each year thereafter); see figure 1 Ⓕ, and figure 1 in secondary prevention of ischaemic cardiac events.[5-7] People with intermittent atrial fibrillation treated with aspirin should be considered at similar risk of stroke, compared with people with sustained atrial fibrillation treated with aspirin (rate of ischaemic stroke/year: 3.2% with intermittent *v* 3.3% with sustained).[8]

Please refer to clinicalevidence.com for full text and references.

Thromboembolism

Search date September 2005

Richard McManus, David Fitzmaurice, and Richard Hobbs

What are the effects of treatments for proximal deep vein thrombosis?

BENEFICIAL

Compression stockings

One systematic review found that elastic compression stockings reduced the incidence of post-thrombotic syndrome after a deep vein thrombosis.

Low molecular weight heparin (reduced mortality, reduced recurrence, and reduced risk of major haemorrhage compared with unfractionated heparin)

One systematic review found that low molecular weight heparin reduced recurrent thromboembolic disease in people with proximal deep vein thrombosis and decreased major haemorrhage over 3–6 months compared with unfractionated heparin. This review also found that low molecular weight heparin reduced overall mortality compared with unfractionated heparin.

LIKELY TO BE BENEFICIAL

Oral anticoagulants*

Consensus based on observational data regards oral anticoagulants as effective for people with proximal deep vein thrombosis. We found no RCTs comparing vitamin K antagonists such as acenocoumarol, flutamide, and warfarin versus placebo. One RCT found that fewer people had recurrence of proximal deep vein thrombosis within 6 months with combined intravenous unfractionated heparin plus acenocoumarol compared with acenocoumarol alone; as a result, the trial was stopped. One systematic review found no significant difference between oral anticoagulation and long term low molecular weight heparin in recurrent thromboembolism, major haemorrhage, or mortality.

*Clinical consensus based on observational data.

TRADE OFF BETWEEN BENEFITS AND HARMS

Prolonged duration of anticoagulation

One systematic review in people with different types of venous thromboembolism found that a prolonged duration of anticoagulation reduced recurrence of venous thromboembolism, but increased major bleeding, compared with shorter durations of anticoagulation. The review found that, although the risk of recurrence drops over time, the risk of bleeding remains stable while anticoagulant treatment continues. The review found no significant difference in mortality between prolonged and shorter duration anticoagulation.

Venae cavae filters

One RCT in people with proximal deep vein thrombosis considered at high risk of pulmonary embolism, all receiving oral anticoagulation, found that venae cavae filters reduced rates of pulmonary embolism at 12 days compared with no filters. However, the difference in rates of pulmonary embolism was not significant at 2 years, and venae cavae filters increased rates of recurrent deep vein thrombosis at 2 years.

UNKNOWN EFFECTIVENESS

Abrupt discontinuation of oral anticoagulation

One RCT in people who had received warfarin for 3–6 months provided insufficient evidence to compare abrupt withdrawal of warfarin versus an additional month of warfarin at a fixed low dose of 1.25 mg daily.

Home treatment with short term low molecular weight heparin

One systematic review of weak RCTs found no significant difference in recurrence of thromboembolism between heparin treatment at home and in hospital.

Low molecular weight heparin versus oral anticoagulation (long term)

One systematic review found no significant difference between long term low molecular weight heparin and oral anticoagulation in recurrent thromboembolism, major haemorrhage, or mortality. One subsequent RCT found no significant difference between low molecular weight heparin and oral anticoagulation in deep venous thrombosis recurrence at 1 year.

Once daily versus twice daily low molecular weight heparin

Systematic reviews found no significant difference between once and twice daily low molecular weight heparin in recurrent thromboembolism or mortality at 10 days or 3 months. However, the reviews may have been underpowered to detect a clinically important difference because of low rates of recurrent thromboembolism and mortality in the trials.

UNLIKELY TO BE BENEFICIAL

High intensity oral anticoagulation

One RCT found that high intensity treatment with warfarin (target international normalised ratio 3.0–4.5) increased bleeding rates compared with lower intensity treatment (target international normalised ratio 2.0–3.0). However, it did not significantly reduce recurrence of thromboembolism.

What are the effects of treatment for isolated calf vein thrombosis?

LIKELY TO BE BENEFICIAL

Warfarin (reduced rate of proximal extension compared with no further treatment in people who had received initial heparin and wore compression stockings)

One RCT, in people who had received initial intravenous unfractionated heparin (international normalised ratio > 2.5–4.2) and wore compression stockings, found that warfarin reduced rates of proximal extension compared with no further treatment.

UNKNOWN EFFECTIVENESS

Prolonged duration of anticoagulation

One open label RCT found no significant difference in recurrent thromboembolism or rates of major haemorrhage between 6 and 12 weeks of warfarin. The absolute risk of recurrent venous thromboembolism decreases with time, but the relative risk reduction with treatment remains constant. Harms of treatment, including major haemorrhage, continue during prolonged treatment. Individuals have different risk profiles and it is likely that the optimal duration of anticoagulation will vary.

Thromboembolism

What are the effects of treatments for pulmonary embolism?

TRADE OFF BETWEEN BENEFITS AND HARMS

Prolonged duration of anticoagulation

In people who had received anticoagulants for 3 months after a pulmonary embolism, one RCT found no significant difference in recurrence of venous thromboembolism between a further 3 months of oral anticoagulation and longer duration treatment (up to 9 months). However, the RCT may have lacked power to detect a clinically important effect. Additional evidence for duration of treatment has been extrapolated from RCTs in people with proximal deep vein thrombosis and any venous thromboembolism, which found that longer courses of anticoagulation reduced recurrence compared with shorter courses but may increase the risk of major haemorrhage.

Warfarin plus heparin

We found no RCTs comparing heparin versus placebo, warfarin versus placebo, or heparin plus warfarin versus heparin alone or versus warfarin alone. One small RCT found that heparin plus warfarin reduced mortality at 1 year compared with no anticoagulation. Anticoagulants are associated with increased risk of haemorrhage.

UNKNOWN EFFECTIVENESS

Low molecular weight heparin (no clear evidence of a difference in mortality or new episodes of thromboembolism or a difference in risk of major haemorrhage compared with unfractionated heparin)

One systematic review in people with symptomatic or asymptomatic pulmonary embolism found no significant difference in recurrent venous thromboembolism or survival between low molecular weight heparin and unfractionated heparin up to 3 months after treatment. The RCTs in the systematic review found no significant difference in major haemorrhage between low molecular weight heparin and unfractionated heparin but may have been underpowered to detect a clinically important difference.

Thrombolysis

One systematic review found no significant difference in mortality or recurrence of pulmonary embolism between thrombolysis (plus anticoagulants) and heparin alone. It found that thrombolysis (plus anticoagulants) increased the incidence of non-major bleeding events, but not major bleeding events, compared with heparin alone. Subgroup analysis suggested a possible benefit in reducing mortality or recurrence of pulmonary embolism for people with major (haemodynamically unstable) pulmonary embolism. RCTs identified by a systematic review found no significant difference in mortality or recurrent pulmonary embolism among different thrombolytics.

UNLIKELY TO BE BENEFICIAL

High intensity anticoagulation

We found no direct evidence in people with pulmonary embolism about the optimum intensity of anticoagulation. Evidence for intensity of treatment has been extrapolated from RCTs in people with proximal deep vein thrombosis and any venous thromboembolism, which found that bleeding rates were increased by higher intensity anticoagulation (target international normalised ratio 3.0–4.5), but recurrence rates were not significantly different compared with a lower intensity anticoagulation (target international normalised ratio 2.0–3.0).

What are the effects of computerised decision support on oral anticoagulation management?

UNKNOWN EFFECTIVENESS

Computerised decision support in oral anticoagulation (increased time spent in target international normalised range, but effect on clinical outcomes unknown)

We found no RCTs comparing computerised decision support versus usual management of oral anticoagulation that used clinically important outcomes (major haemorrhage or death). One systematic review and six subsequent RCTs found that, compared with usual care, the use of computerised decision support in oral anticoagulation increased the time spent in the target international normalised range. Another subsequent RCT found no significant difference between computerised decision support and standard manual support in the time spent in the target international normalised ratio range.

DEFINITION **Venous thromboembolism** is any thromboembolic event occurring within the venous system, including deep vein thrombosis and pulmonary embolism. **Deep vein thrombosis** is a radiologically confirmed partial or total thrombotic occlusion of the deep venous system of the legs sufficient to produce symptoms of pain or swelling. **Proximal deep vein thrombosis** affects the veins above the knee (popliteal, superficial femoral, common femoral, and iliac veins). **Isolated calf vein thrombosis** is confined to the deep veins of the calf and does not affect the veins above the knee. **Pulmonary embolism** is radiologically confirmed partial or total thromboembolic occlusion of pulmonary arteries, sufficient to cause symptoms of breathlessness, chest pain, or both. **Post-thrombotic syndrome** is oedema, ulceration, and impaired viability of the subcutaneous tissues of the leg occurring after deep vein thrombosis. **Recurrence** refers to symptomatic deterioration owing to a further (radiologically confirmed) thrombosis, after a previously confirmed thromboembolic event, where there had been an initial partial or total symptomatic improvement. **Extension** refers to a radiologically confirmed new, constant, symptomatic intraluminal filling defect extending from an existing thrombosis.

INCIDENCE/ PREVALENCE We found no reliable study of the incidence or prevalence of deep vein thrombosis or pulmonary embolism in the UK. A prospective Scandinavian study found an annual incidence of 1.6–1.8/1000 people in the general population.[1,2] One post mortem study estimated that 600 000 people develop pulmonary embolism each year in the USA, of whom 60 000 die as a result.[3]

AETIOLOGY/ RISK FACTORS Risk factors for deep vein thrombosis include immobility, surgery (particularly orthopaedic), malignancy, smoking, pregnancy, older age, and inherited or acquired prothrombotic clotting disorders.[4] The oral contraceptive pill is associated with increased risk of death from venous thromboembolism (ARI with any combined oral contraception: 1–3 deaths per million women a year).[5] The principal cause of pulmonary embolism is a deep vein thrombosis.[4]

PROGNOSIS The annual recurrence rate of symptomatic calf vein thrombosis in people without recent surgery is over 25%.[6,7] Proximal extension develops in 40–50% of people with symptomatic calf vein thrombosis.[8] Proximal deep vein thrombosis may cause fatal or non-fatal pulmonary embolism, recurrent venous thrombosis, and post-thrombotic syndrome. One case series (462 people) published in 1946 found 5.8% mortality from pulmonary emboli in people in a maternity hospital with untreated deep vein thrombosis.[9] One non-systematic review of observational studies found that, in people after recent surgery who have an asymptomatic deep calf vein thrombosis, the rate of fatal pulmonary embolism was 13–15%.[10] The incidence of other complications without treatment is not known. The risk of recurrent venous thrombosis and complications is increased by thrombotic risk factors.[11]

Please refer to clinicalevidence.com for full text and references.

Varicose veins

Search date March 2006

Paul Tisi

What are the effects of treatments in adults with varicose veins?

LIKELY TO BE BENEFICIAL

Surgery (avulsion)*

We found no RCTs comparing avulsion versus no treatment or compression stockings. There is consensus that avulsion is likely to be beneficial for the treatment of varicose veins. One systematic review found that surgery (avulsion, stripping, ligation with or without sclerotherapy) significantly reduced varicose vein recurrence and improved cosmetic appearance compared with injection sclerotherapy alone. However, one subsequent RCT found that saphenofemoral ligation plus foam sclerotherapy reduced time to return to normal activity and improved quality of life compared with saphenofemoral ligation plus stripping plus avulsions. We found conflicting results from three RCTs that compared avulsion plus stripping of the long saphenous vein to the knee versus avulsion, following ligation. The first RCT found that avulsion of the long saphenous vein to the knee increased clinical recurrence, and decreased participant satisfaction compared with avulsion plus stripping. The second RCT found no significant difference between avulsion and avulsion plus stripping in recurrence or participant satisfaction at 5 years. The third RCT found that avulsion decreased pain compared with avulsion plus stripping after 1 week. However, it found no significant difference between treatments in daily activity scores at 1 week. One RCT found no significant difference between avulsion and powered phlebectomy in pain at 8 days, or in participant satisfaction or cosmetic appearance at 6 weeks. It also found no significant difference between treatments in nerve injury or severe bruising after 2 weeks.

Surgery (stripping)*

We found no RCTs comparing stripping (partial or total, with or without avulsion) versus no treatment or compression stockings. There is consensus that stripping is likely to be beneficial for the treatment of varicose veins. One systematic review found that surgery (avulsion, stripping, ligation with or without sclerotherapy) significantly reduced varicose vein recurrence and improved cosmetic appearance compared with injection sclerotherapy alone. However, one subsequent RCT found that saphenofemoral ligation plus foam sclerotherapy reduced time to return to normal activity and improved quality of life compared with saphenofemoral ligation plus stripping plus avulsions. We found conflicting results from three RCTs that compared stripping plus avulsion of the long saphenous vein to the knee versus avulsion. The first RCT found that stripping plus avulsion of the long saphenous vein decreased clinical recurrence, and increased participant satisfaction compared with avulsion alone. The second RCT found no significant difference between stripping plus avulsion and avulsion in recurrence or participant satisfaction at 5 years. The third RCT found that stripping plus avulsion increased pain and bruising compared with avulsion after 1 week. However, it found no significant difference between treatments in daily activity scores at 1 week. One RCT found similar improvements in clinician assessed clinical outcome with both partial stripping of the long saphenous vein to the knee and total stripping to the ankle. However, it found that partial stripping to the knee reduced the incidence of saphenous nerve damage ▶

compared with total stripping to the ankle. One RCT found that inversion stripping reduced pain scores compared with conventional stripping at 1 week. The RCT found no significant difference between treatments in bruising after 1 week.

*Categorisation based on consensus.

UNKNOWN EFFECTIVENESS

Compression stockings

One crossover RCT found no significant difference in symptoms between compression stockings for 4 weeks and no treatment in people with varicose veins. However, the study might have lacked power to detect clinically important effects. One systematic review found that, in pregnant women with varicose veins, sodium tetradecyl sulphate sclerotherapy improved symptoms and cosmetic appearance of varicose veins compared with compression stockings after 6–24 months.

Injection sclerotherapy

One systematic review found no RCTs that compared injection sclerotherapy versus no treatment. One RCT identified by a systematic review found that, in pregnant women with varicose veins, sodium tetradecyl sulphate sclerotherapy improved symptoms and cosmetic appearance of varicose veins compared with compression stockings after 6–24 months. One RCT found no significant difference between sclerotherapy using polidocanol and using sodium tetradecyl sulphate for improving the appearance of varicose veins at 16 weeks. One RCT found that polidocanol plus sodium tetradecyl sulphate improved symptoms and reduced oedema compared with polidocanol or sodium tetradecyl sulphate alone. One RCT reported a similar incidence of new varicose veins at 5 or 10 years with standard dose conventional sclerotherapy, high dose conventional sclerotherapy, and foam sclerotherapy. One systematic review found that surgery (avulsion, stripping, ligation with or without sclerotherapy) significantly reduced varicose vein recurrence and improved cosmetic appearance compared with injection sclerotherapy alone. However, one subsequent RCT found that saphenofemoral ligation plus foam sclerotherapy reduced time to return to normal activity and improved quality of life compared with saphenofemoral ligation plus stripping plus avulsions.

Surgery (powered phlebectomy)

We found no RCTs comparing powered phlebectomy versus no treatment or compression stockings. One RCT found no significant difference between powered phlebectomy and avulsion in pain at 8 days, or in participant satisfaction or cosmetic appearance at 6 weeks. It also found no significant difference between treatments in nerve injury or severe bruising after 2 weeks. A further RCT found that powered phlebectomy increased pain, bruising, and discolouration compared with avulsion.

DEFINITION Although we found no consistent definition of varicose veins,[1] the term is commonly taken to mean veins that are enlarged, twisted, and painful. Varicose veins may appear dark blue or purple in colour and commonly occur on the back of the calves or on the inside of the legs. Any vein may become varicose, but the term "varicose veins" conventionally applies to the superficial veins of the leg. The condition is caused by poorly functioning (incompetent) valves within the veins and decreased elasticity of the vein walls, which allow de-oxygenated blood to be pumped back to the heart to flow backward and pool in the superficial veins, causing them to enlarge and become varicose. This most often occurs in the saphenofemoral and saphenopopliteal junctions and the perforating veins that connect the deep and superficial venous systems along the length of the leg. The presence or absence of reflux due to venous incompetence can be determined by clinical examination, handheld Doppler, or duplex ultrasound. Symptoms of varicose veins include pain, itching, limb heaviness, cramps, and distress about cosmetic appearance. This chapter focuses on uncomplicated, symptomatic varicose veins. We have excluded treatments for chronic venous ulceration and other complications. We have also excluded studies that solely examine treatments for small, dilated veins in the skin of the leg, known as thread veins, spider veins, or superficial telangiectasia.

INCIDENCE/ PREVALENCE One large US cohort study found the biannual incidence of varicose veins to be 2.6% in women and 2.0% in men.[2] The prevalence of varicose veins in Western populations was estimated in one study to be about 25–30% among women and 10–20% in men.[3] A recent Scottish cohort study has, however, found a higher prevalence of varices of the saphenous trunks and their main branches in men than in women (40% men *v* 32% women).[4]

AETIOLOGY/ RISK FACTORS One large case control study found that women with two or more pregnancies were at increased risk of varicose veins compared with women with fewer than two pregnancies (RR about 1.2–1.3 after adjustment for age, height, and weight).[2] It found that obesity was also a risk factor, although only among women (RR about 1.3). One narrative systematic review found insufficient evidence on the effects of other suggested risk factors, including genetic predisposition, prolonged sitting or standing, tight undergarments, low fibre diet, constipation, deep vein thrombosis, and smoking.[3]

PROGNOSIS We found no reliable data on prognosis, or on the frequency of complications, which include chronic inflammation of affected veins (phlebitis), venous ulceration, and rupture of varices.

Please refer to clinicalevidence.com for full text and references.

Ventricular tachyarrhythmias (out of hospital cardiac arrests)

Search date May 2006

Eddy S Lang and Marwan Al Raisi

What are the effects of antiarrhythmic drug treatments for use in out of hospital cardiac arrest associated with shock resistant ventricular tachycardia or ventricular fibrillation?

UNKNOWN EFFECTIVENESS

Amiodarone

One high quality RCT found that more people survived to hospital admission with amiodarone compared with placebo. However, it found no significant difference in survival to hospital discharge. Another RCT found that more people survived to hospital admission with amiodarone compared with lidocaine. However, it also found no significant difference in survival to hospital discharge. Amiodarone was associated with more hypotension and bradycardia than placebo.

Lidocaine

We found no RCTs comparing lidocaine versus placebo in an out of hospital setting. One high quality RCT suggested that lidocaine is inferior to amiodarone for the outcome of admission to the hospital intensive care unit. Two small RCTs found no difference in clinical outcomes between lidocaine and bretylium.

Procainamide

We found no systematic review or RCTs comparing procainamide versus placebo or the other antiarrhythmic drugs included in this chapter (lidocaine, bretylium, amiodarone) for the clinical outcomes of interest.

UNLIKELY TO BE BENEFICIAL

Bretylium

One small RCT comparing bretylium versus placebo in an emergency department setting found no significant difference in survival to discharge from emergency department. Two RCTs found no difference in clinical outcomes between bretylium and lidocaine. One RCT suggested an increase in the rate of hypotension and bradycardia associated with bretylium compared with placebo. We found no studies comparing bretylium with amiodarone or procainamide in this context.

DEFINITION **Ventricular tachyarrhythmias** are defined as abnormal patterns of electrical activity originating within ventricular tissue. The most commonly encountered ventricular tachyarrhythmias of greatest clinical importance to clinicians and which will be the focus of this chapter are ventricular tachycardia and ventricular fibrillation. **Ventricular tachycardia** is further classified as monomorphic when occurring at a consistent rate and amplitude and polymorphic when waveforms are more variable and chaotic. **Torsades de pointes** is a specific kind of polymorphic ventricular tachycardia associated with a prolonged QT interval and a characteristic twisting pattern to the wave signal. It is often associated with drug toxicity and electrolyte disturbances and is commonly treated with intravenous magnesium. Torsades de pointes will not be specifically covered in this chapter. **Pulseless ventricular tachycardia** results in similar clinical manifestations but is diagnosed by a QRS width complex of > 120 milliseconds and electrical rhythm of 150–200 beats a minute. Waveforms in ventricular fibrillation are characterised by an irregular ▶

rate, usually exceeding 300 beats a minute as well as amplitudes generally exceeding 0.2 mV. Ventricular fibrillation usually fades to asystole (flat line) within 15 minutes. Ventricular fibrillation and ventricular tachycardia associated with cardiac arrest and sudden cardiac death (SCD) are abrupt pulseless arrhythmias. **Non-pulseless (stable) ventricular tachycardia** has the same electrical characteristics as ventricular tachycardia but without haemodynamic compromise. The treatment of stable ventricular tachycardia is not covered in this chapter. **Ventricular fibrillation** is characterised by irregular and chaotic electrical activity and ventricular contraction in which the heart immediately loses its ability to function as a pump. Pulseless ventricular tachycardia and ventricular fibrillation are the primary causes of SCD. **Population:** In this chapter we focus on drug treatments, given generally by paramedics, for ventricular tachycardia and ventricular fibrillation associated with cardiac arrest in an out of hospital setting.

INCIDENCE/ PREVALENCE The annual incidence of SCD is believed to approach 2/1000 population but can vary depending on the prevalence of cardiovascular disease in the population.[1] It is estimated that 300 000 SCDs are recorded annually in the US, representing 50% of all cardiovascular mortality in that country.[2] Data from Holter monitor studies suggest that about 85% of SCDs are the result of ventricular tachycardia/ventricular fibrillation.[3]

AETIOLOGY/ RISK FACTORS Ventricular arrhythmias occur as a result of structural heart disease arising primarily from myocardial ischaemia or cardiomyopathies. In developed nations, ventricular tachycardia or ventricular fibrillation associated cardiac arrest is believed to occur most typically in the context of myocardial ischaemia. As a result, major risk factors for SCD reflect those that lead to progressive coronary artery disease. Specific additional risk factors attributed to SCD include dilated cardiomyopathy (especially with ejection fractions of < 30%), age (peak incidence 45–75 years), and male sex.

PROGNOSIS Ventricular fibrillation and ventricular tachycardia associated with cardiac arrest results in lack of oxygen delivery and major ischaemic injury to vital organs. If untreated this condition is uniformly fatal within minutes.

Please refer to clinicalevidence.com for full text and references.

Absence seizures in children

Search date September 2005

Ewa Posner

What are the effects of treatments for typical absence seizures in children?

TRADE OFF BETWEEN BENEFITS AND HARMS

Ethosuximide

We found one systematic review. It found no RCTs comparing ethosuximide versus placebo. There is, however, consensus that ethosuximide is beneficial, although it is associated with rare but serious adverse effects, including aplastic anaemia, skin reactions, and renal and hepatic impairment. The review found three small RCTs comparing ethosuximide versus valproate. It found no significant difference between ethosuximide and valproate in clinical response (as determined by either electroencephalogram or telemetry recordings, or observer reports of seizure frequency). The review found no RCTs comparing ethosuximide versus other anticonvulsants.

Lamotrigine

One RCT in children and adolescents who had previously benefited from lamotrigine found that lamotrigine increased the proportion of children who remained seizure free compared with placebo. However, lamotrigine was associated with serious skin reactions. One small RCT found that lamotrigine was less effective than valproate at preventing seizures at 1 month. We found no RCTs comparing lamotrigine versus other anticonvulsants.

Valproate

We found one systematic review. It found no RCTs comparing valproate versus placebo. There is, however, consensus that valproate (sodium valproate or valproic acid) is beneficial, although it is associated with rare but serious adverse effects, including behavioural and cognitive abnormalities, liver necrosis, and pancreatitis. The review found three small RCTs comparing valproate versus ethosuximide. It found no significant difference between valproate and ethosuximide in clinical response (as determined by either electroencephalogram or telemetry recordings, or observer reports of seizure frequency). One small RCT found that valproate was more effective than lamotrigine at preventing seizures at 1 month. The review found no RCTs comparing valproate versus other anticonvulsants.

UNKNOWN EFFECTIVENESS

Clonazepam

We found no good evidence to assess the effectiveness of clonazepam for the treatment of typical absence seizures in children.

Gabapentin

One RCT found no significant difference between gabapentin and placebo in the frequency of typical absence seizures. However, the study may have lacked power to detect clinically important effects.

DEFINITION Absence seizures are sudden, frequent episodes of unconsciousness lasting a few seconds and are often accompanied by simple automatisms or clonic, atonic, or autonomic components. Typical absence seizures display a characteristic electroencephalogram showing regular symmetrical generalised spike and wave complexes with a frequency of 3 Hz and usually occur in children with normal development and intelligence. Typical absence seizures are often confused with complex partial seizures, especially in cases of prolonged seizure with automatisms. However, the abrupt ending of typical absence seizures, without a postictcal phase, is the most useful clinical feature in distinguishing the two types. Typical absence seizures should not be confused with atypical absence seizures, which differ markedly in electroencephalogram findings and ictal behaviour, and usually present with other seizure types in a child with a background of learning disability and severe epilepsy.[1] Typical absence seizures may be the sole seizure type experienced by a child. If this is the case and the child is of normal development and has no structural lesions, the child is said to have childhood absence epilepsy. Alternatively, typical absence seizures may coexist in children with other epileptic syndromes, such as juvenile myoclonic epilepsy or juvenile absence epilepsy, in which other seizure types are also present. This differentiation into typical versus atypical seizures is important, as the natural history and response to treatment varies in the two groups. Interventions for atypical absence seizures or for absence seizures secondary to structural lesions are not included in this chapter.

INCIDENCE/ PREVALENCE About 10% of seizures in children with epilepsy are typical absence seizures.[1] Annual incidence has been estimated at 0.7–4.6/100 000 people in the general population and 6–8/100 000 in children aged 0–15 years. Prevalence is 5–50/100 000 people in the general population.[2] Similar figures were found in the USA (Connecticut) and Europe (Scandinavia, France) based population studies.[2] Age of onset ranges from 3–13 years, with a peak at 6–7 years.

AETIOLOGY/ RISK FACTORS The cause of childhood absence epilepsy is presumed to be genetic. Seizures can be triggered by hyperventilation in susceptible children. Some anticonvulsants, such as phenytoin,[3] carbamazepine,[4,5] and vigabatrin[6] are associated with an increased risk of absence seizures.

PROGNOSIS In childhood absence epilepsy, in which typical absence seizures are the only type of seizures suffered by the child, seizures generally cease spontaneously by 12 years of age or sooner. Fewer than 10% of children develop infrequent generalised tonic clonic seizures and it is very rare for them to continue having absence seizures.[7] In other epileptic syndromes (in which absence seizures may coexist with other types of seizure) prognosis is varied, depending on the syndrome. Absence seizures have a significant impact on quality of life. The episode of unconsciousness may occur at any time, and usually without warning. Affected children need to take precautions to prevent injury during absences and refrain from activities that would put them at risk if seizures occurred (e.g. climbing heights, swimming unsupervised, or cycling on busy roads). Often, school staff members are the first to notice the recurrent episodes of absence seizures, and treatment is generally initiated because of the adverse impact on learning.

Please refer to clinicalevidence.com for full text and references.

Asthma and other wheezing disorders in children

Search date October 2005

Duncan Keeley and Michael McKean

What are the effects of treatments for acute asthma in children?

BENEFICIAL

Beta$_2$ agonists (high dose nebulised)*

We found no systematic review or RCTs comparing nebulised beta$_2$ agonists versus placebo in acute severe asthma. High dose frequent nebulised beta$_2$ agonists are a standard component of treatment for acute severe asthma, and placebo controlled trials would be unethical. One RCT identified by a systematic review found no significant difference in rates of hospital admission between intermittent and continuous nebulised salbutamol given in the emergency department.

Corticosteroids (high dose inhaled)

We found one systematic review that identified four RCTs comparing high dose inhaled corticosteroids versus oral corticosteroids in children. Three of these RCTs found no significant difference in hospital admissions with nebulised budesonide or dexamethasone compared with oral prednisolone in addition to other routine treatment in children with mild to moderate acute asthma. One RCT in children with moderate to severe acute asthma, identified by the review, found that, compared with inhaled fluticasone, oral prednisolone reduced hospital admissions and improved lung function at 4 hours. A subsequent RCT in children aged 4–16 years found that, compared with oral prednisolone, nebulised fluticasone improved lung function over 7 days. Another RCT in children aged 5–16 years admitted to hospital with severe asthma found no significant difference in lung function at 24 hours or 24 days after admission with nebulised budesonide compared with oral prednisolone.

Corticosteroids (systemic)

One systematic review found that, compared with adding placebo, adding systemic corticosteroids to usual treatment with salbutamol, terbutaline, or theophylline increased the likelihood of discharge after 4 hours and reduced the frequency of relapse within 1–3 months in children admitted to hospital with acute asthma but found no significant difference between treatments in lung function or length of hospital stay. The current consensus is that systemic corticosteroids are beneficial in children with severe acute asthma; therefore, placebo controlled trials in this population would be considered unethical. We found one systematic review that identified four RCTs comparing high dose inhaled corticosteroids versus oral corticosteroids in children. Three of these RCTs found no significant difference in hospital admissions with nebulised budesonide or dexamethasone compared with oral prednisolone in addition to other routine treatment in children with mild to moderate asthma. One RCT in children with moderate to severe asthma found that, compared with inhaled fluticasone, oral prednisolone reduced hospital admissions and improved lung function at 4 hours. A subsequent RCT in children aged 4–16 years found that, compared with oral prednisolone, nebulised fluticasone improved lung function over 7 days. Another RCT in children aged 5–16 years admitted to hospital with ▶

severe asthma found no significant difference in lung function at 24 hours or 24 days after admission with nebulised budesonide compared with oral prednisolone.

Metered dose inhaler plus spacer devices for delivery of beta$_2$ agonists (as effective as nebulisers)

One systematic review, in children with acute but not life threatening asthma, who were old enough to use a spacer, found no significant difference in hospital admission rates with a metered dose inhaler plus a spacer compared with nebulisation for delivery of beta$_2$ agonists (fenoterol, salbutamol, or terbutaline) or beta agonist (orciprenaline). One subsequent RCT in children with acute wheeze found no significant difference in clinical symptoms, oxygen saturation, or lung function 30 minutes after treatment between salbutamol delivered using spacer and salbutamol delivered using a jet nebuliser. Children using a metered dose inhaler with a spacer may have shorter stays in emergency departments, less hypoxia, and lower pulse rates compared with children receiving beta$_2$ agonist by nebulisation.

Multiple dose ipratropium bromide (inhaled) added to beta$_2$ agonists for severe acute asthma (in emergency room)

One systematic review found that, compared with beta$_2$ agonist alone, multiple doses of inhaled ipratropium bromide plus an inhaled beta$_2$ agonist (fenoterol or salbutamol) reduced hospital admissions and improved lung function in children aged 18 months to 17 years with severe asthma exacerbations.

Oxygen*

An RCT comparing oxygen treatment versus no oxygen treatment in acute severe asthma would be considered unethical. One prospective cohort study and clinical experience support the need for oxygen in acute asthma.

*In the absence of RCT evidence, categorisation based on observational evidence and strong consensus.

LIKELY TO BE BENEFICIAL

Theophylline (intravenous)

One systematic review found that, in children aged 1–19 years admitted to hospital with severe asthma and receiving oxygen, bronchodilators, and glucocorticoids, adding intravenous theophylline improved lung function and symptom scores 6–8 hours after treatment compared with adding placebo, but found no significant difference in the number of bronchodilator treatments required or length of hospital stay. It found that adding theophylline increased vomiting. Theophylline can cause serious adverse effects (cardiac arrhythmia or convulsions) if therapeutic blood concentrations are exceeded.

UNKNOWN EFFECTIVENESS

Ipratropium bromide (inhaled) added to salbutamol (after initial stabilisation)

One RCT in children admitted to hospital with initially stabilised severe asthma found no significant difference in clinical asthma scores during the first 36 hours with nebulised ipratropium bromide compared with placebo added to salbutamol (a beta$_2$ agonist) and corticosteroid (hydrocortisone or prednisolone). The RCT found a significant increase in heart rate with the addition of ipratropium bromide to salbutamol compared with placebo.

Asthma and other wheezing disorders in children

Single dose ipratropium bromide (inhaled) added to $beta_2$ agonists (in emergency room)

In children with mild to moderate asthma exacerbations, a single dose of inhaled ipratropium bromide plus a $beta_2$ agonist (fenoterol, salbutamol, or terbutaline), compared with a $beta_2$ agonist alone, improved lung function for up to 2 hours, but did not reduce hospital admissions. The effect on lung function may not be clinically important in children with mild to moderate asthma exacerbations.

What are the effects of single agent prophylaxis in children taking as needed inhaled beta agonists for asthma?

BENEFICIAL

Corticosteroids (inhaled)

One systematic review and two subsequent RCTs found that, compared with placebo, prophylactic inhaled corticosteroids improved symptoms and lung function in children with asthma. Several RCTs found that inhaled corticosteroids slightly reduced growth rate compared with placebo, although one observational study with long term follow up suggested attainment of normal adult height. Inhaled corticosteroids have been associated with rare reports of adrenal suppression. One RCT in children aged 6–16 years found no significant difference in improvement of asthma symptoms between inhaled beclometasone and theophylline, but found less use of bronchodilators and oral corticosteroids with inhaled beclometasone. Small RCTs have found inhaled corticosteroids to be more effective than sodium cromoglycate in improving symptoms and lung function. RCTs in children aged 5–16 years have found that inhaled corticosteroids (beclometasone, budesonide, or fluticasone) were more effective than inhaled long acting $beta_2$ agonist (salmeterol) or inhaled nedocromil at improving symptoms and lung function in children with asthma. Two RCTs compared inhaled corticosteroids versus montelukast and found different results. One RCT found that fluticasone improved lung function at 12 weeks compared with montelukast in children aged 6–12 years with moderate asthma. The second RCT found no significant difference between high or low dose budesonide and montelukast in clinical score or forced expiratory volume in 1 second in children aged 6–18 years with mild asthma.

LIKELY TO BE BENEFICIAL

Leukotriene receptor antagonists (oral montelukast in children over 2 years of age)

Two RCTs in children aged 2–14 years found that montelukast (a leukotriene receptor antagonist) reduced daily $beta_2$ agonist use and the need for rescue oral steroid courses, and improved lung function and day time symptom score compared with placebo. They found no significant difference between montelukast and placebo in night time symptom score or nocturnal awakenings with asthma. One large RCT in children 6–26 months old with mild asthma found no significant difference between montelukast and placebo in asthma or rescue medication usage, asthma attacks, worsening asthma, or physician visits for asthma. One small RCT in children aged 10–26 months with probable asthma found that montelukast improved symptom score and lung function more than placebo, but the significance of this difference was unclear. One RCT in children aged 6–12 years with chronic asthma found that fluticasone improved lung function and night time symptoms and reduced need for rescue medication or salbutamol compared with montelukast. One crossover RCT in children aged

6–17 years with mild to moderate asthma provided limited evidence that fluticasone reduced asthma exacerbations and improved lung function compared with montelukast. One small RCT in children with mild asthma found no significant difference between montelukast and either low or high dose budesonide in symptoms or lung function.

Nedocromil (inhaled)

Two RCTs in children aged 6–12 years taking usual medication found that, compared with placebo, adding inhaled nedocromil reduced asthma symptom scores, asthma severity, and bronchodilator use, and improved lung function. One large RCT in children aged 5–12 years with mild to moderate asthma found no significant difference between nedocromil and placebo in lung function and hospital admission rate, but that nedocromil was superior to placebo in reducing oral corticosteroid use and emergency care visits. It found that nedocromil increased the need for additional asthma medication, admission to hospital, and emergency care compared with budesonide; however, the significance of these differences was unclear.

TRADE OFF BETWEEN BENEFITS AND HARMS

Long acting beta$_2$ agonist (inhaled salmeterol)

Two RCTs in children aged 4–14 years found that, compared with placebo, inhaled salmeterol (a long acting beta$_2$ agonist) improved lung function. The RCTs provided limited evidence that inhaled salmeterol may reduce the need for inhaled salbutamol. One RCT comparing inhaled salmeterol versus beclometasone found that salmeterol was associated with a significant deterioration in bronchial reactivity. Another RCT found that inhaled beclometasone was more effective at increasing lung function and reducing rescue use of salbutamol than salmeterol. Although monotherapy with long acting beta$_2$ adrenergic agonists decreases the frequency of asthma episodes, they may increase the chance of severe asthma episodes and death when those episodes occur.

Theophylline (oral)

One small RCT in children aged 6–15 years receiving usual care found that, compared with placebo, oral theophylline increased mean morning peak expiratory flow rate and reduced the mean number of acute night time attacks and doses of bronchodilator used. Another RCT in children aged 6–16 years found no significant difference in improvement of asthma symptoms with oral theophylline compared with inhaled beclometasone, but found greater use of bronchodilators and oral corticosteroids with theophylline over 1 year. Theophylline has serious adverse effects (cardiac arrhythmia, convulsions) if therapeutic blood concentrations are exceeded.

UNLIKELY TO BE BENEFICIAL

Sodium cromoglycate (inhaled)

One systematic review found no evidence that inhaled sodium cromoglycate for prophylactic treatment was effective in reducing asthma symptoms in children aged 1–18 years. Small RCTs have found sodium cromoglycate to be less effective than inhaled corticosteroids in improving symptoms and lung function.

Asthma and other wheezing disorders in children

What are the effects of additional prophylactic treatments in childhood asthma inadequately controlled by standard dose inhaled corticosteroids?

UNKNOWN EFFECTIVENESS

Adding leukotriene receptor antagonists (montelukast)

One crossover RCT in children aged 6–14 years with persistent asthma who had been taking inhaled budesonide for at least 6 weeks found that, compared with addition of placebo, oral montelukast (a leukotriene receptor antagonist) reduced asthma exacerbations over 4 weeks. This difference was statistically significant but modest in clinical terms.

Adding long acting $beta_2$ agonist

One RCT in children aged 6–16 years found that the addition of inhaled salmeterol (a long acting $beta_2$ agonist) increased peak expiratory flow rates in the first few months of treatment but found no increase after 1 year. A second short term RCT in children aged 4–16 years also found increased morning peak expiratory flow rates and more symptom free days at 3 months with the addition of salmeterol. A third RCT found that the addition of formoterol improved lung function after 3 months of treatment compared with placebo but found no significant difference in symptom scores or use of rescue medication. Long acting $beta_2$ adrenergic agonists may increase the chance of severe asthma episodes and death when those episodes occur.

Adding oral theophylline

One small RCT found that the addition of theophylline to previous treatment, compared with adding placebo, increased the proportion of symptom free days and reduced the use of additional beta agonist (orciprenaline) and additional corticosteroid (beclometasone or prednisolone) over 4 weeks. We found insufficient evidence to weigh these short term benefits against possible harms. A second small RCT using lower dose theophylline showed no benefit.

Increased dose of inhaled corticosteroid (beclometasone)

One RCT in children aged 6–16 years taking inhaled beclometasone comparing a doubling of the dose of inhaled corticosteroid (beclometasone) versus placebo found no significant difference in lung function, symptom scores, exacerbation rates, or bronchial reactivity but found a reduction in growth velocity at 1 year.

What are the effects of treatments for acute wheezing in infants?

LIKELY TO BE BENEFICIAL

Short acting $beta_2$ agonists (salbutamol by nebuliser)

One RCT in infants aged 3 months to 2 years found that nebulised salbutamol improved respiratory rate and clinical symptom score compared with placebo but found no significant difference in hospital admission. Another RCT that included infants aged less than 18 months and children up to 36 months found no significant difference in change from baseline in clinical symptom scores with nebulised salbutamol compared with placebo. Nebulised $beta_2$ agonists may cause tachycardia, tremor, and hypokalaemia.

Short acting $beta_2$ agonists delivered by metered dose inhaler/spacer versus nebuliser

Three RCTs in children aged up to 5 years found no significant difference in hospital admission with delivery of salbutamol through a metered dose inhaler plus spacer compared with nebulised salbutamol. Another RCT in infants aged 1 month to 24 months found no significant difference in improvement of symptoms with delivery of terbutaline through a metered dose inhaler plus spacer compared with nebulised terbutaline. Nebulised $beta_2$ agonists may cause tachycardia, tremor, and hypokalaemia.

UNKNOWN EFFECTIVENESS

Corticosteroids (high dose inhaled)

One systematic review found that high dose inhaled corticosteroids reduced the requirement for oral corticosteroids compared with placebo but the difference was not statistically significant. The review also found a clear preference for the inhaled corticosteroids by the children's parents over placebo. The clinical importance of these results is unclear. One subsequent RCT found no significant difference between high dose inhaled budesonide and placebo in physician rated global assessment of health status.

Corticosteroids (oral prednisolone)

One small RCT found no significant difference in daily symptom scores with oral prednisolone compared with placebo.

Ipratropium bromide (inhaled)

One systematic review of RCTs provided insufficient evidence about the clinical effects of inhaled ipratropium bromide compared with placebo or added to $beta_2$ agonists.

What are the effects of prophylactic treatments for wheezing in infants?

LIKELY TO BE BENEFICIAL

Short acting $beta_2$ agonists (oral salbutamol)

One RCT identified by a systematic review in infants aged 3–14 months found that oral salbutamol (a short acting $beta_2$ agonist) reduced treatment failures compared with placebo.

TRADE OFF BETWEEN BENEFITS AND HARMS

Corticosteroids (inhaled higher dose)

One systematic review and two additional RCTs provided evidence that, compared with placebo, higher dose inhaled corticosteroids reduced the severity and frequency of acute wheezing episodes in infants. Higher doses of inhaled corticosteroids have the potential for adverse effects.

UNKNOWN EFFECTIVENESS

Corticosteroids (inhaled lower dose)

RCTs found insufficient evidence to assess the effectiveness of lower prophylactic doses of inhaled corticosteroids (budesonide, fluticasone, or beclometasone) in children aged 4 months to 6 years with recurrent wheeze.

Asthma and other wheezing disorders in children

Ipratropium bromide (inhaled)

One small RCT identified by a systematic review found no significant difference in relief of symptoms with nebulised ipratropium bromide compared with placebo. The study may have lacked power to exclude a clinically important difference between treatments.

Short acting beta$_2$ agonists (inhaled salbutamol)

Two RCTs identified by a systematic review in infants aged up to 2 years found no significant improvement in symptoms with inhaled salbutamol compared with placebo.

DEFINITION Differentiation between asthma and non-asthmatic viral associated wheeze may be difficult; persisting symptoms and signs between acute attacks are suggestive of asthma, as are a personal or family history of atopic conditions such as eczema and hay fever. **Childhood asthma** is characterised by chronic or recurrent cough and wheeze. The diagnosis is confirmed by demonstrating reversible airway obstruction, preferably on several occasions over time, in children old enough to perform peak flow measurements or spirometry. Diagnosing asthma in children requires exclusion of other causes of recurrent respiratory symptoms. Acute asthma is a term used to describe a severe exacerbation of asthma symptoms accompanied by tachycardia and tachypnoea. The aim of prophylactic treatments in asthma is to minimise persistent symptoms and prevent acute exacerbations. **Wheezing in infants** is characterised by a high pitched purring or whistling sound produced mainly on the out breath, and is commonly associated with an acute viral infection such as bronchiolitis (see bronchiolitis) or asthma. These are not easy to distinguish clinically.

INCIDENCE/ PREVALENCE **Childhood asthma:** Surveys have found an increase in the proportion of children diagnosed with asthma. The increase is higher than can be explained by an increased readiness to diagnose asthma. One questionnaire study from Aberdeen, Scotland, surveyed 2510 children aged 8–13 years in 1964 and 3403 children in 1989. Over the 25 years, the diagnosis of asthma rose from 4% to 10%.[1] The increase in the prevalence of childhood asthma from the 1960s to 1980s was accompanied by an increase in hospital admissions over the same period. In England and Wales, this was a sixfold increase.[2] **Wheezing in infants** is common and seems to be increasing, although the magnitude of any increase is not clear. One Scottish cross-sectional study (2510 children aged 8–13 years in 1964 and 3403 children in 1989) found that the prevalence of wheeze rose from 10% in 1964 to 20% in 1989, and episodes of shortness of breath rose from 5% to 10% over the same period.[1] Difficulties in defining clear groups (phenotypes) and the transient nature of the symptoms, which often resolve spontaneously, have confounded many studies.

AETIOLOGY/ RISK FACTORS **Childhood asthma:** Asthma is more common in children with a personal or family history of atopy, increased severity and frequency of wheezing episodes, and presence of variable airway obstruction or bronchial hyperresponsiveness. Precipitating factors for symptoms and acute episodes include infection, house dust mites, allergens from pets, exposure to tobacco smoke, and anxiety. **Wheezing in infants:** Most wheezing episodes in infancy are precipitated by viral respiratory infections.

PROGNOSIS **Childhood asthma:** A British longitudinal study of children born in 1970 found that 29% of 5 year olds wheezing in the past year were still wheezing at the age of 10 years.[1] Another study followed a group of children in Melbourne, Australia from the age of 7 years (in 1964) into adulthood. The study found that a large proportion (73%) of 14 year olds with infrequent symptoms had few or no symptoms by the age of 28 years, whereas two thirds of those 14 year olds with frequent wheezing still had recurrent attacks at the age of 28 years.[2] **Wheezing in infants:** One cohort study (826 infants followed from birth to 6 years) suggests that there may be at least three different prognostic categories for wheezing in infants: "persistent wheezers" (14% of total, with risk factors for atopic asthma such as elevated immunoglobulin E levels and a maternal history of asthma), who initially suffered wheeze during viral infections and in whom the wheezing persisted into school age; "transient wheezers" (20% of total, with reduced lung function as infants but no early markers of atopy), who also suffered wheeze during viral infections but stopped wheezing after the first 3 years of life; and "late onset wheezers" (15% of total), who did not wheeze when aged under 3 years but had developed wheeze by school age.[3] Another retrospective cohort study found that 14% of children with one attack and 23% of children with four or more attacks in the first year of life had experienced at least one wheezing illness in the past year at the age of 10 years.[1] Administering inhaled treatments to young children can be difficult. Inconsistencies in results could reflect the effects of the differences in the drugs used, delivery devices used, dosages used, and the differences in the pattern of wheezing illnesses and treatment responses among young children.

Please refer to clinicalevidence.com for full text and references.

Attention deficit hyperactivity disorder in children

Search date May 2005

Deborah Pritchard

What are the effects of treatments for attention deficit hyperactivity disorder in children?

LIKELY TO BE BENEFICIAL

Atomoxetine

Six RCTs found that atomoxetine reduced symptoms of attention deficit hyperactivity disorder compared with placebo after up to 12 weeks of treatment. The RCTs found that atomoxetine decreased appetite and increased nausea, vomiting, asthenia, dyspepsia, infection, laryngitis and pruritus compared with placebo. In the light of emerging evidence and consensus on harms data, practitioners should be guided by the recommendations and warnings issued by their national drug regulatory authorities with respect to the prescribing of psycho-active drugs such as atomoxetine to children and adolescents.

Dexamfetamine sulphate

Two systematic reviews and one subsequent RCT found limited evidence that dexamfetamine (dexamphetamine) improved some behavioural outcomes compared with placebo. Another systematic review found insufficient evidence to compare the effects of dexamfetamine versus methylphenidate. One RCT found limited evidence that, in children already taking dexamfetamine or methylphenidate, adding clonidine reduced conduct symptoms of ADHD after 6 weeks compared with adding placebo. Four RCTs found that dexamfetamine reduced appetite, and one RCT found that it increased sleep disturbance, compared with placebo.

Methylphenidate

One systematic review and subsequent RCTs found that methylphenidate reduced core symptoms of attention deficit hyperactivity disorder in the short term compared with placebo, but disturbed sleep and appetite. Two RCTs found limited evidence that once daily dosing was as efficient as conventional three times a day dosing. The review found inconclusive evidence comparing the effects of methylphenidate and dexamfetamine (dexamphetamine). It found limited evidence that methylphenidate improved symptoms in the medium term compared with psychological/behavioural treatment, but the clinical importance of these findings is unclear. One small RCT provided insufficient evidence to compare clonidine alone, methylphenidate alone, and methylphenidate plus clonidine. A second RCT found limited evidence that, in children already taking dexamfetamine (dexamphetamine) or methylphenidate, added clonidine reduced conduct symptoms of ADHD compared with added placebo after 6 weeks. A second systematic review found limited evidence that high dose methylphenidate was no more effective than low dose methylphenidate plus psychological/behavioural treatment.

Methylphenidate plus psychological/behavioural treatment

One systematic review found inconsistent results for methylphenidate plus psychological/behavioural treatment compared with placebo in children with attention deficit hyperactivity disorder. A second systematic review found that methylphenidate plus psychological/behavioural treatment improved ADHD ▶

symptoms compared with psychological/behavioural treatments alone. A third systematic review found limited evidence that low dose methylphenidate plus psychological/behavioural treatment was as effective as high dose methylphenidate alone.

UNKNOWN EFFECTIVENESS

Clonidine

Limited evidence from one systematic review suggested that clonidine reduced core attention deficit hyperactivity disorder symptoms compared with placebo, but the clinical importance of these findings is unclear. One small RCT provided insufficient evidence to compare clonidine alone, methylphenidate alone, and clonidine plus methylphenidate and found limited evidence that clonidine and clonidine plus methylphenidate increased the risk of bradycardia. A second RCT found limited evidence that, in children already taking dexamfetamine (dexamphetamine) or methylphenidate, added clonidine reduced conduct symptoms of ADHD compared with added placebo after 6 weeks.

Psychological/behavioural treatment

One systematic review of two small RCTs provided insufficient evidence to assess the effects of psychological/behavioural treatment compared with standard care. One systematic review of one large RCT found no significant difference between family therapy and standard care in behaviour rating scales. One systematic review found limited evidence that psychological/behavioural treatment was less effective at improving symptoms in the medium term compared with methylphenidate, but the clinical importance of these findings is unclear.

DEFINITION Attention deficit hyperactivity disorder (ADHD) is "a persistent pattern of inattention and hyperactivity and impulsivity that is more frequent and severe than is typically observed in people at a comparable level of development" (APA, DSM-IV).[1] Inattention, hyperactivity, and impulsivity are commonly known as the core symptoms of ADHD. Symptoms must be present for at least 6 months, observed before the age of 7 years, and "clinically important impairment in social, academic, or occupational functioning" must be evident in more than one setting. The symptoms must not be better explained by another disorder, such as an anxiety disorder, mood disorder, psychosis, or autistic disorder.[1] The World Health Organization's *International statistical classification of diseases and related health problems* (ICD-10)[2] uses the term "hyperkinetic disorder" for a more restricted diagnosis. It differs from the DSM-IV classification[3] in that all three problems of attention, hyperactivity, and impulsiveness must be present, more stringent criteria for "pervasiveness" across situations must be met, and the presence of another disorder is an exclusion criterion. The evidence presented in this topic largely relates to children aged 5 years and above. There is a paucity of evidence of efficacy and safety of treatments in pre-school children.

INCIDENCE/ PREVALENCE Prevalence estimates of ADHD vary according to the diagnostic criteria used and the population sampled. DSM-IV prevalence estimates among school children in the US are 3–5%,[1] but other estimates vary from 1.7% to 16.0%.[4,5] No objective test exists to confirm the diagnosis of ADHD, which remains a clinical diagnosis. Other conditions frequently co-exist with ADHD. Oppositional defiant disorder is present in 35% (95% CI 27% to 44%) of children with ADHD, conduct disorder in 26% (95% CI 13% to 41%), anxiety disorder in 26% (95% CI 18% to 35%), and depressive disorder in 18% (95% CI 11% to 27%).[6]

AETIOLOGY/ RISK FACTORS The underlying causes of ADHD are not known.[6] There is limited evidence that

Attention deficit hyperactivity disorder in children

it has a genetic component.[7-9] Risk factors also include psychosocial factors.[10] There is increased risk in boys compared with girls, with ratios varying from 3 : 1[6] to 4 : 1.[3]

PROGNOSIS More than 70% of hyperactive children may continue to meet criteria for ADHD in adolescence, and up to 65% of adolescents may continue to meet criteria for ADHD in adulthood.[5] Changes in diagnostic criteria cause difficulty with interpretation of the few outcome studies that exist. One cohort of boys followed up for an average of 16 years found a ninefold increase in antisocial personality disorder and a fourfold increase in substance misuse disorder.[7]

Please refer to clinicalevidence.com for full text and references.

Autism

Search date August 2004

Jeremy Parr

What are the effects of early intensive multidisciplinary intervention programmes in children with autism?

LIKELY TO BE BENEFICIAL

Autism Pre-school Programme (APP)*

We found no RCTs or cohort studies meeting our inclusion criteria which compared the Autism Preschool Programme (APP) with control or other treatments in children with autism. Despite the lack of robust RCT evidence, there is consensus that the APP is likely to be beneficial in children with autism.

Lovaas therapy (Applied Behavioural Analysis)*

We found no RCTs or cohort studies meeting our inclusion criteria which compared Lovaas therapy with control or other treatments in children with autism. Despite the lack of robust RCT evidence, there is consensus that Lovaas therapy is likely to be beneficial in children with autism.

TEACCH*

We found no RCTs or cohort studies meeting our inclusion criteria which compared TEACCH with control or other treatments in children with autism. Despite the lack of robust RCT evidence, there is consensus that TEACCH is likely to be beneficial in children with autism.

*In the absence of robust RCT evidence in children with autism, categorisation is based on observational evidence and strong consensus belief that these interventions are beneficial.

UNKNOWN EFFECTIVENESS

Rutger's Autism Programme

We found no systematic review or RCTs that compared the effects of the Rutger's Autism Programme with no treatment or other treatments for children with autism.

What are the effects of treatments in children with autism?

LIKELY TO BE BENEFICIAL

Methylphenidate (for hyperactivity only)

There is limited evidence from a small crossover RCT that methylphenidate hydrochloride reduced hyperactivity and irritability in children with autism.

TRADE OFF BETWEEN BENEFITS AND HARMS

Risperidone

Two RCTs found that risperidone improved overall symptoms of autism in children compared with placebo after 8 weeks. The RCTs found that treatment with risperidone was associated with adverse effects such as weight gain, tremors, and drowsiness in children with autism and other pervasive developmental disorders.

Autism

UNKNOWN EFFECTIVENESS

Auditory integration training

We found no RCTs that evaluated the effectiveness of auditory integration training in children with autism. One systematic review included studies that did not meet our inclusion criteria.

Gluten and casein free diet

One small RCT found limited evidence that compared with usual diet, a gluten and casein free diet improved an autistic trait score in children. Owing to the small sample size and potential confounders, results from this study should be treated with caution.

Omega 3 (fish oil)

We found no RCTs evaluating the effects of omega 3 fish oil as a treatment for autism in children.

Selective serotonin re-uptake inhibitors

We found no RCTs examining selective serotonin re-uptake inhibitors in children with autism.

Vitamin A

We found no RCTs evaluating the effects of vitamin A as a treatment for autism in children.

Vitamin B6 (pyridoxine) plus magnesium

Two small RCTs found no evidence that treatment with pyridoxine plus magnesium improved symptoms of autism in children compared with placebo. The RCTs may have been too small to detect a clinically important effect.

Vitamin C

We found no RCTs evaluating the effects of vitamin C as a treatment for autism in children.

DEFINITION Autism is one of the pervasive developmental disorders (PDD), a group of conditions that also includes Asperger syndrome, pervasive developmental disorder not otherwise specified (PDD-NOS), Rett syndrome, and childhood disintegrative disorder (CDD). Collectively, autism, Asperger syndrome and PDD-NOS are often referred to as "autism spectrum disorders", however, Rett syndrome and CDD fall outside the autistic spectrum. Autism is characterised by qualitative impairments in communication, social interaction, and restricted, repetitive, and stereotyped patterns of behaviours and interests. Abnormal development is present before the age of 3 years. The clinical features required for a diagnosis of autism to be made are set out in ICD-10[1] and DSM IV.[2] For ICD-10 criteria see table 1 Ⓣ. Individuals with autism have a history of language delay (single word or phrase speech delay) and a quarter lose previously acquired skills (regression), most commonly in the second year of life.[5] A third of individuals develop epilepsy[6] and three quarters have mental retardation.[7] Males are affected more commonly than females (3.5–4.0 : 1).[8]

INCIDENCE/ PREVALENCE Recent studies suggest that autism has a prevalence of 10/10 000 in the developed world, and the detected prevalence has increased in recent years; the prevalence for studies published between 1977 and 1991 was 4.4/10 000, whereas that for the studies published during the period 1992–2001 was 12.7/10 000.[9] When considering autism spectrum disorders, the prevalence rises to 60/10 000; many of these individuals have PDD-NOS.[8]

AETIOLOGY/ RISK FACTORS Evidence from twin and family studies suggests that most cases of autism arise because of a combination of genetic factors.[10] Family studies indicate the rate of autism in siblings of autistic individuals is about 2.2%,[11] and the sibling recurrence rate for all PDDs is 5–6%,[12] significantly greater than the population prevalence. Monozygotic twin studies show 60–91% concordance for autism, and therefore it is likely that most cases arise on the basis of multiple susceptibility genes, with influence from environmental or other factors.[13] A minority of cases of autism can be attributed to genetic disorders, including chromosomal abnormalities, fragile X syndrome, tuberose sclerosis, neurofibromatosis type 1, and a variety of other medical conditions.[13] Although perinatal factors have been implicated, it is unlikely that they have a causal role.[14] Research evidence suggests that autism is not caused by the MMR vaccine or thimerosal (mercury) in vaccines (See measlesmumps, and rubella: prevention).[14] There is strong evidence supporting a neurobiological basis of autism.[15] Ongoing research into the relationship between neurophysiology, neuroanatomy, neurochemistry, and genetic factors is likely to increase our understanding, and represents the best chance of unravelling the complex aetiology of the autism spectrum disorders. The presence of phenotypic and genetic heterogeneity may have significant implications for studies of interventions/treatments for autism as efficacy may vary with phenotype.

DIAGNOSIS The generally accepted "gold standard" assessment tools for autism are the Autism Diagnostic Interview-Revised (ADI-R),[3] a semistructured, interviewer based schedule administered to the primary caregiver, and the Autism Diagnostic Observational Schedule (ADOS),[4] a semistructured assessment carried out with the individual themselves. Although these schedules are informative for the clinician, autism remains a clinical diagnosis.

PROGNOSIS Autism is a lifelong condition with a highly variable clinical course throughout childhood and adolescence.[16] Many adults with autism require lifelong full time care. About 15% of adults with autism will live independent lives, whereas 15–20% will live alone with community support.[16] Verbal and overall cognitive capacity seem to be the most important predictors of ability to live independently as an adult.[17]

Please refer to clinicalevidence.com for full text and references.

Blood sampling in infants (reducing pain and morbidity)

Search date May 2006

Deborah Pritchard

What are the effects of interventions to reduce pain related distress and morbidity during venepuncture in preterm or term babies under 12 months in a neonatal unit?

LIKELY TO BE BENEFICIAL

Oral sweet solutions

RCTs have found that oral 24–30% sucrose or 25–30% glucose reduce pain responses (particularly the duration of crying) compared with water, topical anaesthetic, or no treatment in term and preterm infants undergoing venepuncture. Less concentrated solutions of sucrose and glucose did not significantly reduce crying time or pain scores compared with water or no treatment. One RCT found that 25% glucose was more effective than 10% glucose. Limited evidence from one RCT suggests that 30% dextrose given orally may be more effective than water.

Pacifiers

One RCT found that pacifiers reduced pain responses compared with no treatment in term infants undergoing venepuncture.

Topical anaesthetics [lidocaine–prilocaine cream, tetracaine]

Three RCTs found limited evidence that lidocaine–prilocaine cream reduced pain responses to venepuncture compared with placebo. Two RCTs found that tetracaine alone reduced pain and crying during venepuncture compared with placebo. Adverse effects were transient and mild with both lidocaine–prilocaine and tetracaine alone.

DEFINITION Methods of sampling blood in infants include heel puncture, venepuncture, and arterial puncture. **Venepuncture** involves aspirating blood through a needle from a peripheral vein. Heel puncture involves lancing of the lateral aspect of the infant's heel, squeezing the heel, and collecting the pooled capillary blood. Heel puncture and arterial blood sampling are not discussed in this review. For this review, we included premature and term infants up to 12 months in a hospital setting.

INCIDENCE/ PREVALENCE Preterm or ill neonates may undergo 1–21 heel punctures or venepunctures per day.[1,2] These punctures are likely to be painful. Heel punctures comprise 61–87% and venepunctures comprise 8–13% of the invasive procedures performed on ill infants. Analgesics are rarely given specifically for blood sampling procedures, but 5–19% of infants receive analgesia for other indications.[1,2] In one study, comfort measures were provided during 63% of venepunctures and 75% of heel punctures.[2]

AETIOLOGY/ RISK FACTORS Blood sampling in infants can be difficult to perform, particularly in preterm or ill infants. Young infants may have increased sensitivity and prolonged response to pain compared with older age groups.[3] Factors that may affect the infant's pain responses include postconceptional age, previous pain experience, and procedural technique.

Blood sampling in infants (reducing pain and morbidity)

PROGNOSIS Pain caused by blood sampling is associated with acute behavioural and physiological deterioration.[3] Experience of pain during heel puncture seems to heighten pain responses during subsequent blood sampling.[4] Other adverse effects of blood sampling include bleeding, bruising, haematoma, and infection.

Please refer to clinicalevidence.com for full text and references.

Bronchiolitis

Search date October 2005

Juan Manuel Lozano

What are the effects of prophylactic measures in high risk children?

BENEFICIAL

Respiratory syncytial virus immunoglobulin or palivizumab (monoclonal antibody) in children at high risk

One systematic review and one subsequent RCT found that, in children with bronchopulmonary dysplasia or congenital heart disease, prophylactic respiratory syncytial virus immunoglobulin or palivizumab (monoclonal antibody) given monthly reduced hospital admissions compared with placebo or no prophylaxis. The systematic review found that immunoglobulin or palivizumab also reduced intensive care admissions. Treatment duration varied between 4 months and 6 months.

What are the effects of measures to prevent transmission in hospital?

LIKELY TO BE BENEFICIAL

Nursing interventions (cohort segregation, handwashing, gowns, masks, gloves, and goggles) in children admitted to hospital

We found no RCTs on the effects of these interventions to prevent spread of bronchiolitis to other children. However, one non-randomised trial and eight observational studies provided limited evidence that nursing interventions (cohort segregation, gowns, and gloves) reduced nosocomial transmission in children.

What are the effects of treatment for children with bronchiolitis?

UNKNOWN EFFECTIVENESS

Bronchodilators (inhaled salbutamol, inhaled adrenaline [epinephrine])

Three systematic reviews found that inhaled bronchodilators improved overall clinical scores in the short term (< 24 hours after treatment) compared with placebo in children (treated as inpatients, outpatients, or in emergency wards), although the clinical importance of these results is uncertain. There is limited evidence that bronchodilators modestly improve oxygenation in outpatients, although, again, the clinical importance of this result is uncertain. The reviews and one subsequent RCT found no evidence that bronchodilators reduced hospital admission rates or duration of stay compared with placebo.

Respiratory syncytial virus immunoglobulins, pooled immunoglobulins, or palivizumab (monoclonal antibody)

Small RCTs provided insufficient evidence to compare immunoglobulins or palivizumab versus control (albumin solution or 0.9% sodium chloride) in children admitted to hospital with bronchiolitis. ▶

Ribavirin

One systematic review found no significant difference between ribavirin and placebo in mortality, risk of respiratory deterioration, or duration of hospital stay in children admitted to hospital with respiratory syncytial virus bronchiolitis. It found limited evidence that ribavirin reduced the duration of mechanical ventilation. Two subsequent RCTs found no significant difference between ribavirin and placebo in duration of hospital stay or admission rate because of lower respiratory tract symptoms during the first year after the acute episode, or in the frequency of recurrent wheezing illness over 1 year of follow up. The RCTs found were small and might have lacked power to detect clinically important differences.

UNLIKELY TO BE BENEFICIAL

Corticosteroids

Three systematic reviews and subsequent RCTs provided evidence that systemic or inhaled corticosteroids did not improve duration of hospital stay, clinical scores, or hospital admission rates compared with placebo or no corticosteroids.

DEFINITION Bronchiolitis is a virally induced acute bronchiolar inflammation that is associated with signs and symptoms of airway obstruction. The diagnosis is based on clinical findings. Clinical manifestations include fever, rhinitis (inflammation of the nasal mucosa), tachypnoea (rapid breathing), expiratory wheezing, cough, rales, use of accessory muscles, apnoea (absence of breathing), dyspnoea (difficulty in breathing), alar flaring (flaring of the nostrils), and retractions (indrawing of the intercostal soft tissues on inspiration). Disease severity of bronchiolitis may be classified clinically as mild, moderate, or severe.

INCIDENCE/ PREVALENCE Bronchiolitis is the most common lower respiratory tract infection in infants, occurring in a seasonal pattern with highest incidence in the winter in temperate climates,[1] and in the rainy season in warmer countries. Each year in the USA about 21% of infants have lower respiratory tract disease and 6–10/1000 infants are admitted to hospital for bronchiolitis (1–2% of children < 12 months of age).[2] The peak rate of admission occurs in infants aged 2–6 months.[3]

AETIOLOGY/ RISK FACTORS Respiratory syncytial virus is responsible for bronchiolitis in 70% of cases. This figure reaches 80–100% in the winter months. However, in early spring parainfluenza virus type 3 is often responsible.[1]

PROGNOSIS **Morbidity and mortality:** Disease severity is related to the size of the infant, and to the proximity and frequency of contact with infective infants. Children at increased risk of morbidity and mortality are those with congenital heart disease, chronic lung disease, history of premature birth, hypoxia, and age less than 6 weeks.[4] Other factors associated with a prolonged or complicated hospital stay include a history of apnoea or respiratory arrest, pulmonary consolidation seen on a chest radiograph, and (in North America) people of Native American or Inuit race.[5] The risk of death within 2 weeks is high for children with congenital heart disease (3.4%) or chronic lung disease (3.5%) as compared with other groups combined (0.1%).[4] Rates of admission to intensive care units (range 31–36%) and need for mechanical ventilation (range 11–19%) are similar among all high risk groups.[4] The percentage of these children needing oxygen supplementation is also high (range 63–80%).[4] In contrast, rates of intensive care unit admission (15%) and ventilation (8%) in children who do not have high risk characteristics are markedly lower.[6] **Long term prognosis:** Information on long term prognosis varies among studies.

Bronchiolitis

One small prospective study of two matched cohorts (25 children with bronchiolitis; 25 children without) found no evidence that bronchiolitis requiring outpatient treatment is associated with an increased risk of asthma in the long term.[7] Possible confounding factors include variation in illness severity, smoke exposure, and being in overcrowded environments.[8] We found one prospective study in 50 randomly selected infants admitted with bronchiolitis, followed up by questionnaires for 5 years and a visit in the fifth year. It found a doubling of asthma incidence compared with that in the general population, although there was large (30%) loss to follow up and no matched control group.[9]

Please refer to clinicalevidence.com for full text and references.

Cardiorespiratory arrest in children

Search date February 2006

Hilary Writer and David Creery

What are the effects of treatments for non-submersion out of hospital cardiorespiratory arrest?

LIKELY TO BE BENEFICIAL

Airway management and ventilation (including bag-mask ventilation and intubation)*

Although we found no direct evidence to support the use of airway management and ventilation, which includes bag-mask ventilation and intubation, widespread consensus based on indirect evidence and extrapolation from adult data holds that this intervention should be universally applied to children who have arrested. Placebo controlled trials would be considered unethical.

Bystander cardiopulmonary resuscitation*

It is widely accepted that cardiopulmonary resuscitation and ventilation should be undertaken in children who have arrested. Placebo controlled trials would be considered unethical. One systematic review of observational studies found that children whose arrest was witnessed were more likely to survive to hospital discharge, but found no consistent association between bystander cardiopulmonary resuscitation and increased rates of survival. One small subsequent prospective observational study found a significant association between bystander cardiopulmonary resuscitation and survival.

Direct current cardiac shock (for ventricular fibrillation or pulseless ventricular tachycardia)*

Although we found no direct evidence to support the use of direct current cardiac shock, widespread consensus based on indirect evidence and extrapolation from adult data suggests that this intervention should be universally applied to children who have arrested. Placebo controlled trials would be considered unethical.

Intravenous adrenaline (epinephrine) at standard dose*

Intravenous adrenaline (epinephrine) at "standard dose" (0.01 mg/kg) is a widely accepted treatment for establishing return of spontaneous circulation, and it would be considered unethical to test its role in a placebo controlled trial.

*Although we found no direct evidence to support their use, widespread consensus holds that, on the basis of indirect evidence and extrapolation from adult data, these interventions should be universally applied to children who have arrested. Placebo controlled trials would be considered unethical.

UNKNOWN EFFECTIVENESS

Intravenous adrenaline at high dose (compared with standard dose)

We found no RCTs or prospective observational studies in children who have arrested in the community comparing adrenaline versus placebo, and such trials would be considered unethical. One RCT found no significant difference between high and standard dose adrenaline in rates of return of spontaneous circulation, survival to 24 hours, survival to hospital discharge, and severe adverse neurological outcomes in survivors, but it may have been too small to detect a difference between groups.

Cardiorespiratory arrest in children

Intravenous sodium bicarbonate

We found no RCTs or prospective observational studies on the effects of intravenous sodium bicarbonate in children who have arrested in the community.

Intubation versus bag–mask ventilation (relative benefits unclear)

We found no RCTs. One non-randomised controlled trial found no significant difference in survival or neurological outcome between endotracheal intubation and bag–mask ventilation in children requiring airway management in the community, including a proportion that had arrested after submersion.

Training parents to perform cardiopulmonary resuscitation

We found no RCTs or prospective observational studies on the effects of training parents to perform cardiopulmonary resuscitation in children who have arrested in the community.

DEFINITION This chapter deals with non-submersion, out of hospital cardiorespiratory arrest in children. The paediatric Utstein style definition[1] is cessation of cardiac mechanical activity, determined by the inability to palpate a central pulse, unresponsiveness, and apnoea occurring outside of a medical facility and not caused by submersion in water.[2]

INCIDENCE/ PREVALENCE We found 14 observational studies (4 prospective, 10 retrospective) reporting the incidence of non-submersion out of hospital cardiorespiratory arrest in children (see table 1) T.[3-16] Two studies reported the incidence in both adults and children,[8,14] and 12 reported the incidence in children alone.[3-7,9-13,15,16] The incidence in the general population ranged from 1.3–5.7/100 000 people a year (mean 2.8, 95% CI 1.4 to 4.2). The incidence in children ranged from 6.3–18.0/100 000 children a year (mean 9.7, 95% CI 5.8 to 13.6). One prospective study (300 children) found that about 50% of out of hospital cardiorespiratory arrests occurred in children aged under 12 months, and about two thirds occurred in children aged under 18 months.[12]

AETIOLOGY/ RISK FACTORS We found 29 observational studies reporting the causes of non-submersion pulseless arrests in a total of 1708 children.[4-13,15-33] The most common causes were undetermined (as in sudden infant death syndrome; 41%), trauma (19%), chronic disease (9.6%), and pneumonia (5.8%) (see table 2) T.

PROGNOSIS We found no observational studies that investigated non-submersion arrests alone. We found one systematic review (search date 2004) of 41 case series and cohort studies (9 prospective, 32 retrospective; total of 5363 children), which reported outcomes for out of hospital cardiopulmonary arrest of any cause, including submersion, in children up to 18 years of age.[34] Studies were excluded if survival (with survival to hospital discharge as a minimum) was not reported as an outcome. The overall survival rate (to hospital discharge) for the children meeting the paediatric Utstein style[1] definition for out of hospital non-submersion arrest was 5.5% (190/3475 children). Of the 190 surviving children, 43/190 (23%) had no or mild neurological disability and 147/190 (77%) had moderate or severe neurological disability. One subsequent retrospective cohort study of 84 children with non-submersion out of hospital cardiac arrest reported a 4.7% survival rate to hospital discharge, with 50% of the survivors sustaining severe neurological deficits.[33] We found one systematic review (search date 1997), which reported outcomes after cardiopulmonary resuscitation for both in hospital and out of hospital arrests in children of any cause, including submersion.[35] Studies were excluded if they did not report on survival. The review found evidence from prospective and retrospective observational studies that out of hospital arrest of any cause in children has a poorer prognosis than arrest within hospital (132/1568 [8%] children survived to hospital discharge after out of hospital arrest v 129/544 [24%] children after in hospital arrests). About half of the survivors were involved in studies that reported neurological outcome. Of these, survival with "good neurological outcome" (i.e. normal or mild neurological deficit) was higher in children who arrested in hospital compared with those who arrested elsewhere (60/77 [78%] surviving children in hospital *v* 28/68 [41%] elsewhere).[35]

Please refer to clinicalevidence.com for full text and references.

Constipation in children

Search date June 2005

Aruna Abhyankar, Iris Carcani, Graham Clayden

What are the effects of treatments for children with chronic constipation?

LIKELY TO BE BENEFICIAL

Fibre *New*

One small RCT found that fibre improved bowel movements and abdominal pain compared with placebo.

Osmotic laxatives *New*

We found no RCTs of any osmotic laxatives (lactulose, lactitol, macrogols, magnesium salts, rectal phosphates, or rectal sodium citrate) compared with placebo. One poor quality RCT found that lactulose was more effective than senna in the number of children passing normal stools. One RCT found that lactulose was as effective as lactitol in number of evacuations a week; another RCT found that lactulose was less effective than lactitol in this outcome. One RCT also found that lactulose was as effective as a macrogol (polyethylene glycol 3350) in increasing stools and decreasing encopresis frequencies.

UNKNOWN EFFECTIVENESS

Behavioural treatments (biofeedback, diaries, or toilet training) *New*

One systematic review of poor quality, small RCTs found no significant difference between groups when adding biofeedback to conventional treatment in the number of children cured or improved from encopresis. We found no systematic review or RCTs of behavioural treatment compared with no treatment or a sham treatment. One RCT found no significant difference between groups when adding anorectal manometry to conventional treatment in treatment success and number of evacuations.

Bulk forming laxatives *New*

We found no systematic review or RCTs on bulk forming laxatives (methylcellulose, ispaghula husk, or sterculia).

Faecal softeners *New*

One RCT found that mineral oil (liquid paraffin) was more effective than senna in the number of children reporting daily bowel movement and daily soiling. We found no systematic review or RCTs on faecal softeners (arachis oil or mineral oil [liquid paraffin]) compared with placebo.

UNLIKELY TO BE BENEFICIAL

Anal dilatation *New*

One RCT found no significant difference between anal dilatation and no dilatation in symptom severity in children who also received anorectal manometry, evacuation of faeces, intensified medical treatment, and toilet training.

Oral fluids *New*

One RCT found similar results in stool frequency and passing difficulty between increased water, hyperosmolar fluid, and normal fluid intake.

Stimulant laxatives *New*

We found no RCTs that compared stimulant laxatives (bisacodyl, dantron, senna, docusate, sodium picosulfate, or glycerol) with placebo. One poor quality RCT found that senna was less effective than lactulose in the number of children passing normal stools. Another RCT found that senna was less effective than mineral oil (liquid paraffin) in the number of children reporting daily bowel movement and daily soiling. One RCT found no benefit to adding senna to behavioural treatment in faecal soiling.

What are the effects of treatments for clearing the bowel in children with faecal impaction?

UNKNOWN EFFECTIVENESS

Enemas *New*

We found no systematic review or RCTs that compared enemas versus placebo or each other. We found one review of complications of phosphate enema administration which reported various adverse effects in a population with mainly intestinal or renal system abnormalities.

Macrogols (by oral or nasogastric tube) *New*

One RCT found that polyethylene glycol (PEG) 3350 was more effective in reducing abdominally palpable faecal masses and in producing more frequent bowel movements compared with mineral oil. It also reported more problems with compliance in the PEG 3350 group because of the higher volume required compared with mineral oil. In another RCT, PEG 3350 was found to be more effective in disimpaction in higher doses than lower doses.

Surgical disimpaction *New*

We found no systematic review or RCTs of surgical disimpaction compared with another type of surgical disimpaction or enema.

DEFINITION According to the **Rome II criteria**, functional childhood constipation is defined as at least 2 weeks of: scybalous, pebble-like, hard stools for most of the stools; or firm stools two or fewer times a week and no evidence of structural endocrine or metabolic disease.[1] These criteria are not necessarily comprehensive and found to be restrictive by some researchers.[2] (There are now Rome III criteria, which have yet to be responded to by the PACCT [Paris Consensus on Childhood Constipation Terminology] group.) The **PACCT group** has defined childhood constipation as the occurrence of two or more of the following six criteria in the previous 8 weeks: frequency of movements less than 3 a week; more than one episode of faecal incontinence a week; large stools in the rectum or palpable on abdominal examination; passing of stools so large that they may obstruct the toilet; retentive posturing and withholding behaviour; painful defecation.[3] In selecting studies for this chapter, we did not use a singular definition owing to no clear agreement over the definitions (see methods).

INCIDENCE/ PREVALENCE Constipation accounts for about 3% of consultations in an average paediatric outpatient clinic in the USA.[4] In the UK population 5% of school children aged 4–11 years experience constipation lasting more than 6 months.[5] In an inner city population in Brazil the incidence of constipation has been reported as 28%,[6] and 1–2% of healthy school children in the USA.[7]

AETIOLOGY/ RISK FACTORS No aetiological factors can be found in most children. Hirschsprung's disease, cystic fibrosis, anorectal abnormalities, and metabolic conditions such as hypothyroidism are rare organic causes of childhood constipation. An episode

Constipation in children

of painful defecation has been noted in more than 50% of people who were suffering from faecal soiling or chronic faecal impaction.[8] **Risk factors:** One study found higher incidence of constipation among children with birth weight under 750 g associated with neurodevelopment impairment.[9] Low fibre intake may be associated with childhood constipation.[10] Constipation and soiling are more prevalent in obese children.[11] We found no evidence for a difference between bottle fed and breast fed babies although it is generally accepted that bottle fed babies are more at risk of relative water deficiency and breast fed babies frequently have delays of many days between passing normal stools.

PROGNOSIS Childhood constipation continues beyond puberty in up to a third of the children followed up beyond that age.[12] Children aged 2–4 years seem to have a higher recurrence rate and a need for prolonged medication and support than younger infants.[4] One follow up study has noted increased risk of persistent constipation in children who developed constipation early in infancy and who have a family history of constipation.[13] **Faecal impaction:** Disimpaction is necessary if the amount and character of faeces in the colon is of such magnitude that spontaneous expulsion in unlikely, or if it is causing discomfort and affecting normal feeding. Some children with a large rectosigmoid faecaloma may have difficulty passing urine.

Please refer to clinicalevidence.com for full text and references.

Croup

Search date November 2004

David Johnson

What are the effects of treatments in children with mild croup?

BENEFICIAL

Dexamethasone (oral single dose)

Two RCTs found that, compared with placebo, a single oral dose of dexamethasone (0.15–0.6 mg/kg) reduced the proportion of children with mild croup seeking additional medical attention for ongoing croup symptoms within 7–10 days. One of the RCTs also found that dexamethasone reduced the duration of croup symptoms compared with placebo. We found no RCTs evaluating single versus multiple doses of dexamethasone or other corticosteroids in children with mild croup.

UNKNOWN EFFECTIVENESS

Decongestants (oral)

We found no systematic review, RCTs, or observational studies of sufficient quality on oral decongestants in children with mild croup.

Humidification

We found no systematic review, RCTs, or observational studies of sufficient quality evaluating the effects of humidification in children with mild croup.

UNLIKELY TO BE BENEFICIAL

Antibiotics

We found no systematic review, RCTs, or observational studies of sufficient quality evaluating any type of antibiotic in children with mild croup. However, there is widespread consensus that antibiotics do not shorten the clinical course of a disease that is predominantly viral in origin.

What are the effects of treatments in children with moderate to severe croup?

BENEFICIAL

Adrenaline (epinephrine), nebulised

Three RCTs found that, compared with placebo, nebulised racemic adrenaline (epinephrine) 2.25% improved croup score within 30 minutes after starting treatment. One of these RCTs found that, by 2 hours, the treatment effect of adrenaline (epinephrine) had largely disappeared. None of the RCTs reported adverse complications suggesting myocardial insufficiency, nor any evidence suggesting that treatment increases cardiac demand. However, we found one well documented case report of a previously normal child with severe croup who sustained a small myocardial infarction after being treated with three adrenaline (epinephrine) nebulisations within 1 hour. One small RCT found no significant difference between nebulised racemic adrenaline (epinephrine) and heliox (helium–oxygen mixture) in overall mean change in croup scores over 4 hours in children already treated with humidified oxygen and intramuscular dexamethasone 0.6 mg/kg.

Croup

Budesonide, nebulised (compared with placebo)

One systematic review found that, compared with placebo, nebulised budesonide improved croup score at 6, 12, and 24 hours and reduced return hospital visits and readmissions in children with moderate to severe croup. Two RCTs identified by the review found that nebulised budesonide (1 or 4 mg) was less effective than intramuscular dexamethasone 0.6 mg/kg at improving croup score at up to 12 hours, but one of the RCTs found no significant difference in hospital admissions. Two further RCTs identified by the review found no significant difference in croup score improvement at 4 hours or hospital admission at up to 1 week, between nebulised budesonide 2 mg and oral dexamethasone 0.6 mg/kg. Although nebulised budesonide and oral dexamethasone appear to have similar efficacy, there is consensus that it is preferable to use oral dexamethasone because nebulisation usually causes prolonged agitation and crying, which worsens the child's respiratory distress, and it takes on average 15 minutes to deliver nebulised budesonide compared with 1–2 minutes with oral dexamethasone. One RCT found no significant difference in improvement in croup score at 4 hours between nebulised budesonide 2 mg plus oral dexamethasone 0.6 mg/kg and either oral dexamethasone alone or nebulised budesonide alone.

Dexamethasone, intramuscular or oral (compared with placebo)

One systematic review found that, compared with placebo, intramuscular or oral dexamethasone improved croup score at 12 and 24 hours in children with moderate to severe croup.

LIKELY TO BE BENEFICIAL

Dexamethasone, intramuscular (compared with nebulised budesonide for croup scores)

Two RCTs identified by a systematic review found that, compared with nebulised budesonide (1 or 4 mg), intramuscular dexamethasone 0.6 mg/kg improved croup score at up to 12 hours, but one of the RCTs found no significant difference in hospital admissions.

Dexamethasone, oral (compared with nebulised budesonide)*

Two RCTs identified by a systematic review found no significant difference in croup score improvement at 4 hours or hospital admission at up to 1 week, between oral dexamethasone 0.6 mg/kg and nebulised budesonide 2 mg. Although oral dexamethasone and nebulised budesonide appear to have similar efficacy, there is consensus that it is preferable to use oral dexamethasone because nebulisation usually causes prolonged agitation and crying, which worsens the child's respiratory distress, and it takes on average 15 minutes to deliver nebulised budesonide compared with 1–2 minutes with oral dexamethasone.

Oxygen*

We found no systematic review, RCTs, or observational studies of sufficient quality evaluating the effects of oxygen in children with moderate to severe croup. An RCT of oxygen versus no oxygen in children with severe croup would be considered unethical. There is widespread consensus that oxygen is beneficial in children with severe respiratory distress. One small RCT provided insufficient evidence to compare heliox (helium 70%, oxygen 30%) versus oxygen 30% alone.

UNKNOWN EFFECTIVENESS

Adrenaline (epinephrine) (nebulised) plus intermittent positive pressure breathing (compared with nebulised adrenaline alone)

One small crossover RCT provided insufficient evidence to compare nebulised adrenaline (epinephrine) plus intermittent positive pressure breathing versus nebulised adrenaline (epinephrine) alone.

Beta$_2$ agonists, short acting (nebulised)

We found no systematic review, RCTs, or observational studies of sufficient quality evaluating the effects of nebulised short acting beta$_2$ agonists in children with moderate to severe croup.

Decongestants (oral)

We found no systematic review, RCTs, or observational studies of sufficient quality evaluating the effects of any oral decongestants in children with moderate to severe croup.

Dexamethasone (different doses and routes of administration)

One RCT identified by a systematic review found no significant difference between single oral dexamethasone doses of 0.6 mg/kg and 0.3 mg/kg or between 0.3 mg/kg and 0.15 mg/kg in croup score or in return visit or readmission to hospital. A systematic review (including studies using several different corticosteroids other than dexamethasone) provided limited evidence that the higher the dose administered, the greater the difference in the proportion of children reported to be improved between the corticosteroid and placebo groups. Two RCTs identified by the review found no significant difference between intramuscular and oral dexamethasone 0.6 mg/kg for return visit or readmission to hospital.

Dexamethasone (oral) plus budesonide (nebulised)

One RCT found no significant difference in improvement in croup score at 4 hours between nebulised budesonide 2 mg plus oral dexamethasone 0.6 mg/kg and either oral dexamethasone alone or nebulised budesonide alone.

Heliox (helium–oxygen mixture)

One small RCT provided insufficient evidence to compare heliox (helium 70%, oxygen 30%) versus oxygen 30% alone. Another RCT found no significant difference between nebulised racemic adrenaline (epinephrine) and heliox in overall mean change in croup scores over 4 hours in children already treated with humidified oxygen and intramuscular dexamethasone 0.6 mg/kg.

Humidification

One RCT found no significant difference between humidified oxygen (via a "mist stick") and no humidified oxygen in mean change in croup scores at 2 hours in children who had already received a single oral dose of dexamethasone 0.6 mg/kg. Another RCT found no significant difference in improvement in croup scores at 12 hours between placing children with croup in a high humidity atmosphere (87–95%) in a humidified tent, and room air. One small case series of children with croup reported scalds from hot humidified air.

L-adrenaline (epinephrine) compared with racemic adrenaline (epinephrine)

One small RCT found no significant difference in overall improvement in croup scores between L-adrenaline (epinephrine) (1 : 1000, 5 mL) and racemic adrenaline (epinephrine) (2.25%, 5 mL).

Croup

UNLIKELY TO BE BENEFICIAL

Antibiotics

We found no systematic review, RCTs, or observational studies of sufficient quality on antibiotics in children with moderate to severe croup. However, there is strong consensus that antibiotics do not shorten the clinical course of a disease that is predominantly viral in origin. This does not apply if bacterial tracheitis is suspected.

What are the effects of treatments in children with impending respiratory failure due to severe croup?

BENEFICIAL

Adrenaline (epinephrine), nebulised*

We found no RCTs comparing adrenaline (epinephrine) versus no adrenaline (epinephrine) in children with impending respiratory failure due to severe croup. Such an RCT would be considered unethical, as there is widespread consensus that adrenaline (epinephrine) is beneficial in children with impending respiratory failure due to severe croup. One cohort study in children with acute upper airway obstruction found that nebulised L adrenaline (epinephrine) improved mean croup score and reduced carbon dioxide levels. Another cohort study found that nebulised racemic adrenaline (epinephrine) reduced both stridor and paradoxical breathing.

Corticosteroids

One systematic review found that, compared with placebo, treatment with corticosteroids reduced the rate of endotracheal intubation. One RCT in intubated children showed that, compared with placebo, treatment with prednisolone (1 mg/kg via nasogastric tube every 12 hours until 24 hours after extubation) reduced the duration of intubation and the need for reintubation.

LIKELY TO BE BENEFICIAL

Oxygen*

We found no systematic review, RCTs, or observational studies of sufficient quality evaluating the effects of oxygen in children with impending respiratory failure due to severe croup. An RCT of oxygen versus no oxygen in children with severe croup would be considered unethical, as there is widespread consensus that oxygen is likely to be beneficial in children with severe respiratory distress.

UNKNOWN EFFECTIVENESS

Heliox (helium–oxygen mixture)

We found no systematic review, RCTs, or observational studies of sufficient quality evaluating the effects of heliox (helium–oxygen mixture) in children with impending respiratory failure due to severe croup.

UNLIKELY TO BE BENEFICIAL

Antibiotics

We found no systematic review, RCTs, or observational studies of sufficient quality on antibiotics in children with impending respiratory failure due to severe croup. However, there is strong consensus that antibiotics do not shorten the clinical course of a disease that is predominantly viral in origin. This does not apply if bacterial tracheitis is suspected.

◀ **Sedatives**

We found no systematic review or RCTs evaluating the effects of sedatives in children with impending respiratory failure in severe croup. One prospective cohort study found that children with severe croup treated with sedatives had decreased croup scores, but found no corresponding decrease in transcutaneous carbon dioxide pressure. This suggests that sedatives decrease respiratory effort without improving ventilation.

*Based on consensus.

DEFINITION Croup is characterised by the abrupt onset, most commonly at night, of a barking cough, inspiratory stridor, hoarseness, and respiratory distress due to upper airway obstruction. Croup symptoms are often preceded by symptoms of upper respiratory tract infection-like symptoms. The most important diagnoses to differentiate from croup include bacterial tracheitis, epiglottitis, and the inhalation of a foreign body. Some investigators distinguish subtypes of croup;[1-3] the subtypes most commonly distinguished are acute laryngotracheitis and spasmodic croup. Children with acute laryngotracheitis have an antecedent upper respiratory tract infection, are usually febrile, and are thought to have more persistent symptoms. Children with spasmodic croup do not have an antecedent upper respiratory tract infection, are afebrile, have recurrent croup, and are thought to have more transient symptoms. However, there is little empirical evidence justifying the view that spasmodic croup responds differently from acute laryngotracheitis. **Population:** In this chapter, we have included children up to the age of 12 years with croup; no attempt has been made to exclude spasmodic croup. We could not find definitions of clinical severity that are either widely accepted or rigorously derived. For this chapter, we have elected to use definitions derived by a committee consisting of a range of specialists and subspecialists during the development of a clinical practice guideline from Alberta Medical Association (Canada).[4] The definitions of severity have been correlated with the Westley croup score (see table 1Ⓣ),[5] since it is the most widely used clinical score, and its validity and reliability have been well demonstrated.[6,7] However, RCTs included in the chapter use a variety of croup scores. **Mild croup:** Occasional barking cough, no stridor at rest, and none to mild suprasternal and/or intercostal indrawing (retractions of the skin of the chest wall), corresponding to a Westley croup score of 0–2. **Moderate croup:** Frequent barking cough, easily audible stridor at rest, and suprasternal and sternal wall retraction at rest, but no or little distress or agitation, corresponding to a Westley croup score of 3–5. **Severe croup:** Frequent barking cough, prominent inspiratory and — occasionally — expiratory stridor, marked sternal wall retractions, decreased air entry on auscultation, and significant distress and agitation, corresponding to a Westley croup score of 6–11. **Impending respiratory failure:** Barking cough (often not prominent), audible stridor at rest (occasionally can be hard to hear), sternal wall retractions (may not be marked), usually lethargic or decreased level of consciousness, and often dusky complexion without supplemental oxygen, corresponding to a Westley croup score of > 11. During severe respiratory distress, a young child's compliant chest wall "caves in" during inspiration, causing unsynchronised chest and abdominal wall expansion (paradoxical breathing). Approximately 85% of children attending general emergency departments, by this classification scheme, have mild croup, and less than 1% have severe croup (unpublished prospective data obtained from 21 Alberta general emergency departments).

INCIDENCE/ PREVALENCE Croup has an average annual incidence of 3% and accounts for 5% of emergent admissions to hospital in children under 6 years of age in North America (unpublished population based data from Calgary Health Region, Alberta, Canada, 1996–2000).[8] One retrospective Belgian study found that 16% of 5–8 year old children had suffered from croup at least once during ▶

their life, and 5% had experienced recurrent croup (3 or more episodes).[9] We are not aware of epidemiological studies establishing the incidence of croup in other parts of the world.

AETIOLOGY/ RISK FACTORS Croup occurs most commonly in children between 6 months and 3 years of age, but can also occur in children as young as 3 months and as old as 12–15 years of age.[8] It is extremely rare in adults.[10] Infections occur predominantly in late autumn, but can occur during any season, including summer.[8] Croup is caused by a variety of viral agents and, occasionally, by *Mycoplasma pneumoniae*.[8] Parainfluenza accounts for 75% of all cases, with the most common type being parainfluenza type 1. The remaining proportion of cases are largely accounted for by respiratory syncytial virus, metapneumovirus, influenza A and B, adenovirus, and mycoplasma.[8,11-13] Viral invasion of the laryngeal mucosa leads to inflammation, hyperaemia, and oedema.[1] This leads to narrowing of the subglottic region. Children compensate for this narrowing by breathing more quickly and deeply. In children with more severe illness, as the narrowing progresses, their increased effort at breathing becomes counterproductive, airflow through the upper airway becomes turbulent (stridor), their compliant chest wall begins to cave in during inspiration, resulting in paradoxical breathing, and consequently the child becomes fatigued. With these events — if untreated — the child becomes hypoxic and hypercapnoeic, which eventually results in respiratory failure and arrest.[14,15]

PROGNOSIS Croup symptoms resolve in the majority of children within 48 hours.[16] However, a small percentage of children with croup have symptoms that persist for up to 1 week.[16] Hospitalisation rates vary significantly between communities but, on average, less than 5% of all children with croup are admitted to hospital.[17-20] Of those admitted to hospital, only 1–3% are intubated.[21-24] Mortality is low; in one 10-year study, less than 0.5% of intubated children died.[22] Uncommon complications of croup include pneumonia, pulmonary oedema, and bacterial tracheitis.[25-27]

Please refer to clinicalevidence.com for full text and references.

Depression in children and adolescents

Search date April 2005

Philip Hazell

What are the effects of treatments for depression in children and adolescents?

BENEFICIAL

Fluoxetine (prevents acute remission and relapse)

One systematic review found that, in children and adolescents, fluoxetine increased remission rates and improved depressive symptoms compared with placebo after 7– 12 weeks, although did not significantly improve functioning. One RCT found that fluoxetine increased time to relapse compared with placebo. The review found that fluoxetine led to greater improvement in depressive symptoms compared with cognitive behaviour therapy. In the light of emerging evidence and consensus on harms data, practitioners should be guided by the recommendations and warnings issued by their national drug regulatory authorities with respect to the prescribing of antidepressants to children and adolescents.

Fluoxetine plus cognitive therapy (in adolescents)

One large RCT found that, in adolescents, fluoxetine combined with cognitive behaviour therapy improved depressive symptoms compared with placebo, fluoxetine alone, and cognitive behaviour therapy alone, although benefits compared with fluoxetine alone were small.

Interpersonal therapy (in adolescents with mild to moderate depression)

One systematic review found that interpersonal therapy increased remission rates and improved self-rated and clinician-rated depressive symptoms compared with inactive control treatment (in adolescents). We found no evidence that interpersonal therapy is more effective than standard care in the treatment of depression (in adolescents).

LIKELY TO BE BENEFICIAL

Cognitive behaviour therapy (group; in children and adolescents with mild to moderate depression)

One systematic review found that group cognitive behaviour therapy improved self-rated and clinician-rated symptoms of depression compared with waiting list control. We found no RCTs that compared group cognitive behaviour therapy with other active treatments.

UNKNOWN EFFECTIVENESS

Citalopram (in children or adolescents)

The review found limited evidence that citalopram improved depressive symptoms after 8 weeks compared with placebo, although there was no evidence that rates of remission were improved. Citalopram was more likely than placebo to cause adverse events in general. The regulatory authority in the UK has recommended that selective serotonin reupake inhibitors (except fluoxetine) should not be prescribed to people under 18 years old, whereas the regulatory authority in the USA requires a safety warning in bold text about suicide risk in package inserts for all antidepressants.

Depression in children and adolescents

Cognitive behaviour therapy (individual; in children and adolescents with mild to moderate depression)

One systematic review found limited evidence from one small RCT that individual cognitive behaviour therapy improved self-rated depressive symptoms. The review found no significant difference in symptoms of depression between individual cognitive behaviour therapy and interpersonal therapy (in adolescents), family therapy (in adolescents), non-directive supportive therapy (in children and adolescents) or standard care.

Fluoxetine plus cognitive therapy (in children)

We found no evidence of the effectiveness of fluoxetine plus cognitive therapy in children.

Fluvoxamine (in children or adolescents)

We found no evidence of the effectiveness of fluvoxamine on depression in children or adolescents. The regulatory authority in the UK has recommended that selective serotonin reuptake inhibitors (except fluoxetine) should not be prescribed to people under 18 years old, whereas the regulatory authority in the USA requires a safety warning in bold text about suicide risk in package inserts for all antidepressants.

Group therapeutic support (other than cognitive behaviour therapy)

We found no evidence about the effects of group therapeutic support (other than cognitive behaviour therapy) on symptoms of depression in children and adolescents.

Guided self-help

We found no evidence about the effects of guided self-help on symptoms of depression or remission in children and adolescents.

Individual psychodynamic psychotherapy

One RCT found no significant difference in remission rates, depressive symptoms, or functioning between family therapy and individual psychodynamic psychotherapy in children and adolescents.

Interpersonal therapy (in children)

We found no RCTs that examined the effectiveness of interpersonal therapy in children under the age of 12 years.

Monoamine oxidase inhibitors

We found insufficient evidence from one small RCT to compare the reversible monoamine oxidase inhibitor, moclobemide, versus placebo in children aged 9–15 years with major depression, some of whom had a comorbid disorder. We found no RCTs of non-reversible monoamine oxidase inhibitors in children or adolescents. In the light of emerging evidence and consensus on harms data, practitioners should be guided by the recommendations and warnings issued by their national drug regulatory authorities with respect to the prescribing of antidepressants to children and adolescents.

Paroxetine (in children)

We found no RCTs examining the effectiveness of paroxetine on depression in children under 12 years old. The regulatory authority in the UK has recommended that SSRIs (except fluoxetine) should not be prescribed to people under 18 years old, whereas the regulatory authority in the USA requires a safety warning in bold text about suicide risk in package inserts for all antidepressants.

St John's Wort (*Hypericum perforatum*)

We found no RCTs on St John's Wort (*Hypericum perforatum*) in children or adolescents with depression.

UNLIKELY TO BE BENEFICIAL

Cognitive behaviour therapy (for relapse prevention)

One systematic review found no significant difference in relapse rates between individual cognitive behaviour therapy and waiting list control, interpersonal therapy, or clinical management. The review found limited evidence that individual cognitive behaviour therapy reduced relapse rates compared with family therapy and non-directive supportive therapy (in children and adolescents). The review found limited evidence that group cognitive therapy reduced relapse rates compared with waiting list control, although booster sessions of group cognitive behaviour therapy were of no benefit in maintaining remission from depression (in adolescents).

Family therapy (in children and adolescents)

We found no evidence from one systematic review that family therapy is of greater benefit than inactive control treatment (in adolescents), non-specific supportive therapy (in adolescents) or individual psychodynamic psychotherapy for the treatment of depression (in children and adolescents). We found limited evidence that family therapy increased relapse rates compared with cognitive behaviour therapy, but had no effect on symptoms of depression in adolescents.

Paroxetine (in adolescents)

The systematic review found limited evidence that paroxetine improved remission rate but had no effect on symptoms of depression compared with placebo. One RCT found no significant difference in improvement of depression between tricyclic antidepressants and paroxetine. Paroxetine is more likely than placebo to cause adverse events in general. The regulatory authority in the UK has recommended that selective serotonin reuptake inhibitors (except fluoxetine) should not be prescribed to people under 18 years old, whereas the regulatory authority in the USA requires a safety warning in bold text about suicide risk in package inserts for all antidepressants.

Sertraline (in children or adolescents)

The review found no significant difference between sertraline and placebo in rates of remission, improved symptoms of depression or improved functioning in children and adolescents. The regulatory authority in the UK has recommended that selective serotonin reuptake inhibitors (except fluoxetine) should not be prescribed to people under 18 years old, whereas the regulatory authority in the USA requires a safety warning in bold text about suicide risk in package inserts for all antidepressants.

LIKELY TO BE INEFFECTIVE OR HARMFUL

Tricyclic antidepressants (oral)

One systematic review found no significant difference between tricyclic antidepressants and placebo in depressive symptoms, remission rates, or functional status after 6–10 weeks. One RCT found no significant difference between imipramine and placebo in rates of severe adverse events. Single case reports and case series have reported rare occurrences of toxicity and mortality from overdose. Although very rare, any such risk has been considered unacceptable when there are safer alternatives. In the light of emerging evidence and

Depression in children and adolescents

consensus on harms data, practitioners should be guided by the recommendations and warnings issued by their national drug regulatory authorities with respect to the prescribing of antidepressants to children and adolescents.

Venlafaxine

One systematic review found limited evidence that venlafaxine was more effective than placebo in improving depressive symptoms. Venlafaxine was more likely than placebo to cause suicidal behaviour/ideation.

What are the effects of treatments for refractory depression in children and adolescents?

UNKNOWN EFFECTIVENESS

Electroconvulsive therapy

We found no RCTs on electroconvulsive therapy in children and adolescents with depression.

Lithium

One small RCT in children with depression and a family history of bipolar affective disorder found no significant difference between lithium and placebo in global assessment or depression scores after 6 weeks. However, the study may have lacked power to detect clinically important effects.

DEFINITION Compared with adult depression (see depressive disorders), depression in children (6–12 years) and adolescents (13–18 years) may have a more insidious onset, may be characterised more by irritability than sadness, and occurs more often in association with other conditions such as anxiety, conduct disorder, hyperkinesis, and learning problems.[1] The term "major depression" is used to distinguish discrete episodes of depression from mild, chronic (1 year or longer) low mood, or irritability, which is known as "dysthymia".[1] The severity of depression may be defined by the level of impairment and the presence or absence of psychomotor changes and somatic symptoms (see depressive disorders). In some studies, severity of depression is defined according to cut-off scores on depression rating scales. A manic episode is defined by abnormally and persistently elevated, expansive, or irritable mood. Additional symptoms may include grandiosity, decreased need for sleep, pressured speech, flight of ideas, distractibility, psychomotor agitation, and impaired judgement.[2] Refractory depression, also known as treatment resistant depression, refers to depression that has failed to respond or has only partially responded to an adequate trial of at least one recognised treatment.

INCIDENCE/ PREVALENCE Estimates of prevalence of depression among children and adolescents in the community range from 2–6%.[3,4] Prevalence tends to increase with age, with a sharp rise at around the onset of puberty. Pre-adolescent boys and girls are affected equally by the condition, but, in adolescents, depression is more common among girls than boys.[5]

AETIOLOGY/ RISK FACTORS The cause is uncertain, but may include genetic vulnerability,[6] childhood events, and current psychosocial adversity.[1]

PROGNOSIS In children and adolescents, the recurrence rate after a first depressive episode is 40%.[7] Young people experiencing a moderate to severe depressive episode may be more likely than adults to have a manic episode within the following few years.[1,8] Trials of treatments for child and adolescent depression have found high rates of response to placebo (as much as two thirds of people in some inpatient studies), suggesting that episodes of depression may be self limiting in many cases.[9] A third of young people who experience a depressive episode will make a suicide attempt at some stage, and 3–4% will die from suicide.[1]

Please refer to clinicalevidence.com for full text and references.

Febrile seizures

Search date July 2005

Leena D Mewasingh

What are the effects of treatments given during episodes of fever in children with one or more previous simple febrile seizure?

UNKNOWN EFFECTIVENESS

Antipyretic treatments

Two RCTs provided insufficient evidence to assess the routine use of regular antipyretics in children with one previous simple febrile seizure. The RCTs found no significant difference in recurrent febrile seizures at 1–2 years between paracetamol or ibuprofen and placebo. We found no systematic review or RCTs of physical methods of temperature reduction in children with simple febrile seizures.

LIKELY TO BE INEFFECTIVE OR HARMFUL

Anticonvulsants (intermittent)

Two systematic reviews found inconsistent results about the effects of intermittent diazepam compared with placebo in children with a history of simple or complex febrile seizures. The first review found that intermittent diazepam reduced the risk of febrile seizure recurrence, the second review found no significant difference in recurrence of febrile seizures. The contrasting results may be owing to differences in reporting event rates of one of the RCTs identified by both reviews. RCTs identified by the review found that diazepam increased hyperactivity compared with placebo and was associated with lethargy, irritability, or difficulties with speech, activity level, or sleep. One additional RCT found that clobazam reduced the risk of recurrence of febrile seizure compared with placebo. We found no RCTs comparing intermittent versus continuous anticonvulsants in children with previous febrile seizures.

What are the effects of long term (daily, > 1 month) anticonvulsant treatment in children with a history of simple febrile seizures?

TRADE OFF BETWEEN BENEFITS AND HARMS

Anticonvulsants (continuous)

Two systematic reviews found that continuous phenobarbital reduced febrile seizure recurrence in children with a history of simple febrile seizures or complex febrile seizures compared with placebo or no treatment. However, phenobarbital is associated with cognitive impairment and behavioural problems, including hyperactivity, irritability, and aggressiveness. One systematic review found no significant difference in febrile seizure recurrence between continuous sodium valproate and placebo or no treatment in children with simple or complex febrile seizures. Serious adverse events associated with sodium valproate include hepatotoxicity and haematologic toxicity, both of which may be occasionally fatal. One RCT found no significant difference between continuous phenobarbital and sodium valproate in the recurrence of simple febrile seizures.

What are the effects of treatments on reducing the risk of subsequent epilepsy in children with a history of simple febrile seizures?

UNLIKELY TO BE BENEFICIAL

Anticonvulsants (intermittent and continuous)

One RCT found no significant decrease in risk of epilepsy up to 12 years later between intermittent diazepam and no treatment in children with a history of simple febrile seizures. One RCT found no significant decrease in risk of epilepsy in children who had received daily phenobarbital.

DEFINITION Febrile seizures are divided up into three types: simple febrile seizures, complex febrile seizures, and febrile status epilepticus. **This chapter focuses on children with simple febrile seizures.** The National Institutes of Health (NIH) definition of a febrile seizure is as "An event in infancy or childhood usually occurring between 3 months and 5 years of age associated with a fever, but without evidence of intracranial infection or defined cause for their seizure",[1] after having excluded children with previous afebrile seizures. Another definition from the International League Against Epilepsy (ILAE) is that of 'a seizure occurring in childhood after 1 month of age associated with a febrile illness not caused by an infection of the central nervous system (CNS), without previous neonatal seizures or a previous unprovoked seizure, and not meeting the criteria for other acute symptomatic seizures.'[2] In working practice the lower age limits for febrile seizures is generally taken to be 6 months, given concerns regarding possibility of an underlying serious but treatable infection in younger infants masquerading as a febrile seizure eg meningitis. A simple febrile seizure is a generalised seizure, lasting less than 15 minutes in duration, which does not occur more than once in 24 hours, and is followed by full recovery within 1 hour. Treatment for the actual seizure is generally not indicated, given the short duration. Often by the time the child presents to hospital, the seizure has already stopped. A febrile seizure may be the presenting sign of a fever episode. **This chapter does not include children experiencing complex febrile seizures,** which are characterised by any of the following features: greater than 15 minutes in duration, focal symptoms, recurrence within 24 hours, and not followed by full consciousness within 1 hour. Diagnosis often requires neuroimaging and metabolic evaluation and treatment is usually required. **Also excluded are children experiencing febrile status epilepticus** which lasts for greater than 30 minutes and will require treatment.

INCIDENCE/ PREVALENCE About 2–5% of children in the US and Western Europe and 6–9% of infants and children in Japan will have experienced at least one febrile seizure, simple or complex, by the age of 5 years. Elsewhere the incidence varies, being 5–10% in India and as high as 14% in Guam.[2] There are no specific data available for simple febrile seizures.

AETIOLOGY/ RISK FACTORS The exact cause of simple febrile seizures is unknown. In some cases, there is a genetic predisposition, with febrile seizures occurring in families. However, the exact mode of inheritance is not known and seems to vary between families. A "febrile seizure susceptibility trait" has been described with an autosomal dominant pattern of inheritance with reduced penetrance.[3] In addition, mutations in several genes have been found that account for enhanced susceptibility to febrile seizures.[4-8] Febrile seizures are more frequent in children attending day care centres and those having a first or second degree relative with a history of febrile seizures.[9] The risk of another child having febrile seizures is one in five if one sibling is affected and one in three if both parents and a previous child have had febrile seizures.[10] Other risk factors associated with an increased rate of febrile seizure recurrence include young age at onset (< 12 months), history of simple or complex febrile seizures, and body temperature at onset of less than 40 °C.[9,11] Among these, age at onset seems to be the most constant predictive factor, with 50% of children aged less than 12 months and 30% of children aged more than 12 months presenting with a recurrent febrile seizure. Positive family history of epilepsy is not consistently associated with increased simple febrile seizure recurrence.[11]

PROGNOSIS Simple febrile seizures may slightly increase the risk of developing epilepsy,[12] but have no adverse effects on behaviour, scholastic performance, or neurocognition. The risk of developing epilepsy is increased further in children with a history of complex febrile seizures.[13-16] A strong association exists between febrile status epilepticus or febrile seizures characterised by focal symptoms and later development of temporal lobe epilepsy.[12,17]

Please refer to clinicalevidence.com for full text and references.

Gastroenteritis in children

Search date August 2005

Jacqueline Dalby-Payne and Elizabeth Elliott

What are the effects of treatments for acute gastroenteritis?

BENEFICIAL

Enteral rehydration solutions (as effective as intravenous fluids)

One systematic review, which included studies in children with mild to severe dehydration, found that enteral (oral or nasogastric) rehydration reduced hospital stay compared with intravenous rehydration, and found no significant difference between treatments in weight gain or duration of diarrhoea. Enteral rehydration reduced major adverse events compared with intravenous rehydration; this was largely based on the results of one large RCT in children with severe gastroenteritis. One additional RCT also found no significant difference in successful rehydration between oral rehydration and intravenous rehydration.

LIKELY TO BE BENEFICIAL

Lactose-free feeds (reduces duration of diarrhoea)

One systematic review and three of five subsequent RCTs found limited evidence that lactose-free feeds reduced the duration of diarrhoea in children with mild to severe dehydration compared with feeds containing lactose. The remaining two subsequent RCTs found no significant difference between lactose-free and lactose-containing feeds in duration of diarrhoea.

Loperamide (reduces duration of diarrhoea, but adverse effects unclear)

Two RCTs found that, in children with mild to moderate dehydration, loperamide reduced the duration of diarrhoea compared with placebo. Another RCT found no significant difference between loperamide and placebo in the duration of diarrhoea. We found insufficient evidence to assess the risk of adverse effects.

UNKNOWN EFFECTIVENESS

Clear fluids (other than oral rehydration solutions)

We found no systematic review or RCTs comparing "clear fluids" (water, carbonated drinks, and translucent fruit juices) versus oral rehydration solutions for treatment of acute gastroenteritis.

DEFINITION Acute gastroenteritis results from infection of the gastrointestinal tract, most commonly with a virus. It is characterised by rapid onset of diarrhoea with or without vomiting, nausea, fever, and abdominal pain.[1] In children the symptoms and signs can be non-specific.[2] Diarrhoea is defined as the frequent passage of unformed liquid stools.[3] Regardless of the cause, the mainstay of management of acute gastroenteritis is provision of adequate fluids to prevent and treat dehydration. In this chapter we examine the benefits and harms of different treatments for gastroenteritis irrespective of its cause.

INCIDENCE/ PREVALENCE Worldwide, about 3–5 billion cases of acute gastroenteritis occur each year in children under 5 years of age, resulting in nearly 2 million deaths.[4,5] In the UK, acute gastroenteritis accounts for 204/1000 general practitioner consultations in children under 5 years of age.[6] Gastroenteritis leads to hospital admission in 7/1000 children under 5 years of age each year in the UK[6] and 13/1000 in the USA.[7] In Australia, gastroenteritis accounts for 6% of all hospital admissions in children under 15 years of age.[8]

Gastroenteritis in children

AETIOLOGY/ RISK FACTORS In developed countries, acute gastroenteritis is predominantly caused by viruses (87%), of which rotavirus is most common.[8-12] Bacteria, predominantly *Campylobacter*, *Salmonella*, *Shigella*, and *Escherichia coli*, cause most of the remaining cases. In developing countries, where bacterial pathogens are more frequent, rotavirus is also a major cause of gastroenteritis.

PROGNOSIS Acute gastroenteritis is usually self limiting but if untreated it can result in morbidity and mortality secondary to water loss and electrolyte and acid–base disturbance. Acute diarrhoea causes 4 million deaths each year in children aged under 5 years in Asia (excluding China), Africa, and Latin America, and more than 80% of deaths occur in children under 2 years of age.[13] Although death is uncommon in developed countries, dehydration secondary to gastroenteritis is a significant cause of morbidity and need for hospital admission.[7-9]

Please refer to clinicalevidence.com for full text and references.

Gastro-oesophageal reflux in children

Search date July 2005

Yadlapalli Kumar and Rajini Sarvananthan

What are the effects of treatment for symptomatic gastro-oesophageal reflux?

LIKELY TO BE BENEFICIAL

Feed thickeners in infants

One systematic review found limited evidence from small RCTs that thickened feeds reduced the regurgitation severity and frequency of emesis, but not reflux index, compared with unthickened feed. One subsequent RCT in infants aged 14–120 days found that a pre-thickened infant formula reduced regurgitation, choking and gagging, and coughing within 1 week without causing constipation. Another subsequent RCT in infants aged 3–5 months found that formula thickened with locust bean gum reduced episodes of regurgitation compared with standard infant formula. A third subsequent RCT of infants with a mean age of 93 days found that a casein dominant formula thickened with cornstarch reduced regurgitation and vomiting.

Sodium alginate

Two RCTs in infants and in children under 2 years found that sodium alginate reduced the frequency of regurgitation at 8–14 days compared with placebo. A third small RCT of children under 17 years of age comparing sodium alginate versus metoclopramide and placebo found no significant difference between treatments in regurgitation episodes or reflux index. One small crossover RCT found no significant difference between sodium plus magnesium alginate and placebo in frequency of reflux events. The high sodium content of sodium alginate may be inappropriate in preterm babies.

TRADE OFF BETWEEN BENEFITS AND HARMS

Left lateral or prone positioning

We found no systematic reviews or RCTs that assessed clinical outcomes. One systematic review of children aged under 6 months and one additional RCT found limited evidence that prone or left lateral positioning improved oesophageal pH variables compared with supine or right lateral positioning. One additional crossover RCT found evidence that prone or left lateral positioning improved oesophageal pH variables significantly compared with right lateral positioning. Both prone and side lateral positions may be associated with a higher risk of sudden infant death syndrome compared with supine positioning.

Metoclopramide

One systematic review found limited evidence from small RCTs that metoclopramide reduced symptom frequency and reflux index, but may increase adverse effects compared with placebo or no treatment. One additional small RCT of children under 17 years of age found no significant difference between metoclopramide and sodium alginate or placebo in regurgitation episodes or reflux index.

UNKNOWN EFFECTIVENESS

Domperidone

One small RCT provided insufficient evidence about the effects of domperidone in children with gastro-oesophageal reflux.

Gastro-oesophageal reflux in children

H_2 antagonists

Two small RCTs provided insufficient evidence about the effects of H_2 antagonists on children with gastro-oesophageal reflux.

Head elevated positioning

We found no systematic reviews or RCTs that assessed clinical outcomes. One systematic review found no consistent evidence of a difference in oesophageal pH variables between head elevated and horizontal positions in children under 6 months.

Proton pump inhibitors

One small RCT of infants aged 3–12 months found that omeprazole improved oesophageal pH variables. However, the clinical importance of this result is unclear.

Surgery

We found no RCTs of surgery for gastro-oesophageal reflux in children.

DEFINITION Gastro-oesophageal reflux disease is the passive transfer of gastric contents into the oesophagus owing to transient or chronic relaxation of the lower oesophageal sphincter.[1] A survey of 69 children (median age 16 months) with gastro-oesophageal reflux disease attending a tertiary referral centre found that presenting symptoms were recurrent vomiting (72%), epigastric and abdominal pain (36%), feeding difficulties (29%), failure to thrive (28%), and irritability (19%).[2] However, results may not be generalisable to younger children or children presenting in primary care, who make up the most of the cases. Over 90% of children with gastro-oesophageal reflux disease have vomiting before 6 weeks of age.[1]

INCIDENCE/ PREVALENCE Gastro-oesophageal regurgitation is considered a problem if it is frequent, persistent, and is associated with other symptoms such as increased crying, discomfort with regurgitation, and frequent back arching.[1,3] A cross-sectional survey of parents of 948 infants attending 19 primary care paediatric practices found that regurgitation of at least one episode a day was reported in 51% of infants aged 0–3 months. "Problematic" regurgitation occurred in significantly fewer infants (14% with problematic regurgitation *v* 51% with regurgitation of at least 1 episode a day; $P < 0.001$).[3] Peak regurgitation reported as "problematic" was reported in 23% of infants aged 6 months.[3]

AETIOLOGY/ RISK FACTORS Risk factors for gastro-oesophageal reflux disease include immaturity of the lower oesophageal sphincter, chronic relaxation of the sphincter, increased abdominal pressure, gastric distension, hiatus hernia, and oesophageal dysmotility.[1] Premature infants and children with severe neurodevelopmental problems or congenital oesophageal anomalies are particularly at risk.[1]

PROGNOSIS Regurgitation is considered benign, and most cases resolve spontaneously by 12–18 months of age.[4] In a cross-sectional survey of 948 parents, the peak age for reporting four or more episodes of regurgitation was at 5 months of age (23%), which decreased to 7% at 7 months ($P < 0.001$). One cohort study found that infants with frequent spilling in the first 2 years of life ($\geq$ 90 days in the first 2 years) were more likely to have symptoms of gastro-oesophageal reflux at 9 years of age than those with no spilling (RR 2.3, 95% CI 1.3 to 4.0).[5] The prevalence of "problematic" regurgitation also reduced from 23% in infants aged 6 months to 3.25% in infants aged 10–12 months.[3] Rare complications of gastro-oesophageal reflux disease include oesophagitis with haematemesis and anaemia, respiratory problems (such as cough, apnoea, and recurrent wheeze), and failure to thrive.[1] A small comparative study (40 children) suggested that, when compared with healthy children, infants with gastro-oesophageal reflux disease had slower development of feeding skills and had problems affecting behaviour, swallowing, food intake, and mother–child interaction.[6]

Please refer to clinicalevidence.com for full text and references.

Infantile colic

Search date September 2005

Sally Wade

What are the effects of treatments for infantile colic?

LIKELY TO BE BENEFICIAL

Whey hydrolysate milk

One small RCT found that replacing cows' milk formula with whey hydrolysate formula reduced crying recorded in a parental diary.

UNKNOWN EFFECTIVENESS

Advice to reduce stimulation

One RCT found limited evidence that advice to reduce stimulation (by not patting, lifting, or jiggling the baby, or by reducing auditory stimulation) reduced crying after 7 days in infants under 12 weeks compared with an empathetic interview giving no advice. However, we were unable to draw reliable conclusions from this small study.

Car ride simulation

One RCT found no significant difference between car ride simulation plus reassurance, counselling mothers about specific management techniques (responding to crying with gentle soothing motion, avoiding over stimulation, using a pacifier, and prophylactic carrying) plus reassurance, and reassurance alone, in terms of maternal anxiety or hours of infant crying over 2 weeks.

Casein hydrolysate milk

Two RCTs provided insufficient evidence to assess the effects of replacing cows' milk formula with casein hydrolysate hypoallergenic formula. Another small RCT found that substituting soya or cows' milk with casein hydrolysate formula was less effective at reducing the duration and extent of crying than focused counselling.

Cranial osteopathy

We found no systematic review or RCTs on the effects of cranial osteopathy in infants with colic.

Focused counselling

One RCT found no significant difference between counselling mothers about specific management techniques (responding to crying with gentle soothing motion, avoiding over stimulation, using a pacifier, and prophylactic carrying) plus reassurance, car ride simulation plus reassurance, and reassurance alone, in terms of maternal anxiety or hours of infant crying over 2 weeks. Another small RCT found that counselling decreased the duration of crying compared with substitution of soya or cows' milk with casein hydrolysate formula.

Gripe water

We found no systematic review or RCTs on the effects of gripe water in infants with colic.

Infant massage

One RCT found no significant difference between massage and a crib vibrator for colic related crying or parental rating of symptoms of infantile colic, but it may have lacked power to detect a clinically important difference. ▶

Low lactose milk

Four small crossover RCTs provided insufficient evidence on the effects of low lactose milk in infants with colic.

Simethicone (activated dimeticone)

One RCT found no significant difference between simethicone and placebo in colic rated by carers. Another RCT found no significant difference between simethicone and placebo in improvement as rated by parental interview, 24 hour diary, or behavioural observation. Another poor quality RCT found that simethicone reduced the number of crying attacks on days 4–7 of treatment compared with placebo.

Soya based infant feeds

One small RCT found that soya based infant feeds reduced the duration of crying in infants with colic compared with standard cows' milk formula. However, we were unable to draw reliable conclusions from this small study.

Spinal manipulation

Two RCTs found insufficient evidence about the effects of spinal manipulation in infants with colic.

UNLIKELY TO BE BENEFICIAL

Advice to increase carrying

One RCT found no significant difference in daily crying time between advice to carry the infant, even when not crying, for at least an additional 3 hours a day and general advice (to carry, check baby's nappy, feed, offer pacifier, place baby near mother, or use background stimulation such as music).

DEFINITION Infantile colic is defined as excessive crying in an otherwise healthy baby. The crying typically starts in the first few weeks of life and ends by 4–5 months. Excessive crying is defined as crying that lasts at least 3 hours a day, for 3 days a week, for at least 3 weeks.[1] Due to the natural course of infantile colic, it can be difficult to interpret trials which do not include a placebo or have no treatment group for comparison.

INCIDENCE/ PREVALENCE Infantile colic causes one out of six families (17%) to consult a health professional. One systematic review of 15 community based studies found a wide variation in prevalence, which depended on study design and method of recording.[2] Two prospective studies identified by the review yielded prevalence rates of 5% and 19%.[2] One RCT (89 breast and formula fed infants) found that, at 2 weeks of age, the prevalence of crying more than 3 hours a day was 43% among formula fed infants and 16% among breast fed infants. The prevalence at 6 weeks was 12% among formula fed infants and 31% among breast fed infants.[3] A national survey of 3345 infants found that maternal smoking was associated with colic (OR 1.34, 95% CI 0.88 to 2.04).[4]

AETIOLOGY/ RISK FACTORS The cause is unclear and, despite its name, infantile colic may not have an abdominal cause. It may reflect part of the normal distribution of infantile crying. Other possible explanations are painful intestinal contractions, lactose intolerance, gas, or parental misinterpretation of normal crying.[1]

PROGNOSIS Infantile colic improves with time. One self reporting parent questionnaire on crying patterns found that 29% of infants aged 1–3 months cried for more than 3 hours a day, but by 4–6 months of age the prevalence had fallen to 7–11%.[5]

Please refer to clinicalevidence.com for full text and references.

Measles, mumps, and rubella: prevention

Search date July 2005

Robert Booy, Nitu Sengupta, Helen Bedford, and David Elliman

What are the effects of measles vaccination?

BENEFICIAL

Monovalent measles vaccine or combined MMR vaccine versus placebo or no vaccine

We found no systematic review or RCTs comparing the protective efficacy against measles of combined measles, mumps, and rubella (MMR) versus no vaccine or placebo. RCTs using a control group who received no vaccine or placebo are now deemed unethical because of the existing evidence of efficacy of MMR vaccine and the harms associated with naturally acquired measles, mumps, and rubella. One quasi-randomised trial, one large retrospective cohort study, and several large observational studies found that measles vaccine (monovalent or MMR) reduced the incidence of measles. Mass population cohort studies and other observational studies also consistently found important reductions in child mortality after measles vaccination. Observational studies found that measles vaccination programmes were followed by a reduction in the incidence of subacute sclerosing panencephalitis. Several features of measles infection occur or are suspected to occur after the vaccine, but we found no studies comparing rates of occurrence between people with naturally acquired measles and those who have been vaccinated. Severe complications are rare with measles immunisation. Observational studies found that, compared with placebo or no vaccine, MMR vaccination increased the incidence of fever and febrile seizures, although febrile seizures were uncommon and did not progress into afebrile seizures. Observational studies also found that aseptic meningitis, a rare complication, increased after mass vaccination with the Leningrad-Zagreb (L-Z) and Urabe strains of MMR, but no increased incidence has been reported with Jeryl Lynn, Hoshino, or Rubini strains. Observational studies found that both MMR vaccination and naturally acquired measles increased the incidence of idiopathic thrombocytopenic purpura. Observational studies found no association between the incidence of asthma and MMR vaccination. They also found no significant increase in the incidence of Guillain–Barré syndrome, autism, diabetes, gait disturbance, demyelinating disorders, or inflammatory bowel disease as a result of measles vaccination. Anaphylaxis has been reported after vaccination with MMR, but this is extremely rare.

UNKNOWN EFFECTIVENESS

Comparative effects of MMR versus monovalent measles vaccine

We found no systematic review or RCTs comparing the clinical effects of measles, mumps, and rubella (MMR) versus monovalent measles vaccines in children. RCTs found that seroconversion rates and rates of adverse effects were similar with both vaccines.

What are the effects of mumps vaccination?

BENEFICIAL

Monovalent mumps vaccine or combined MMR vaccine versus placebo or no vaccine

We found no systematic review or RCTs comparing the clinical effects of combined measles, mumps, and rubella (MMR) vaccine versus no vaccine or placebo. RCTs using a control group who received no vaccine or placebo are now deemed unethical because of the existing evidence of efficacy of MMR vaccine and the harms associated with naturally acquired measles, mumps, and rubella. Two RCTs found that monovalent mumps vaccine reduced the incidence of mumps compared with placebo. Population based surveillance studies and other observational studies also have consistently found important reductions in the incidence of mumps and admission to hospital owing to mumps after MMR or monovalent mumps vaccination. For harms of MMR vaccination see question on MMR for preventing measles.

UNKNOWN EFFECTIVENESS

Comparative effects of MMR versus monovalent mumps vaccine

We found no systematic review or RCTs comparing the clinical effects of measles, mumps, and rubella (MMR) versus monovalent mumps vaccine in children. One RCT found similar seroconversion rates for mumps when comparing a monovalent mumps vaccine versus two different MMR vaccines. More children having MMR had rash, whereas more children having monovalent mumps vaccine had local reactions.

What are the effects of rubella vaccination?

BENEFICIAL

Monovalent rubella vaccine or combined MMR vaccine versus placebo or no vaccine

One RCT undertaken in 1968 found that both measles, mumps, and rubella (MMR) vaccine and monovalent rubella vaccines provided high levels of protection against rubella disease compared with placebo or no vaccine. Another RCT undertaken in the 1960s also found high protective efficacy of monovalent rubella vaccines. Population based surveillance studies and other observational studies have also consistently found important reductions in the incidence of rubella after vaccination. For harms of MMR vaccination, see question on MMR for preventing measles.

UNKNOWN EFFECTIVENESS

Comparative effects of MMR versus monovalent rubella vaccine

We found no systematic review or RCTs comparing clinical effects of measles, mumps, and rubella (MMR) versus monovalent vaccine in children. One RCT found similar seroconversion rates for rubella and similar rates of adverse effects when comparing a monovalent mumps vaccine versus two different MMR vaccines.

DEFINITION Measles, mumps, and rubella are infectious diseases. **Measles** is caused by a ribonucleic acid [RNA] paramyxovirus. The illness is characterised by an incubation period of 6–19 days (median 13 days);[1] a prodromal period of 2–4 days with upper respiratory tract symptoms; conjunctivitis, Koplik's spots on mucosal membranes, and high fever; followed by a widespread maculopapular rash that persists, with fever, for 5–6 days. **Mumps** is caused by a RNA virus classified as a rubulavirus in the *Paramyxoviridae* family.[1] The illness is characterised by an incubation period of 15–24 days (median 19 days), with a prodromal period of non-specific flu-like symptoms preceding the development of parotitis. This swelling, which is frequently bilateral and accompanied by abdominal pain and headache, usually resolves within 7–10 days. About one third of mumps infections are subclinical or mild non-specific illnesses not recognised as mumps.[2] **Rubella** is caused by rubivirus, a RNA enveloped

Measles, mumps, and rubella: prevention

togavirus in the *Togaviridae* family. There are no animal reservoirs and only one serotype.[1] The incubation period is 15–20 days (median 17 days). Although virus is shed from 7 days before to 6 days after the appearance of the rash, the period of infectivity with rubella is not known. The infection is frequently subclinical.[1] In clinical infection, there are often no prodromal symptoms. A generalised lymphadenopathy is followed by a rash up to 7 days later. Babies with congenital rubella syndrome (CRS) may excrete virus for years and therefore be a source of infection.

INCIDENCE/ PREVALENCE Incidence of measles, mumps, and rubella varies according to vaccination coverage. **Measles:** Worldwide, there are an estimated 30 million cases of measles each year,[3] but the incidence is only 0–10/100 000 people in countries with widespread vaccination programmes such as the USA, UK, Mexico, India, China, Brazil, and Australia.[4] In the USA, before licensing of effective vaccines, more than 90% of people were infected by the age of 15 years. After licensing in 1963, incidence fell by about 98%.[5] The mean annual incidence in Finland was 366/100 000 in 1970,[6] but declined to about zero by the late 1990s.[7] Similarly, the annual incidence declined to about zero in Chile, the English speaking Caribbean, and Cuba during the 1990s when vaccination programmes were introduced.[8,9] **Mumps** predominately affects children, with 32% of reported cases worldwide in children aged 0–4 years and 53% in children aged 5–14 years.[10] In the pre-vaccine era, by 10 years of age, 87% of the population in England had serological evidence of mumps infection.[11] After introduction of measles, mumps, and rubella (MMR) vaccine there has been a decrease in incidence of disease such that in some countries, for example Finland, there is no longer any indigenous disease.[6] Those cases that still occur are usually in an older age group, who are unvaccinated. There has been an increase in the proportion of cases in people aged 15 years and over in England and Wales from 12% in 1989 to 90% in 2004.[12] **Rubella:** In the pre-vaccine era in the UK, rubella was uncommon under the age of 5 years with the peak incidence being 5–10 years of age.[13] Serological surveys around the world found that by late adolescence/early adulthood 80% of women had been infected.[14]

AETIOLOGY/ RISK FACTORS Measles is highly contagious, with mumps and rubella being less so. As with most other infectious diseases, risk factors include overcrowding and low herd immunity. **Measles** spreads through airborne droplets.[1] Newborn babies have a lower risk of measles than do older infants, owing to protective maternal antibodies, although in recent US outbreaks maternal antibody protection was lower than expected.[5] Antibody levels are lower in babies born to immunised mothers compared with offspring of naturally infected mothers.[15,16] **Mumps** spreads through respiratory droplets, saliva, and possibly urine.[1] The period of infectivity extends from a few days before the salivary glands become enlarged to about 5 days after. As with measles, the risk of mumps is lower in the first 9–12 months of age owing to the presence of maternal antibodies, although this pattern may change in a largely vaccinated maternal population. **Rubella** spreads through direct contact or airborne droplets.[1]

PROGNOSIS **Measles:** The World Health Organization estimated that measles caused 777 000 deaths and 27.5 million disability adjusted life years in 2000.[17] **Measles in healthy people:** In developed countries, most prognostic data come from the pre-vaccination era and from subsequent outbreaks in unvaccinated populations. The overall rate of complications in the UK was 6.7% before the introduction of measles vaccination. Encephalitis affected 1.2/1000 diseased people, and respiratory complications in 38/1000 diseased people.[18] Other complications before the introduction of the vaccine included seizures, with or without fever, affecting 5/1000 people with measles.[19] Idiopathic thrombocytopenic purpura (ITP) has been reported, but the frequency is not known. Subacute sclerosing panencephalitis (SSPE) is an inevitably fatal, progressive degenerative disorder of the central nervous system with a mean onset 7–10 years after measles infection. It is more common when measles occurs under the age of 1 year (18/100 000 in children < 1 year of age *v* 4/100 000 overall), as identified by a passive reporting system set up in England and Wales to monitor the incidence of SSPE.[20] Between 1989 and 1991 in the USA, measles resurgence among young children (aged < 5 years) who had not been immunised led to 55 622 cases, with more than 11 000 hospital admissions and 166 deaths.[21-23] Measles complications also include diarrhoea (9%) and pneumonia (6%).[23] Measles during pregnancy results in higher risk of premature labour[24] but no proved increase in congenital anomalies.[25] **Measles in malnourished or immunocompromised people:** In malnourished people, particularly those with vitamin A deficiency, measles case fatality can be as high as 25%. Immunocompromised people have a higher morbidity and mortality. Children younger than 5 years, and adults older than 20 years, have a higher risk of severe complications and death.[21,26] In the period 1974–1984, four UK centres reported that 15/51 (29%) deaths in children in their first remission from leukaemia resulted from measles.[27] Another report reviewing cases from the same four UK centres between 1973 and 1986 found that 5/17 cases of measles in children with malignancies proved fatal.[28] At least 5/36 (14%) measles associated deaths in 1991 in the USA were in HIV infected persons.[21] Worldwide, measles is a major cause of blindness, and causes 5% of deaths in young children (aged < 5 years).[29] **Mumps:** Deaths following mumps are uncommon with about five a year registered in the pre-vaccine era in England and Wales, although only half of these were judged to be directly because of mumps.[10] Deaths occurred mainly in people aged over 40 years. The most important complications of mumps are those relating to the central nervous system, the gonads, and the pancreas. Before the introduction of MMR vaccine in the UK, mumps was one of the most common causes of aseptic meningitis, accounting for about 20% of cases.[30] The outcome was usually benign. Mumps encephalitis is less common and the outcome more serious.[31] A case series (41 children) in Finland found that that 2/40 (5%) children had continuing ataxia and 7/42 (17%) had behavioural disturbances at 4 months to 2 years after mumps encephalitis.[32] Sensorineural hearing loss, usually unilateral, occurs after mumps infection, but its prevalence is unknown, although paediatricians in Israel who had observed cases of hearing loss following a mumps epidemic in 1984 suggested it may be as common as 1/3400.[33] A large population based study of mumps undertaken in the USA (1310 cases from 1935–1974) found orchitis in 10% of males overall, being much more common in adults.[34] Orchitis was bilateral in 17% of men. The study found testicular atrophy in 47/132 (36%) men of whom two developed testicular neoplasms. A smaller population based study of mumps in a virgin population (561 Eskimos on St Lawrence Island) found that 52/205 (25%) of men with mumps had orchitis, of which 26 cases were unilateral, 19 bilateral, and seven unknown.[35] Most cases (73%) occurred in men aged 15 years or over of whom 37% had bilateral disease. In women who had mumps, 15% had mastitis, a third of whom were aged 15 years or over.[35] In a community based study in the USA (342 cases), the most frequent complication of mumps was pancreatitis occurring in 12/342 (4%) people,[2] while in a case series, 50/109 (46%) people admitted to hospital had clinical signs of pancreatitis.[36] There is an increase in the rate of spontaneous abortion following mumps infection in the first trimester,[25] but no increase in congenital anomalies or prematurity.[24] **Rubella:** Complications of rubella are rare in children. In an epidemic in Japan in 1987, 8250 children under 15 years of age were estimated to have suffered rubella infection.[37] Five children developed encephalitis (1 with adverse sequelae), three had meningitis, four had idiopathic thrombocytopenic purpura (ITP), four vascular purpura, two haemolytic anaemia, and eight pneumonia. Retrospective observational data suggest that ITP may occur at a rate of about 1/3000.[38] Rubella encephalopathy occurs, but rarely, and a case series suggested that long term sequelae were less frequent than after measles encephalopathy.[39] In children, arthralgia is infrequent, however in adults, especially women, it is common. A review of hospital records

Measles, mumps, and rubella: prevention

(74 adults with rubella) in London found that most had arthralgia and 11/74 (15%) had arthritis.[13] Arthritis may be recurrent, but is usually self limiting. The most serious consequence of rubella infection is congenital rubella syndrome (CRS) first described by Gregg in 1941.[40] Almost any system can be affected by CRS depending on the stage of pregnancy at which the infection occurs. In a prospective cohort study of over 1000 pregnant women in England and Wales with confirmed rubella infection, the frequency of congenital infection after maternal rubella with a rash during the first 12 weeks of pregnancy was more than 80%, declining to 25% when the infection occurred at the end of the second trimester.[41] Rubella defects occurred in all infants infected before the 11th week, in 35% of those infected at 13–16 weeks, and in no infants infected later in pregnancy.[41] The earlier the infection occurred, the more serious the defects, for example, children infected before the 11th week had both congenital heart disease and deafness, whereas children with later infections only had deafness.

Please refer to clinicalevidence.com for full text and references.

Migraine headache in children

Search date August 2005

Nick Barnes, Guy Millman, and Elizabeth James

What are the effects of treatments for acute attacks of migraine headache in children?

UNKNOWN EFFECTIVENESS

$5HT_1$ antagonists (e.g. Triptans)

Two RCTs provided insufficient evidence that nasal sumatriptan reduced symptoms of migraine, but found that sumatriptan increased taste disturbance compared with placebo. One RCT found no significant difference in pain relief between oral rizatriptan and placebo.

Antiemetics

We found no RCTs of antiemetics in children with migraine headache.

Codeine phosphate

We found no RCTs addressing the effects of codeine phosphate in children or adolescents with migraine headache.

Non-steroidal anti-inflammatory drugs

We found no reliable RCTs assessing the effects of non-steroidal anti-inflammatory drugs in children and adolescents with migraine headache.

Paracetamol

We found no RCTs of sufficient quality addressing the effects of paracetamol (acetaminophen) in children or adolescents with migraine headache.

What are the effects of prophylaxis for migraine in children?

LIKELY TO BE BENEFICIAL

Stress management

One small RCT provided limited evidence that a stress management programme improved headache severity and frequency compared with no stress management at 1 month.

UNKNOWN EFFECTIVENESS

Beta-blockers

One RCT found that propranolol increased perception of benefit compared with placebo. However, one RCT found no significant difference in migraine episodes, and another RCT found that propranolol increased headache duration compared with placebo.

Dietary manipulation

We found no RCTs of sufficient quality in children and adolescents with migraine headache.

Pizotifen

We found no RCTs of sufficient quality.

Migraine headache in children

Progressive muscle relaxation

We found no RCTs of sufficient quality examining effects of progressive muscle relaxation in children with migraine headache.

Thermal biofeedback

We found no RCTs of sufficient quality examining effects of thermal biofeedback in children with migraine headache.

DEFINITION Migraine is defined by the International Headache Society (IHS) as a recurrent headache that occurs with or without aura and lasts 2–48 hours.[1] It is usually unilateral in nature, pulsating in quality, of moderate or severe intensity, and is aggravated by routine physical activity. Nausea, vomiting, photophobia, and phonophobia are common accompanying symptoms. This topic focuses on children younger than 18 years. Diagnostic criteria for children are broader than criteria for adults, allowing for a broader range of duration and a broader localisation of the pain (see table 1)Ⓣ.[2] Diagnosis is difficult in young children because the condition is defined by subjective symptoms. Studies that do not explicitly use criteria that are congruent with IHS diagnostic criteria (or revised IHS criteria in children $<$ 15 years of age) have been excluded from this topic.

INCIDENCE/ PREVALENCE Migraine occurs in 3–10% of children,[3-7] and currently affects 50/1000 school age children in the UK and an estimated 7.8 million children in the European Union.[8] Studies in developed countries suggest that migraine is the most common diagnosis among children presenting with headache to a medical practitioner. It is rarely diagnosed in children under 2 years of age because of the symptom based definition, but increases steadily with age thereafter.[1,9,10] It affects boys and girls similarly before puberty, but after puberty girls are more likely to suffer from migraine.[4,6,10] See incidence/ prevalence of migraine headache [web only].

AETIOLOGY/ RISK FACTORS The cause of migraine headaches is unknown. We found few reliable data identifying risk factors or measuring their effects in children. Suggested risk factors include stress, foods, menses, and exercise in genetically predisposed children and adolescents.[10,11]

PROGNOSIS We found no reliable data about prognosis of childhood migraine headache diagnosed by IHS criteria. It has been suggested that more than half the children will have spontaneous remission after puberty.[10] It is believed that migraine that develops during adolescence tends to continue in adult life, although attacks tend to be less frequent and severe in later life.[12] We found one longitudinal study from Sweden (73 children with "pronounced" migraine and mean age of onset of 6 years) with over 40 years follow up, which predated the IHS criteria for migraine headache.[13] It found that migraine headaches had ceased before the age of 25 years in 23% of people. However, by the age of 50 years, more than 50% of people continued to have migraine headaches. We found no prospective data examining long term risks in children with migraine.

Please refer to clinicalevidence.com for full text and references.

Neonatal infection: group B streptococcus

Search date March 2006

James Hanley

What are the effects of prophylactic treatment of asymptomatic neonates < 7 days old with known risk factors for group B streptococcal infection?

UNKNOWN EFFECTIVENESS

Different antibiotics

We found no systematic review or RCTs comparing different antibiotics versus each other for routine prophylaxis against group B streptococcal infection in neonates with known risk factors for group B streptococcal infection.

UNLIKELY TO BE BENEFICIAL

Routine antibiotic prophylaxis (no more effective than monitoring and selective treatment)

Two RCTs identified by a systematic review found no significant difference between routine early penicillin prophylaxis and delayed selective antibiotic treatment in the incidence of early onset group B streptococcal infection or neonatal mortality. One RCT in low birth weight, preterm infants identified by a second systematic review found no significant difference between routine early penicillin prophylaxis and monitoring, and selective antibiotics in early onset group B streptococcal infection, mortality in infants with neonatal infection, or overall neonatal mortality.

DEFINITION Early onset neonatal sepsis usually occurs within the first 7 days of life, and is typically due to infection with group B streptococcus; about 90% of cases present within 24 hours of birth.[1] One in three women carries group B streptococcus, which exists as part of the normal bacterial flora in the vaginal and anal areas. Infection can be transmitted by aspiration of group B streptococcus positive amniotic fluid by the fetus.[2] Symptoms of early onset group B streptococcal infection may be non-specific, including temperature instability, poor feeding, excessive crying or irritability, and respiratory distress. Early onset group B streptococcal infection typically presents with sepsis (69% of cases), leukopenia (31% of cases), pneumonia (26% of cases), respiratory distress (13% of cases), and, rarely, meningitis (11% of cases).[3-5] Late onset group B streptococcus infection occurs from 7–9 days of age, through to the end of the second month of life, and differs from early onset group B streptococcal infection in terms of group B streptococcus serotype, clinical manifestations, and outcome. Late onset infection typically presents with fever (100% of cases) and meningitis (60% of cases).[3,4] This chapter deals with full term and premature asymptomatic babies born with a known risk factor for group B streptococcal infection, but in whom a specific diagnosis of group B streptococcus (either by blood, urine, or cerebrospinal fluid) has not yet been made. The antenatal or intrapartum treatment of women with known group B streptococcal colonisation or infection is outside the scope of this chapter.

INCIDENCE/ PREVALENCE The overall incidence of neonatal bacterial infections is between one and eight infants per 1000 live births and between 160 and 300 per 1000 in very low birth weight infants.[6] Group B streptococcal infection accounts for nearly 50% of serious neonatal bacterial infections.[7] One survey conducted in 2000–2001 estimated that there were 0.72 cases of group B streptococcal infection per 1000 live births in the UK and Ireland, and, of these, 0.48 cases ▶

Neonatal infection: group B streptococcus

per 1000 live births were early onset and 0.24 cases per 1000 live births were late onset infection.[5] One population based study (427 000 live births) carried out in the USA in 2004 found that of the 308 reported cases of neonatal group B streptococcus infections, the prevalence of early onset group B streptococcus infections in the USA has decreased from 2.0 per 1000 live births in 1990 to 0.3 per 1000 live births in 2004.[1] This is thought to be as a result of the increasing use of maternal intrapartum antibiotic prophylaxis.

AETIOLOGY/ RISK FACTORS The main risk factor for group B streptococcal infection in the baby is maternal group B streptococcal infection, which is transmitted in utero.[8] Bacteria originating from the maternal genital tract can infect the amniotic fluid via intact or ruptured membranes. Neonatal infection can result from fetal aspiration or ingestion of the infected amniotic fluid.[1] Infection of the neonate can also occur during birth, when the neonate moves through the vagina, with systemic infection occurring via the umbilical cord, respiratory tract, or skin abrasions.[1] Other risk factors for group B streptococcal infection include prematurity, low birth weight, prolonged rupture of membranes, intrapartum fever, chorioamnionitis, maternal ethnicity (black and hispanic mothers are at increased risk compared with white mothers), and frequent vaginal examinations during labour and delivery.[1,9-11] Lower maternal age (< 20 years) and cigarette smoking have been suggested to be associated with an increased risk of early onset group B streptococcal infection; however, this association has not been proven.[10] Other factors that may increase the risk of group B streptococcal infection include lower socioeconomic status and maternal urinary tract infection during the third trimester (quantitative estimates of the increase in risk are not available). The role of group B streptococcal colonisation of fathers, siblings, and close household contacts in the development of late onset group B streptococcal infection is unclear.[12] For further details of risk factors for early onset group B streptococcal infection, see table 1 Ⓣ.

PROGNOSIS Group B streptococcal infection is a frequent cause of neonatal morbidity and mortality. Untreated, mortality from symptomatic early onset group B streptococcal infection approaches 100%. The combined morbidity and mortality in early onset group B streptococcal infection exceeds 50%, despite the use of appropriate antibiotics and supportive treatment.[7] In the UK, one study has estimated that early onset group B streptococcus infection causes more than 40 neonatal deaths and around 25 cases of long term disability every year, whereas late onset group B streptococcus infection causes around 16 deaths and 40 cases of long term disability every year.[1] Even with immediate initiation of antibiotic treatment, mortality with early onset group B streptococcal infection has been reported to be as high as about 30%.[13] Mortality is particularly high among babies born prematurely, with low birth weight; after prolonged rupture of membranes; or who develop respiratory distress, sepsis, meningitis, or leukopenia. Even with aggressive interventions, premature infants have a 4–15 times higher risk of mortality compared with term infants with early onset group B streptococcus disease.[14] One population based study (427 000 live births) carried out in the USA in 2004 found that the mortality rate for preterm infants with early onset group B streptococcus infection was 23%.[15] The morbidity rate in late onset group B streptococcal infection has been estimated at 4–6%.[3,4] Late onset group B streptococcal infection tends to have a less fulminant onset and is less frequently fatal than is early onset infection.[13] One recent observational study reported a mortality rate of 14% with early onset group B streptococcal infection compared with 4% with late onset infection.[3] Infants with a blood pH of < 7.25, birth weight < 2500 grams, absolute neutrophil count of < 1500 cells per mm^3, hypotension, apnoea, and pleural effusion may be at higher risk of mortality. Little information is available concerning long term sequelae for survivors of neonatal group B streptococcal infection.

Please refer to clinicalevidence.com for full text and references.

Neonatal jaundice

Search date November 2005

David Evans

What are the effects of treatments for unconjugated hyperbilirubinaemia in term and preterm infants?

BENEFICIAL

Exchange transfusion*

We found no RCTs on the effects of exchange transfusion versus no treatment or versus phototherapy. There is general consensus that exchange transfusion is effective in reducing serum bilirubin levels and in preventing neurodevelopmental sequelae.

Hospital phototherapy

One systematic review with two RCTs and one subsequent RCT found that conventional or fibreoptic phototherapy reduced neonatal jaundice more effectively than no treatment. One systematic review (which included quasi-randomised as well as randomised controlled trials) and one subsequent RCT found that conventional phototherapy was more effective than fibreoptic phototherapy, although subgroup analysis in the systematic review found no significant difference between groups in preterm infants. No trials included in the review evaluated the impact of either phototherapy method on parent–infant bonding. One RCT found a greater effect with double conventional compared with single conventional phototherapy, whereas another RCT found no significant difference between double fibreoptic and single conventional phototherapy. One systematic review (which included quasi-randomised as well as randomised controlled trials) found no significant difference between fibreoptic plus conventional and conventional phototherapy alone in additional phototherapy, exchange transfusion, or percentage change in bilirubin after 24 hours, although it noted a trend favouring the fibreoptic plus conventional group. Most trials did not report kernicterus as an outcome. We found insufficient evidence on the adverse effects of phototherapy.

*Although we found no RCTs, there is a general consensus that exchange transfusion is effective in reducing serum bilirubin levels.

UNKNOWN EFFECTIVENESS

Albumin infusion

We found no RCTs on the effects of albumin infusion versus no treatment or versus other treatment.

Home versus hospital phototherapy

We found no RCTs on the effects of home phototherapy versus no treatment or versus hospital phototherapy.

DEFINITION Neonatal jaundice refers to the yellow colouration of the skin and sclera of newborn babies that results from hyperbilirubinaemia.

INCIDENCE/ PREVALENCE Jaundice is the most common condition requiring medical attention in newborn babies. About 50% of term and 80% of preterm babies develop jaundice in the first week of life.[1] Jaundice is also a common cause of readmission to hospital after early discharge of newborn babies.[2] Jaundice usually appears 2–4 days after birth and disappears 1–2 weeks later, usually without the need for treatment.

AETIOLOGY/ RISK FACTORS In most infants with jaundice, there is no underlying disease and the jaundice is termed physiological. Physiological jaundice occurs when there is accumulation of unconjugated bilirubin in the skin and mucous membranes. It typically presents on the second or third day of life and results from the increased production of bilirubin (due to increased circulating red cell mass and a shortened red cell lifespan) and the decreased excretion of bilirubin (due to low concentrations of the hepatocyte binding protein, low activity of glucuronyl transferase, and increased enterohepatic circulation) that normally occur in newborn babies. In some infants, unconjugated hyperbilirubinaemia may be associated with breast feeding (breast milk jaundice), and this typically occurs after the third day of life. Although the exact cause of breast milk jaundice is not clear, it is *generally* believed to be due to an unidentified factor in breast milk. Non-physiological causes include blood group incompatibility (Rhesus or ABO problems), other causes of haemolysis, sepsis, bruising, and metabolic disorders. Gilbert's and Crigler-Najjar syndromes are rare causes of neonatal jaundice.

DIAGNOSIS Jaundice is usually seen first in the face and progresses caudally to the trunk and extremities. However, visual estimation of the bilirubin levels can lead to errors, and a low threshold should exist for measuring serum bilirubin. There are devices that measure transcutaneous bilirubin, but these are generally for screening purposes.[3]

PROGNOSIS In the newborn baby, unconjugated bilirubin can penetrate the blood–brain barrier and is potentially neurotoxic. Acute bilirubin encephalopathy comprises initial lethargy and hypotonia, followed by hypertonia (retrocollis and opisthotonus), irritability, apnoea and seizures. Kernicterus refers to the yellow staining of the deep nuclei of the brain – namely, the basal ganglia (globus pallidus); however, the term is also used to describe the chronic form of bilirubin encephalopathy, which includes symptoms such as athetoid cerebral palsy, hearing loss, failure of upward gaze and dental enamel dysplasia. The exact level of bilirubin that is neurotoxic is unclear, and kernicterus at autopsy has been reported in infants in the absence of markedly elevated levels of bilirubin.[4] Recent reports suggest a resurgence of kernicterus in countries in which this complication had virtually disappeared.[5] This has been attributed mainly to early discharge of newborns from hospital.

Please refer to clinicalevidence.com for full text and references.

Nocturnal enuresis in children

Search date March 2005

John Makari and H. Gil Rushton

What are the effects of interventions for relief of symptoms?

BENEFICIAL

Desmopressin (while treatment continues)

One systematic review found that desmopressin reduced wet nights and increased initial treatment success (14 consecutive dry nights) compared with placebo. The review found insufficient evidence comparing either intranasal versus oral administration of desmopressin or desmopressin versus tricyclic drugs. There was limited evidence that higher doses of desmopressin reduced wet nights during treatment compared with lower doses. One systematic review found insufficient evidence to compare desmopressin versus tricyclic drugs. The review found no significant difference between desmopressin and enuresis alarms in the number of children achieving initial success, although it found limited evidence that desmopressin reduced wet nights compared with alarm during the first week of treatment. A subsequent RCT found that desmopressin reduced wet nights during 12 weeks of treatment compared with alarm. One RCT found no significant difference between laser acupuncture and intranasal desmopressin in the number of wet nights in children after 3 months. We found no RCTs comparing the effects of adding desmopressin to the anticholinergic drugs oxybutynin, tolterodine, and hyoscyamine.

Dry bed training plus enuresis alarm

The addition of an enuresis alarm to dry bed training increased the success of treatment (14 consecutive dry nights) and decreased relapse rates.

Enuresis alarm

One systematic review found that enuresis alarms decreased the number of wet nights during treatment and increased treatment success rates compared with no treatment after 10–20 weeks. One review found no significant difference in treatment success rates between enuresis alarm and dry bed training after 4-20 weeks. The review found that alarm treatment combined with dry bed training increased treatment success and reduced relapse after 8–20 weeks compared with no treatment. There were no significant differences between alarm plus dry bed training and alarm only in success of treatment or relapse when treatment ended. Another systematic review found no significant difference between desmopressin and enuresis alarms in the number of children achieving initial success, although it found limited evidence that desmopressin reduced wet nights compared with alarm during the first week of treatment. A subsequent RCT found that desmopressin significantly reduced wet nights during 12 weeks of treatment compared with alarm. One systematic review found that desmopressin plus alarm reduced the number of wet nights per week during treatment compared with alarm alone or alarm plus placebo, although there was no significant difference between alarm plus desmopressin and alarm alone in treatment success rate (14 consecutive dry nights) after 6–24 weeks or in the rate of relapse after treatment discontinuation. RCTs found that enuresis alarms reduced treatment failure and relapse after treatment ended compared with tricyclic drugs after 8–14 weeks. One RCT found no evidence that an enuresis alarm was more effective in combination with tricyclic drugs after 5–6 weeks. ▶

TRADE OFF BETWEEN BENEFITS AND HARMS

Tricyclic drugs (imipramine, desipramine)

One systematic review found that tricyclic drugs (imipramine, desipramine) increased the chance of attaining 14 consecutive dry nights compared with placebo, although this benefit did not continue after treatment ended. Tricyclic drugs are associated with adverse effects such as anorexia, anxiety, constipation, depression, diarrhoea, dizziness, drowsiness, dry mouth, headache, irritability, lethargy, sleep disturbance, upset stomach, and vomiting compared with placebo. RCTs found that enuresis alarms reduced treatment failure and relapse after treatment ended compared with tricyclic drugs after 8–14 weeks. One RCT found no evidence that an enuresis alarm was more effective in combination with tricyclic drugs after 5–6 weeks. One systematic review found insufficient evidence to compare desmopressin versus tricyclic drugs. One small RCT found that a combination of oxybutynin and imipramine (a tricyclic drug) increased treatment success compared with placebo.

UNKNOWN EFFECTIVENESS

Anticholinergic drugs (oxybutynin, tolterodine, hyoscyamine)

One small RCT provided insufficient evidence to assess the anticholinergic drugs oxybutynin, tolterodine, and hyoscyamine for the treatment of nocturnal enuresis. We found no RCTs comparing oxybutynin, tolterodine, or hyoscyamine versus desmopressin, tricyclic drugs, alarms, or dry bed training. One small RCT found that a combination of oxybutynin and imipramine (a tricyclic drug) increased treatment success compared with placebo.

Desmopressin plus enuresis alarm

One systematic review found that desmopressin plus alarm reduced the number of wet nights per week during initial treatment compared with alarm alone or alarm plus placebo, although there was no significant difference between alarm plus desmopressin and alarm alone in treatment success rate (14 consecutive dry nights) after 6–24 weeks or in the rate of relapse after treatment discontinuation.

Dry bed training

One systematic review found insufficient evidence to determine whether dry bed training alone for 8–24 weeks was superior to no intervention. The review found that use of an enuresis alarm increased dry nights after 4–20 weeks compared with dry bed training alone.

Laser acupuncture (as effective as desmopressin in one RCT)

One RCT found no significant difference between laser acupuncture and intranasal desmopressin in the number of wet nights after 3 months.

Standard home alarm clock

One RCT found that a higher proportion of children achieved 14 consecutive dry nights during treatment for 4 months with a standard home alarm clock compared with waking every 3 hours but no significant difference in relapse rates 3 months after treatment ended.

Nocturnal enuresis in children

UNLIKELY TO BE BENEFICIAL

Desmopressin (following treatment discontinuation)

Small RCTs found limited evidence that after treatment was discontinued, there was no significant difference in the rate of treatment success between desmopressin and placebo. Two RCTs found that desmopressin was less effective than alarm when treatment ended.

DEFINITION Nocturnal enuresis is the involuntary discharge of urine at night in a child aged 5 years or older in the absence of congenital or acquired defects of the central nervous system or urinary tract.[1] Disorders that have bedwetting as a symptom (termed "nocturnal incontinence") can be excluded by a thorough history, examination, and urinalysis. "Monosymptomatic" nocturnal enuresis is characterised by night time symptoms only and accounts for 85% of cases. Nocturnal enuresis is defined as primary if the child has not been dry for a period of more than 6 months, and secondary if such a period of dryness preceded the onset of wetting. Most management strategies are aimed at children aged $\geq$ 7 years.

INCIDENCE/ PREVALENCE Between 15% and 20% of 5 year olds, 7% of 7 year olds, 5% of 10 year olds, 2–3% of 12–14 year olds, and 1–2% of people aged 15 years and over wet the bed twice per week on average.[2]

AETIOLOGY/ RISK FACTORS Nocturnal enuresis is associated with several factors, including small functional bladder capacity, nocturnal polyuria, and, most commonly, arousal dysfunction. Linkage studies have identified associated genetic loci on chromosomes 8q, 12q, 13q, and 22q11.[3-6]

PROGNOSIS Nocturnal enuresis has widely differing outcomes, from spontaneous resolution to complete resistance to all current treatments. About 1% of children remain enuretic until adulthood. Without treatment, about 15% of children with enuresis become dry each year.[7] We found no RCTs on the best age at which to start treatment in children with nocturnal enuresis. Behavioural treatments, such as moisture or wetting alarms, require motivation and commitment from the child and a parent. Anecdotal experience suggests that reassurance is sufficient below the age of 7 years, since children under this age may not exhibit the commitment needed.

Please refer to clinicalevidence.com for full text and references.

Nosebleeds in children

Search date January 2006

Gerald McGarry

What are the effects of treatments for recurrent idiopathic epistaxis in children?

LIKELY TO BE BENEFICIAL

Antiseptic cream

One RCT found that chlorhexidine/neomycin cream reduced nosebleeds compared with no treatment at 8 weeks. One small RCT found no significant difference in nosebleeds between chlorhexidine/neomycin cream and silver nitrate cautery at 8 weeks, although the study may have lacked power to detect a clinically important effect. Some children found the smell and taste of antiseptic cream unpleasant. All children found cautery painful, despite the use of local anaesthesia. One small RCT found insufficient evidence about the effects of silver nitrate cautery plus chlorhexidine/neomycin cream versus chlorhexidine/neomycin cream alone.

UNKNOWN EFFECTIVENESS

Cautery

We found no RCTs comparing silver nitrate cautery with no treatment. One small RCT found no significant difference in nosebleeds between silver nitrate cautery and antiseptic cream at 8 weeks, although the study may have lacked power to detect a clinically important effect. Some children found the smell and taste of antiseptic cream unpleasant. All children found cautery painful, despite the use of local anaesthesia. One small RCT found insufficient evidence about the effects of silver nitrate cautery plus chlorhexidine/neomycin cream versus chlorhexidine/neomycin cream alone.

Petroleum jelly

One RCT found no significant difference in complete resolution of recurrent bleeding between petroleum jelly and no treatment at 8 weeks.

DEFINITION Recurrent idiopathic epistaxis is recurrent, self limiting, nasal bleeding for which no specific cause is identified. There is no consensus on the frequency or severity of recurrences.

INCIDENCE/ PREVALENCE A cross-sectional study of 1218 children (aged 11–14 years) found that 9% had frequent episodes of epistaxis.[1] It is likely that only the most severe episodes are considered for treatment.

AETIOLOGY/ RISK FACTORS In children, most epistaxis occurs from the anterior part of the septum in the region of Little's area.[2] Initiating factors include local inflammation, mucosal drying, and local trauma (including nose picking).[2] Epistaxis caused by other specific local (e.g. tumours) or systemic (e.g. clotting disorders) factors is not considered here.

PROGNOSIS Recurrent epistaxis is less common in people over 14 years old, and many children "grow out" of this problem.

Please refer to clinicalevidence.com for full text and references.

Otitis media in children (acute)

Search date January 2006

Paddy O'Neill, Tony Roberts, and Clare Bradley-Stevenson

What are the effects of treatments for acute otitis media?

LIKELY TO BE BENEFICIAL

Analgesics (reduced earache)

One RCT in children aged 1–6 years receiving antibiotic treatment found that ibuprofen or paracetamol reduced earache as assessed by parental observation after 2 days compared with placebo.

TRADE OFF BETWEEN BENEFITS AND HARMS

Antibiotics (compared with placebo)

We found four systematic reviews comparing antibiotics versus placebo in acute otitis media. The reviews used different inclusion criteria and outcome measures. One review in children aged 4 months to 18 years found a reduction in symptoms with a range of antibiotics (cephalosporins, erythromycin, penicillins, trimethoprim–sulfamethoxazole [co-trimoxazole]) after 7–14 days of treatment compared with placebo. A second review in children younger than 2 years found no significant difference in clinical improvement after 7 days between antibiotics (penicillins, sulphonamides, amoxicillin/clavulanic acid [co-amoxiclav]) and placebo alone or placebo plus myringotomy. A third review in children aged 4 weeks to 18 years found that antibiotics (ampicillin, amoxicillin) reduced clinical failure rate within 2–7 days compared with placebo or observational treatment. The fourth review in children aged 6 months to 15 years found that, compared with placebo, the early use of antibiotics (erythromycin, penicillins) reduced the proportion of children still in pain 2–7 days after presentation, and reduced the risk of developing contralateral acute otitis media. One review also found that antibiotics increased the risk of vomiting, diarrhoea, or rashes compared with placebo.

Choice of antibiotic regimen

One systematic review in children aged 4 months to 18 years found no significant difference between a range of antibiotics in rate of treatment success at 7–14 days or of middle ear effusion at 30 days. A second systematic review in children aged 4 weeks to 18 years found no significant difference between antibiotics in clinical failure rates within 3–14 days. The second review also found that adverse effects, primarily gastrointestinal, were more common with cefixime than with amoxicillin or ampicillin, and were more common with amoxicillin/clavulanate (original formulation) than with azithromycin. One systematic review of placebo controlled RCTs found that antibiotics increase the risk of vomiting, diarrhoea, and rashes.

Immediate compared with delayed antibiotic treatment

One RCT in children aged 6 months to 10 years found that immediate antibiotic treatment reduced the number of days of earache, ear discharge, and amount of daily paracetamol used after the first 24 hours of illness compared with delayed antibiotic treatment, but found no significant difference between groups in daily pain scores. It also found that immediate antibiotic treatment increased diarrhoea compared with delayed antibiotic treatment. One systematic review of placebo controlled RCTs found that antibiotics increase the risk of vomiting, diarrhoea, and rashes.

Longer compared with short courses of antibiotics

One systematic review and two subsequent RCTs found that 8 to 10 day courses of antibiotics reduced treatment failure (lack of clinical resolution, relapse, or re-infection) at 8–19 days compared with 5 day courses, but found no significant difference between groups at 20–42 days. One systematic review of placebo controlled RCTs found that antibiotics increased the risk of vomiting, diarrhoea, and rashes.

LIKELY TO BE INEFFECTIVE OR HARMFUL

Myringotomy

One RCT in infants aged 3 months to 1 year found higher rates of persistent infection and lower rates of otoscopic recovery in children treated with myringotomy plus placebo compared with children receiving antibiotic alone. A second RCT in children aged 2–12 years found no significant difference between myringotomy alone, amoxicillin alone, and no treatment in reduction of pain at 24 hours or 7 days. A third RCT found higher rates of initial treatment failure (resolution of symptoms within 12 hours) with myringotomy plus placebo than with antibiotic alone for severe episodes of acute otitis media in children aged 2–12 years.

What are the effects of interventions to prevent recurrence of acute otitis media?

TRADE OFF BETWEEN BENEFITS AND HARMS

Antibiotic prophylaxis (long term)

One systematic review in children and adults found that long term antibiotic prophylaxis reduced recurrence of acute otitis media compared with placebo. One subsequent RCT in children aged 3 months to 6 years found no significant difference between antibiotic prophylaxis and placebo in prevention of recurrence. A second subsequent RCT found that amoxicillin, but not sulfisoxazole, reduced recurrence of acute otitis media within 6 months compared with placebo. The systematic review provided insufficient evidence on adverse effects of long term antibiotic prophylaxis. However, systematic reviews of placebo controlled RCTs of short term antibiotic treatment found that antibiotics increased the risk of vomiting, diarrhoea, and rashes. One subsequent RCT of antibiotic prophylaxis also reported that adverse effects included thrombocytopenia. We found insufficient evidence on which antibiotic to use, for how long, and how many episodes of acute otitis media justify starting preventive treatment.

UNLIKELY TO BE BENEFICIAL

Vaccination (pneumococcal) *New*

One systematic review in children aged from 2 months to 7 years concluded that, based on currently available results, a large scale use of pneumococcal polysaccharide and conjugate vaccines for prevention of acute otitis media was not yet recommended. Harm caused by vaccination was not quantified, and an analysis of the cost effectiveness of an immunisation programme with pneumoccocal vaccine to prevent acute otitis media has yet to be done. Further ongoing trials may clarify the position with regard to specific high risk populations.

Otitis media in children (acute)

LIKELY TO BE INEFFECTIVE OR HARMFUL

Tympanostomy (ventilation tubes)

One small RCT found that tympanostomy tube insertion reduced the mean number of episodes of acute otitis media during the first 6 month period after treatment compared with myringotomy alone or no surgery, but not during the subsequent 18 months. It also found a non-significant trend toward more recurrent infections and worse hearing after tube extrusion in those treated with tympanostomy. It found more tympanosclerosis in ears that received ventilation tubes compared with those that received myringotomy alone or no surgery.

DEFINITION Otitis media is an inflammation in the middle ear. Subcategories include acute otitis media (AOM), recurrent AOM, and chronic suppurative otitis media. AOM is the presence of middle ear effusion in conjunction with rapid onset of one or more signs or symptoms of inflammation of the middle ear. AOM presents with systemic and local signs, and has a rapid onset. The diagnosis is made on the basis of signs and symptoms, principally ear pain in the presence of a cloudy or bulging eardrum (and immobility of the eardrum if pneumatic otoscopy is performed). Erythema is a moderately useful sign for helping to establish the diagnosis. If the eardrum has a normal colour, then risk of AOM is low.[1] Uncomplicated AOM is limited to the middle ear cleft.[2] The persistence of an effusion beyond 3 months without signs of infection defines otitis media with effusion (also known as "glue ear"; see otitis media with effusion), which can arise as a consequence of AOM but can also occur independently. Chronic suppurative otitis media is characterised by continuing inflammation in the middle ear causing discharge (otorrhoea) through a perforated tympanic membrane (see chronic suppurative otitis media). This chapter only deals with AOM in children.

INCIDENCE/ PREVALENCE AOM is common and has a high morbidity and low mortality in otherwise healthy children. In the UK, about 30% of children under 3 years of age visit their general practitioner with AOM each year, and 97% receive antimicrobial treatment.[3] By 3 months of age, 10% of children have had an episode of AOM. It is the most common reason for outpatient antimicrobial treatment in the USA.[4]

AETIOLOGY/ RISK FACTORS The most common bacterial causes of AOM in the USA and UK are *Streptococcus pneumoniae*, *Haemophilus influenzae*, and *Moraxella catarrhalis*.[3] Similar pathogens are found in Colombia.[5] The incidence of penicillin resistant *S pneumoniae* has risen, but rates differ between countries. The most important risk factors for AOM are young age and attendance at day care centres, such as nursery schools. Other risk factors include being white; male sex; a history of enlarged adenoids, tonsillitis, or asthma; multiple previous episodes; bottle feeding; a history of ear infections in parents or siblings; and use of a soother or pacifier. The evidence for an effect of environmental tobacco smoke is controversial.[3]

PROGNOSIS Without antibiotic treatment AOM symptoms improve in 24 hours in about 60% of children, and in about 80% of children the condition resolves in about 3 days. Suppurative complications occur in about 0.12% of children if antibiotics are withheld.[6] Serious complications are rare in otherwise healthy children but include hearing loss, mastoiditis, meningitis, and recurrent attacks.[3] The World Health Organization estimates that each year 51 000 children under the age of 5 years die from complications of otitis media in developing countries.[7]

Please refer to clinicalevidence.com for full text and references.

Perinatal asphyxia

Search date June 2005

William McGuire

What are the effects of interventions in term or near term newborns with perinatal asphyxia?

UNKNOWN EFFECTIVENESS

Antioxidants

One systematic review found insufficient evidence from two small RCTs about the effects of antioxidants in infants with perinatal asphyxia.

Calcium channel blockers

We found no systematic review or RCTs on the effects of calcium channel blockers in infants with perinatal asphyxia.

Corticosteroids

We found no systematic review or RCTs on the effects of corticosteroids in infants with perinatal asphyxia.

Fluid restriction

One systematic review found no RCTs on the effects of fluid restriction in infants with perinatal asphyxia.

Head and/or whole body hypothermia

One systematic review and two subsequent RCTs found no significant effect of hypothermia on mortality or neurodevelopmental disability in infants with perinatal asphyxia. We found inconclusive evidence on the incidence of sinus bradycardia, coagulopathy, or need for inotrope support, and no significant effect of hypothermia on other adverse outcomes.

Hyperventilation

We found no systematic review or RCTs on the effects of hyperventilation in infants with perinatal asphyxia.

Inotrope support

One systematic review found no RCTs of sufficient size to assess the effects of dopamine or other inotropic agents in infants with perinatal asphyxia.

Magnesium sulphate

One systematic review found no RCTs on the effects of magnesium sulphate in infants with asphyxia. Limited evidence from one small RCT found no significant difference in mortality, blood pressure, or heart rate between a magnesium sulphate/dopamine combination and no drug treatment. However, it found that the combination treatment improved survival with normal cranial computed tomography and electroencephatography results, and establishment of oral feeding by 14 days of age.

Mannitol

One small RCT provided insufficient evidence on the effects of mannitol in infants with asphyxia.

Opiate antagonists

One systematic review found no RCTs assessing the effects of opiate antagonists on mortality or neurodevelopmental outcomes in infants with perinatal asphyxia.

Resuscitation in air (compared with resuscitation using pure oxygen)

Two systematic reviews found lower mortality in infants resuscitated in air compared with 100% oxygen, but no significant difference in rates of hypoxic-ischaemic encephalopathy. We found no RCTs of sufficient quality comparing the effects of resuscitation in air and using pure oxygen on neurodevelopmental outcomes.

UNLIKELY TO BE BENEFICIAL

Prophylactic anticonvulsants

One systematic review of three small, methodologically flawed RCTs found no significant difference in mortality or neurodevelopmental outcomes between barbiturates and no drug treatment in infants with perinatal asphyxia.

DEFINITION The clinical diagnosis of perinatal asphyxia is based on several criteria, the two main ones being evidence of cardiorespiratory and neurological depression, defined as an Apgar score remaining less than 7 at 5 minutes after birth; and evidence of acute hypoxic compromise with acidaemia, defined as an arterial blood pH of less than 7 or base excess greater than 12 mmol/L.[1] In many settings, especially in resource poor countries, it may be impossible to assess fetal or neonatal acidaemia. In the immediate postpartum period when resuscitation is being undertaken, it may not be possible to determine whether the neurological and cardiorespiratory depression is secondary to hypoxia-ischaemia, or to another condition such as feto-maternal infection or metabolic disease. Consequently, resuscitation and early management will often be of suspected rather than confirmed perinatal asphyxia.[2-4]

INCIDENCE/ PREVALENCE Estimates of the incidence of perinatal asphyxia vary depending on the definitions used. In resource rich countries, the incidence of severe perinatal asphyxia (causing death or severe neurological impairment) is about 1/1000 live births.[5,6] In resource poor countries, perinatal asphyxia is probably much more common. Data from hospital based studies in such settings suggest an incidence of 5–10/1000 live births.[7-9] However, this probably represents an underestimate of the true community incidence of perinatal asphyxia in resource poor countries.

AETIOLOGY/ RISK FACTORS Perinatal asphyxia may occur *in utero*, during labour and delivery, or in the immediate postnatal period. There are numerous causes, including placental abruption, cord compression, transplacental anaesthetic or narcotic administration, intrauterine pneumonia, severe meconium aspiration, congenital cardiac or pulmonary anomalies, and birth trauma. Postnatal asphyxia can be caused by an obstructed airway, maternal opiates, which can cause respiratory depression, or congenital sepsis.

PROGNOSIS Worldwide, perinatal asphyxia is a major cause of death and of acquired brain damage in newborn infants.[9] The prognosis depends on the severity of the asphyxia. Only a minority of infants with severe encephalopathy after perinatal asphyxia survive without handicap.[5] However, there are limited population based data on long term outcomes after perinatal asphyxia, such as cerebral palsy, developmental delay, visual and hearing impairment, and learning and behavioural problems. After an asphyxial event, there may be an opportunity to intervene to minimise brain damage. The first phase of brain damage, early cell death, results from primary exhaustion of the cellular energy stores. Early cell death can occur within minutes. Immediate resuscitation to restore oxygen supply and blood circulation aims to limit the extent of this damage. A secondary phase of neuronal injury may occur several hours after the initial insult. The mechanisms believed to be important in this process include oxygen free radical production, intracellular calcium entry, and apoptosis. Treatments during the post-resuscitation phase aim to block these processes thereby limiting secondary cell damage and minimising the extent of any brain damage.

Please refer to clinicalevidence.com for full text and references.

Sleep disorders in children

Search date June 2005

Paul Montgomery and Danielle Dunne

What are the effects of treatments for dysomnias in children?

LIKELY TO BE BENEFICIAL

Extinction and graded approaches New

One systematic review and one additional RCT found that both extinction and graduated extinction interventions improved settling and reduced night wakes compared with placebo in otherwise healthy children. RCTs found that graduated extinction based interventions either alone or in combination with sleep hygiene improved sleep scores in children with a severe learning disability. One RCT identified by the systematic review compared graduated extinction and sleep hygiene and found similar benefits in reducing bedtime tantrums in otherwise healthy children.

Sleep hygiene (in otherwise healthy children) New

One RCT identified by a systematic review found that sleep hygiene interventions reduced bedtime tantrums in otherwise healthy children compared with placebo. It found similar benefits with graduated extinction and sleep hygiene in reducing bedtime tantrums.

TRADE OFF BETWEEN BENEFITS AND HARMS

Melatonin (in otherwise healthy children) New

One RCT identified by a systematic review found that melatonin improved sleep onset and sleep time compared with placebo in otherwise healthy children. The RCT found no significant difference in sleep latency and wake up time. The second RCT identified by the review found that melatonin improved sleep outcomes; however, the RCT did not report significance and there was heterogeneity between groups. Little is known about the long term effects of melatonin and the quality of the product purchased could be variable.

UNKNOWN EFFECTIVENESS

Antihistamines New

We found no systematic review or RCTs on antihistamines in children with dysomnia.

Behavioural therapy plus benzodiazepines, or plus chloral and derivatives New

We found no systematic review or RCTs on behavioural therapy plus benzodiazepines, or behavioural therapy plus chloral and derivatives (chloral hydrate, diclofos sodium) in children with dysomnia.

Exercise New

We found no systematic review or RCTs on exercise in children with dysomnia.

Light therapy New

We found no systematic review or RCTs on light therapy in children with dysomnia.

Melatonin (in children with physical or learning disabilities) *New*

One RCT found that melatonin improved sleep scores compared with placebo in children with epilepsy through change in sleep scores from baseline. There was no significant difference between groups in the actual median sleep scores. Little is known about the long term effects of melatonin and the quality of the product purchased could be variable.

Sleep hygiene (in children with physical or learning disabilities) *New*

We found no systematic review or RCTs of sleep hygiene alone in children with physical or learning disabilities. One RCT found that sleep hygiene in combination with graduated extinction based interventions improved sleep scores in children with a severe learning disability.

Sleep restriction *New*

We found no systematic review or RCTs on sleep restriction in children with dysomnia.

What are the effects of treatments for parasomnias in children?

UNKNOWN EFFECTIVENESS

Antihistamines *New*

We found no systematic review or RCTs on antihistamines in children with parasomnia.

Behavioural therapy plus benzodiazepines, or plus chloral and derivatives *New*

We found no systematic review or RCTs on behavioural therapy plus benzodiazepines, or behavioural therapy plus chloral and derivatives (chloral hydrate, diclofos sodium) in children with parasomnia.

Exercise *New*

We found no systematic review or RCTs on exercise in children with parasomnia.

Extinction and graded approaches *New*

We found no systematic review or RCTs on extinction and graded approaches in children with parasomnia.

Light therapy *New*

We found no systematic review or RCTs on light therapy in children with parasomnia.

Melatonin *New*

One RCT found that melatonin decreased parasomnia score in children with epilepsy; however, the RCT selected children by their epilepsy and not by sleep disorder. We found no systematic review or RCTs examining the effect of melatonin on otherwise healthy children with parasomnia. Little is known about the long term effects of melatonin and the quality of the product purchased could be variable.

Safety/protective interventions *New*

We found no systematic review or RCTs on safety/protective interventions in children with parasomnia.

Sleep disorders in children

Scheduled waking *New*

We found no systematic review or RCTs on scheduled waking in children with parasomnia.

Sleep hygiene *New*

We found no systematic review or RCTs on sleep hygiene in children with parasomnia.

Sleep restriction *New*

We found no systematic review or RCTs on sleep restriction in children with parasomnia.

DEFINITION The International Classification of Sleep Disorders-2 (ICSD-2) defines more than 80 sleep disorders, many of which apply to children – although often in different ways – as much as adults.[1] Sleep problems can be divided into three broad areas: too much sleep or too little sleep (dysomnias), and parasomnias. **Dysomnias** are disorders that produce either excessive daytime sleepiness or difficulty initiating or maintaining sleep. They can be intrinsic, extrinsic, or circadian rhythm sleep disorders. Dysomnias include: primary insomnia, primary hypersomnia, narcolepsy, breathing related sleep disorders, and circadian rhythm sleep disorder. **Parasomnias** are undesirable phenomena that occur predominantly during sleep. They are caused by inappropriately timed activation of physiological systems. Parasomnias include: nightmare disorder, sleep terror disorder, and sleepwalking disorder. **Children with physical or learning disabilities:** Sleep problems tend to be greater in prevalence and severity in this population. For example, pain is related to sleep disturbance and attention paid to helping the child sleep better is likely to improve recovery. Across a range of physical problems, there are reports in the literature of sleep disturbance associated with them. In most cases, research is limited and the mechanisms are unclear. Children with visual impairment are prone to circadian rhythm problems: their light perception is poor and the primary cue for sleep onset is lost. Many medications are known to cause sleep problems such as severe drowsiness with many antiepileptic drugs. Learning disabilities vary considerably in the range of conditions covered by this global term. However, some conditions such as Smith-Magenis, Prader-Willi, and Williams syndrome have sleep disturbance as cardinal features. Others, such as Down's syndrome and mucopolysaccharidoses are associated with sleep related breathing problems. Treatment for these groups of children needs to be tailored to their particular problems and may be problematic for anatomical and neurological reasons. Nevertheless, in large part, these sleep problems should be regarded as treatable and careful investigation of these problems is required.[2,3]

INCIDENCE/ PREVALENCE Sleep problems, primarily settling problems and frequent night wakings, are experienced by about 20–30% of children aged 1–5 years old but cultural differences would seem to play at least some role.[4-7] These sleep disturbances often persist in later childhood:[8] 40–80% of children displaying sleep problems when aged 15–48 months were found to have persistent sleep disorders 2–3 years later.[9] In toddlers, settling and night waking problems are dominant with rates about 20–25%.[10] A second peak in sleep problems occurs in adolescence where sleep timing problems including delayed sleep phase syndrome occurs. Such children have difficulty getting off to sleep and then problems getting up in the morning for school. Across the age range, sleep related breathing problems occur at rates about 2%.[11] Narcolepsy is thought to occur with a prevalence of 4–6/10 000 in the USA in adults with the onset of symptoms tending to occur in the second decade.[12] **Children with physical or learning disabilities:** Prevalence of sleep disorders tends to be even greater in children with physical or learning disabilities: about 86%

of children aged up to 6 years old, 81% of children aged 6–11 years, and 77% of children aged 12–16 years with physical or learning disabilities suffer from severe sleep problems.[13] We found no separate data for dysomnias and parasomnias.

AETIOLOGY/ RISK FACTORS Evidence of the aetiology of sleep disorders in children is generally limited; however, the proportion of rapid eye movement (REM – active sleep) is greater in infants than in adults. REM is frequently associated with awakenings and infants with a sleep disorder often need assistance to resume sleep after such arousals.[14] Factors related to sleep disorders are having had colic,[15] the child being the first born,[16] and the child having a difficult temperament (e.g. low sensory threshold, negative mood, decreased adaptability).[17] Other factors have been suggested, such as being born prematurely and low birth weight; however, evidence of such associations is contradictory.[14] These factors may influence the onset of a sleep disorder, but the factors influencing the maintenance of a sleep problem are likely to be different. Increased maternal responsiveness is associated with the maintenance of sleep disorders in children.[18]

PROGNOSIS Children with excessive daytime sleepiness or night waking are likely to suffer from impaired daytime functioning without treatment and their parents are likely to have increased stress. In addition to these effects, children with parasomnias are at serious risk of accidental injuries. Between 40% to 80% of children aged 15–48 months displaying sleep problems had persistent sleep problems 2–3 years later.[9] **Children with physical or learning disabilities:** Children with learning disabilities and sleep disorders are more likely to have greater challenging behaviour than those without sleep problems.[19] This naturally affects the quality of life of the parents, frequently resulting in maternal stress, mothers displaying less affection for their children, and marital discord.[13,20] For children with epilepsy, sleep disorders may exacerbate their condition: a persistent lack of sleep has been associated with an increased frequency of seizures.[21]

Please refer to clinicalevidence.com for full text and references.

Sudden infant death syndrome

Search date July 2005

David Creery and Angelo Mikrogianakis

What are the effects of interventions to reduce the risk of sudden infant death syndrome?

BENEFICIAL

Advice to avoid prone sleeping*

One non-systematic review and 12 observational studies found that eight campaigns encouraging non-prone positioning and seven campaigns involving, among other recommendations, advice to encourage non-prone sleeping positions, were followed by a reduced incidence of sudden infant death syndrome.

LIKELY TO BE BENEFICIAL

Advice to avoid tobacco smoke exposure*

One non-systematic review and four observational studies found limited evidence that campaigns to reduce several risk factors for sudden infant death, which included tobacco smoke exposure, were followed by a reduced incidence of sudden infant death syndrome. One observational study found that smoking was associated with an increased risk of sudden infant death. Two of the observational studies found that national campaigns that advised mothers to avoid tobacco smoke exposure were followed by a reduction in maternal smoking rates.

UNKNOWN EFFECTIVENESS

Advice to avoid bed sharing*

One observational study found that a campaign to reduce several risk factors for sudden infant death, which included advice to avoid bed sharing, was followed by a reduced incidence of sudden infant death syndrome. However, it is not clear whether effects were specifically due to the advice to avoid bed sharing.

Advice to avoid overheating or overwrapping*

One non-systematic review and one observational study found limited evidence that campaigns to reduce several risk factors for sudden infant death, which included overwrapping and overheating, were followed by a reduced incidence of sudden infant death syndrome. However, it is not clear whether effects were specifically due to the advice to avoid overwrapping or overheating.

Advice to avoid soft sleeping surfaces*

We found no evidence on the effects of advice to avoid soft sleeping surfaces in the prevention of sudden infant death syndrome.

Advice to breastfeed*

One non-systematic review and three observational studies found that campaigns to reduce several risk factors for sudden infant death, which included advice to breastfeed, were followed by a reduced incidence of sudden infant death syndrome. However, it is not clear whether effects were specifically due to the advice to breastfeed.

Advice to promote soother use*

One systematic review found insufficient evidence on the effects of advice to promote soother use in the prevention of sudden infant death syndrome. ▶

*Observational evidence only; RCTs unlikely to be conducted.

DEFINITION Sudden infant death syndrome (SIDS) is the sudden death of an infant aged under 1 year that remains unexplained after review of the clinical history, examination of the scene of death, and postmortem.

INCIDENCE/ PREVALENCE The incidence of SIDS has varied over time and among nations (incidence per 1000 live births of SIDS in 1996: The Netherlands 0.3, Japan 0.4, Canada 0.5, England and Wales 0.7, USA 0.8, and Australia 0.9).[1]

AETIOLOGY/ RISK FACTORS By definition, the cause of SIDS is not known. Observational studies have found an association between SIDS and several risk factors, including prone sleeping position,[2,3] prenatal or postnatal exposure to tobacco smoke,[4] soft sleeping surfaces,[5,6] hyperthermia/overwrapping (see tables A, B, and C on web extra),[7,8] bed sharing (particularly with mothers who smoke),[9,10] lack of breastfeeding,[11,12] and lack of soother use.[7,13] The incidence of SIDS is increased in the siblings of that infant.[14,15]

PROGNOSIS Prognosis is not applicable.

Please refer to clinicalevidence.com for full text and references.

Urinary tract infection in children

Search date December 2005

James Larcombe

What are the effects of treatment of acute urinary tract infection in children?

LIKELY TO BE BENEFICIAL

Antibiotics (more effective than placebo)*

There is consensus that antibiotics are likely to be beneficial in children with urinary tract infection compared with placebo. Placebo controlled trials of antibiotics for symptomatic acute urinary tract infection in children are considered unethical.

Oral antibiotics (as effective as initial intravenous antibiotics in children without severe vesicoureteric reflux or renal scarring)

One RCT identified by a systematic review found no significant difference between oral cephalosporins alone and a regimen of 3 days of intravenous cephalosporins plus continued oral cephalosporins, in duration of fever, reinfection rate, renal scarring, or extent of scarring at 6 months in children aged 2 years or younger with a first confirmed urinary tract infection. The RCT found weak evidence that, in children with grades III–IV vesicoureteric reflux, initial intravenous treatment plus oral treatment may reduce renal scarring at 6 months compared with oral treatment alone.

*Based on consensus. Placebo controlled RCTs would be considered unethical.

UNKNOWN EFFECTIVENESS

Immediate empirical antibiotic treatment (unclear benefit compared with delayed treatment, based on microscopy and culture)

We found no RCTs comparing early empirical treatment with delayed treatment based on the results of microscopy or culture in acute urinary tract infection in children. Retrospective analysis of one RCT found no significant difference in risk of renal scarring between cephalosporin treatment within 24 hours compared with 24 hours after the onset of fever in children under 2 years of age with urinary tract infections.

UNLIKELY TO BE BENEFICIAL

Longer (7–14 days) courses of initial intravenous antibiotics (no more effective than shorter [3–4 days] courses of intravenous antibiotics in children with acute pyelonephritis)

One systematic review found no significant difference between long (7–14 days) and short (3–4 days) courses of initial intravenous antibiotics in persistence of bacteriuria after treatment, recurrent urinary tract infection at 6–12 months, or renal scarring at 3–6 months in children with acute pyelonephritis.

Longer (7–14 days) courses of oral antibiotics (no more effective than shorter [2–4 days] courses for non-recurrent lower urinary tract infections in the absence of renal tract abnormality)

One systematic review found no significant difference between longer courses (7–14 days) and shorter courses (2–4 days) of the same oral antibiotic in cure rate at 7 days after treatment in children with no history of renal tract abnormality and judged not to have acute pyelonephritis. Another systematic ▶

review found no significant difference between 7–14 day courses and 3 day courses of any antibiotic in cure rate. However, longer courses may be associated with more adverse effects.

LIKELY TO BE INEFFECTIVE OR HARMFUL

Prolonged delay in antibiotic treatment (> 4 days)

We found no RCTs. Five retrospective studies found that medium to long term delays (4 days to 7 years) in treatment may be associated with an increased risk of renal scarring.

Single dose of oral antibiotics (less effective than longer course [7–10 days])

One systematic review found that single dose oral amoxicillin decreased cure rate at 3–30 days compared with a longer (10 days) course of oral amoxicillin. Another systematic review found that single day or single dose regimens increased treatment failure compared with 7–14 day courses of any antibiotic.

What are the effects of interventions to prevent recurrence of urinary tract infection in children?

LIKELY TO BE BENEFICIAL

Immunotherapy

One RCT in children with recurrent urinary tract infection found that adding pidotimod (an immunotherapeutic agent) to antibiotic treatment reduced recurrence compared with adding placebo. A second RCT found no significant difference between an antigenic extract of *E Coli* and antibiotics in the incidence of urinary tract infection in girls after 6 months.

Prophylactic antibiotics

One systematic review found that prophylactic antibiotics (co-trimoxazole, nitrofurantoin, given for 10 weeks to 12 months) reduced urinary tract infection recurrence in children compared with placebo or no treatment. One RCT found that nitrofurantoin reduced recurrence of urinary tract infection over 6 months compared with trimethoprim. However, more children discontinued treatment with nitrofurantoin because of adverse effects. We found no RCTs evaluating the optimum duration of prophylactic antibiotics. For antibiotics versus immunotherapeutic agents, see immunotherapy option.

UNLIKELY TO BE BENEFICIAL

Surgical correction of minor functional anomalies

We found no RCTs. One observational study suggested that children with minor anomalies do not develop renal scarring and therefore may not benefit from surgery.

Surgical correction of moderate to severe vesicoureteric reflux (grades III-IV, as effective as medical management but with surgical risks)

One systematic review in children with moderate to severe vesicoureteric reflux found no significant difference in numbers of urinary tract infections or their complications between surgical and medical management (prophylactic antibiotic treatment) at 1–5 years after treatment, although surgery abolished reflux. Long term follow up of one RCT included in the review found that new renal scars rarely occurred with either management strategy after 5 years. One RCT found a non-significantly greater decline in glomerular filtration rate over 10 years with

Urinary tract infection in children

medical treatment compared with surgery in children with moderate to severe bilateral vesicoureteric reflux and bilateral nephropathy. This RCT was too small to detect a clinically important effect of surgery in children with bilateral nephropathy.

DEFINITION Urinary tract infection (UTI) is defined by the presence of a pure growth of more than 10^5 colony forming units of bacteria per millilitre of urine. Lower counts of bacteria may be clinically important, especially in boys and in specimens obtained by urinary catheter. Any growth of typical urinary pathogens is considered clinically important if obtained by suprapubic aspiration. In practice, three age ranges are usually considered on the basis of differential risk and different approaches to management: children under 1 year; young children (1–4, 5, or 7 years, depending on the information source); and older children (up to 12–16 years). Recurrent UTI is defined as a further infection by a new organism. Relapsing UTI is defined as a further infection with the same organism.

INCIDENCE/ PREVALENCE Boys are more susceptible to urinary tract infection (UTI) before the age of 3 months; thereafter, the incidence is substantially higher in girls. Estimates of the true incidence of UTI depend on rates of diagnosis and investigation. At least 8% of girls and 2% of boys will have a UTI in childhood.[1]

AETIOLOGY/ RISK FACTORS The normal urinary tract is sterile. Contamination by bowel flora may result in urinary infection if a virulent organism is involved or if the child is immunosuppressed. In neonates, infection may originate from other sources. **Escherichia coli** accounts for about 75% of all pathogens. **Proteus** is more common in boys (about 30% of infections). **Obstructive anomalies** are found in 0–4% and **vesicoureteric reflux** in 8–40% of children being investigated for their first UTI.[2] One meta-analysis of 12 cohort studies (537 children admitted to hospital for UTI, 1062 kidneys) found that 36% of all kidneys had some scarring on DMSA scintigraphy, and that 59% of children with vesicoureteric reflux on micturating cystourethography had at least one scarred kidney (pooled positive likelihood ratio 1.96, 95% CI 1.51 to 2.54; pooled negative likelihood ratio 0.71, 95% CI 0.58 to 0.85). There was evidence of heterogeneity in likelihood ratios among studies. The authors concluded that vesicoureteric reflux is a weak predictor of renal damage in children admitted to hospital.[3] Thus, although vesicoureteric reflux is a major risk factor for adverse outcome, other factors, some of which have not yet been identified, are also important. **Family history:** Vesicoureteric reflux itself runs in families: in one review article, the incidence of reflux in siblings ranged from 26% (a cohort of asymptomatic siblings) to 86% (siblings with a history of urinary tract infection) compared with a rate of less than 1% in the normal population.[4] Although some gene variants seem to be more common in children who suffer renal damage, no clear link has yet been established between specific genes and an adverse outcome.[5] Local or systemic immune problems are also likely to be factors in the development of UTI.

PROGNOSIS **Recurrence:** A study in the UK found that 78% of girls and 71% of boys presenting with UTI within the first year of life experienced recurrence, and that 45% of girls and 39% of boys presenting after their first year of life developed further infections.[6] **Vesicoureteric reflux:** In a longitudinal study, 84% of children (572 children with UTI and vesicoureteric reflux) had spontaneous resolution during medical follow up at between 5–15 years.[7] **Renal scarring:** A systematic review of imaging in childhood UTI suggested that renal scarring (assessed with intravenous pyelogram [IVP] or dimercaptosuccinic acid [DMSA] scan) occurs in 5–15% of children within 1–2 years of their first diagnosed UTI.[2] Between 32–70% of these scars were noted at the time of initial assessment, suggesting a high level of pre-existing scarring, perhaps due to previously unrecognised infection.[2] This percentage did not substantially alter, despite an increasing referral rate, during the 3 years studied. One meta-analysis of 12 cohort studies (537 children admitted to hospital for UTI, 1062 kidneys) found that 36% of all kidneys had some scarring on DMSA scintigraphy, and that 59% of children with vesicoureteric reflux on micturating cystourethography had at least one scarred kidney (pooled positive likelihood ratio 1.96, 95% CI 1.51 to 2.54; pooled negative likelihood ratio 0.71, 95% CI 0.58 to 0.85). However, there was evidence of heterogeneity in likelihood ratios among studies. The authors concluded that vesicoureteric reflux is a weak predictor of renal damage in children admitted to hospital.[3] A retrospective population based study in the UK suggested that 4.3% of boys and 4.7% of girls develop scarring (assessed using DMSA scans after their first referral for UTI).[8] **New or progressive renal scarring and recurrent UTI:** The systematic review reported on four studies that provided at least 2 years' follow up: new renal scars developed in 1.6–23% of children, and existing renal scars progressed in 6–34%.[2] It is unclear whether figures for new scars included any children who were previously unscarred. The highest rates of scarring were associated with the highest rates of recurrent UTI.[2] A further study showed that, in children aged 5 years and over, abnormal DMSA scans were noted in 64/118 (55%) children presenting with recurrent UTI, whereas 7/44 (15%) who presented with "first UTI" had scarring (OR for recurrences causing scarring: OR 6.3; 95% CI 2.6 to 15.2).[9] However, recurrent UTI may be less important as a risk factor for scarring in older children: one study[10] showed that, in children with initially normal scans at 3 or 4 years of age, 5/176 (3%) children aged 3 years at presentation, and 0/179 (0%) aged 4 years at presentation had developed scarring between 2 and 11 years later. Of those children that developed scarring, 4/5 (80%) had a definite history of recurrent UTI, in all cases ≥3 episodes (OR for recurrences causing scarring: 11.5; 95% CI 1.3 to 106.1).[10] Another study (287 children with severe vesicoureteric reflux treated either medically or surgically for any UTI) used serial DMSA scintigraphy to evaluate the risk of renal scarring over 5 years. It found that younger children (aged < 2 years) were at greater risk of renal scarring than older children, regardless of treatment for the infection (AR for deterioration in DMSA scan over 5 years: 21/86 (24%) for younger children *v* 27/201 (13%) for older children; RR 1.82, 95% CI 1.09 to 3.03).[11] It is likely that children who present when older, and are found to have scarring, will have had one or more previous UTI that remained undiagnosed. Many children seem to lose their susceptibility to renal damage with age. **Consequences for longer term:** One long term follow up study in the UK found that children with renal scarring and vesicoureteric reflux at presentation, or just one of these followed by documented UTI, were associated with an increased risk of progressive renal damage compared with children presenting without these features (RR of progressive renal damage: 17, 95% CI 2.5 to 118).[6] Renal scarring may be associated with future complications: poor renal growth, recurrent adult pyelonephritis, impaired glomerular function, early hypertension, and end stage renal failure.[12-15] A combination of recurrent UTI, severe vesicoureteric reflux, and the presence of renal scarring at first presentation is associated with the worst prognosis.

Please refer to clinicalevidence.com for full text and references.

Diabetic nephropathy

Search date November 2005

Michael Shlipak

What are the effects of treatments in people with type 1 diabetes and early nephropathy?

BENEFICIAL

Angiotensin converting enzyme inhibitors (reduced progression to late nephropathy)

One systematic review found that, compared with placebo or controls, angiotensin converting enzyme inhibitors (captopril, lisinopril, enalapril, perindopril, and ramipril) reduced progression to macroalbuminuria and increased regression to normoalbuminuria in normotensive people with type 1 diabetes and microalbuminuria. We found no RCTs comparing angiotensin converting enzyme inhibitors versus angiotensin II receptor antagonists or assessing combined angiotensin converting enzyme inhibitors plus angiotensin II receptor antagonists in people with type 1 diabetes and early nephropathy.

Glycaemic control (reduced progression to late nephropathy)

One systematic review found that, compared with conventional control, intensive glycaemic control reduced progression of nephropathy in people with type 1 diabetes and either normal albumin excretion or microalbuminuria. The review found no significant difference between intensive glycaemic control and conventional control in the incidence of severe hypoglycaemia. It found a higher incidence of diabetic ketoacidosis in people treated with continuous subcutaneous insulin infusion compared with conventional multiple injection treatment.

UNKNOWN EFFECTIVENESS

Angiotensin II receptor antagonists

We found no systematic review or RCTs comparing the effects of angiotensin II receptor antagonists versus placebo in people with type 1 diabetes and early nephropathy on outcomes of all cause mortality, incidence of end stage renal disease, or incidence of cardiovascular events (stroke, heart failure, and myocardial infarction). Long term placebo controlled RCTs would not be ethical because of the established benefits of angiotensin converting enzyme inhibitors and similarity between these two drug classes. We found no RCTs comparing angiotensin II receptor antagonists versus angiotensin converting enzyme inhibitors or assessing combined angiotensin II receptor antagonists plus angiotensin converting enzyme inhibitors in people with type 1 diabetes and early nephropathy.

Protein restriction

We found no systematic review or RCTs comparing the effects of low protein diet versus usual diet in people with type 1 diabetes and early nephropathy on the outcomes of progression to late nephropathy, all cause mortality, incidence of end stage renal disease, or incidence of cardiovascular events (stroke, heart failure, and myocardial infarction).

Tight control of blood pressure

We found no systematic review or RCTs comparing the effects of tight control of blood pressure versus conventional control in people with type 1 diabetes and ▶

early nephropathy on the outcomes of progression to late nephropathy, all cause mortality, incidence of end stage renal disease, or incidence of cardiovascular events (stroke, heart failure, and myocardial infarction).

What are the effects of treatments in people with type 1 diabetes and late nephropathy?

BENEFICIAL

Captopril

One RCT in people with type 1 diabetes and late nephropathy found that, compared with placebo, captopril (an angiotensin converting enzyme inhibitor) reduced the combined outcome of renal transplant, end stage renal disease, or death over 3 years. We found no RCTs comparing angiotensin II receptor antagonists versus angiotensin converting enzyme inhibitors or assessing combined angiotensin converting enzyme inhibitors plus angiotensin II receptor antagonists in people with type 1 diabetes and late nephropathy.

UNKNOWN EFFECTIVENESS

Angiotensin II receptor antagonists

We found no RCTs comparing the effects of angiotensin II receptor antagonists versus placebo in people with type 1 diabetes and late nephropathy on outcomes of all cause mortality, incidence of end stage renal disease, or incidence of cardiovascular events (stroke, heart failure, and myocardial infarction). Long term placebo controlled RCTs would not be ethical because of the established benefits of angiotensin converting enzyme inhibitors and similarity between these two drug classes. We found no RCTs comparing angiotensin II receptor antagonists versus angiotensin converting enzyme inhibitors or assessing combined angiotensin II receptor antagonists plus angiotensin converting enzyme inhibitors in people with type 1 diabetes and late nephropathy.

Glycaemic control

We found no systematic review or RCTs comparing the effects of intensive glycaemic control versus conventional glycaemic control in people with type 1 diabetes and late nephropathy on the outcomes of all cause mortality, incidence of end stage renal disease, or incidence of cardiovascular events (stroke, heart failure, and myocardial infarction).

Protein restriction

One small RCT found that, compared with usual protein intake, a low protein diet reduced the cumulative incidence of end stage renal disease or death over 4 years in people with type 1 diabetes and late nephropathy. This RCT was small, and neither participants nor study investigators could be blinded to the randomisation owing to the nature of the intervention.

Tight control of blood pressure

We found no systematic review or RCTs comparing the effects of tight blood pressure control versus conventional control in people with type 1 diabetes and late nephropathy on the outcomes of all cause mortality, incidence of end stage renal disease, or incidence of cardiovascular events (stroke, heart failure, and myocardial infarction).

Diabetic nephropathy

What are the effects of treatments in people with type 2 diabetes and early nephropathy?

BENEFICIAL

Angiotensin converting enzyme inhibitors

One RCT found that, compared with placebo, enalapril reduced progression to late nephropathy in people with type 2 diabetes and early nephropathy. One RCT comparing ramipril versus placebo with subgroup analysis in people with diabetes and early nephropathy found that ramipril reduced the combined outcome of myocardial infarction, stroke, or cardiovascular death. One RCT found no significant difference in mortality, end stage renal disease, stroke, heart failure, or myocardial infarction between very low dose ramipril and placebo. One systematic review in people with diabetes and nephropathy, which did not stratify the results by the type of diabetes, found that, compared with placebo, angiotensin converting enzyme inhibitors reduced progression to late nephropathy in people with diabetes and microalbuminuria over 3 years. One RCT in people with type 2 diabetes and early nephropathy found no significant difference in change in glomerular filtration rate, mortality, stroke, heart failure, or myocardial infarction between an angiotensin converting enzyme inhibitor, enalapril, and an angiotensin II receptor blocker, telmisartan, over 5 years. We found no systematic review or RCTs assessing combined angiotensin converting enzyme inhibitors plus angiotensin II receptor antagonists in people with type 2 diabetes and early nephropathy.

Angiotensin II receptor antagonists

One RCT in people with type 2 diabetes, hypertension, and microalbuminuria found that, compared with placebo, an angiotensin II receptor antagonist, irbesartan 300 mg, reduced progression from early to late nephropathy over 2 years. However, it found no significant decrease with irbesartan 150 mg. One RCT in people with type 2 diabetes and early nephropathy found no significant difference in change in glomerular filtration rate, mortality, stroke, heart failure, or myocardial infarction between an angiotensin II receptor antagonist, telmisartan, and an angiotensin converting enzyme inhibitor, enalapril, over 5 years. We found no systematic review or RCTs assessing combined angiotensin II receptor antagonists plus angiotensin converting enzyme inhibitors in people with type 2 diabetes and early nephropathy.

Tight control of blood pressure (reduced progression to late nephropathy)

One RCT found that, in people with type 2 diabetes, early nephropathy, and baseline blood pressure within the normal range, a lower diastolic blood pressure target (10 mm Hg below baseline) reduced progression from microalbuminuria to overt albuminuria over 5 years compared with a moderate diastolic blood pressure target (80–89 mm Hg).

UNKNOWN EFFECTIVENESS

Glycaemic control

We found no systematic review or RCTs evaluating the effects of glycaemic control in people with type 2 diabetes and early nephropathy on the outcomes of progression to late nephropathy, all cause mortality, incidence of end stage renal disease, or incidence of cardiovascular events (stroke, heart failure, and myocardial infarction).

Protein restriction

We found no systematic review or RCTs evaluating the effects of protein restriction in people with type 2 diabetes and early nephropathy on the outcomes of progression to late nephropathy, all cause mortality, incidence of end stage renal disease, or incidence of cardiovascular events (stroke, heart failure, and myocardial infarction).

What are the effects of treatments in people with type 2 diabetes and late nephropathy?

BENEFICIAL

Angiotensin II receptor antagonists

We found two RCTs comparing the effects of angiotensin II receptor antagonists versus placebo or versus angiotensin converting enzyme inhibitors on the outcomes of progression to end stage renal disease, cardiovascular events, and all cause mortality. One RCT in people with type 2 diabetes and late nephropathy found that, compared with placebo, losartan reduced progression to end stage renal disease over 3.4 years. It found no significant difference in fatal or non-fatal cardiovascular events or death from any cause. Another RCT in people with type 2 diabetes and late nephropathy found no significant difference between irbesartan and placebo in progression to end stage renal disease or death from any cause over 2.6 years. It found that irbesartan reduced the incidence of congestive heart failure compared with placebo. It found no significant difference in a composite cardiovascular outcome, cardiovascular death, myocardial infarction, cerebrovascular accident, or cardiac revascularisation. In both RCTs, angiotensin II receptor antagonist was discontinued if hyperkalaemia occurred. We found no systematic review or RCTs assessing combined angiotensin II receptor antagonists plus angiotensin converting enzyme inhibitors in people with type 2 diabetes and late nephropathy.

UNKNOWN EFFECTIVENESS

Angiotensin converting enzyme inhibitors

We found no systematic review or RCTs comparing the effects of angiotensin converting enzyme inhibitors versus placebo or versus angiotensin II receptor antagonists, or assessing combined angiotensin converting enzyme inhibitors plus angiotensin II receptor antagonists in people with type 2 diabetes and late nephropathy that assessed the outcomes of all cause mortality, incidence of end stage renal disease, or incidence of cardiovascular events (stroke, heart failure, and myocardial infarction).

Glycaemic control

We found no systematic review or RCTs on glycaemic control in people with type 2 diabetes and late nephropathy on the outcomes of all cause mortality, incidence of end stage renal disease, or incidence of cardiovascular events (stroke, heart failure, and myocardial infarction).

Protein restriction

We found no systematic review or RCTs evaluating the effects of protein restriction in people with type 2 diabetes and late nephropathy on the outcomes of all cause mortality, incidence of end stage renal disease, or incidence of cardiovascular events (stroke, heart failure, and myocardial infarction).

Diabetic nephropathy

Tight control of blood pressure

We found no systematic review or RCTs evaluating the effects of tight blood pressure control in people with type 2 diabetes and late nephropathy on the outcomes of all cause mortality, incidence of end stage renal disease, or incidence of cardiovascular events (stroke, heart failure, and myocardial infarction).

DEFINITION Diabetic nephropathy is a clinical syndrome characterised by albuminuria on at least two occasions that are separated by 3–6 months, in people with diabetes. Diabetic nephropathy is usually accompanied by hypertension, progressive rise in proteinuria, and decline in renal function. In type 1 diabetes, five stages (see table 1)Ⓣ have been proposed. Of these stages, stages 1 and 2 are equivalent to preclinical nephropathy and are detected only by imaging or biopsy. Stage 3 is synonymous with early nephropathy, the clinical term used in this chapter. Stage 4 nephropathy is also known clinically as late nephropathy, and this term will be used for the remainder of this chapter. Stage 5 represents the progression to end stage renal disease. **Population:** For the purpose of this review, we have included people with diabetes and both early nephropathy, synonymous with microalbuminuria, usually defined by albuminuria level of 30–300 mg/day (or albumin/creatinine ratio of 30–300 mg/g [3.4–34.0 mg/mmol]), and late nephropathy, synonymous with macroalbuminuria, characterised by albuminuria > 300 mg/day (or albumin/creatinine ratio > 300 mg/g [34 mg/mmol]). The treatment of people with diabetes and end stage renal disease is not covered in this chapter.

INCIDENCE/ PREVALENCE In 1997, the worldwide prevalence of diabetes was 124 million and is expected to increase to 221 million in 2010.[1] In the UK, 1.4 million people had been diagnosed with diabetes in 1998, and estimates suggest 1 million more have diabetes, but have not yet been diagnosed.[2] After 20 years of diabetes, the cumulative risk of proteinuria is 27% in type 2 and 28% in type 1.[3] In both type 1 and type 2 diabetes, the overall prevalence of microalbuminuria and macroalbuminuria is about 30–35%.[4] In addition, the incidence of diabetic nephropathy is increasing, in part owing to the growing epidemic of type 2 diabetes and increased life expectancies; for example, in the USA, the incidence has increased by 150% in the past decade.[5]

AETIOLOGY/ RISK FACTORS Duration of diabetes, older age, male gender, smoking, and poor glycaemic control have all been found to be risk factors in the development of nephropathy.[6,7] In addition, certain ethnic groups seem to be at greater risk for developing diabetic nephropathy (see prognosis). Microalbuminuria is less pathognomonic among type 2 diabetics, because hypertension, which commonly complicates type 2 diabetes, can also cause microalbuminuria. Hypertension can also cause renal insufficiency, so the time to development of renal insufficiency can be shorter in type 2 diabetes than in type 1. For people who have an atypical course, renal biopsy may be advisable. In addition, there are some differences in the progression of type 1 and type 2 diabetic nephropathy. In type 2 diabetics, albuminuria is more often present at diagnosis. Hypertension is also more common in type 2 diabetic nephropathy. Finally, microalbuminuria is less predictive of late nephropathy in type 2 diabetics compared with type 1.[8]

PROGNOSIS People with microalbuminuria are at increased risk for progression to macroalbuminuria and end stage renal disease. The course of renal function is similar between type 1 and type 2 diabetes. The natural history of diabetic nephropathy is better defined in type 1 than type 2 diabetes. In type 2 diabetes, the course can be more difficult to predict, primarily because the date of onset of diabetes is less commonly known and comorbid conditions can contribute to renal disease. Without specific interventions, about 80% of people with type 1 diabetes and 20–40% of people with type 2 diabetes with microalbuminuria will progress to macroalbuminuria.[9] Diabetic nephropathy is associated with poor outcomes. It is the most common cause of end stage renal disease in the UK, accounting for 20% of all cases[10] whereas, in the USA, diabetes accounts for 48% of all new cases of end stage renal disease.[11] People with type 1 diabetes and proteinuria have been found to have a 40-fold greater risk of mortality than people without proteinuria.[12] The prognostic significance of proteinuria is less extreme in type 2 diabetes, although people with proteinuria do have a four-fold risk of death compared with people without proteinuria.[13] In addition, increased cardiovascular risk has been associated with albuminuria in people with diabetes.[14] African Americans, Native Americans, and Mexican Americans have a much higher risk of developing end stage renal disease in the setting of diabetes compared with white people.[9,15] In the USA, African American people with diabetes progress to end stage renal disease at a considerably more rapid rate than white people with diabetes.[16] In England, the rates for initiating treatment for end stage renal disease are 4.2 and 3.7 times higher for African Caribbeans and Indo Asians than they are for white people.[17] The Pima tribe of Native Americans, located in southwestern USA, have much higher rates of diabetic nephropathy than white people, and also progress to end stage renal disease at a faster rate.[18]

Please refer to clinicalevidence.com for full text and references.

Diabetic retinopathy

Search date November 2004

Simon Harding

What are the effects of treatments in people with diabetic retinopathy?

BENEFICIAL

Macular photocoagulation to macular microaneurysms in people with clinically significant macular oedema

RCTs found that, compared with no treatment, laser photocoagulation to macular microaneurysms reduced visual loss at 2–3 years in eyes with macular oedema plus mild to moderate diabetic retinopathy. There was some evidence of greater benefit in eyes with better vision. Subgroup analysis found that the benefits increased further in eyes with clinically significant macular oedema, particularly in people in whom the centre of the macula was involved or imminently threatened. We found no evidence that one type of laser was better than another.

Peripheral retinal laser photocoagulation in people with preproliferative (*moderate/severe non-proliferative*) retinopathy and maculopathy

RCTs in eyes with preproliferative retinopathy and maculopathy found that peripheral retinal photocoagulation reduced the risk of severe visual loss at 5 years compared with no treatment. We found no evidence that one type of laser was better than another.

Peripheral retinal laser photocoagulation in people with proliferative retinopathy

RCTs in eyes with proliferative retinopathy found that peripheral retinal photocoagulation reduced the risk of severe visual loss at 2–3 years compared with no treatment. One RCT in eyes with high risk proliferative diabetic retinopathy found that low intensity argon laser reduced vitreous haemorrhage and macular oedema compared with standard intensity argon laser. It found no significant difference between treatments in visual acuity, although it may have lacked power to detect clinically important effects. We found no evidence that one type of laser was better than another.

LIKELY TO BE BENEFICIAL

Grid photocoagulation to zones of retinal thickening in people with maculopathy

One RCT found that grid photocoagulation to zones of retinal thickening improved visual acuity in eyes with diffuse maculopathy with or without clinically important macular oedema at 12 months and at 24 months compared with no treatment. Photocoagulation reduced the risk of moderate visual loss by 50–70% compared with no treatment. We found no evidence that one type of laser was better than another.

UNKNOWN EFFECTIVENESS

Peripheral retinal laser photocoagulation in people with background or preproliferative (*non-proliferative) retinopathy without maculopathy**

We found no systematic review or RCTs of peripheral retinal photocoagulation in people with background or preproliferative retinopathy without maculopathy. ►

Photocoagulation to macular microaneurysms in people with maculopathy but without clinically significant macular oedema

We found no systematic review or RCTs of laser photocoagulation to macular microaneurysms in people with maculopathy without clinically significant macular oedema.

What are the effects of treatments for vitreous haemorrhage?

LIKELY TO BE BENEFICIAL

Vitrectomy in people with severe vitreous haemorrhage and proliferative retinopathy (if performed early)

One RCT found that early vitrectomy reduced visual loss at 1, 2, and 3 years in eyes with severe vitreous haemorrhage and proliferative retinopathy compared with deferred (for 1 year) vitrectomy.

UNKNOWN EFFECTIVENESS

Vitrectomy in people with maculopathy

We found no systematic review or RCTs of vitrectomy in people with both vitreous haemorrhage and maculopathy.

DEFINITION Diabetic retinopathy is characterised by varying degrees of microaneurysms, haemorrhages, exudates (*hard exudates**), venous changes, new vessel formation, and retinal thickening. It can involve the peripheral retina, the macula, or both. The range of severity of retinopathy includes background (*mild non-proliferative*), preproliferative (*moderate/severe non-proliferative*), proliferative and advanced retinopathy. Involvement of the macula can be focal, diffuse, ischaemic, or mixed.

INCIDENCE/ PREVALENCE Diabetic eye disease is the most common cause of blindness in the UK, responsible for 12% of registrable blindness in people aged 16–64 years.[1]

AETIOLOGY/ RISK FACTORS Risk factors include age, duration and control of diabetes, raised blood pressure, and raised serum lipids.[2]

PROGNOSIS Natural history studies from the 1960s found that at least half of people with proliferative diabetic retinopathy progressed to Snellen visual acuity of less than 6/60 (*20/200*) within 3–5 years.[3-5] After 4 years' follow up, the rate of progression to less than 6/60 (*20/200*) visual acuity in the better eye was 1.5% in people with type 1 diabetes, 2.7% in people with non-insulin requiring type 2 diabetes, and 3.2% in people with insulin requiring type 2 diabetes.[6]

Please refer to clinicalevidence.com for full text and references.

Dyslipidaemia in diabetes

Search date April 2005

Jigisha Patel

What are the effects of interventions in people with diabetes and lower risk for macrovascular complications?

UNKNOWN EFFECTIVENESS

Lifestyle management

We found no systematic review or RCTs in people with diabetes and lower risk for macrovascular complications comparing structured lifestyle management programmes with either advice to make lifestyle changes or usual care for clinical outcomes of interest. Structured lifestyle management programmes would entail making specific lifestyle changes such as dietary changes including the use of food products containing plant stanols, increased exercise, smoking cessation and reduced alcohol intake.

Statins

We found no systematic review or RCTs in people with diabetes and lower risk for macrovascular complications comparing statins versus either placebo or lifestyle management, or comparison between different statins, or different doses of statins for clinical outcomes of interest. Some studies were excluded because the authors did not report sufficient data to calculate risk.

What are the effects of interventions in people with diabetes and higher risk for macrovascular complications?

BENEFICIAL

Statins (for cardiovascular mortality and morbidity)

One meta-analysis of diabetic specific data from several large lipid lowering trials, and subsequent separate subgroup analysis for people with diabetes from two of these large RCTs and one RCT of people with diabetes alone found that, compared with placebo, statins (pravastatin, simvastatin, atorvastatin, lovastatin, and fluvastatin) improve cardiovascular outcomes in people with diabetes. This beneficial effect is seen in people without a past history of cardiovascular disease and without raised low density lipoprotein cholesterol or total cholesterol. Myalgia and significant changes in liver enzymes or creatine kinase were found to be rare.

Statins (for improving lipids profile)

RCTs found that, compared with placebo, statins improve total cholesterol and low density lipoprotein cholesterol and high density lipoprotein cholesterol and also improve triglycerides at higher doses.

LIKELY TO BE BENEFICIAL

Combined treatments (for lipid modification)

One RCT compared statin alone with statin plus ezetimibe. The addition of ezetimibe reduced low density lipoprotein cholesterol further and this combination may be of benefit in achieving lower low density lipoprotein cholesterol levels in people with diabetes already on statins. One RCT compared a statin alone with a statin plus fibrate. The combination was effective at improving all ▶

four lipid parameters compared with statin alone and may be an option for treating mixed dyslipidaemia in diabetes. Both combinations were well tolerated with few adverse effects.

Fibrates (for cardiovascular morbidity)

RCTs found that, compared with placebo, fibrates may have a beneficial effect on cardiovascular mortality and morbidity. There are few data on adverse effects.

Fibrates (for improving triglycerides)

RCTs found that, compared with placebo, fibrates improve triglyceride levels.

Intensive multiple intervention treatment programmes (for lipid modification)

One RCT found that, compared with usual care, intensive intervention by a nurse led hyperlipidaemia clinic improved achievement of target total cholesterol level of less than 5.0 mmol/L (< 193 mg/dL) in a mixed group of people with type 1 and type 2 diabetes and higher risk for macrovascular complications. However, given that the nature of the intervention precluded any blinding, and the ethical restrictions to including a placebo arm, it is difficult to determine which aspect of the intervention (i.e. increased frequency of visits to a health professional or changes in medication) was beneficial.

TRADE OFF BETWEEN BENEFITS AND HARMS

Fish oil (for lipid modification)

One systematic review found that, compared with controls, fish oil reduced plasma triglyceride concentration. This effect was most marked in hypertriglyceridaemic people. However, in these people, the use of fish oil was associated with an increase in low density lipoprotein cholesterol. Although fish oil may be beneficial in people with normotriglyceridaemia, its use may be limited in hypertriglyceridaemic individuals. No serious adverse effects were reported.

Nicotinic acid (for lipid modification)

One RCT found that, compared with placebo, nicotinic acid had a beneficial effect on the surrogate outcome of lipid modification. However, a significant proportion of people in this study were also taking a statin. Although serious adverse effects were rare, the relatively high incidence of flushing, especially among female patients, may limit its use.

UNKNOWN EFFECTIVENESS

Anion exchange resins

We found no systematic review or RCTs in people with diabetes and higher risk for macrovascular complications comparing anion exchange resins (colestyramine, colestipol) versus placebo or comparisons of different anion exchange resins, or different doses for clinical outcomes of interest.

Ezetimibe

We found no systematic review or RCTs in people with diabetes and higher risk for macrovascular complications comparing ezetimibe versus placebo, or comparisons of different doses for clinical outcomes of interest.

DEFINITION The term dyslipidaemia is used to describe a group of conditions in which there are abnormal levels of lipids and lipoproteins in the blood. Abnormalities of lipid metabolism are present in both type 1 and type 2 diabetes. The nature of these abnormalities is complex, but the core components of diabetic dyslipidaemia are elevated circulating levels of triglycerides (TG) and

Dyslipidaemia in diabetes

decreased circulating levels of high density lipoprotein cholesterol (HDL-C). In addition the number of small dense lipoprotein particles is raised. As a consequence, although the cholesterol content of these particles may be low, low density lipoprotein cholesterol (LDL-C) is raised. Total cholesterol and LDL-C may be normal if glycaemic control is adequate.[1,2] Triglycerides and cholesterol are the main lipids of interest. The main classes of lipoprotein considered in this chapter are low density lipoproteins (LDL) and high density lipoproteins (HDL). **Diagnosis:** A diagnosis of diabetic dyslipidaemia requiring drug treatment is determined by the person's lipid profile and level of cardiovascular risk. The classification of cardiovascular risk and lipid targets for drug treatment differ between the UK[3] and USA,[4] and the rest of Europe.[5] While it is accepted that people with diabetes are at high risk of cardiovascular disease,[6,7] in the UK and USA this high risk group is stratified further in an attempt to target those people most likely to benefit from therapeutic intervention. However, the European guidelines on cardiovascular disease prevention classify all people with type 2 diabetes, and type 1 diabetes and microalbuminuria as high risk. Treatment targets for the UK and USA and the rest of Europe are shown in Table 1 Ⓣ. These targets apply to people with type 2 diabetes. Both in the UK[8] and USA[9] it is acknowledged that there is a case for offering drug treatment at lower lipid levels in people who are at high cardiovascular risk. In the USA, an "optional" goal for LDL-C of 1.81 mmol/L (70 mg/dL) is considered in people with high cardiovascular risk.[9] Although these targets apply to type 2 diabetes, in clinical practice, they are often extrapolated to people with type 1 diabetes. **Population:** For the purposes of this chapter we have included studies of adults with type 1 and type 2 diabetes including those with concurrent hypertension and have used UK (NICE) guidelines to determine level of risk. The UKPDS (United Kingdom Prospective Diabetes Study) tool, which includes data from people with diabetes, was used to calculate level of cardiovascular risk only.[10] Subpopulations are described in detail in the description of individual studies where appropriate. Studies of adults with diabetes and microalbuminuria or nephropathy (see Diabetic nephropathy) and children are excluded.

INCIDENCE/ PREVALENCE **Type 1 diabetes mellitus:** In well controlled type 1 diabetes dyslipidaemia is not considered to be more common compared with the general population.[6] However, there are no detailed data on the incidence and prevalence of dyslipidaemia in type 1 diabetes mellitus. **Type 2 diabetes mellitus:** Dyslipidaemia is common in people with type 2 diabetes. A survey of 498 adults with type 2 diabetes[11] (representing a projected population size of 13 369 754 in the general US population of adults) estimated that over 70% of people have an LDL-C greater than the US treatment goal of less than 2.6 mmol/L (< 100 mg/dL; some have estimated this figure to be greater than 80%[12]). Over half of men and two thirds of women have an HDL-C level below US recommended goals while over half have elevated triglyceride levels. Only 28.2% of people with diabetes were on lipid modifying drugs and only 3% were controlled to US targets for all lipids.[11]

AETIOLOGY/ RISK FACTORS In diabetes mellitus, insulin insufficiency or insulin resistance can have an effect on lipid metabolism.[7] **Type 1 diabetes mellitus:** Little is understood about the cause of dyslipidaemia in type 1 diabetes. In poorly controlled type 1 diabetes and in those with nephropathy the typical cluster of abnormalities seen in diabetic dyslipidaemia does occur and is associated with a much greater cardiovascular risk than in people without diabetes.[6] **Type 2 diabetes mellitus:** Impaired insulin action may not be the only cause of dyslipidaemia. Central /visceral obesity may increase the amount of free fatty acids released into the portal circulation increasing hepatic triglyceride production, while high fat meals, typical of a Western diet, may exacerbate postprandial hypertriglyceridaemia.[7] Impaired insulin action in type 2 diabetes is thought to result in the loss of suppression of lipolysis (the breakdown of triglycerides into free fatty acids and glycerol) in adipose tissue. This leads to an increased release of free fatty acids into the portal circulation and consequently, increased delivery of free fatty acids to the liver. The effect of this process is increased production of triglycerides by the liver and a decreased production of HDL-C. In addition there is impaired clearance of triglycerides from the circulation. This resulting hypertriglyceridaemia alters the activity of other enzymes, which leads to the formation of small dense LDL particles and increased catabolism of HDL.

PROGNOSIS Cardiovascular disease is 2–6 times more frequent in people with diabetes compared with those without diabetes and progresses more rapidly when it occurs. Overall it is the most common cause of death in people with diabetes with at least 50% of deaths in type 2 diabetes caused by coronary heart disease (CHD).[7] Dyslipidaemia is one of the major contributors to this increased cardiovascular risk. Lipid abnormalities are important predictors of CHD in type 2 diabetes. High LDL-C, high triglycerides, and low HDL-C have all been reported as predictors for cardiovascular risk. A 1.57 fold increase in CHD risk has been reported to be associated with a 1 mmol/L increase in LDL-C and a 15% decrease in risk with a 0.1 mmol/L increase in HDL-C concentration.[7]

Please refer to clinicalevidence.com for full text and references.

Foot ulcers and amputations in diabetes

Search date September 2005

Dereck Hunt

What are the effects of preventive interventions in people with diabetes?

LIKELY TO BE BENEFICIAL

Screening and referral to foot care clinics

One RCT identified by a systematic review found that a diabetes screening and protection programme (involving referral to a foot clinic if high risk features were present) reduced the risk of major amputation compared with usual care after 2 years.

UNKNOWN EFFECTIVENESS

Education

One systematic review provided insufficient evidence to assess the effects of patient education for preventing foot ulcers, serious foot lesions, or amputation.

Therapeutic footwear

One RCT identified by a systematic review in people with previous diabetic foot ulcer but without severe foot deformity found no significant difference in rates of foot ulceration between therapeutic footwear and usual footwear.

What are the effects of treatments in people with diabetes with foot ulceration?

BENEFICIAL

Pressure off-loading with non-removable cast

Four RCTs found that pressure off-loading with total contact casting or non-removable fibreglass casts improved healing of non-infected diabetic foot ulcers compared with traditional dressing changes, removable cast walkers or half shoes, or specialised cloth shoes. One RCT in people with non-infected diabetic foot ulcers found no significant difference in ulcer healing between a standard total contact cast and a removable cast walker rendered non-removable at 12 weeks

LIKELY TO BE BENEFICIAL

Human skin equivalent

One RCT in people with chronic neuropathic non-infected foot ulcers found that human skin equivalent increased ulcer healing rates compared with saline moistened gauze.

Systemic hyperbaric oxygen (for infected ulcers)

One RCT identified by a systematic review found that systemic hyperbaric oxygen plus usual care reduced amputation rates at 10 weeks compared with usual care alone in people with severely infected diabetic foot ulcers. One small RCT found no significant difference between systemic hyperbaric oxygen plus usual care and usual care alone in major amputation rates, but may have been too small to detect a clinically important difference.

◀ **Topical growth factors**

Four RCTs identified by a systematic review and one subsequent RCT found that topical growth factors increased healing rates compared with placebo and control in people with non-infected diabetic foot ulcers. Another subsequent RCT in people with non-infected foot ulcers found no significant difference in healing rates between beclapermin plus dressing and dressing alone after 20 weeks.

UNKNOWN EFFECTIVENESS

Human cultured dermis

One systematic review provided insufficient evidence on the effects of human cultured dermis on ulcer healing in people with non-infected diabetic foot ulcers.

Pressure off-loading with felted foam or pressure relief half shoe

One RCT found no significant difference in time to ulcer healing between a pressure off-loading felted foam dressing and a pressure relief half shoe.

Systemic hyperbaric oxygen (for non-infected non-ischaemic ulcers)

One small RCT found no significant difference between hyperbaric oxygen plus usual care and usual care alone in ulcer healing at 4 weeks in people with non-infected, neuropathic, non-ischaemic ulcers, but may have been too small to detect a clinically important difference.

DEFINITION Diabetic foot ulceration is full thickness penetration of the dermis of the foot in a person with diabetes. Ulcer severity is often classified using the Wagner system.[1] **Grade 1** ulcers are superficial ulcers involving the full skin thickness but no underlying tissues. **Grade 2** ulcers are deeper, penetrating down to ligaments and muscle, but not involving bone or abscess formation. **Grade 3** ulcers are deep ulcers with cellulitis or abscess formation, often complicated with osteomyelitis. Ulcers with localised gangrene are classified as **Grade 4**, and those with extensive gangrene involving the entire foot are classified as **Grade 5**.

INCIDENCE/ PREVALENCE Studies conducted in Australia, Finland, the UK, and the USA, have reported the annual incidence of foot ulcers among people with diabetes as 2.5–10.7%, and the annual incidence of amputation for any reason as 0.25–1.80%.[2-11]

AETIOLOGY/ RISK FACTORS Long term risk factors for foot ulcers and amputation include duration of diabetes, poor glycaemic control, microvascular complications (retinopathy, nephropathy, and neuropathy), peripheral vascular disease, foot deformities, and previous foot ulceration or amputation. Strong predictors of foot ulceration are altered foot sensation, foot deformities, and previous foot ulcer or amputation (altered sensation: RR 2.2, 95% CI 1.5 to 3.1; foot deformity: RR 3.5, 95% CI 1.2 to 9.9); previous foot ulcer: RR 1.6, 95% CI 1.2 to 2.3; previous amputation: RR 2.8, 95% CI 1.8 to 4.3).[1-11]

PROGNOSIS In people with diabetes, foot ulcers frequently co-exist with vascular insufficiency and may be complicated by infection. Amputation is indicated if disease is severe or does not improve with conservative treatment. As well as affecting quality of life, these complications of diabetes account for a large proportion of the health care costs of dealing with diabetes. For people with healed diabetic foot ulcers, the 5 year cumulative rate of ulcer recurrence is 66% and of amputation is 12%.[12]

Please refer to clinicalevidence.com for full text and references.

Glycaemic control in type 1 diabetes

Search date December 2005

Amaryllis Campbell

What are the effects of interventions in adolescents with type 1 diabetes?

LIKELY TO BE BENEFICIAL

Educational interventions (compared with controls)

We found no systematic review or RCTs evaluating a specific type of education or using HbA1c as the only method for measuring glycated haemoglobin. One systematic review found that, compared with controls, different educational and psychosocial interventions in adolescents with type 1 diabetes produced a small improvement in quality of life and glycated haemoglobin (measured using a variety of methods). However, most of the RCTs in the review were small, most of the interventions lacked any theoretical basis, and many of the outcome measures were not validated or standardised. We found no systematic review or RCTs evaluating the effects of education in adolescents with type 1 diabetes on the incidence of hypoglycaemia, diabetic ketoacidosis, neuropsychological impairment, weight gain, or fluid retention.

UNKNOWN EFFECTIVENESS

Different frequencies of insulin administration

We found no systematic review or RCTs specifically evaluating the effects of frequency of insulin administration in adolescents with type 1 diabetes for the outcomes of rate of rise of glycated haemoglobin (measured as HbA1c), quality of life, incidence of and mortality from hypoglycaemia or diabetic ketoacidosis, weight gain, fluid retention, neuropsychological impairment, or all cause mortality.

Different frequencies of self blood glucose monitoring

We found no systematic review or RCTs specifically evaluating the effects of frequency of self blood glucose monitoring in adolescents with type 1 diabetes for the outcomes of rate of rise of glycated haemoglobin (measured as HbA1c), quality of life, incidence of and mortality from hypoglycaemia or diabetic ketoacidosis, weight gain, fluid retention, neuropsychological impairment, or all cause mortality.

Intensive treatment programmes (compared with conventional treatment programmes)

We found no systematic review or RCTs specifically in adolescents comparing intensive treatment programmes with conventional treatment programmes for the outcomes of rate of rise of glycated haemoglobin (measured as HbA1c), quality of life, incidence of and mortality from hypoglycaemia or diabetic ketoacidosis, weight gain, fluid retention, neuropsychological impairment, or all cause mortality.

What are the effects of interventions in adults with type 1 diabetes?

TRADE OFF BETWEEN BENEFITS AND HARMS

Continuous subcutaneous insulin infusion (compared with multiple daily subcutaneous insulin injections)

One RCT found that continuous subcutaneous infusion of insulin improved glycated haemoglobin levels and quality of life compared with multiple daily subcutaneous injections at 16 weeks, but one smaller RCT found no significant difference between groups in either outcome at 9 months. The two RCTs found inconclusive evidence on mild and severe hypoglycaemia. The potential disadvantages of continuous subcutaneous insulin infusion include the risk of diabetic ketoacidosis owing to disconnection or malfunction of the pump and infection.

Intensive treatment programmes (compared with conventional treatment programmes)

One RCT identified by a systematic review, one additional RCT, and one subsequent RCT found that, compared with conventional treatment programmes, intensive treatment programmes reduced glycated haemoglobin levels at follow up varying from 1 to 10 years. The additional RCT found no significant difference between intensive and conventional treatment programmes in diabetes related quality of life but found an increase in the incidence of severe hypoglycaemia with intensive treatment programmes. The subsequent RCT found that, compared with conventional treatment, intensive treatment improved diabetes dependent quality of life but found no significant difference in the perceived frequency of hypoglycaemia. A second systematic review found that, compared with conventional treatment, intensive treatment increased hypoglycaemia, diabetic ketoacidosis (when the treatment programme involved the use of insulin pumps), and mortality associated with acute complications of intensive treatment, but found no significant difference in all cause mortality.

UNKNOWN EFFECTIVENESS

Different frequencies of self blood glucose monitoring

We found no systematic review or RCTs specifically evaluating the effects of frequency of self blood glucose monitoring in adults with type 1 diabetes for the outcomes of rate of rise of glycated haemoglobin (measured as HbA1c), quality of life, incidence of and mortality from hypoglycaemia or diabetic ketoacidosis, weight gain, fluid retention, neuropsychological impairment, or all cause mortality.

Educational interventions (compared with controls)

One small RCT identified by a systematic review found no significant difference in glycated haemoglobin (measured as HbA1c) levels at 18 months between education in self monitoring of blood glucose, self management education, or usual care, but was incompletely reported and may have lacked power to detect clinically important differences. We found no systematic review or RCTs specifically comparing the effects of group versus individual educational interventions or secondary care versus primary care educational interventions in adults with type 1 diabetes for the outcomes of interest. Given the nature of type 1 diabetes and the central importance of self management of the condition, all individuals with type 1 diabetes will have received some education at diagnosis; most

Glycaemic control in type 1 diabetes

studies of the effects of education will therefore be examining the impact of subsequent educational interventions. It may be difficult to separate out the effects of individual components of what typically will be a complex package of care, including elements of education, self management training, psychological support, and optimisation of insulin regimens.

DEFINITION The term diabetes mellitus encompasses a group of disorders characterised by chronic hyperglycaemia with disturbances of carbohydrate, fat, and protein metabolism resulting from defects of insulin secretion, insulin action, or both. The World Health Organization definition recognises diabetes as a progressive disorder of glucose metabolism in which individuals may move between normoglycaemia, impaired glucose tolerance or impaired fasting glycaemia, and frank hyperglycaemia. Type 1 diabetes occurs when the pancreas produces too little insulin or no insulin at all, because of destruction of the pancreatic islet beta cells, usually attributable to an autoimmune process. Markers of autoimmune destruction (autoantibodies to islet cells, autoantibodies to insulin, or autoantibodies to both islet cells and insulin, and to glutamic acid decarboxylase) can be found in 85–90% of individuals with type 1 diabetes when fasting diabetic hyperglycaemia is first detected.[1] The definition of type 1 diabetes also includes individuals with beta cell destruction who are prone to ketoacidosis but for which no specific cause can be found. However, it excludes those forms of beta cell destruction for which a specific cause can be found (e.g. cystic fibrosis, pancreatitis, cancer of the pancreas).[2] Type 2 diabetes results from defects in both insulin secretion and insulin action. The risk of type 2 diabetes increases with age and lack of physical activity, and occurs more frequently in individuals with obesity, hypertension, and dyslipidaemia (the metabolic syndrome). It occurs more frequently in women with previous gestational diabetes. There is also evidence of a familial predisposition. Type 2 diabetes is not covered in this chapter. **Diagnosis:** In the presence of symptoms (such as thirst, passing increased volumes of urine, blurring of vision, and weight loss), diabetes may be diagnosed on the basis of a single random elevated plasma glucose (≥ 11.1 mmol/L). In the absence of symptoms, the diagnosis should be based on at least one additional blood glucose result in the diabetic range, either from a random or fasting (plasma blood glucose ≥ 7.0 mmol/L) sample, or from the oral glucose tolerance test (plasma blood glucose (≥ 11.1 mmol/L 2 hours after a 75 g glucose load).[2] **Population:** For the purpose of this chapter, we have included adolescents and adults with type 1 diabetes, but excluded pregnant women and people who are acutely unwell, for example after surgery or myocardial infarction.

INCIDENCE/ PREVALENCE It is estimated that slightly more than 218 000 people develop type 1 diabetes worldwide annually, of whom about 40% are children. The incidence varies considerably between populations, with 60 000 new cases occurring annually in Europe, 45 000 new cases in South East Asia, 36 000 new cases in North America, and the lowest number of new cases, 6900 annually, in Africa.[3] There seems to be a worldwide increase in the incidence of type 1 diabetes in both high and low incidence populations.[4] The prevalence of type 1 diabetes is currently estimated at 5.3 million people worldwide, and also varies between populations, reflecting both the variation in incidence rates and differing population structures and mortality.[3]

AETIOLOGY/ RISK FACTORS Two main aetiological forms of type 1 diabetes are recognised. Autoimmune diabetes mellitus results from autoimmune mediated destruction of the beta cells of the pancreas. The rate of destruction varies, but all individuals with this form of diabetes eventually become dependent on insulin for survival. Peak incidence of autoimmune diabetes is during childhood and adolescence but it may occur at any age. There is a genetic predisposition and people with this type of diabetes may have other autoimmune disorders.[5] Certain viruses have also been associated with beta cell destruction, including rubella, Coxsackie B, and cytomegalovirus. Other environmental factors are probably also contributory, but these are poorly defined and understood. Idiopathic diabetes (in which the cause is unidentified) is more common in individuals of African and Asian origin.[2]

PROGNOSIS Untreated, most people with type 1 diabetes, particularly those with autoimmune diabetes mellitus, will experience increasing blood glucose levels, progressing to ketoacidosis or non-ketotic hyperosmolar states resulting in coma and death. The course of idiopathic diabetes may be more varied, with some people experiencing permanent lack of insulin and a tendency to ketoacidosis, although in others the requirement for insulin treatment may fluctuate.[2] However, most people with type 1 diabetes require insulin for survival, and are described as insulin dependent. The long term effects of diabetes include retinopathy, nephropathy, and neuropathy. Individuals with diabetes mellitus are also at increased risk of cardiovascular, cerebrovascular, and peripheral vascular disease. Good glycaemic control can reduce the risk of developing diabetic complications.[6]

Please refer to clinicalevidence.com for full text and references.

Glycaemic control in type 2 diabetes

Search date June 2005

Amaryllis Campbell

What are the effects of interventions in adults with type 2 diabetes?

BENEFICIAL

Metformin (compared with diet alone or placebo)

One systematic review found that, compared with diet alone or placebo, metformin reduced glycated haemoglobin. It found no significant difference in mean weight between groups. One RCT found a lower median HbA1c over 10 years, a lower risk of all cause mortality, and a higher rate of hypoglycaemia in people taking metformin compared with diet alone. Two RCTs found that, compared with placebo, metformin reduced HbA1c and found no significant difference in body weight between groups. Systematic reviews and one large RCT have found that lactic acidosis, an often cited adverse effect of metformin treatment, is a rare occurrence provided that recognised contraindications to metformin treatment are observed. Quality of life was not assessed.

Sulphonylureas (reduce HbA1c compared with placebo or diet alone; newer sulphonylureas reduce hypoglycaemia compared with older sulphonylureas)

One RCT found that, compared with diet alone, older sulphonylureas (chlorpropamide, glibenclamide) reduced HbA1c over 10 years but also found a higher rate of hypoglycaemia and weight gain in people taking sulphonylureas compared with diet alone. One RCT found that glibenclamide reduced HbA1c compared with placebo after 15 months. Four RCTs found that, compared with placebo, newer sulphonylureas (glimepiride, glipizide) improved HbA1c levels over 12–14 weeks. These RCTs found that newer sulphonylureas did not increase the incidence of hypoglycaemia but one RCT found an increase in weight over 14 weeks with glimepiride. Two RCTs found no significant difference in HbA1c levels between glimepiride and glibenclamide and found a lower incidence of hypoglycaemia with glimepiride. One RCT found no significant difference in HbA1c at 27 weeks between modified release gliclazide and glimepiride, but found that gliclazide reduced the proportion of people with confirmed hypoglycaemia.

LIKELY TO BE BENEFICIAL

Education (compared with usual care)

We found limited evidence that intensive educational programmes reduced HbA1c in the short term (< 24 months) compared with usual care. We found no good quality studies on educational interventions that reported on quality of life using validated outcome measures. Group education seems to be more effective than standard care and as effective as individual educational programmes. Otherwise there is insufficient evidence to identify specific educational programmes or approaches as effective. No harmful effects of intensive education have been identified.

Intensive treatment programmes (compared with usual care)

One large RCT (Japan Diabetes Complications Study) found a statistically significant but clinically unimportant difference in reduction from baseline HbA1c of 0.05% at 3 years with an intensive treatment programme compared with usual care. The smaller reduction in HbA1c seen with an intensive treatment programme in this large RCT compared with other large trials may have been the result of the longer duration of diabetes in the participants in this study and their good control at baseline (mean HbA1c 7.74 ± 1.35%). A second RCT found that, compared with usual care, a patient participation programme reduced HbA1c over 4 years. Participants in this RCT were highly educated and the level of education and motivation in this population may not be representative of the diabetic population as a whole.

Meglitinides (nateglinide, repaglinide)

RCTs found that nateglinide reduced HbA1c levels compared with placebo over 12–24 weeks with an increase in symptomatic and confirmed hypoglycaemia but without affecting body weight. Two RCTs found similar HbA1c levels and incidences of hypoglycaemic episodes with repaglinide and glibenclamide at up to 12 months. One RCT found comparable HbA1c levels and body weight at 12 months with repaglinide and glimepiride.

TRADE OFF BETWEEN BENEFITS AND HARMS

Combined oral drug treatment (compared with monotherapy)

RCTs have found that combinations of sulphonylureas (chlorpropamide, glibenclamide, or glimepiride) plus metformin, or meglitinides (nateglinide, repaglinide) plus metformin, reduced HbA1c compared with monotherapy but with an increase in symptomatic hypoglycaemia. One RCT found an increased risk of death from all causes for combination treatment with sulphonylurea (chlorpropamide or glibenclamide) plus metformin, but the reason for this is unclear.

Insulin (compared with continuation of oral drug treatment where HbA1c is inadequately controlled)

Four RCTs found that, compared with continuation of oral hypoglycaemic agents (sulphonylureas with or without metformin), insulin reduced HbA1c levels over 12 – 52 weeks. Three of these RCTs found an increase in frequency of hypoglycaemic symptoms or weight gain with insulin compared with continuing oral hypoglycaemic agents. One smaller RCT found no significant difference in the number of hypoglycaemic symptoms. Two RCTs found no significant difference between treatments for quality of life.

UNKNOWN EFFECTIVENESS

Different frequencies of self blood glucose monitoring

One RCT identified by a systematic review found no significant difference between blood glucose monitoring and no monitoring in HbA1c or weight gain in people with type 2 diabetes not treated with insulin. We found no systematic review or RCTs specifically evaluating the effects of different frequencies of blood glucose monitoring in people with type 2 diabetes treated with insulin for our outcomes of interest.

Insulin delivered by continuous subcutaneous infusion

One RCT found no significant difference in HbA1c levels at 24 weeks with insulin (insulin aspart) delivered by continuous subcutaneous insulin infusion compared with multiple daily injections (basal isophane insulin and bolus insulin aspart). This RCT found a similar percentage of hypoglycaemic episodes over 24 weeks in people treated with continuous subcutaneous insulin infusion compared with multiple daily insulin injections but also found a higher incidence of hyperglycaemia in people treated with multiple daily injections. The RCT did not assess quality of life outcomes.

Glycaemic control in type 2 diabetes

UNLIKELY TO BE BENEFICIAL

Insulin compared with sulphonylureas as initial treatment (no added benefit and with more hypoglycaemic episodes and more weight gain)

One RCT comparing insulin versus sulphonylureas (chlorpropamide, glibenclamide, or glipizide) or diet alone as preferred treatment in people with newly diagnosed type 2 diabetes found no significant difference in HbA1c levels between insulin and sulphonylureas. It found a reduction in HbA1c with insulin or sulphonylureas compared with diet alone and found a higher rate of major hypoglycaemic episodes and weight gain at 10 years in people taking insulin compared with diet alone or sulphonylureas. This RCT assessed quality of life outcomes using two cross-sectional studies and a longitudinal study of people enrolled in the RCT and found no significant difference in quality of life with insulin compared with diet alone or sulphonylurea.

DEFINITION The term diabetes mellitus encompasses a group of disorders characterised by chronic hyperglycaemia with disturbances of carbohydrate, fat, and protein metabolism resulting from defects of insulin secretion, insulin action, or both. Type 2 diabetes is the most common form of diabetes and defects of both insulin action and insulin secretion are usually present by the time of diagnosis. The WHO now recognises diabetes as a progressive disorder of glucose metabolism in which individuals may move between normoglycaemia (fasting plasma venous glucose < 6.1 mmol/L), impaired glucose tolerance (fasting plasma venous glucose < 7.0 mmol/L or ≥ 7.8 mmol/L 2 hours after 75 g oral glucose load), or impaired fasting glycaemia (fasting venous plasma glucose ≥ 6.1–< 7.0 mmol/L), and frank hyperglycaemia (fasting plasma venous glucose ≥ 7.0 mmol/L or ≥ 11.1 mmol/L 2 hours after 75 g oral glucose load).[1] As a consequence of the inability of the body to use glucose as an energy source, blood glucose levels rise and symptoms such as thirst, polyuria, blurring of vision, or weight loss may develop.[1] **Diagnosis:** In the presence of symptoms, diabetes may be diagnosed on the basis of a single random elevated plasma glucose (≥ 11.1 mmol/L). In the absence of symptoms the diagnosis should be based on at least one additional blood glucose result in the diabetic range, either from a random sample, or fasting (plasma blood glucose ≥ 7.0 mmol/L) or from the oral glucose tolerance test (plasma blood glucose ≥ 11.1 mmol/L 2 hours after 75 g glucose load).[1] **Population:** For the purpose of this chapter, we have excluded pregnant women and acutely unwell adults (e.g. after surgery or myocardial infarction).

INCIDENCE/ PREVALENCE The estimated prevalence of diabetes worldwide for the year 2000 was 177 million people aged 20–79 years, of whom 85–95% had type 2 diabetes,[2] an increase in prevalence from 135 million in 1995 (WHO data). Incidence and prevalence figures for children and adolescents are unreliable, but there is some evidence that type 2 diabetes is becoming more common in adolescents and young adults especially in developing countries. The overall estimated prevalence of 5.1% for type 2 diabetes conceals considerable variation in prevalence which ranges from less than 2% in some African countries to over 14% in some populations.[2]

AETIOLOGY/ RISK FACTORS By definition, the specific reasons for the development of the defects of insulin secretion and insulin action that characterise type 2 diabetes are unknown.[1] The risk of type 2 diabetes increases with age and lack of physical activity, and occurs more frequently in individuals with obesity, hypertension, and dyslipidaemia (the Metabolic Syndrome). Features of the Metabolic Syndrome can be present for up to 10 years before disorders of glycaemic control become apparent and are powerful predictors of cardiovascular disease and abnormal glucose tolerance (impaired glucose tolerance or diabetes).[3] Type 2 diabetes also occurs more frequently in women with previous gestational diabetes. There is also evidence of a familial, probably genetic, predisposition.[1]

Glycaemic control in type 2 diabetes

◀ **PROGNOSIS** People with type 2 diabetes have blood glucose levels which have been shown to rise progressively from the time of diagnosis, with or without treatment and irrespective of the type of treatment given.[4] Blood glucose levels above the normal range have been shown to be associated not only with the presence of symptoms but also with an increased risk of long term microvascular and macrovascular complications.[1]

Please refer to clinicalevidence.com for full text and references.

Hypertension in diabetes

Search date February 2004

Sandeep Vijan

What are the effects of antihypertensives to control blood pressure in people with diabetes?

BENEFICIAL

Angiotensin converting enzyme inhibitors

One RCT found that ramipril (an angiotensin convertin enzyme [ACE] inhibitor) reduced cardiovascular events and nephropathy compared with placebo. One RCT found that chlorthalidone (a diuretic) was at least as effective as lisinopril (an ACE inhibitor) at reducing cardiovascular events. One RCT found no significant difference in cardiovascular events, microvascular events, or diabetes related death between atenolol (a beta-blocker) and captopril (an ACE inhibitor), although atenolol led to greater weight gain and a greater need for glucose lowering therapy. Two RCTs found that ACE inhibitors (fosinopril and enalapril) reduced cardiovascular events compared with calcium channel blockers (amlodipine and nisoldipine). We found no RCTs comparing ACE inhibitors versus alpha-blockers, angiotensin II receptor antagonists, or combinations including ACE inhibitors.

Diuretics

One RCT found that chlorthalidone reduced cardiovascular events compared with placebo plus usual care in people with diabetes and isolated systolic hypertension. One RCT found that chlorthalidone was at least as effective as lisinopril (an ACE inhibitor) for reducing cardiovascular events. Two RCTs found no significant difference in overall cardiovascular events between diuretics (chlorthalidone or co-amilozide) and calcium channel blockers (nifedipine or amlodipine). However, one of the RCTs found that chlorthalidone reduced heart failure compared with amlodipine. One RCT found that doxazosin (an alpha-blocker) increased cardiovascular events compared with chlorthalidone (a diuretic). We found no RCTs comparing diuretics versus beta-blockers, angiotensin II receptor antagonists, or combinations including diuretics.

LIKELY TO BE BENEFICIAL

Angiotensin II receptor antagonists (reduce cardiovascular events compared with beta-blockers)

We found no RCTs comparing angiotensin II receptor antagonists versus placebo in people with diabetes and hypertension but without nephropathy. One RCT found that, in people with diabetes, hypertension, and left ventricular hypertrophy, losartan (an angiotensin II receptor antagonist) reduced cardiovascular events compared with atenolol (a beta-blocker). We found no RCTs comparing angiotensin II receptor antagonists versus alpha-blockers, ACE inhibitors, calcium channel blockers, or combinations including angiotensin II receptor antagonists.

Beta-blockers (similar reduction in cardiovascular and microvascular events to ACE inhibitors)

We found no RCTs comparing beta-blockers versus placebo. One RCT found no significant difference in cardiovascular events, microvascular events, or diabetes related death between atenolol (a beta-blocker) and captopril (an angiotensin converting enzyme inhibitor), although atenolol led to greater weight ▶

gain and a greater need for glucose lowering therapy. One RCT found that losartan (an angiotensin II receptor antagonist) reduced cardiovascular events compared with atenolol in people with diabetes, hypertension, and left ventricular hypertrophy. We found no RCTs comparing beta-blockers versus alpha-blockers, diuretics, calcium channel blockers, or combinations including beta-blockers.

Calcium channel blockers (similar reduction in cardiovascular events to diuretics but less effective than ACE inhibitors)

Two RCTs found that angiotensin converting enzyme inhibitors (fosinopril and enalapril) reduced cardiovascular events compared with calcium channel blockers (amlodipine and nisoldipine). Two RCTs found no significant difference in overall cardiovascular events between diuretics (chlorthalidone or co-amilozide) and calcium channel blockers (nifedipine or amlodipine). However, one of the RCTs found that amlodipine was less effective at reducing heart failure than chlorthalidone. We found no RCTs comparing calcium channel blockers versus alpha-blockers, angiotensin II receptor anatagonists, or combinations including alpha-blockers.

UNKNOWN EFFECTIVENESS

Alpha-blockers

We found no RCTs comparing alpha-blockers versus placebo in people with diabetes. One RCT found that doxazosin (an alpha-blocker) was less effective than chlorthalidone (a diuretic) for preventing cardiovascular events. We found no RCTs comparing alpha-blockers versus beta-blockers, angiotensin converting enzyme inhibitors, calcium channel blockers, angiotensin II receptor antagonists, or combinations including alpha-blockers.

What are the effects of different blood pressure targets in people with diabetes?

BENEFICIAL

Lower blood pressure targets

Three RCTs found that more intensive (lower) blood pressure targets reduced cardiovascular events or overall mortality compared with non-intensive blood pressure targets. We found no RCTs examining targets lower than 150 mm Hg systolic and 75 mm Hg diastolic.

DEFINITION Hypertension in diabetes is classically defined as a systolic blood pressure of 140 mm Hg or greater or a diastolic blood pressure of 90 mm Hg or greater.[1] Hypertension is broken into three stages. **Pre-hypertension** is a systolic blood pressure between 120–139 mm Hg or a diastolic blood pressure between 80–89 mm Hg. **Stage 1 hypertension** is a systolic blood pressure of 140–159 mm Hg or diastolic blood pressure of 90–99 mm Hg. **Stage 2 hypertension** is a systolic blood pressure of 160 mm Hg or greater or a diastolic blood pressure of 100 mm Hg or greater.[1] However, guidelines now suggest that pharmacologic therapy should be instituted in any person with diabetes and hypertension, regardless of stage. This chapter focuses on adults with diabetes with stage 1 or 2 hypertension but no diagnosis of coronary heart disease or diabetic retinopathy. Most studies on the topic do

Hypertension in diabetes

not differentiate between type 1 and type 2 diabetes, but the underlying epidemiology and ages of the populations studied suggest that more than 95% of study participants are likely to have type 2 diabetes. The control of hypertension in people with diabetic retinopathy (see p 000) and those with diabetic nephropathy (p 000) is described in separate chapters.

INCIDENCE/ PREVALENCE Hypertension is highly prevalent among people with diabetes. It is about 1.5–3 times more common in people with type 2 diabetes than in the age matched general population.[2] Using a diagnostic threshold of 140/90 mm Hg, about 40% of people with diabetes have hypertension at age 45 years and more than 60% have hypertension by age 75 years. About 30% of people with type 1 diabetes eventually develop hypertension, usually after they develop diabetic nephropathy.[2] The prevalence of hypertension varies depending on the population studied (see aetiology/risk factors below).

AETIOLOGY/ RISK FACTORS The aetiology of hypertension is multifactorial, complex, and not fully understood. In the general population, there are several major risk factors for hypertension; specific risk factors are not clearly different in the diabetic population. Age is the predominant factor; recent data suggest that prevalence increases with age, and the cumulative lifetime risk of hypertension in the general population is nearly 90%.[3,4] People with at least one parent with hypertension are about twice as likely to develop hypertension.[5] African-Americans have a 7–10% increase in prevalence compared with non-Hispanic American whites.[4] Those who are obese also have greater risk; for each unit increase in body mass index, the prevalence increases by about 1–1.5%.[4] Insulin resistance is associated with development of hypertension.[6-8]

PROGNOSIS Untreated hypertension in people with diabetes is associated with high rates of cardiovascular disease (such as myocardial infarction, heart failure, and stroke) and microvascular disease (such as renal disease [including albuminuria, renal insufficiency, and end-stage renal disease] and diabetic retinopathy).[9-12] In the placebo groups of major trials of hypertension control in type 2 diabetes, major cardiac events occurred in about 4–6% of people annually, and were substantially higher in populations with additional risk factors such as diabetic nephropathy.[9-12]

Please refer to clinicalevidence.com for full text and references.

Prevention of cardiovascular events in diabetes

Search date November 2004

Ronald Sigal, Janine Malcolm, and Amel Arnaout

What are the effects of promoting smoking cessation in people with diabetes?

LIKELY TO BE BENEFICIAL

Smoking cessation*

We found no RCTs on promoting smoking cessation specifically in people with diabetes. Observational evidence and extrapolation from people without diabetes suggest that promotion of smoking cessation is likely to reduce cardiovascular events.

*No RCT but observational evidence suggests some benefit.

What are the effects of controlling blood pressure in people with diabetes?

BENEFICIAL

Antihypertensive treatment (compared with no antihypertensive treatment)

Systematic reviews and subsequent RCTs found that, in adults with diabetes and hypertension or previous cardiovascular disease, blood pressure lowering with antihypertensive agents (angiotensin converting enzyme inhibitors, angiotensin receptor blockers, beta-blockers, calcium channel blockers, or diuretics) reduced cardiovascular morbidity and mortality compared with no antihypertensive treatment. One systematic review found that beta-blockers reduced mortality in people with diabetes and congestive heart failure, but to a lesser extent than in non-diabetic people with congestive heart failure.

Lower target blood pressures

Large RCTs, primarily including people with hypertension, found that tighter control of blood pressure to a target diastolic blood pressure of 80 mm Hg or lower reduces the risk of major cardiovascular events. One RCT in normotensive people with diabetes found that intensive blood pressure lowering reduced cerebral vascular accidents but found no significant difference in cardiovascular death, myocardial infarction, congestive heart failure, or all cause mortality.

TRADE OFF BETWEEN BENEFITS AND HARMS

Different antihypertensive drugs

Systematic reviews and RCTs found that angiotensin converting enzyme inhibitors, angiotensin II receptor antagonists, beta-blockers, and calcium channel blockers were all effective in reducing cardiovascular morbidity and mortality in older people with diabetes and hypertension; most RCTs found no significant difference between different antihypertensive drugs. However, some RCTs found a lesser degree of protection against heart failure with calcium channel blockers compared with other antihypertensive agents and an increase in the risk of stroke or congestive heart failure with the angiotensin converting enzyme inhibitor lisinopril compared with the diuretic chlorthalidone. There was also an increase in the risk of cardiovascular morbidity and mortality with angiotensin II ▶

receptor antagonists compared with beta-blockers or diuretics. Different anti-hypertensive drugs were associated with different adverse effects. RCTs found that people taking atenolol gained more weight than those taking captopril, had a higher frequency of headache and constipation with diltiazem than with diuretics or beta-blockers, and had a higher rate of withdrawal from treatment because of adverse effects with atenolol than with losartan.

What are the effects of treating dyslipidaemia in people with diabetes?

BENEFICIAL

Statins

One systematic review and a subsequent RCT found that statins reduced cardiovascular events compared with placebo. The RCT found that in people without high LDL cholesterol, atorvastatin 10 mg daily reduced cardiovascular events compared with placebo at 3.9 years.

LIKELY TO BE BENEFICIAL

Aggressive versus moderate lipid lowering with statins

One RCT found that, compared with usual care, treatment with atorvastatin to achieve a target low density lipoprotein concentration below 2.6 mmol/L (< 100 mg/dL) reduced cardiovascular morbidity and mortality. Another RCT found no significant difference between a lower target low density lipoprotein (1.55–2.20 mmol/L) using lovastatin, plus cholestyramine if needed, and a moderate target low density lipoprotein (3.36–3.62 mmol/L) in 4 year event rate for myocardial infarction and death.

Fibrates

One RCT found that gemfibrozil reduced cardiovascular events over 5 years compared with placebo. Another, smaller RCT found no significant difference. One RCT found that bezafibrate reduced cardiovascular events over 3 years compared with placebo. One RCT found no significant difference between fenofibrate and placebo in the frequency of myocardial infarction or death over 39 months.

Low versus standard statin dose in older people

One RCT found no significant difference in cardiovascular events between low dose pravastatin (5 mg/day) and standard dose pravastatin (10–20 mg/day) over 4 years.

What are the effects of antiplatelet drugs in people with diabetes?

LIKELY TO BE BENEFICIAL

Adding glycoprotein IIb/IIIa inhibitors to heparin in acute coronary syndromes

We found no RCTs comparing glycoprotein IIb/IIIa inhibitors versus no antiplatelet treatment. One RCT in people presenting with unstable angina or acute myocardial infarction without ST segment elevation found that adding tirofiban (a glycoprotein IIb/IIIa inhibitor) to heparin reduced the composite outcome of death, myocardial infarction, or refractory ischaemia at 180 days compared with heparin alone. This RCT found no significant difference between tirofiban plus heparin versus heparin alone in risk of bleeding in people already taking aspirin. RCTs in people undergoing percutaneous transluminal coronary angioplasty found that the combination of glycoprotein IIb/IIIa inhibitor plus stent reduced cardiovascular morbidity and mortality compared with placebo plus stent. One RCT in people with acute ST segment elevation myocardial infarction found that a combination of abciximab plus half dose reteplase reduced recurrent myocardial infarction compared with full dose reteplase alone at 7 days. It also found that abciximab plus half dose reteplase increased bleeding.

Clopidogrel

We found no RCTs comparing clopidogrel versus placebo. One RCT in people with diabetes and with recent ischaemic stroke, myocardial infarction, or established peripheral arterial disease found no significant difference in cardiovascular events between clopidogrel and aspirin at 28 days. This RCT also found a lower proportion of people hospitalised for a bleeding event with clopidogrel than with aspirin.

TRADE OFF BETWEEN BENEFITS AND HARMS

Aspirin

One systematic review found that, compared with controls, antiplatelet treatment mainly with aspirin did not reduce the combined risk of non-fatal myocardial infarction, non-fatal stroke, death from a vascular cause, or death from an unknown cause in people with diabetes and cardiovascular disease diagnosis. The review found that antiplatelet treatment was associated with an increase in the risk of major extracranial haemorrhage and haemorrhagic stroke, but the results for people with diabetes were not reported separately. One subsequent RCT comparing aspirin with placebo found no significant reduction in the composite endpoint of death, stroke, or acute myocardial infarction. One additional RCT found that aspirin reduced the risk of acute myocardial infarction over 5 years compared with placebo. Both of these RCTs also found that aspirin increased bleeding. One RCT in people with diabetes and with recent stroke, myocardial infarction, or established arterial disease found no significant difference in cardiovascular events between aspirin and clopidogrel at 28 days. This RCT also found that that aspirin increased hospitalisation for a bleeding event. One RCT in people presenting with unstable angina or non-Q wave myocardial infarction and also taking aspirin found no significant reduction in cardiovascular events after 12 months with the addition of clopidogrel compared with placebo. This RCT also found that adding clopidogrel increased the proportion of people who had major bleeds compared with placebo.

UNLIKELY TO BE BENEFICIAL

Adding clopidogrel to heparin in acute coronary syndromes

One RCT in people presenting with unstable angina or non-Q wave myocardial infarction and also taking aspirin found no significant reduction in cardiovascular events after 12 months with the addition of clopidogrel compared with placebo. This RCT also found that adding clopidogrel increased the proportion of people who had major bleeds compared with adding placebo.

Prevention of cardiovascular events in diabetes

What are the effects of blood glucose control in prevention of cardiovascular disease in people with diabetes?

LIKELY TO BE BENEFICIAL

Intensive versus conventional glycaemic control

One systematic review found that, compared with conventional glycaemic control, intensive glycaemic control for more than 2 years reduced the occurrence of a first major cardiovascular event in people with type 1 diabetes. Two RCTs found no significant difference in cardiovascular morbidity and mortality with intensive compared with conventional glycaemic control in people with type 2 diabetes. These RCTs also found an increase in weight gain and hypoglycaemic episodes with intensive compared with conventional treatment.

Metformin versus diet alone as initial treatment in overweight or obese people with type 2 diabetes

One RCT in overweight or obese people with type 2 diabetes found that intensive treatment with metformin compared with conventional treatment with diet alone reduced the incidence of myocardial infarction and stroke over 5 years, but this did not reach significance for stroke. One RCT suggested that metformin increased the incidence of mild and moderate hypoglycaemic events compared with diet alone.

What are the effects of treating multiple risk factors in prevention of cardiovascular disease in people with diabetes?

BENEFICIAL

Intensive multiple risk factor treatment

We found no systematic review or RCTs comparing treating multiple risk factors versus treating a single risk factor for cardiovascular outcomes. One RCT found that, compared with conventional treatment according to clinical guidelines, intensive treatment of multiple risk factors with strict treatment goals in people with type 2 diabetes and microalbuminuria reduced cardiovascular disease over 8 years. Multiple risk factor treatment included simultaneously targeting diet, exercise, glycaemic control, blood pressure, treatment of microalbuminuria, and antiplatelet treatment.

What are the effects of revascularisation procedures in people with diabetes?

BENEFICIAL

Coronary artery bypass graft compared with percutaneous transluminal coronary angioplasty

One systematic review found that, in people with diabetes, CABG reduced all cause mortality at 4 years after initial revascularisation compared with PTCA, but found no significant difference at 6.5 years. One large RCT in people with diabetes and multivessel coronary artery disease found that CABG reduced mortality or myocardial infarction within 8 years compared with PTCA. Another, smaller RCT found a non-significant reduction in mortality with CABG compared with PTCA at 4 years.

Stent plus glycoprotein IIb/IIIa inhibitors in people undergoing percutaneous transluminal coronary angioplasty

RCTs in people with diabetes undergoing percutaneous transluminal coronary angioplasty found that the combination of stent and a glycoprotein IIb/IIIa inhibitor reduced cardiovascular morbidity and mortality compared with stent plus placebo.

LIKELY TO BE BENEFICIAL

Percutaneous transluminal coronary angioplasty compared with thrombolysis

One systematic review suggested that percutaneous transluminal coronary angioplasty reduced the risk of death or recurrent myocardial infarction at 30 days in diabetic people presenting with acute myocardial infarction compared with thrombolysis.

TRADE OFF BETWEEN BENEFITS AND HARMS

Coronary artery bypass graft compared with percutaneous transluminal coronary angioplasty plus stent

One RCT in people with diabetes and multivessel coronary artery disease found that CABG reduced death, myocardial infarction, and revascularisation at 1 and 3 years compared to PTCA plus stenting. However, it found an increased risk of stroke with CABG in the short term up to discharge.

DEFINITION **Diabetes mellitus:** Diabetes mellitus is a group of disorders characterised by hyperglycaemia, defined as a fasting plasma glucose ≥ 7.0 mmol/L or ≥ 11.1 mmol/L 2 hours after a 75 g oral glucose load, on two or more occasions. Intensive treatment is designed to achieve blood glucose values as close to the non-diabetic range as possible. The components of such treatment are education, counselling, monitoring, self management, and pharmacological treatment with insulin or oral anti-diabetic agents to achieve specific glycaemic goals. **Cardiovascular disease:** Atherosclerotic disease of the heart and/or the coronary, cerebral, or peripheral vessels leading to clinical events such as acute myocardial infarction, congestive heart failure, sudden cardiac death, stroke, gangrene, and/or need for revascularisation procedures. **Population:** In previous versions of *Clinical Evidence*, we attempted to differentiate between primary and secondary prevention in this topic. However, in middle aged and older people with type 2 diabetes, this distinction may not be clinically important. We are not aware of any intervention that has been shown to be effective in secondary prevention but ineffective in primary prevention, or vice versa, in people with diabetes. In most cases, a large proportion of people with diabetes entered into cardiovascular disease prevention trials are middle aged and older, with additional cardiovascular risk factors, and a large portion of these actually have undiagnosed cardiovascular disease.

INCIDENCE/ PREVALENCE Diabetes mellitus is a major risk factor for cardiovascular disease. In the USA, a survey of deaths in 1986 suggested that 60–75% of people with diabetes die from cardiovascular causes.[1] The annual incidence of cardiovascular disease is increased in people with diabetes (men: RR 2–3; women: RR 3–4, adjusted for age and other cardiovascular risk factors).[2] About 45% of middle aged and older white people with diabetes have evidence of coronary artery disease compared with about 25% of people without diabetes in the same populations. In a Finnish population based cohort study (1059 people with diabetes and 1373 people without diabetes, aged 45–64 years), the 7 year risk of acute myocardial infarction was as high in adults with diabetes without

Prevention of cardiovascular events in diabetes

previous cardiac disease (20.2/100 person years) as it was in people without diabetes with previous cardiac disease (18.8/100 person years).[3]

AETIOLOGY/ RISK FACTORS Diabetes mellitus increases the risk of cardiovascular disease. Cardiovascular risk factors in people with diabetes include conventional risk factors (age, prior cardiovascular disease, cigarette smoking, hypertension, dyslipidaemia, sedentary lifestyle, family history of premature cardiovascular disease) and more diabetes specific risk factors (elevated urinary protein excretion, poor glycaemic control). Conventional risk factors for cardiovascular disease contribute to an increase in the relative risk of cardiovascular disease in people with diabetes to about the same extent as in those without diabetes. One prospective cohort study (164 women and 235 men with diabetes [mean age 65 years] and 437 women and 1099 men without diabetes [mean age 61 years] followed for mortality for a mean of 3.7 years after acute myocardial infarction) found that significantly more people with diabetes died compared with people without diabetes (116/399 [29%] with diabetes *v* 204/1536 [13%] without diabetes; RR 2.2, 95% CI 1.8 to 2.7).[4] It also found that the mortality risk after myocardial infarction associated with diabetes was higher for women than for men (adjusted HR 2.7, 95% CI 1.8 to 4.2 for women *v* 1.3, 95% CI 1.0 to 1.8 for men). Physical inactivity is a considerable risk factor for cardiovascular events in both men and women. Another cohort study (5125 women with diabetes) found that participation in little (< 1 hour a week) or no physical activity compared with physical activity for at least 7 hours a week was associated with a doubling of the risk of a cardiovascular event.[5] A third cohort study (1263 men with diabetes, mean follow up 12 years) found that low baseline cardiorespiratory fitness increased overall mortality compared with moderate or high fitness (RR 2.9, 95% CI 2.1 to 3.6), and overall mortality was higher in those reporting no recreational exercise in the previous 3 months than in those reporting any recreational physical activity in the same period (RR 1.8, 95% CI 1.3 to 2.5).[6] The absolute risk of cardiovascular disease is almost the same in women as in men with diabetes. Diabetes specific cardiovascular risk factors include the duration of diabetes during adulthood (the years of exposure to diabetes before age 20 years add little to the risk of cardiovascular disease); raised blood glucose concentrations (reflected in fasting blood glucose or HbA1c); and any degree of microalbuminuria (albuminuria 30–299 mg/24 hours).[7] People with diabetes and microalbuminuria have a higher risk of coronary morbidity and mortality than do people with normal levels of urinary albumin and a similar duration of diabetes (RR 2–3).[8,9] Clinical proteinuria increases the risk of mortality from cardiac events in people with type 2 diabetes (RR 2.61, 95% CI 1.99 to 3.43)[10] and type 1 diabetes (RR 9)[7,11,12] compared with people with the same type of diabetes who have normal albumin excretion. An epidemiological analysis of people with diabetes enrolled in the Heart Outcomes Prevention Evaluation cohort study (3498 people with diabetes and at least 1 other cardiovascular risk factor, age > 55 years, of whom 1140 [32%] had microalbuminuria at baseline; 5 years' follow up) found a higher risk for major cardiovascular events in those with microalbuminuria (albumin : creatinine ratio [ACR] ≥ 2.0 mg/mmol) than in those without microalbuminuria (adjusted RR 1.97, 95% CI 1.68 to 2.31), and for all cause mortality (RR 2.15, 95% CI 1.78 to 2.60).[13] It also found an association between ACR and the risk of major cardiovascular events (ACR 0.22–0.57 mg/mmol: RR 0.85, 95% CI 0.63 to 1.14; ACR 0.58–1.62 mg/mmol: RR 1.11, 95% CI 0.86 to 1.43; ACR 1.62–1.99 mg/mmol: RR 1.89, 95% CI 1.52 to 2.36).

PROGNOSIS Diabetes mellitus increases the risk of mortality or serious morbidity after a coronary event (RR 1.5–3.0).[2,3,14,15] This excess risk is partly accounted for by increased prevalence of other cardiovascular risk factors in people with diabetes. A systematic review (search date 1998, 15 prospective cohort studies) found that, in people with diabetes admitted to hospital for acute myocardial infarction, "stress hyperglycaemia" was associated with significantly higher mortality in hospital compared with lower blood glucose levels (RR 1.7, 95% CI 1.2 to 2.4).[16] One large prospective cohort study (91 285 men aged 40–84 years) found that, compared with men with no diabetes and no coronary heart disease (CHD), there was higher all cause and CHD mortality at 5 years' follow up in men with diabetes with or without CHD, in men with coronary artery disease alone, with the highest risk in men with both risk factors, see table 1 (T).[17] Multivariate analysis did not materially alter these associations. Diabetes mellitus alone is associated with a twofold increase in risk for all cause death, with a threefold increase in risk of death from CHD, and, in people with pre-existing CHD, with a 12-fold increase in risk of death from CHD compared with people with neither risk factor.[17]

Please refer to clinicalevidence.com for full text and references.

Anal fissure (chronic)

Search date January 2006

Rick Nelson

What are the effects of treatments for chronic anal fissure?

BENEFICIAL

Internal anal sphincterotomy

One systematic review found that internal anal sphincterotomy improved fissure healing compared with topical glyceryl trinitrate after 6 weeks to 2 years. One subsequent RCT found that sphincterotomy reduced time to pain reduction and healing compared with topical glyceryl nitrate, although there was no significant difference in treatments after 6 weeks. One systematic review and two subsequent RCTs found that anal sphincterotomy reduced fissure persistence compared with botulinum A toxin–haemagglutinin complex from 6 to 12 months. One systematic review and three subsequent RCTs found no difference in fissure healing between open and closed sphincterotomy after 1 week to 2 years. One RCT found that lateral anal sphincterotomy increased healing compared with oral nifedipine after 4 months, although this difference was not significant after 4 weeks.

LIKELY TO BE BENEFICIAL

Nitric oxide donors (topical glyceryl trinitrate, isosorbide mononitrate, isosorbide dinitrate)*

One systematic review and two subsequent RCTs found limited evidence from heterogeneous RCTs that topical glyceryl trinitrate reduced persistence of fissures compared with placebo. Results were difficult to interpret because of differing durations and doses of treatments. Consensus regards glyceryl trinitrate as an effective first line treatment for chronic anal fissure. One small RCT found that anal dilation increased healing rates compared with topical glyceryl trinitrate after 30 days. One systematic review found that internal anal sphincterotomy improved fissure healing compared with topical glyceryl trinitrate after 6 weeks to 2 years. One subsequent RCT found that sphincterotomy reduced time to pain reduction and healing compared with topical glyceryl trinitrate, although there was no significant difference between the treatments after 6 weeks. One systematic review found no significant difference in fissure persistence between topical glyceryl trinitrate ointment and botulinum A toxin–haemagglutinin complex injection after 2 months. Two RCTs found no significant difference between glyceryl trinitrate ointment and a glyceryl trinitrate patch in fissure healing after 8–12 weeks. Two RCTs found no significant difference between topical glyceryl trinitrate and topical diltiazem in healing after 8 weeks. One RCT found no significant difference between topical glyceryl trinitrate and oral nifedipine in rate of fissure persistence after 30 days. A second RCT found that topical nifedipine significantly increased healing rate compared with topical glyceryl trinitrate after 6 months. We found no systematic reviews or RCTs comparing isosorbide mononitrate or isosorbide dinitrate versus placebo. One RCT found that sphincterotomy improved healing compared with isosorbide dinitrate after 10 weeks.

*Categorisation is based on limited evidence and consensus that nitric oxide donors are beneficial.

UNKNOWN EFFECTIVENESS

Anal advancement flap (as effective as internal anal sphincterotomy based on one small RCT)

One small RCT found no difference between lateral internal anal sphincterotomy and anal advancement flap in patient satisfaction or fissure healing.

Botulinum A toxin-haemagglutinin complex (botulinum A toxin-hc)

One systematic review and one additional RCT found no significant difference in fissure persistence between botulinum A toxin–haemagglutinin complex and placebo or topical glyceryl nitrate at up to 2 months. One RCT found no significant difference between botulinum A toxin–haemagglutinin complex injection and nifedipine in rate of fissure persistence after 30 days. One systematic review and one additional RCT found no significant difference between high and low dose botulinum A toxin–haemagglutinin complex after 2–3 months. One systematic review and two subsequent RCTs found that botulinum A toxin–haemagglutinin complex increased fissure persistence compared with anal sphincterotomy from 6–12 months.

Botulinum A toxin–haemagglutinin complex (botulinum A toxin-hc) plus nitrates

We found no RCTs comparing botulinum A toxin–haemagglutinin complex plus nitrates versus placebo. One small RCT found that botulinum A toxin–haemagglutinin complex plus topical isosorbide dinitrate three times daily increased fissure healing at 6 weeks compared with botulinum A toxin–haemagglutinin complex alone. It found no significant difference at 8 or 12 weeks.

Calcium channel blockers (diltiazem, nifedipine)

We found no placebo controlled RCTs. Two RCTs found no significant difference between topical glyceryl trinitrate and topical diltiazem in healing after 8 weeks. One RCT found no significant difference between topical glyceryl trinitrate and oral nifedipine in rate of fissure persistence after 30 days. A second RCT found that topical nifedipine significantly increased healing rate compared with topical glyceryl trinitrate after 6 months. One small RCT identified by a systematic review found no significant difference in fissure persistence after 8 weeks between oral diltiazem and topical diltiazem, but found that adverse events were more common with oral diltiazem. One RCT found that lateral anal sphincterotomy increased healing compared with oral nifedipine after 4 months, although this difference was not significant after 4 weeks.

Indoramin

One RCT found no significant difference between oral indoramin, a beta blocker, and placebo in fissure healing after 6 weeks, but it may have been too small to detect a clinically important difference.

Minoxadil *New*

One RCT found no significant difference in healing rate between minoxadil and lignocaine in complete healing rates after 6 weeks.

Anal fissure (chronic)

UNLIKELY TO BE BENEFICIAL

Anal stretch (compared with internal anal sphincterotomy)

One systematic review found limited evidence that internal anal sphincterotomy may reduce persistence of fissures compared with anal stretch. Anal stretch increased rates of flatus incontinence compared with internal anal sphincterotomy.

DEFINITION An anal fissure is an ulcer or tear in the squamous epithelium of the distal anal canal, usually in the posterior midline. People with an anal fissure usually experience pain during defecation and for 1–2 hours afterwards. Multiple fissures, large and/or irregular fissures, or fissures off the midline are considered atypical. Atypical fissures may be caused by malignancy, chemotherapy, sexually transmitted infection, inflammatory bowel disease, or other traumas. Treatments for atypical fissures are not included in this review. It is not clear what the best treatment strategy is in people who present with a painless anal fissure, and in whom an atypical aetiology has been ruled out. **Acute anal fissures** have sharply demarcated, fresh mucosal edges, often with granulation tissue at the base. Acute fissures are believed to often heal spontaneously. **Chronic anal fissures:** Fissures persisting for longer than 4 weeks or recurrent fissures are generally defined as chronic. Chronic anal fissures have distinct anatomical features, such as visible sphincter fibres at the fissure base, anal papillae, sentinel piles, and indurated margins.[1] Most published studies only require the presence of one of these signs or symptoms of chronicity to classify a fissure as chronic.[2] This chapter deals only with chronic anal fissures.

INCIDENCE/ PREVALENCE Anal fissures are a common cause of anal pain in all age groups, but we found no reliable evidence about precise incidence.

AETIOLOGY/ RISK FACTORS The aetiology of anal fissure is not fully understood. Low intake of dietary fibre may be a risk factor for the development of acute anal fissure.[3] People with anal fissure often have raised resting anal canal pressures with anal spasm, which may give rise to ischaemia.[1,4,5]

PROGNOSIS Chronic fissure typically has a cyclical pain history with intermittent healing and then recurrence. One systematic review found healing rates of approximately 35% without intervention, depending on the length of study follow up.[1]

Please refer to clinicalevidence.com for full text and references.

Appendicitis

Search date October 2005

John Simpson, David Humes, and William Speake

What are the effects of treatments for acute appendicitis?

BENEFICIAL

Surgery plus antibiotics

One systematic review and one subsequent RCT in children and adults with simple or complicated appendicitis undergoing appendicectomy found that surgery plus antibiotics reduced wound infections and intra-abdominal abscesses compared with surgery alone. Subgroup analysis from the systematic review found that in children with complicated appendicitis, surgery plus antibiotics reduced the number of wound infections compared with surgery alone, but in children with simple appendicitis it found no significant difference in the number of wound infections whether or not antibiotics were added. One subsequent RCT in children with simple appendicitis found no significant difference in wound infections between adding antibiotics and not adding antibiotics, but the RCT might have been too small to detect a clinically important difference.

LIKELY TO BE BENEFICIAL

Laparoscopic surgery versus open surgery (in children)

One systematic review found that, in children, laparoscopic surgery reduced the number of wound infections and the length of hospital stay compared with open surgery, but found no significant difference in postoperative pain, time to mobilisation, or proportion of intra-abdominal abscesses. One subsequent quasi-RCT in children provided limited evidence of no significant difference in rates of infection or postoperative complications, or in length of hospital stay between laparoscopic surgery and open surgery.

TRADE OFF BETWEEN BENEFITS AND HARMS

Antibiotics versus surgery

One small RCT in adults with suspected appendicitis found that conservative treatment with antibiotics reduced pain and morphine consumption for the first 10 days compared with appendicectomy. However, the RCT found that 35% of people treated with antibiotics were readmitted within 1 year with acute appendicitis and subsequently underwent appendicectomy.

Laparoscopic surgery versus open surgery (in adults)

One systematic review and one subsequent RCT provided evidence that laparoscopic surgery in adults reduced wound infections, postoperative pain, duration of hospital stay, and time taken to return to work compared with open surgery. However, the systematic review found that laparoscopic surgery increased postoperative intra-abdominal abscesses compared with open surgery. One RCT in adult men provided limited evidence of no significant difference between treatments in need for pain relieving medication, length of hospital stay, or complication rates.

BMJ Clin Evid Concise 2006;16:187–188.

Appendicitis

UNKNOWN EFFECTIVENESS

Antibiotics (versus no treatment/placebo)

We found no RCTs comparing antibiotics versus no treatment or placebo. Such RCTs are unlikely to be conducted because of ethical concerns.

Surgery (versus no treatment)

We found no RCTs comparing surgery versus no treatment, and such studies are unlikely to be conducted because of ethical concerns. One small RCT in adults with suspected appendicitis found that appendicectomy was less effective at reducing pain and morphine consumption for the first 10 days compared with conservative treatment with antibiotics. However, the RCT found that 35% of people treated with antibiotics were readmitted within 1 year with acute appendicitis and subsequently underwent appendicectomy.

LIKELY TO BE INEFFECTIVE OR HARMFUL

Stump inversion at open appendicectomy versus simple ligation

Two RCTs provided insufficient evidence on the effects of stump inversion in people undergoing appendicectomy.

DEFINITION Acute appendicitis is acute inflammation of the vermiform appendix.

INCIDENCE/PREVALENCE The incidence of acute appendicitis is falling, although the reason for this is unclear. The reported lifetime risk of appendicitis in the USA is 8.7% in men and 6.7% in women,[1] and about 35 000 cases are reported annually in England.[2] Appendicitis is the most common abdominal surgical emergency requiring operation.

AETIOLOGY/RISK FACTORS The cause of appendicitis is uncertain, although various theories exist. Most relate to luminal obstruction, which prevents escape of secretions and inevitably leads to a rise in intraluminal pressure within the appendix. This can lead to subsequent mucosal ischaemia, and the stasis provides an ideal environment for bacterial overgrowth. Potential causes of the obstruction are faecoliths (often because of constipation), lymphoid hyperplasia, or caecal carcinoma.[3]

PROGNOSIS The prognosis of untreated appendicitis is unknown, although spontaneous resolution has been reported in at least 1/13 (8%) episodes.[4] The recurrence of appendicitis after conservative management,[4,5] and recurrent abdominal symptoms in certain people[6] suggest that chronic appendicitis and recurrent acute or subacute appendicitis may also exist.[7] The standard treatment for acute appendicitis is appendicectomy. RCTs comparing treatment versus no treatment would be regarded as unethical. The mortality from acute appendicitis is less than 0.3%, rising to 1.7% after perforation.[8] The most common complication of appendicectomy is wound infection, occurring in 5–33% of cases.[9] Intra-abdominal abscess formation occurs less frequently, in 2% of appendicectomies.[10] A perforated appendix in childhood does not appear to have subsequent negative consequences for female fertility.[11]

Please refer to clinicalevidence.com for full text and references.

Cholecystitis (acute)

Search date December 2005

Li Ern Chen, Valerie Halpin, and Robb Whinney

Digestive system disorders

What are the effects of treatments for acute cholecystitis?

BENEFICIAL

Early cholecystectomy (reduces hospital stay and the need for emergency surgery compared with delayed cholecystectomy)

Two systematic reviews found that early (at the time of diagnosis or within 7 days of onset of symptoms) open or laparoscopic cholecystectomy reduced the duration of hospital stay compared with delayed (≥ 6 weeks after onset of symptoms) open or laparoscopic cholecystectomy. They found no significant differences in operative or perioperative complications and postoperative mortality. The first systematic review found that unplanned urgent operation was necessary in 23% of people scheduled to undergo delayed cholecystectomy because of recurrent or worsening symptoms.

Laparoscopic cholecystectomy (reduced hospital stay and may improve intraoperative and postoperative outcomes compared with open cholecystectomy)

Four RCTs found that laparoscopic cholecystectomy reduced hospital stay, but found limited evidence that it reduced duration of surgery and intraoperative/postoperative complications compared with open cholecystectomy. One RCT found no difference between conventional laparoscopic cholecystectomy and minilaparoscopic cholecystectomy in use of analgesics, hospital stay, and rates of conversion to open cholecystectomy. However, the trial may have lacked power to detect clinically important differences between techniques. Duration of surgery was marginally shorter with conventional laparoscopic cholecystectomy than with minilaparoscopic cholecystectomy.

TRADE OFF BETWEEN BENEFITS AND HARMS

Observation alone (resulting in a 30% failure rate and a 36% rate of gallstone related complications)

One RCT found that observation alone had a failure rate after 8 years of 30%, but found no difference in the rate of gallstone related complications (recurrent cholecystitis, pancreatitis, intractable pain) or emergency admissions for pain compared with cholecystectomy (open or laparoscopic).

Open cholecystectomy (conversion from laparoscopic to open cholecystectomy necessary in 4–27% of people but may increase intraoperative and postoperative complications)

One RCT found that observation alone had a failure rate after 8 years of 30% but found no difference in the rate of gallstone related complications (recurrent cholecystitis, pancreatitis, intractable pain) or emergency admissions for pain compared with cholecystectomy (open or laparoscopic). Four RCTs found that open cholecystectomy increased hospital stay and found limited evidence that it increased duration of surgery and intraoperative/postoperative complications compared with laparoscopic cholecystectomy. The RCTs found conversion from laparoscopic to open cholecystectomy necessary in 4–27% of people. ▶

Cholecystitis (acute)

UNKNOWN EFFECTIVENESS

Minilaparoscopic cholecystectomy

One RCT found no difference between minilaparoscopic and conventional laparoscopic cholecystectomy in use of analgesics, hospital stay, and rates of conversion to open cholecystectomy. However, it may have lacked power to detect clinically important differences between the techniques. Duration of surgery was marginally longer with minilaparoscopic cholecystectomy than with conventional cholecystectomy.

DEFINITION **Acute cholecystitis** results from obstruction of the cystic duct, usually by a gallstone, followed by distension and subsequent chemical or bacterial inflammation of the gallbladder. People with acute cholecystitis usually have unremitting right upper quadrant pain, anorexia, nausea, vomiting, and fever. About 95% of people with acute cholecystitis have gallstones (calculous cholecystitis) and 5% lack gallstones (acalculous cholecystitis).[1] Severe acute cholecystitis may lead to necrosis of the gallbladder wall, known as gangrenous cholecystitis. This review does not include people with acute cholangitis, which is a severe complication of gallstone disease and generally a result of bacterial infection.

INCIDENCE/ PREVALENCE The incidence of acute cholecystitis among people with gallstones is unknown. Of people admitted to hospital for biliary tract disease 20% have acute cholecystitis.[1] The number of cholecystectomies carried out for acute cholecystitis has increased from the mid-1980s to the early 1990s, especially in elderly people.[2] Acute calculous cholecystitis is three times more common in women than in men up to the age of 50 years, and is about 1.5 times more common in women than in men thereafter.[1]

AETIOLOGY/ RISK FACTORS Acute calculous cholecystitis seems to be caused by obstruction of the cystic duct by a gallstone or local mucosal erosion and inflammation caused by a stone, but cystic duct ligation alone does not produce acute cholecystitis in animal studies. The role of bacteria in the pathogenesis of acute cholecystitis is not clear; positive cultures of bile or gallbladder wall are found in 50–75% of cases.[3,4] The cause of acute acalculous cholecystitis is uncertain and may be multifactorial, including increased susceptibility to bacterial colonisation of static gallbladder bile.[1]

PROGNOSIS Complications of acute cholecystitis include perforation of the gallbladder, pericholecystic abscess, and fistula caused by gallbladder wall ischaemia and infection. In the USA the overall mortality from untreated complications is about 20%.[5]

Please refer to clinicalevidence.com for full text and references.

Colonic diverticular disease

Search date March 2006

John Simpson, David Humes and Robin Spiller

What are the effects of treatments for uncomplicated diverticular disease?

LIKELY TO BE BENEFICIAL

Rifaximin (plus dietary fibre supplementation v dietary fibre supplementation alone)

Two RCTs in people with uncomplicated diverticular disease found that rifaximin (400 mg twice daily) plus dietary fibre supplementation improved symptoms compared with dietary fibre supplementation alone after 12 months of treatment. One methodologically flawed RCT provided insufficient evidence about the effects of rifaximin compared with mesalazine.

UNKNOWN EFFECTIVENESS

Bran and ispaghula husk

One small RCT in people with uncomplicated diverticular disease found no significant difference between bran or ispaghula husk and placebo in symptom relief after 16 weeks.

Elective surgery

We found no systematic review or RCTs of elective open or laparoscopic colonic resection in people with uncomplicated diverticular disease.

Lactulose

One small RCT in people with uncomplicated diverticular disease found no significant difference between lactulose and a high fibre diet in self rated improvement after 12 weeks.

Mesalazine *New*

One methodologically flawed RCT provided insufficient evidence about the effects of mesalazine compared with rifaximin.

Methylcellulose

One small RCT in people with uncomplicated diverticular disease found no significant difference between methylcellulose and placebo in mean symptom scores after 3 months.

What are the effects of treatments to prevent complications of diverticular disease?

UNKNOWN EFFECTIVENESS

Advice to increase fibre intake

We found no systematic review or RCTs examining complication rates after advice to consume a high fibre diet or of dietary fibre supplementation.

Mesalazine (after an attack of acute diverticulitis)

One methodologically flawed RCT provided insufficient evidence about the effects of mesalazine compared with no treatment in people previously treated for an episode of acute diverticulitis.

Colonic diverticular disease

What are the effects of treatments for acute diverticulitis?

UNKNOWN EFFECTIVENESS

Medical treatment

We found no systematic review or RCTs comparing medical treatment versus placebo in people with acute diverticulitis. One small RCT found no significant difference between intravenous cefoxitin and intravenous gentamicin plus intravenous clindamycin in rates of clinical cure or toxicity. Observational studies in people with acute diverticulitis have found low mortality with medical treatment, but found that recurrence rates may be high.

Surgery (for diverticulitis complicated by generalised peritonitis)

We found no systematic review or RCTs comparing surgery versus no surgery or versus medical treatment. One RCT found no significant difference in mortality and complication rates between acute resection and transverse colostomy of the sigmoid colon. A second RCT found no significant difference in mortality and rates of wound or extra-abdominal complications between primary and secondary sigmoid colonic resection, but found that primary resection reduced rates of postoperative peritonitis and emergency reoperation. We found no RCTs comparing open versus laparoscopic surgery.

DEFINITION Colonic diverticula are mucosal outpouchings through the large bowel wall. They are often accompanied by structural changes (elastosis of the taenia coli, muscular thickening, and mucosal folding). They are usually multiple and occur most frequently in the sigmoid colon. The majority of people with colonic diverticula are asymptomatic, with little to find on clinical examination, while 20% develop symptoms at some point in their life.[1] If diverticula are associated with symptoms, then this is termed diverticular disease. If asymptomatic, then the condition is known as diverticulosis. People who go on to develop complications associated with diverticula (inflammation, perforation, fistulae, abscess formation, obstruction, or haemorrhage) are referred to as having complicated diverticular disease. People with uncomplicated diverticular disease may report abdominal pain (principally colicky left iliac fossa pain), bloating, and altered bowel habit, and may have mild left iliac fossa tenderness on examination. Acute diverticulitis occurs when a diverticulum becomes acutely inflamed. People with acute diverticulitis typically present with severe left iliac fossa pain associated with fever, malaise, and altered bowel habit with left iliac fossa tenderness, associated with general signs of infection, such as fever and tachycardia.

INCIDENCE/ PREVALENCE In the UK the incidence of diverticulosis increases with age; about 5% of people are affected in their fifth decade of life and about 50% by their ninth decade.[2] Diverticulosis is common in developed countries, although there is a lower prevalence of diverticulosis in Western vegetarians consuming a diet high in roughage.[3] Diverticulosis is almost unknown in rural Africa and Asia.[4]

AETIOLOGY/ RISK FACTORS There is an association between low fibre diets and diverticulosis of the colon.[4] Prospective observational studies have found that both physical activity and a high fibre diet are associated with a lower risk of developing diverticular disease.[5,6] Case control studies have found an association between perforated diverticular disease and non-steroidal anti-inflammatory drugs, corticosteroids, and opiate analgesics, and have found that calcium antagonists have a protective effect.[7-10] People in Japan, Singapore, and Thailand develop diverticula that affect mainly the right side of the colon.[11]

PROGNOSIS Inflammation will develop in 10–25% of people with diverticula at some point in their lives.[2] It is unclear why some people develop symptoms and some do not. Even after successful medical treatment of acute diverticulitis, almost two thirds of people suffer recurrent pain in the lower abdomen.[12] Recurrent diverticulitis is observed in 7–42% of people with diverticular disease, and after recovery from the initial attack the calculated yearly risk of suffering a further episode is 3%.[13] About 50% of recurrences occur within 1 year of the initial episode and 90% occur within 5 years.[14] Complications of diverticular disease (perforation, obstruction, haemorrhage, and fistula formation) are each seen in about 5% of people with colonic diverticula when followed up for 10–30 years.[15] In the UK the incidence of perforation is four cases per 100 000 people a year, leading to approximately 2000 cases annually.[16] Intra-abdominal abscess formation is also a recognised complication.

Please refer to clinicalevidence.com for full text and references.

Colorectal cancer

Search date August 2005

Praveen Roy and Reuben Last

What are the effects of treatments?

BENEFICIAL

Adjuvant chemotherapy

Three systematic reviews and one subsequent RCT found that adjuvant chemotherapy reduced mortality compared with surgery alone in people with Dukes' A, B, and C colorectal cancer. One RCT found that adding levamisole to adjuvant fluorouracil did not reduce mortality or recurrence rate compared with adjuvant fluorouracil alone in people with Dukes' A, B, and C colorectal cancer. One RCT found that mortality and recurrence rates were similar with adjuvant fluorouracil plus high or low dose folinic acid in people with Dukes' A, B, and C colorectal cancer.

LIKELY TO BE BENEFICIAL

Routine intensive follow up

One systematic review found that intensive follow up reduced time to detection of recurrence and increased detection rates for isolated local recurrence compared with less intensive follow up, in people with colorectal cancer treated surgically with curative intent. One systematic review found that intensive follow up increased survival compared with less intensive follow up.

TRADE OFF BETWEEN BENEFITS AND HARMS

Preoperative radiotherapy

Two systematic reviews and two subsequent RCTs found that adding preoperative radiotherapy to surgery is at least as effective as surgery alone for mortality and recurrence in people with rectal cancer. One RCT found no significant difference in mortality between preoperative and postoperative radiotherapy. However, it found that preoperative radiotherapy reduced local tumour recurrence. One systematic review found that preoperative radiotherapy increased early postoperative morbidity.

UNKNOWN EFFECTIVENESS

Total mesorectal excision

We found no systematic review or RCTs of total mesorectal excision in people with rectal cancer. Observational studies suggest that total mesorectal excision may reduce the rate of local recurrence compared with conventional surgery.

DEFINITION Colorectal cancer is a malignant neoplasm arising from the lining (mucosa) of the large intestine (colon and rectum). Nearly two thirds of colorectal cancers occur in the rectum or sigmoid colon. Colorectal cancer may be categorised as A, B, or C Dukes'.

INCIDENCE/ PREVALENCE Colorectal cancer is the third most common malignancy in the developed world. It accounts for about 20 000 deaths each year in the UK and 60 000 deaths each year in the USA. Although the incidence of, and mortality from, colorectal cancer has changed little over the past 40 years, the incidence of the disease has fallen recently in both the UK and the USA.[1,2] In the UK, about a quarter of people with colorectal cancer present with either intestinal obstruction or perforation.[3,4]

AETIOLOGY/ RISK FACTORS Colon cancer affects almost equal proportions of men and women, most commonly between the ages of 60 and 80 years. Rectal cancer is more common in men.[1] The pathogenesis of colorectal cancer involves genetic and environmental factors. The most important environmental factor is probably diet.[5]

PROGNOSIS Overall 5 year survival is about 50% and has not changed over the past 40 years. Disease specific mortality in both USA and UK cancer registries is decreasing but the reasons for this are unclear.[1,2] Surgery is undertaken with curative intent in over 80% of people, but about half experience cancer recurrence.

Please refer to clinicalevidence.com for full text and references.

Colorectal cancer screening

Search date November 2005

Carmen Lewis and Michael Pignone

What are the effects of screening for colorectal cancer?

BENEFICIAL

Faecal occult blood test (annual or biennial testing, followed by further investigation if positive)

A systematic review of RCTs found that annual or biennial faecal occult blood testing, followed by further investigation in people with a positive test, decreased colorectal cancer related mortality compared with no screening after 8–18 years.

LIKELY TO BE BENEFICIAL

Flexible sigmoidoscopy (single test, followed by colonoscopy if positive)

A systematic review found one small RCT comparing flexible sigmoidoscopy versus no screening. It found that single test flexible sigmoidoscopy (followed by colonoscopy if positive) reduced colorectal cancer rates, but not mortality from colorectal cancer, compared with no screening. Some people found the flexible sigmoidoscopy procedure painful.

UNKNOWN EFFECTIVENESS

Colonoscopy

One systematic review found no RCTs comparing colonoscopy versus no screening for colorectal cancer. Colonoscopy is associated with rare but serious morbidity, including perforation and bleeding.

Combination of faecal occult blood test and flexible sigmoidoscopy

One systematic review found no RCTs comparing combined screening with faecal occult blood testing plus flexible sigmoidoscopy versus no screening.

Computed tomography colography

We found no systematic review or RCTs comparing computed tomography colography versus no screening.

Double contrast barium enema

One systematic review found no RCTs comparing double contrast barium enemas versus no screening.

DEFINITION Colorectal cancer is a malignant neoplasm arising from the lining (mucosa) of the large intestine (colon and rectum). Nearly two thirds of colorectal cancers occur in the rectum or sigmoid colon. Colorectal cancer may be classified as A, B, or C Dukes'. Screening is defined (and distinguished from testing on demand) as any organised or systematic testing of asymptomatic people. In this chapter, we have included studies of screening in men and women over 45 years of age (with no upper age limit) who are not known to be at high risk for colorectal cancer. High risk people are defined as those with one or more first degree relatives with colorectal cancer or personal history of inflammatory bowel disease, polyps, or colorectal cancer.

INCIDENCE/ PREVALENCE Colorectal cancer is the third most common malignancy in the developed world. It accounts for about 20 000 deaths each year in the UK and 60 000 deaths each year in the USA. Over most of the last 40 years, the incidence of, ▶

and mortality from, colorectal cancer has changed little. However, recently, both the incidence and mortality have fallen in the UK and the USA.[1,2] In the UK, about a quarter of people with colorectal cancer present with either intestinal obstruction or perforation.[3,4]

AETIOLOGY/ RISK FACTORS Colon cancer affects almost equal proportions of men and women, most commonly between the ages of 60 and 80 years. Rectal cancer is more common in men.[1] The pathogenesis of colorectal cancer involves genetic and environmental factors. The most important environmental factor is probably diet.[5] People with a personal or family history of colorectal cancer or polyps, or a personal history of inflammatory bowel disease, are at high risk.

PROGNOSIS Overall 5 year survival after colorectal cancer is about 50% and has not changed over the past 40 years. Disease specific mortality in both the UK and the USA cancer registries is decreasing but the reasons for this are unclear.[1,2] Surgery is undertaken with curative intent in over 80% of people, but about half experience cancer recurrence.

Please refer to clinicalevidence.com for full text and references.

Constipation in adults

Search date October 2005

Frank Frizelle and Murray Barclay

What are the effects of lifestyle interventions in adults with idiopathic chronic constipation?

UNKNOWN EFFECTIVENESS

Advice to consume a high fibre diet

We found no systematic review or RCTs of advice to consume a high fibre diet in adults with idiopathic chronic constipation.

Advice to exercise

We found no systematic review or RCTs of sufficient quality assessing advice to exercise in adults with idiopathic chronic constipation.

Advice to increase fluids

We found no systematic review or RCTs of advice to increase oral fluids in adults with idiopathic chronic constipation.

Biofeedback *New*

We found no systematic review or RCTs of biofeedback in adults with idiopathic chronic constipation.

What are the effects of other treatments in adults with idiopathic chronic constipation?

BENEFICIAL

Macrogols (polyethylene glycols)

Four RCTs found that macrogols (polyethylene glycols) improved symptoms after 2–20 weeks compared with placebo in adults with idiopathic chronic constipation. One RCT found insufficient evidence to compare macrogol 3350 versus ispaghula husk. Two RCTs found that macrogols improved global satisfaction and severity of constipation at 4 weeks compared with lactulose. Two RCTs found no significant difference between macrogols and placebo in the frequency of adverse effects. One RCT found no difference in bowel frequency between four different macrogol dosing regimens.

LIKELY TO BE BENEFICIAL

Ispaghula husk (psyllium)

One RCT found that ispaghula husk increased the frequency of bowel movements and improved overall symptoms compared with placebo after 2 weeks in adults with chronic idiopathic constipation. We found limited evidence from two RCTs that ispaghula husk improved frequency of bowel movements and reduced hard stools compared with lactulose at 4 weeks. However, one of the RCTs found that both ispaghula husk and lactulose produced similar physician rated clinical improvement. One RCT provided insufficient evidence to compare ispaghula husk versus macrogol 3350. One poor quality RCT found no clinically important difference between ispaghula husk and docusate in frequency of bowel movements, stool consistency, straining, or pain after 2 weeks.

Lactitol

One small crossover RCT found that lactitol increased the frequency of bowel movements compared with placebo after 4 weeks in adults with chronic idiopathic constipation. Three RCTs found no significant difference in frequency of bowel movements at 2–4 weeks between lactitol and lactulose.

Lactulose

Two RCTs found limited evidence that lactulose improved symptoms compared with placebo in adults with chronic idiopathic constipation. Two RCTs provided limited evidence that lactulose was less effective than ispaghula husk in improving the frequency of bowel movements and reducing hard stools at 4 weeks. However, one of the RCTs found that both lactulose and ispaghula husk produced similar physician rated clinical improvement. Three RCTs found no significant difference in frequency of bowel movements at 2–4 weeks between lactulose and lactitol. Two RCTs found that lactulose was less effective than macrogols in improving global satisfaction and severity of constipation at 4 weeks.

UNKNOWN EFFECTIVENESS

Bisacodyl

We found no systematic review or RCTs of the effects of bisacodyl in adults with idiopathic chronic constipation.

Cascara *New*

We found no systematic review or RCTs of the effects of cascara in adults with idiopathic chronic constipation.

Docusate

One systematic review identified no RCTs of sufficient quality comparing docusate versus placebo in adults with chronic idiopathic constipation. One poor quality RCT found no clinically important difference between docusate and ispaghula husk in frequency of bowel movements, stool consistency, straining, or pain after 2 weeks.

Glycerol/glycerin suppositories

We found no systematic review or RCTs of the effects of glycerol/glycerin suppositories in adults with idiopathic chronic constipation.

Magnesium salts

We found no systematic review or RCTs of magnesium salts in adults with idiopathic chronic constipation.

Methylcellulose *New*

We found no systematic review or RCTs of methylcellulose in adults with idiopathic chronic constipation.

Paraffin

We found no systematic review or RCTs on paraffin in adults with idiopathic chronic constipation.

Phosphate enemas

We found no systematic review or RCTs of phosphate enemas in adults with idiopathic chronic constipation.

Constipation in adults

Seed oils/arachis oil

We found no systematic review or RCTs of seed oils/arachis oil in adults with idiopathic chronic constipation.

Senna

We found no systematic review or RCTs of the effects of senna in adults with idiopathic chronic constipation.

Sodium citrate enemas

We found no systematic review or RCTs of sodium citrate enemas in adults with idiopathic chronic constipation.

Sterculia *New*

We found no systematic review or RCTs of sterculia in adults with idiopathic chronic constipation.

DEFINITION Bowel habits and perception of bowel habit vary widely within and among populations, making constipation difficult to define strictly. Constipation may also be divided into two main categories; those where the patient has difficulty defecating (but normal frequency) and those who have a transit abnormality, (i.e. infrequent defecation). The Rome II criteria is a standardised tool that diagnoses chronic constipation on the basis of two or more of the following symptoms for at least 12 weeks in the preceding year: straining at defecation on at least a quarter of occasions; stools that are lumpy/hard on at least a quarter of occasions; sensation of incomplete evacuation on at least a quarter of occasions; and three or fewer bowel movements a week.[1] In practice, however, diagnostic criteria are less rigid and are in part dependent on perception of normal bowel habit. Typically, chronic constipation might be diagnosed when a person has bowel actions twice a week or less, for two consecutive weeks, especially in the presence of features such as straining at stool, abdominal discomfort, and sensation of incomplete evacuation. **Population:** For the purposes of this review we included all RCTs that stated that all participants had chronic constipation, whether or not this diagnosis was made according to strict Rome II criteria. Where the definitions of constipation in the RCTs differ markedly from those presented here, we have made this difference explicit. In this chapter, we deal with chronic constipation that is not caused by a specific underlying disease (sometimes known as idiopathic constipation) in adults aged over 18 years. We excluded studies in pregnant women and in people with constipation associated with underlying specific organic diseases such as autonomic neuropathy, spinal cord injury, bowel obstruction, and paralytic ileus. This chapter does not cover interventions, such as dantron, which are recommended for use only in people who are terminally ill. **Diagnosis:** The diagnosis of constipation is initially based on history (see above). Specific tests available for further investigation include thyroid function tests, calcium concentration, barium enema or colonoscopy, defecation proctogram, anorectal manometry, and colon transit time studies.

INCIDENCE/ PREVALENCE Twelve million general practitioner prescriptions were written for laxatives in England in 2001.[2] Prevalence data are limited by small samples and problems with definition. One UK survey of 731 women found that 8.2% had constipation meeting Rome II criteria, and 8.5% defined themselves as being constipated.[3] A larger survey (1892 adults) found that 39% of men and 52% of women reported straining at stool on more than a quarter of occasions.[4] Prevalence rises in the elderly. Several surveys from around the world suggest that in a community setting, prevalence among the elderly is about 20%.[4-7]

AETIOLOGY/ RISK FACTORS One systematic review suggested that factors associated with increased risk of constipation included low fibre diet, low fluid intake, reduced mobility, and consumption of drugs such as opioids and anticholinergic antidepressants.[8]

PROGNOSIS Untreated constipation may lead to faecal impaction, particularly in elderly and confused people.[9] Constipation has been suggested as a risk factor for haemorrhoids and diverticular disease; however, evidence of causality is lacking.[9]

Please refer to clinicalevidence.com for full text and references.

Crohn's disease

Search date March 2006

Alexander C. von Roon, George E. Reese, Timothy R. Orchard, and Paris P. Tekkis

---

What are the effects of medical treatments in adults to induce remission in Crohn's disease?

LIKELY TO BE BENEFICIAL

Aminosalicylates New

Four RCTs have found that, compared with placebo, mesalazine significantly reduced Crohn's Disease Activity Index scores at doses greater than 3 g daily. Meta-analysis has shown the improvement in Crohn's Disease Activity Index to be only marginally better than with placebo. Lower mesalazine doses (1 g/day or 2 g/day) were not significantly different from placebo in terms of efficacy. There is insufficient evidence to assess different mesalazine formulations for different disease locations. One RCT found sulfasalazine to be better than placebo. Four RCTs described adverse effects with mesalazine, which were not analysed for significance. There is insufficient evidence to assess different sulfasalazine formulations for different disease locations.

Corticosteroids (oral) New

One systematic review and two additional RCTs found that, compared with placebo, corticosteroids increased remission rates in active Crohn's disease, although remission rates for budesonide were slightly lower than for methylprednisolone and prednisolone. The optimal budesonide dose and whether this should be given in a single or in two divided daily doses remain unclear. One small RCT found similar remission rates between a 7 week and a 15 week tapering regimen of methylprednisolone. No evidence was found on the relative efficacy of methylprednisolone and prednisolone or different routes of administration. Two RCTs demonstrated significant adverse effects with methylprednisolone and prednisolone compared with placebo. One systematic review found no significant difference in adverse effects of budesonide compared with placebo. The same review found budesonide to have significantly fewer adverse effects than methylprednisolone and prednisolone. One RCT found no significant difference in bone mineral density reduction between budesonide and prednisolone.

Infliximab New

One RCT found that a single dose of infliximab increased remission rates in moderate to severe Crohn's disease after 4 weeks compared with placebo. A dose of 5 mg/kg had similar effects to 10 mg/kg or 20 mg/kg. No difference was found in the incidence of adverse events between the treatment and placebo groups.

Methotrexate New

One RCT found evidence that intramuscular methotrexate is beneficial in induction of remission in chronic active Crohn's disease. Adverse events were significantly more frequent than with placebo.

TRADE OFF BETWEEN BENEFITS AND HARMS

Azathioprine/mercaptopurine *New*

A systematic review found evidence that azathioprine and mercaptopurine significantly increase remission rates and have significant corticosteroid sparing effects. However, a minimum treatment period of 17 weeks was necessary for maximal benefit. Adverse effects are dose related and may be severe.

UNLIKELY TO BE BENEFICIAL

Antibiotics *New*

One small RCT reported that monotherapy with metronidazole in active Crohn's disease achieved the same remission rates as treatment with sulfasalazine. A further RCT found that remission rates for treatment with metronidazole were no different from those with placebo. Therapy was well tolerated in both RCTs, although common adverse events included nausea, fatigue, and anorexia. No RCTs that met our inclusion criteria were found for monotherapy with ciprofloxacin. One small RCT found that combination therapy with ciprofloxacin and metronidazole achieved similar remission rates to treatment with methylprednisolone. A further RCT demonstrated no difference in remission rates between ciprofloxacin plus metronidazole combination therapy and placebo when given as an adjunct to oral budesonide therapy. Participant withdrawal rates because of adverse events were high in both trials, at 20% and 27% respectively. One small RCT found similar remission rates between antimycobacterial therapy with clofazimine and placebo when given in conjunction with oral prednisolone. Adverse reactions were skin pigmentation and rash.

What are the effects of lifestyle interventions in adults with Crohn's disease to maintain remission?

BENEFICIAL

Smoking cessation *New*

Nine cohort studies provided good evidence that people with Crohn's disease who smoke experience significantly more episodes of clinical relapse and surgery rates compared with non-smokers. One intervention study found strong evidence that people with Crohn's disease who stop smoking experience significantly fewer relapses and require significantly less immunosuppressive therapy than those who continue to smoke.

UNKNOWN EFFECTIVENESS

Enteral nutrition *New*

No RCTs that met our inclusion criteria were found on the effectiveness of elemental diet for maintaining remission in Crohn's disease.

Fish oil *New*

One RCT has found that treatment with enteric coated fish oil capsules reduced relapse rates and increased the proportion of people with Crohn's disease in remission after 1 year compared with placebo. Another RCT found no evidence that treatment with non-enteric coated fish oil capsules increased the proportion of people with Crohn's disease in remission after 1 year compared with placebo. Adverse events were diarrhoea with enteric coated capsules and belching or heartburn with non-enteric coated capsules.

Crohn's disease

Probiotics *New*

One RCT that compared *Lactobacillus johnsonii* LA1 versus placebo in people with Crohn's disease in remission found no evidence that treatment with *L. johnsonii* reduces recurrence rates. No adverse effects were reported with *L. johnsonii* administration.

What are the effects of surgical interventions in adults with small bowel Crohn's disease to induce remission?

LIKELY TO BE BENEFICIAL

Resection *New*

One RCT found similar incidence of Crohn's disease recurrence with limited resection margins compared with extended resection margins.

UNKNOWN EFFECTIVENESS

Strictureplasty *New*

A systematic review found evidence that Finney strictureplasty may be superior to the Heineke-Mikulicz procedure in inducing remission and reoperation rate in Crohn's disease. However, the review was of low quality and it is therefore difficult to draw reliable conclusions.

What are the effects of surgical interventions in adults with colonic Crohn's disease to induce remission?

LIKELY TO BE BENEFICIAL

Segmental colectomy *New*

A systematic review found segmental and subtotal colectomy to have similar remission rates. There is some evidence that recurrence occurs earlier after segmental colectomy than after subtotal colectomy.

What are the effects of medical interventions to maintain remission in adults with Crohn's disease?

LIKELY TO BE BENEFICIAL

Infliximab *New*

Two RCTs found good evidence that in people with refractory Crohn's disease who went into remission following an initial dose of infliximab, further doses of infliximab result in higher rates of maintaining remission than placebo. One of the RCTs found that continued infliximab therapy reduced the need for conventional corticosteroid treatment and improved quality of life compared with placebo. A dosage regimen of 5 mg/kg every 8 weeks was as effective at maintaining remission as 10 mg/kg. Scheduled treatment every 8 weeks as opposed to episodic (on-demand) treatment did not increase long term remission rates. However, scheduled treatment did result in improved rates of endoscopic mucosal healing, fewer hospitalisations, and fewer abdominal operations than did episodic therapy after 1 year. No significant difference in adverse events was reported between groups of people receiving a single dose of infliximab followed by regular placebo over 1 year and those who continued to receive infliximab every 8 weeks, regardless of the dose used. Serious adverse events included infusion reactions, serum sickness, drug induced lupus syndrome, fatal sepsis, and tuberculosis.

Methotrexate *New*

One RCT found evidence that intramuscular methotrexate 15 mg weekly was beneficial in maintaining remission in Crohn's disease compared with placebo. Adverse effects were frequent, but no severe adverse effects were reported.

TRADE OFF BETWEEN BENEFITS AND HARMS

Azathioprine *New*

One systematic review and one RCT found that azathioprine was effective in maintaining remission in Crohn's disease. Adverse effects included pancreatitis, leukopenia and myelodysplastic syndrome, and benefits and risks must be discussed on an individual basis. A dose of 2.0–2.5 mg/kg daily is required to achieve adequate response. We found no evidence on mercaptopurine for maintaining remission in Crohn's disease.

LIKELY TO BE INEFFECTIVE OR HARMFUL

Aminosalicylates *New*

One systematic review found similar recurrence and remission rates between aminosalicylates and placebo for maintenance of remission in Crohn's disease.

Ciclosporin *New*

Two RCTs found no evidence that oral ciclosporin increased remission rates in people with quiescent or mildly active Crohn's disease compared with placebo after 1 year. People treated with ciclosporin had more adverse effects compared with placebo, and both trials reported a significantly higher withdrawal rate with ciclosporin than with placebo because of adverse events.

What are the effects of medical interventions in adults with Crohn's disease to maintain remission following surgery?

LIKELY TO BE BENEFICIAL

Azathioprine/mercaptopurine *New*

One RCT found good evidence that mercaptopurine reduced clinical and endoscopic recurrence rates in people with Crohn's disease of the ileocaecal segment 2 years after surgical resection, with a low incidence of adverse events. No evidence was found on the relative efficacy of different dosing regimens or on azathioprine.

UNKNOWN EFFECTIVENESS

Ciclosporin *New*

We found no systematic review or RCTs on the effects of ciclosporin in adults with Crohn's disease to maintain remission following surgery.

Methotrexate *New*

We found no systematic review or RCTs on the effects of methotrexate in adults with Crohn's disease to maintain remission following surgery.

Crohn's disease

UNLIKELY TO BE BENEFICIAL

Aminosalicylates *New*

A meta-analysis found mesalazine to be beneficial in maintaining remission after surgery. Two further large RCTs found a trend toward but no statistically significant benefit. We found no evidence that 4.0 g/day mesalazine is different from 2.4 g/day mesalazine in maintaining clinical remission after 12 months of therapy. There were no reports of severe adverse events.

DEFINITION Crohn's disease is a chronic inflammatory condition of the gastrointestinal tract that is characterized by transmural granulomatous inflammation, a discontinuous pattern of distribution, and fistulae.[1] Although any part of the digestive tract from mouth to anus may be affected, Crohn's disease most frequently occurs in the terminal ileum, ileocaecal region, colon, and perianal region. The disease may be further classified into inflammatory, fistulating, and stricturing disease.[2] The symptoms vary, but commonly include diarrhoea, abdominal pain, weight loss, blood or mucus in the stool, perineal pain, discharge, and irritation resulting from perianal fistulae. Extraintestinal manifestations of the disease include arthritis, uveitis, and skin rash.[3] **Diagnosis:** There is no single gold standard for the diagnosis of Crohn's disease. The diagnosis is made by clinical evaluation and a combination of endoscopic, histological, radiological, and biochemical investigations. Internationally accepted criteria for the diagnosis of Crohn's disease have been defined by Lennard-Jones.[4] After exclusion of infection, ischaemia, irradiation, and malignancy as causes for intestinal inflammation, a combination of three or more of the following findings on clinical examination, radiological investigation, endoscopy, and histological examination of endoscopic biopsies or excised specimens is considered diagnostic: chronic inflammatory lesions of the oral cavity, pylorus or duodenum, small bowel or anus; a discontinuous disease distribution (areas of abnormal mucosa separated by normal mucosa); transmural inflammation (fissuring ulcer, abscess, or fistula); fibrosis (stricture); lymphoid aggregates or aphthoid ulcers; retention of colonic mucin on biopsy in the presence of active inflammation; and granulomata (of the non-caseating type and not caused by foreign bodies). Further macroscopic findings not included in the Lennard-Jones classification that are considered diagnostic for Crohn's disease include fat wrapping, cobblestoning, and thickening of the intestinal wall. Laboratory findings that are consistent with Crohn's disease include anaemia, thrombocytosis, raised C-reactive protein levels, and a raised erythrocyte sedimentation rate.[3] It may be difficult to distinguish Crohn's disease from ulcerative colitis, particularly when only the colon is affected. In 10–15% of patients originally diagnosed as having Crohn's disease, the diagnosis changes to ulcerative colitis during the first year.[3]

INCIDENCE/ PREVALENCE Estimates of the incidence of Crohn's disease worldwide vary considerably. In Europe incidence rates range from 0.7 (Croatia) to 9.8 (Scotland) new cases per 100 000 people per year, whereas in North America these range from 3.6 (California) to 15.6 (Manitoba, Canada). The incidence of Crohn's disease is increasing, with incidence rates in the UK, Italy, Iceland, Finland, and the USA having doubled between 1955 and 1995.[5] Crohn's disease is most commonly diagnosed in late adolescence and early adulthood, but the mean age at diagnosis in North American studies ranges from 33.4 to 45 years.[6] Crohn's disease appears to affect women more commonly than men. In a systematic review of North American cohort studies of Crohn's disease, the percentage of females affected by the disease varied from 48% to 66%, and was above 50% in nine out of 11 studies.[6]

AETIOLOGY/ RISK FACTORS The true aetiology of Crohn's disease remains unknown. Current aetiological theories suggest that the disease results from a genetic predisposition, regulatory defects in the gut mucosal immune system, and environmental triggers.[7] Defects in the gut mucosal immune system are mainly related to disordered activity of T cells (a type of white blood cell). Environmental triggers that have been linked with Crohn's disease include smoking, diet (high sugar intake), and the balance of beneficial and harmful bacteria in the gut.[5] Finally, debate has raged since *Mycobacterium avium paratuberculosis* was cultured from intestinal tissue of people with Crohn's disease, with little agreement as to whether this bacterium is an infective cause of Crohn's disease.[8]

PROGNOSIS Crohn's disease is a lifelong condition, with periods of active disease alternating with periods of remission. The disease causes significant disability, with only 75% of sufferers being fully capable of work in the year of diagnosis, and 15% of people unable to work after 5–10 years of disease.[2] At least 50% of people with Crohn's disease require surgical treatment during the first 10 years of disease, and approximately 70–80% will require surgery during their lifetime.[9] People with Crohn's disease are at higher risk of developing colorectal and small bowel cancer than the normal population.[10] **Mortality:** Mortality rates among people with Crohn's disease are slightly higher than in the normal population. A systematic review of seven population-based cohort studies found that estimates of standardized mortality ratios were greater than 1 in six of the seven studies, with estimates ranging from 0.72 (95% CI 0.49 to 1.01) to 2.16 (95% CI 1.54 to 2.94).[11] The review also found that mortality rates in Crohn's disease have not changed during the past 40 years.

Please refer to clinicalevidence.com for full text and references.

Gastro-oesophageal reflux disease

Search date July 2005

Paul Moayyedi, Brendan Delaney, and David Forman

What are the effects of initial treatment of gastro-oesophageal reflux disease associated with oesophagitis?

BENEFICIAL

H_2 receptor antagonists

One systematic review found that H_2 receptor antagonists reduced the risk of persistent oesophagitis compared with placebo, but they were not as effective as proton pump inhibitors. One RCT found no significant difference in endoscopic healing between cimetidine and antacids at 8 weeks. Another RCT found that ranitidine improved heartburn symptoms more than antacids at 12 weeks.

Proton pump inhibitors

One systematic review, one additional RCT, and three subsequent RCTs found evidence that proton pump inhibitors increased healing compared with placebo or H_2 receptor antagonists. One systematic review found that esomeprazole 40 mg daily increased healing at 4 weeks compared with omeprazole 20 mg daily. One RCT found that esomeprazole 40 mg daily increased healing at 8 weeks compared with pantoprazole 40 mg once daily. RCTs found no significant differences in clinical benefit among other proton pump inhibitors.

UNKNOWN EFFECTIVENESS

Antacids/alginates

Two RCTs provided limited evidence that antacids reduced symptom scores at 4–8 weeks compared with placebo, but neither found a significant difference in endoscopic healing. We found limited evidence on the effects of antacids compared with H_2 receptor antagonists. One RCT found no significant difference between antacids and cimetidine in endoscopic healing at 8 weeks. A second RCT found that antacids were less effective than ranitidine for heartburn symptoms at 12 weeks.

Lifestyle advice/modification

Small RCTs provided insufficient evidence on the effects of raising the head of the bed or weight loss for the treatment of reflux oesophagitis. We found no RCTs on the effects of reducing coffee intake, stopping smoking, reducing alcohol intake, or reducing fatty food intake.

LIKELY TO BE INEFFECTIVE OR HARMFUL

Motility stimulants

We found one RCT investigating cisapride, but no RCTs of other motility stimulants (domperidone or metoclopramide). The use of cisapride has been restricted in some countries because of concerns about heart rhythm abnormalities. The RCT found that cisapride increased endoscopic healing compared with placebo at 12 weeks.

What are the effects of maintenance treatment of gastro-oesophageal reflux disease associated with oesophagitis?

BENEFICIAL

Proton pump inhibitors

One systematic review and one subsequent RCT found that standard or low dose proton pump inhibitors (omeprazole, lansoprazole, pantoprazole rabeprazole, and esomeprazole) reduced relapse of oesophagitis and reflux symptoms compared with placebo or H_2 receptor antagonist at 6–12 months. One systematic review and one subsequent RCT found that standard dose proton pump inhibitor reduced relapse of oesophagitis or relapse symptoms compared with low dose proton pump inhibitor at 6–12 months. The systematic review found no consistent evidence of a difference between different dosage schedules for proton pump inhibitors, between high versus standard dose proton pump inhibitors, or between different proton pump inhibitors in relapse.

LIKELY TO BE BENEFICIAL

H_2 receptor antagonists

One systematic review and one additional RCT found no significant difference between H_2 receptor antagonists and placebo in relapse of oesophagitis, although the review found a non-significant trend toward a reduction in relapse with H_2 receptor antagonists. The review found that H_2 receptor antagonists reduced relapse of reflux symptoms compared with placebo. RCTs found that H_2 receptor antagonists are less effective than proton pump inhibitors for maintaining remission at up to 12 months. One RCT found that nizatidine increased maintenance of remission compared with famotidine.

TRADE OFF BETWEEN BENEFITS AND HARMS

Laparoscopic surgery

One systematic review identified no fully published RCTs comparing laparoscopic surgery versus medical treatment for maintenance of remission. One systematic review and one subsequent RCT found no significant difference in recurrence rate between laparoscopic fundoplication and open fundoplication. However, they found that laparoscopic fundoplication was associated with lower operative morbidity and a shorter postoperative hospital stay. The benefit of antireflux surgery in controlling symptoms must be balanced against the small risk of operative mortality (< 1%) associated with this procedure.

Open surgery

RCTs found that open Nissen fundoplication improved the endoscopic grade of oesophagitis compared with medical treatment in people with chronic gastro-oesophageal reflux disease and oesophagitis at 3–38 months. However, longer term follow up from one RCT found no significant difference in endoscopic appearance between surgery and medical treatment at 10 years. One systematic review and one subsequent RCT found no significant difference in recurrence rate between laparoscopic fundoplication and open fundoplication. However, they found that laparoscopic fundoplication was associated with lower operative morbidity and a shorter postoperative hospital stay. The benefit of antireflux surgery in controlling symptoms must be balanced against the small risk of operative mortality (< 1%) associated with this procedure.

Gastro-oesophageal reflux disease

UNKNOWN EFFECTIVENESS

Antacids/alginates

We found no RCTs on the effects of antacids/alginates on the long term management of reflux oesophagitis.

Lifestyle advice/modification

We found no RCTs on the effects of lifestyle advice/modification (reducing coffee intake, stopping smoking, reducing alcohol intake, reducing fatty food intake, or raising the head of the bed) on the long term management of reflux oesophagitis.

LIKELY TO BE INEFFECTIVE OR HARMFUL

Motility stimulants

We found one systematic review investigating cisapride, but found no RCTs of other motility stimulants (domperidone or metoclopramide). The use of cisapride has been restricted in some countries because of concerns about heart rhythm abnormalities. The review found that cisapride significantly reduced relapse of oesophagitis. It found no significant difference in relapse of reflux symptoms between cisapride and placebo.

DEFINITION Gastro-oesophageal reflux disease (GORD) is defined as reflux of gastroduodenal contents into the oesophagus, causing symptoms that are sufficient to interfere with quality of life.[1] People with GORD often have symptoms of heartburn and acid regurgitation.[2] GORD can be classified according to the results of upper gastrointestinal endoscopy. Currently, the most validated method is the Los Angeles classification, in which an endoscopy showing mucosal breaks in the distal oesophagus indicate the presence of oesophagitis, which is graded in severity from grade A (mucosal breaks of < 5 mm in the oesophagus) to grade D (circumferential breaks in the oesophageal mucosa).[1,3] Alternatively, severity may be graded according to the Savary–Miller classification (grade I: linear, non-confluent erosions, to grade IV: severe ulceration or stricture).[4]

INCIDENCE/ PREVALENCE Surveys from Europe and the USA suggest that 20–25% of the population have symptoms of GORD, and 7% have heartburn daily.[5,6] In primary care settings, about 25–40% of people with GORD have oesophagitis on endoscopy, but most have endoscopy negative reflux disease.[3]

AETIOLOGY/ RISK FACTORS We found no evidence of clear predictive factors for GORD. Obesity is reported to be a risk factor for GORD but epidemiological data are conflicting.[7,8] Smoking and alcohol are also thought to predispose to GORD, but observational data are limited.[8,9] It has been suggested that some foods, such as coffee, mints, dietary fat, onions, citrus fruits, or tomatoes, may predispose to GORD.[10] However, we found insufficient data on the role of these factors. We found limited evidence that drugs that relax the lower oesophageal sphincter, such as calcium channel blockers, may promote GORD.[11] Twin studies suggest that there may be a genetic predisposition to GORD.[9]

PROGNOSIS GORD is a chronic condition, with about 80% of people relapsing once medication is discontinued.[12] Many people therefore require long term medical treatment or surgery. Endoscopy negative reflux disease remains stable, with a minority of people developing oesophagitis over time.[13] However, people with severe oesophagitis may develop complications such as oesophageal stricture or Barrett's oesophagus.[1]

Please refer to clinicalevidence.com for full text and references.

Haemorrhoids

Search date March 2005

R Justin Davies

What are the effects of treatments for haemorrhoidal disease?

BENEFICIAL

Rubber band ligation

One RCT found that fewer people with second degree haemorrhoids had persistent symptoms after rubber band ligation compared with no treatment at 48 months. Rubber band ligation was found to be similarly effective in control of symptoms in three RCTs as infrared coagulation in people with mainly first and second degree haemorrhoids. A fourth RCT found that rubber band ligation was more effective in control of bleeding. The four RCTs found conflicting results with regards to postoperative pain. Three RCTs found that rubber band ligation was better than injection sclerotherapy in a variety of outcomes (pain, repeat treatment, prolapse, bleeding) in people with mainly second degree haemorrhoids; however, rubber band ligation was associated with more immediate adverse effects. One RCT found that more people who had rubber band ligation had bleeding in the short term compared with stapled haemorrhoidectomy in people with mainly third degree haemorrhoids, although there was no significant difference after 2 months; however, it found that there were less adverse effects with rubber band ligation. Two RCTs found no significant difference between rubber band ligation and open excisional haemorrhoidectomy in bleeding; one of the RCTs found that rubber band ligation was less effective for prolapse in third degree haemorrhoids, but found no significant difference in prolapse in second degree haemorrhoids.

LIKELY TO BE BENEFICIAL

Closed haemorrhoidectomy

One RCT found no significant difference between closed haemorrhoidectomy and haemorrhoidal artery ligation in relief of symptoms in people with first to fourth degree haemorrhoids; however, length of hospital stay and postoperative complications were increased with closed haemorrhoidectomy. One systematic review and four subsequent RCTs comparing conventional surgery (open excisional and closed) with stapled haemorrhoidectomy found mixed results for symptom reduction and length of hospital stay. However, the systematic review and RCTs found that postoperative pain and complications were greater with conventional surgery (open excisional and closed haemorrhoidectomy). Seven RCTs found no significant difference in length of hospital stay and symptom relief between closed haemorrhoidectomy and open excisional haemorrhoidectomy in people with mainly third and fourth degree haemorrhoids; the RCTs also found mixed results with postoperative pain.

Infrared coagulation/photocoagulation

One RCT found no significant difference between infrared coagulation and injection sclerotherapy in reduction of symptoms or adverse effects for people with first and second degree haemorrhoids. Another RCT found that infrared coagulation was more effective at reducing symptoms than injection sclerotherapy, and caused less immediate postoperative pain. Infrared coagulation was found to be similarly effective in control of symptoms in three RCTs than ▶

Haemorrhoids

rubber band ligation in people with mainly first and second degree haemorrhoids. However, a fourth RCT found that infrared coagulation was less effective in control of bleeding. The four RCTs found conflicting results with regards to postoperative pain.

Open excisional (Milligan-Morgan/diathermy) haemorrhoidectomy

Two RCTs found no significant difference between open excisional haemorrhoidectomy and rubber band ligation in bleeding; one of the RCTs found that open excisional haemorrhoidectomy was more effective for prolapse in third degree haemorrhoids, but found no significant difference in prolapse in second degree haemorrhoids. Two RCTs found that there were longer hospital stays with open excisional haemorrhoidectomy compared with radiofrequency ablation in people with third degree haemorrhoids, and that postoperative pain was worse. One RCT also found longer hospital stays and worse postoperative pain with open excisional haemorrhoidectomy compared with semi-open haemorrhoidectomy (degree of haemorrhoids unknown). Seven RCTs found no significant difference in length of hospital stay and symptom relief between open excisional haemorrhoidectomy and closed haemorrhoidectomy in people with mainly third and fourth degree haemorrhoids; the RCTs also found mixed results with postoperative pain. Two RCTs which compared open excisional haemorrhoidectomy by conventional procedures with other procedures (LigaSure™, Harmonic scalpel®, bipolar scissors) found conflicting results for length of hospital stay. They found no significant difference with postoperative pain. One systematic review and four subsequent RCTs comparing conventional surgery (open excisional and closed) with stapled haemorrhoidectomy found mixed results for symptom reduction and length of hospital stay. However, the systematic review and RCTs found that postoperative pain and complications were greater with conventional haemorrhoidectomy (open excisional and closed).

TRADE OFF BETWEEN BENEFITS AND HARMS

Stapled haemorrhoidectomy

One RCT found that people who had stapled haemorrhoidectomy had less bleeding in the short term compared with rubber band ligation in those with mainly third degree haemorrhoids, although there was no significant difference after 2 months; however, it found that there were more adverse effects with stapled haemorrhoidectomy. One systematic review and four subsequent RCTs comparing stapled haemorrhoidectomy and conventional surgery (open excisional and closed) found mixed results for the outcomes of reduction in symptoms and length of hospital stay. However, the systematic review and RCTs found that postoperative pain and complications were less with stapled haemorrhoidectomy.

UNKNOWN EFFECTIVENESS

Haemorrhoidal artery ligation

One RCT found no significant difference between haemorrhoidal artery ligation and closed haemorrhoidectomy in relief of symptoms in people with first to fourth degree haemorrhoids; however, length of hospital stay and postoperative complications were improved with haemorrhoidal artery ligation.

Injection sclerotherapy

One RCT found no significant difference between injection sclerotherapy and education and advice in bleeding in people with first and second degree haemorrhoids; however, less people were given bulk forming evacuant with injection sclerotherapy. One RCT found no significant difference between injection sclerotherapy and infrared coagulation in reduction of symptoms or adverse events for people with first and second degree haemorrhoids. Another RCT found that injection sclerotherapy was less effective at reducing symptoms than infrared coagulation and caused more immediate postoperative pain. Three RCTs found that injection sclerotherapy was worse than rubber band ligation in a variety of outcomes (pain, repeat treatment, prolapse, and bleeding) in people with mainly second degree haemorrhoids; however, injection sclerotherapy was associated with less immediate adverse effects.

DEFINITION Haemorrhoids are cushions of submucosal vascular tissue located in the anal canal starting just distal to the dentate line. These vascular cushions are a normal anatomical structure of the anal canal, and their existence does not necessarily indicate actual haemorrhoidal disease. Haemorrhoidal disease occurs when there are symptoms such as bleeding, prolapse, pain, thrombosis, mucus discharge, and pruritus. Rectal bleeding is the most common manifestation of haemorrhoidal disease. The bleeding tends to be bright red in nature and occurs on the toilet tissue or drips into the toilet bowl. Haemorrhoids can occur internally, externally, or can be mixed (internal and external components). If prolapse occurs, a perianal mass may be evident with defecation. Haemorrhoids are traditionally graded into four degrees. **First degree (or grade):** The haemorrhoids bleed with defecation but do not prolapse. First degree haemorrhoids associated with mild symptoms are usually secondary to leakage of blood from mildly inflamed, thin walled veins or arterioles. Conservative management with dietary manipulation (addition of fibre) and attention to anal hygiene is often adequate. Recurrent rectal bleeding may require ablation of the vessels with non-surgical ablative techniques, such as injection sclerotherapy, infrared coagulation, or rubber band ligation. Infrared coagulation is used infrequently in clinical practice in the UK today, whereas rubber band ligation and injection sclerotherapy are very commonly used. **Second degree:** The haemorrhoids prolapse with defecation and reduce spontaneously. Second degree haemorrhoids can be treated with rubber band ligation or other non-surgical ablative techniques. **Third degree:** The haemorrhoids prolapse and require manual reduction. In third degree haemorrhoids, where there is significant destruction of the suspensory ligaments, relocation and fixation of the mucosa to the underlying muscular wall is generally necessary. Prolapse can be treated with rubber band ligation initially, but haemorrhoidectomy may be required, especially if prolapse is seen in more than one position. **Fourth degree:** The haemorrhoids prolapse and cannot be reduced. If treatment is necessary, fourth degree haemorrhoids require haemorrhoidectomy. Haemorrhoids are thought to be associated with chronic constipation, straining to defecate, pregnancy, and low dietary fibre. Frequency, duration, and severity of haemorrhoidal symptoms, such as bleeding, prolapse, or both, determine the type of treatment. Often, absent or episodic symptoms do not require treatment, and the presence of symptoms does not mandate invasive treatment. Some people choose to decline treatment if they can be appropriately reassured that there is no other more serious cause for their symptoms.

INCIDENCE/ PREVALENCE Haemorrhoids are thought to be common in the general population, but we found no reliable data regarding incidence. Data from the National Center for Health Statistics found that 10 million people in the USA complained of haemorrhoids, leading to a prevalence rate of 4.4%.[1] However, a true figure for prevalence of haemorrhoids is unknown, as there will be many people with the condition who never consult with a medical practitioner.

AETIOLOGY/ RISK FACTORS The cause of haemorrhoids remains unknown, but it is thought that the downward slide of the anal vascular cushions is the most likely explanation.[2]

Haemorrhoids

Other possible causes include straining to defecate, erect posture, and obstruction of venous return from raised intra-abdominal pressure, for example, in pregnancy. It is thought that there may be a hereditary predisposition in some individuals, thought possibly to be owing to a congenital weakness of the venous wall.

DIAGNOSIS Accurate diagnosis requires a detailed history, thorough examination, and proctoscopic inspection of the anal canal and distal rectum. In those with symptoms not typical of haemorrhoids, it is important to exclude other conditions such as colorectal cancer or inflammatory bowel disease.

PROGNOSIS The prognosis is generally excellent, as many symptomatic episodes will often settle with conservative measures only. If further intervention is required, the prognosis remains very good, although recurrent symptoms may occur. Early in the clinical course of haemorrhoids, prolapse reduces spontaneously. Later, the prolapse may require manual reduction and might result in mucus discharge which can cause pruritus ani. Pain is usually not a symptom of internal haemorrhoids unless the haemorrhoids are prolapsed. Pain may be associated with thrombosed external haemorrhoids. Death from bleeding haemorrhoids is an incredibly rare event.

Please refer to clinicalevidence.com for full text and references.

Helicobacter pylori infection

Search date September 2005

Brendan Delaney, Paul Moayyedi, and David Forman

What are the effects of H pylori *eradication treatment in people with a proven duodenal ulcer?*

BENEFICIAL

H pylori eradication for healing and preventing recurrence of duodenal ulcer

One systematic review found that *H pylori* eradication treatment increased duodenal ulcer healing compared with no treatment, and that *H pylori* eradication treatment plus 1 month of antisecretory drug treatment increased duodenal ulcer healing compared with antisecretory drugs alone for 1 month. It also found that eradication treatment reduced recurrence compared with no treatment, although there was no significant difference in recurrence between eradication treatment plus antisecretory drug treatment for 1 month and ongoing antisecretory maintenance treatment alone in people with healed duodenal ulcers. One systematic review found that *H pylori* eradication treatment reduced the risk of bleeding compared with short term antisecretory treatment alone, or compared with short term antisecretory treatment plus subsequent antisecretory maintenance treatment in people with duodenal or gastric ulcer.

What are the effects of H pylori *eradication treatment for people with a proven gastric ulcer?*

BENEFICIAL

H pylori eradication for preventing recurrence of gastric ulcer

One systematic review found no significant difference in endoscopic healing between *H pylori* eradication treatment plus antisecretory drugs and antisecretory drugs alone. It found that *H pylori* eradication treatment reduced recurrence compared with no treatment. One systematic review found that *H pylori* eradication treatment reduced the risk of bleeding compared with short term antisecretory treatment alone, or compared with short term antisecretory treatment plus subsequent antisecretory maintenance treatment in people with duodenal or gastric ulcer.

What are the effects of H pylori *eradication treatment in people with non-steroidal anti-inflammatory drug (NSAID) related peptic ulcers?*

UNKNOWN EFFECTIVENESS

H pylori eradication for healing of NSAID related peptic ulcers

One RCT found no significant difference between *H pylori* eradication and antisecretory treatment alone in healing of peptic ulcer in people who were taking non-steroidal anti-inflammatory drugs and had bleeding peptic ulcers. ▶

Helicobacter pylori infection

What are the effects of H pylori *eradication treatment for preventing non-steroidal anti-inflammatory drug (NSAID) related peptic ulcers in people with previous ulcers or dyspepsia?*

UNKNOWN EFFECTIVENESS

***H pylori* eradication for prevention of NSAID related peptic ulcers in people with previous ulcers or dyspepsia**

One RCT found that, in people with *H pylori* infection and taking non-steroidal anti-inflammatory drugs who had previous ulcers or dyspepsia, *H pylori* eradication treatment reduced the risk of developing new peptic ulcers compared with omeprazole at 6 months. Another RCT found that, in people with *H pylori* infection and with a previous bleeding ulcer, *H pylori* eradication was less effective than maintenance treatment with omeprazole in preventing a recurrent bleeding peptic ulcer in people taking naproxen, but there was no significant difference between treatments in people taking low dose aspirin.

What are the effects of H pylori *eradication treatment for preventing non-steroidal anti-inflammatory drug (NSAID) related peptic ulcers in people without previous ulcers?*

LIKELY TO BE BENEFICIAL

***H pylori* eradication for the prevention of non-steroidal anti-inflammatory drug (NSAID) related peptic ulcers in people without previous ulcers (more effective than placebo and as effective as antisecretory treatment)**

One RCT found that *H pylori* eradication treatment reduced the risk of non-steroidal anti-inflammatory drug related peptic ulcers compared with no treatment in people without previous ulcers. Another RCT found that *H pylori* eradication reduced the risk of non-steroidal anti-inflammatory drug related peptic ulcers compared with placebo, but was not significantly different from antisecretory treatment alone.

What are the effects of H pylori *eradication treatment in people with proved gastro-oesophageal reflux disease?*

UNLIKELY TO BE BENEFICIAL

***H pylori* eradication in *H pylori* positive people with gastro-oesophageal reflux disease**

Two RCTs in *H pylori* positive people with gastro-oesophageal reflux disease found no significant difference between *H pylori* eradication treatment and placebo in symptoms over 2 years.

What are the effects of H pylori eradication treatment in people with B cell lymphoma of the stomach?

UNKNOWN EFFECTIVENESS

H pylori eradication for gastric B cell lymphoma

We found no RCTs of *H pylori* eradication treatment in people with B cell gastric lymphoma. Observational studies provided limited evidence that 60–93% of people with localised low grade B cell lymphoma experience tumour regression in response to *H pylori* eradication treatment, possibly avoiding, or delaying, the need for radical surgery, radiotherapy, or chemotherapy.

What are the effects of H pylori eradication treatment on the risk of developing gastric cancer?

UNKNOWN EFFECTIVENESS

H pylori eradication for prevention of gastric cancer (adenocarcinoma)

One RCT in people positive for *H pylori* found no significant difference in the risk of gastric cancer between eradication treatment and placebo at 7.5 years. In people with gastric atrophy or intestinal metaplasia, one RCT found that *H pylori* eradication increased the regression of high risk lesions compared with no eradication. However, the RCT did not assess the effects of eradication treatment on development of gastric cancer. We found consistent evidence from observational studies of an association between *H pylori* infection and increased risk of distal gastric adenocarcinoma.

What are the effects of H pylori eradication treatment in people with proved non-ulcer dyspepsia?

BENEFICIAL

H pylori eradication for non-ulcer dyspepsia

One systematic review in people with non-ulcer dyspepsia found that *H pylori* eradication reduced dyspeptic symptoms at 3–12 months compared with placebo.

What are the effects of H pylori eradication treatment in people with uninvestigated dyspepsia?

BENEFICIAL

H pylori eradication in people with uninvestigated dyspepsia (more effective than placebo)*

One RCT in people with *H pylori* found that *H pylori* eradication increased relief from dyspeptic symptoms at 1 year compared with placebo. One systematic review in people at low risk of gastrointestinal malignancy found a small reduction in dyspeptic symptoms at 1 year with management based on initial endoscopy compared with *H pylori* testing plus eradication. Delaying endoscopy is not safe in people at increased risk of gastrointestinal malignancy.

*Endoscopy should not be delayed in people at risk of malignancy.

Helicobacter pylori infection

Do H pylori *eradication treatments differ in their effects?*

LIKELY TO BE BENEFICIAL

Quadruple regimen (as effective as triple regimen)

Two RCTs found that quadruple treatments were as effective as triple treatments for eradication of *H pylori* in people with or without a history of duodenal ulcer.

Three day quadruple regimen (as effective as 1 week triple regimen but with fewer adverse effects)

One RCT comparing a 3 day quadruple regimen versus a 1 week triple regimen found no significant difference in *H pylori* eradication at 6 weeks. However, it found that people taking the 3 day quadruple regimen experienced fewer days of adverse effects.

Triple regimen (more effective than dual regimen)

We found no systematic review or RCTs of the effects of triple regimens compared with dual regimens on dyspeptic symptom scores, proportion of individuals with symptoms, quality of life, or mortality. One systematic review found that triple regimens eradicated *H pylori* from more people than dual regimens.

Two week triple regimen (more effective than 1 week triple regimen)

One systematic review found that 14 days of treatment with proton pump inhibitor based triple regimens increased *H pylori* eradication rates compared with 7 days of treatment with the same regimen.

UNKNOWN EFFECTIVENESS

Different triple regimens (relative effects of different drug combinations on clinical outcomes unclear)

We found no systematic review or RCTs of the effects of different triple regimens on dyspeptic symptom scores, proportion of individuals with symptoms, quality of life, or mortality. One systematic review found that increasing the clarithromycin dose in a triple regimen containing amoxicillin increased *H pylori* eradication. However, increasing the clarithromycin dose in a triple regimen containing metronidazole had no significant additional effect on *H pylori* eradication. Another systematic review found that a triple regimen of metronidazole plus clarithromycin plus ranitidine bismuth increased eradication at 5–7 days compared with a triple regimen containing amoxicillin plus clarithromycin plus ranitidine bismuth.

DEFINITION *Helicobacter pylori* is a Gram negative flagellated spiral bacterium found in the stomach. Infection with *H pylori* is predominantly acquired in childhood. *H pylori* infection is not associated with a specific type of dyspeptic symptom. The organism is associated with lifelong chronic gastritis and may cause other gastroduodenal disorders.[1] *H pylori* can be identified indirectly by serology or by the C13 urea breath test. The urea breath test is more accurate than serology, with a sensitivity and specificity greater than 95%, and indicates active infection, whereas serology may lack specificity and cannot be used reliably as a test of active infection. Thus, the urea breath test is the test of choice where prevalence, and hence predictive value of serology may be low, or where a "test of cure" is required. In some areas stool antigen tests that have a similar performance to the urea breath test are now available. **Population:** This chapter focuses on *H pylori* positive people throughout.

Helicobacter pylori infection

INCIDENCE/ PREVALENCE In the developed world, *H pylori* prevalence rates vary with year of birth and social class. Prevalence in many developed countries tends to be much higher (50–80%) in individuals born before 1950 compared with prevalence (< 20%) in individuals born more recently.[2] In many developing countries, the infection has a high prevalence (80–95%) irrespective of the period of birth.[3] Adult prevalence is believed to represent the persistence of a historically higher rate of infection acquired in childhood, rather than increasing acquisition of infection during life.

AETIOLOGY/ RISK FACTORS Overcrowded conditions associated with childhood poverty lead to increased transmission and higher prevalence rates. Adult reinfection rates are low — less than 1% a year.[3]

PROGNOSIS *H pylori* infection is believed to be causally related to the development of duodenal and gastric ulceration, B cell gastric lymphoma, and distal gastric cancer. About 15% of people infected with *H pylori* will develop a peptic ulcer, and 1% of people will develop gastric cancer during their lifetime.[4] One systematic review of observational studies (search date 2000, 16 studies, 1625 people) found that the frequency of peptic ulcer disease in people taking non-steroidal anti-inflammatory drugs (NSAIDs) was greater in those who were *H pylori* positive than in those who were *H pylori* negative (peptic ulcer: 341/817 [41.7%] in *H pylori* positive NSAID users *v* 209/808 [25.9%] in *H pylori* negative NSAID users, OR 2.12, 95% CI 1.68 to 2.67).[5]

Please refer to clinicalevidence.com for full text and references.

Inguinal hernia

Search date September 2005

Sanjay Purkayastha, Andre Chow, Thanos Athanasiou, Paris Tekkis, Ara Darzi

What are the effects of elective treatment for primary unilateral inguinal hernia in adults?

BENEFICIAL

Open mesh repair (reduced recurrence compared with open suture repair, with no increase in surgical complications)

We found no systematic review, RCTs, or cohort studies of sufficient quality comparing open mesh repair versus expectant management. One systematic review found that open mesh repair reduced inguinal hernia recurrence and slightly reduced the length of hospital stay compared with open suture repair. The review and one subsequent RCT found no significant difference in surgical complications between open mesh repair and open suture repair. One systematic review found that open mesh repair increased persisting pain, length of hospital stay, time to return to normal activity, haematoma, and persisting numbness compared with totally extraperitoneal (TEP) laparoscopic repair. It found no significant difference between open mesh repair and TEP laparoscopic repair in recurrence, seroma, or postoperative superficial infection. A subsequent RCT found no difference between TEP laparoscopic repair and open mesh repair in recurrence, postoperative analgesic requirements, or postoperative complications. It found that open mesh repair increased the time taken to return to work compared with TEP laparoscopic repair. One systematic review found that open mesh repair increased persisting pain at 1 year, and time to return to usual activities compared with transabdominal preperitoneal (TAPP) laparoscopic repair. It found no significant difference in recurrence between TAPP laparoscopic repair and open mesh repair. Two subsequent RCTs found that open mesh repair increased postoperative pain and length of hospital stay compared with TAPP. Adverse effects of open mesh repair and TAPP laparoscopic repair were similar, although TAPP laparoscopic repair increased the risk of seroma and decreased postoperative numbness and superficial infection compared with open mesh repair.

Totally extraperitoneal (TEP) laparoscopic repair (reduced pain and time to return to usual activities compared with open repair)

We found no systematic review, RCTs, or cohort studies of sufficient quality comparing totally extraperitoneal (TEP) laparoscopic repair versus expectant management. One systematic review found that TEP laparoscopic repair reduced pain after 3 months and slightly reduced length of hospital stay compared with open suture repair. It found no significant difference in risk of recurrence or time to return to normal activities. One subsequent RCT found no significant difference between TEP laparoscopic repair and open suture repair in recurrence, length of hospital stay, or groin pain. Adverse effects were similar for TEP laparoscopic repair and open suture repair, although the review found that TEP laparoscopic repair increased the risk of seroma but decreased the risk of infection compared with open suture repair. One systematic review found that TEP laparoscopic repair reduced length of hospital stay, time to return to normal activity, persisting pain, persisting numbness, and haematoma compared with open mesh repair. The review found no significant difference between TEP laparoscopic repair and open mesh repair in hernia recurrence, seroma, or postoperative superficial infection. A subsequent RCT found no difference ▶

between TEP laparoscopic repair and open mesh repair in recurrence, postoperative analgesic requirements, or postoperative complications. It found that TEP laparoscopic repair reduced time to return to work compared with open mesh repair.

Transabdominal preperitoneal (TAPP) laparoscopic repair (reduced pain and time to return to usual activities compared with open repair)

We found no systematic review, RCTs, or cohort studies of sufficient quality comparing transabdominal preperitoneal (TAPP) laparoscopic repair versus expectant management. One systematic review and subsequent RCTs found that TAPP laparoscopic repair decreased postoperative pain and time to return to usual activities compared with open suture repair. The systematic review found limited evidence that TAPP laparoscopic repair reduced recurrence compared with open suture repair; however, two subsequent RCTs found no significant difference in recurrence. Adverse effects of TAPP laparoscopic repair and open suture repair were similar. One systematic review found that TAPP laparoscopic repair reduced persisting pain at 1 year and time to return to usual activities compared with open mesh repair. It found no significant difference in recurrence between TAPP laparoscopic repair and open mesh repair. Two subsequent RCTs found that TAPP reduced postoperative pain and length of hospital stay compared with open mesh repair. Adverse effects of open mesh repair and TAPP laparoscopic repair were similar, although TAPP laparoscopic repair increased the risk of seroma and decreased postoperative numbness and superficial infection compared with open mesh repair.

LIKELY TO BE BENEFICIAL

Open suture repair (conventional, well established surgical technique but less effective for improving clinically important outcomes than open mesh repair, laparoscopic repair)*

Clinical experience and consensus opinion suggest that surgery is effective for primary unilateral inguinal hernia. Open suture repair is a well established surgical technique. However, we found no systematic review, RCTs, or cohort studies of sufficient quality comparing open suture repair versus expectant management. One systematic review found that open suture repair was less effective at reducing inguinal hernia recurrence than open mesh repair and that it increased length of hospital stay. The review and one subsequent RCT found no significant difference in surgical complications between open suture repair and open mesh repair. One systematic review found that open suture repair increased pain after 3 months and increased length of hospital stay slightly compared with totally extraperitoneal (TEP) laparoscopic repair. It found no significant difference in risk of recurrence or time to return to normal activities. One subsequent RCT found no significant difference between TEP laparoscopic repair and open suture repair in recurrence, length of hospital stay, or groin pain. Adverse effects were similar for TEP laparoscopic repair and open suture repair, although the review found that open suture repair decreased the risk of seroma but increased the risk of infection compared with TEP laparoscopic repair. One systematic review and subsequent RCTs found that open suture repair increased postoperative pain, and time to return to usual activities compared with transabdominal preperitoneal (TAPP) laparoscopic repair. The systematic review found limited evidence that open suture repair was less effective at reducing recurrence compared with TAPP laparoscopic repair; however, two subsequent RCTs found no significant difference. Adverse effects of open suture repair and TAPP laparoscopic repair were similar.

Inguinal hernia

UNKNOWN EFFECTIVENESS

Expectant management

We found no systematic review, RCTs, or cohort studies of sufficient quality of expectant management in people with unilateral inguinal hernia.

What are the effects of elective treatment for primary bilateral inguinal hernia in adults?

LIKELY TO BE BENEFICIAL

Open mesh repair (may reduce length of hospital stay compared with open suture repair)

We found no systematic review, RCTs, or cohort studies of sufficient quality comparing open mesh repair versus expectant management in people with bilateral inguinal hernia. One systematic review found limited evidence that open mesh repair slightly reduced length of hospital stay compared with open suture repair but found insufficient evidence to compare other clinical effects. One systematic review found no significant difference between open mesh repair and totally extraperitoneal (TEP) laparoscopic repair in return to usual activities, hernia recurrence, persisting pain, seroma, haematoma, superficial infection, or persisting numbness. One systematic review found limited evidence that open mesh repair increased time taken to return to normal activities, persisting numbness, and superficial infection compared with transabdominal preperitoneal (TAPP) laparoscopic repair. It found no significant difference between open mesh repair and TAPP laparoscopic repair in length of hospital stay, persisting pain, haematoma, seroma, or hernia recurrence.

Open suture repair (conventional, well established surgical technique but may be less effective in improving clinically important outcomes than open mesh repair or transabdominal preperitoneal (TAPP) laparoscopic repair)*

Clinical experience and consensus opinion suggest that surgery is an effective treatment for bilateral inguinal hernia. Open suture repair is a well established surgical technique. However, we found no systematic review, RCTs, or cohort studies of sufficient quality comparing open suture repair versus expectant management. One systematic review found limited evidence that open suture repair slightly increased length of hospital stay compared with open mesh repair but found insufficient evidence to compare other clinical effects. One systematic review found limited evidence that open suture repair increased the time taken to return to normal activities compared with transabdominal preperitoneal (TAPP) laparoscopic repair. It found insufficient evidence to compare other clinical effects and insufficient data to compare benefits of open suture repair versus totally extraperitoneal (TEP) laparoscopic repair.

Totally extraperitoneal (TEP) laparoscopic repair (similar outcomes to open mesh repair)

We found no systematic review, RCTs, or cohort studies of sufficient quality comparing totally extraperitoneal laparoscopic (TEP) repair versus expectant management in people with bilateral inguinal hernia. One systematic review found insufficient evidence to compare clinical effects of TEP laparoscopic repair versus open suture repair. One systematic review found no significant difference between TEP laparoscopic repair and open mesh repair in return to usual activities, hernia recurrence, persisting pain, seroma, haematoma, superficial infection, or persisting numbness.

Transabdominal preperitoneal (TAPP) laparoscopic repair (may reduce time to return to normal activities compared with open repair)

We found no systematic review, RCTs, or cohort studies of sufficient quality comparing transabdominal preperitoneal (TAPP) laparoscopic repair versus expectant management in people with bilateral inguinal hernia. One systematic review found limited evidence that TAPP laparoscopic repair reduced the time taken to return to normal activities compared with open suture repair. It found insufficient evidence to compare other clinical effects. One systematic review found limited evidence that TAPP laparoscopic repair reduced time taken to return to normal activities, persisting numbness, and superficial infection compared with open mesh repair. It found no significant difference between TAPP laparoscopic repair and open mesh repair in length of hospital stay, persisting pain, haematoma, seroma, or hernia recurrence.

UNKNOWN EFFECTIVENESS

Expectant management

We found no systematic review, RCTs, or cohort studies of sufficient quality of expectant management in people with bilateral inguinal hernia.

What are the effects of elective treatment for recurrent inguinal hernia in adults?

LIKELY TO BE BENEFICIAL

Open mesh repair (slightly reduced length of hospital stay compared with open suture repair; other effects uncertain)

We found no systematic review, RCTs, or cohort studies of sufficient quality comparing open mesh repair versus expectant management. One systematic review found limited evidence that open mesh repair slightly reduced length of hospital stay compared with open suture repair in people with recurrent inguinal hernia. However, the review found insufficient evidence to compare effects on pain, time to return to usual activities, further recurrence, or other complications of surgery. One systematic review found that open mesh repair increased haematoma formation compared with totally extraperitoneal (TEP) laparoscopic repair. It also found limited evidence that open mesh repair increased the time taken to return to usual activities compared with TEP laparoscopic repair. However, it found no significant difference in hernia recurrence, length of hospital stay, seroma, persisting numbness, or persisting pain. The review found that open mesh repair increased the time taken to return to usual activities compared with transabdominal preperitoneal (TAPP) laparoscopic repair. However, it found no significant difference between open mesh repair and TAPP laparoscopic repair in haematoma, seroma, superficial infection, visceral injury, length of hospital stay, persisting pain, or hernia recurrence.

Totally extraperitoneal (TEP) laparoscopic repair (may reduce time to return to normal activities compared with open mesh repair)

We found no systematic review, RCTs, or cohort studies of sufficient quality comparing totally extraperitoneal (TEP) laparoscopic repair versus expectant management in people with recurrent inguinal hernia. One systematic review found limited evidence that TEP laparoscopic repair reduced the time taken to return to usual activities compared with open mesh repair. It also found that TEP laparoscopic repair reduced haematoma formation. However, it found no significant difference in hernia recurrence, length of hospital stay, seroma, persisting numbness, or persisting pain. One systematic review found insufficient data to compare the effects of TEP laparoscopic repair versus open suture repair.

Transabdominal preperitoneal (TAPP) laparoscopic repair (may reduce time to return to normal activities compared with open repair; other effects uncertain)

We found no systematic review, RCTs, or cohort studies of sufficient quality comparing transabdominal preperitoneal (TAPP) laparoscopic repair versus expectant management. One systematic review found that although there was a trend towards a reduction in time taken to return to normal activities with TAPP laparoscopic repair compared with open suture repair, this reduction did not reach statistical significance. However, the analysis was based on few data and lacked power to detect clinically important differences in outcomes. The review found insufficient evidence to compare other clinical effects. One systematic review found that TAPP laparoscopic repair reduced the time taken to return to usual activities compared with open mesh repair. However, it found no significant difference between TAPP laparoscopic repair and open mesh repair in haematoma, seroma, superficial infection, visceral injury, length of hospital stay, persisting pain, or hernia recurrence.

TRADE OFF BETWEEN BENEFITS AND HARMS

Open suture repair (conventional, well established surgical technique but may be less effective in improving clinically important outcomes than open mesh repair or transabdominal preperitoneal (TAPP) laparoscopic repair)*

Clinical experience and consensus opinion suggest that surgery is an effective treatment for recurrent inguinal hernia. Open suture repair is a well established surgical technique. However, we found no systematic review, RCTs, or cohort studies of sufficient quality comparing open suture repair versus expectant management. One systematic review found limited evidence that open suture repair slightly increased length of hospital stay compared with open mesh repair in people with recurrent inguinal hernia. However, the review found insufficient evidence to compare effects on pain, time to return to usual activities, further recurrence, or complications of surgery. One systematic review found that although there was a trend towards a reduction in time taken to return to normal activities with transabdominal preperitoneal (TAPP) laparoscopic repair compared with open suture repair, this reduction did not reach statistical significance. However, the analysis was based on few data and lacked power to detect clinically important differences in outcomes. The review found insufficient evidence to compare other clinical effects. One systematic review found insufficient data to compare the effects of totally extraperitoneal (TEP) laparoscopic repair versus open suture repair.

UNKNOWN EFFECTIVENESS

Expectant management

We found no systematic review, RCTs, or cohort studies of sufficient quality of expectant management in adults with recurrent inguinal hernia.

*Based on clinical experience and consensus

DEFINITION Inguinal hernia is an out-pouching of peritoneum, with or without its contents, which occurs through the muscles of the anterior abdominal wall at the level of the inguinal canal in the groin. It almost always occurs in men, because of the inherent weakness of the abdominal wall where the spermatic cord passes through the inguinal canal. A portion of bowel may become caught in the peritoneal pouch, and present as a lump in the groin. The hernia may extend into the scrotum, and can cause discomfort or ache. Primary hernias relate to the first presentation of a hernia and are distinct from recurrent hernias. A hernia is described as reducible if it occurs intermittently (e.g. on straining or standing) and can be pushed back into the abdominal cavity and is irreducible if it remains permanently outside the abdominal cavity. Inguinal hernia is usually a long standing condition and diagnosis is made clinically, on the basis of these typical symptoms and signs. The condition may occur in one groin (unilateral hernia) or both groins simultaneously (bilateral hernia), and may recur after treatment (recurrent hernia). Occasionally, hernia may present acutely because of complications (see prognosis below). Clinical experience and consensus opinion suggest that surgical intervention is an effective treatment for inguinal hernia. However, surgery is associated with complications (see outcomes below), therefore, much of this chapter examines the relative effectiveness and safety of different surgical techniques. Inguinal hernias are frequently classified as direct or indirect, depending on whether the hernia sac bulges directly through the posterior wall of the inguinal canal (direct hernia), or rather passes through the internal inguinal ring alongside the spermatic cord, and follows the course of the inguinal canal (indirect hernia). However, none of the studies that we identified distinguished between these two types of inguinal hernia. Identified studies gave little detail about the severity of hernia among included participants. In general, studies explicitly excluded people with irreducible or complicated hernia, large hernia (extending into the scrotum), or serious co-morbidity, and those at high surgical risk (e.g. because of coagulation disorders). In this chapter we deal only with non-acute, uncomplicated inguinal hernias in adults.

INCIDENCE/ PREVALENCE Inguinal hernia is usually repaired surgically in resource rich countries. Surgical audit data therefore provide reasonable estimates of incidence, and support estimates of this order of magnitude. We found one nationally mandated guideline, which reported that in 2001–2002 there were about 70 000 inguinal hernia surgeries performed in England, involving 0.14% of the population and requiring over 100 000 National Health Service hospital bed-days.[1] Of these procedures, 62 969 were for the repair of primary hernias and 4939 for the repair of recurrent hernias.[1] A similar number of inguinal hernia repairs were undertaken in public health care settings in England in 2002–2003.[2] In the USA, estimates based on cross-sectional data suggest that about 700 000 inguinal hernia repairs were undertaken in 1993.[3] A national survey of general practices covering about 1% of the population of England and Wales in 1991–1992 found that about 95% of people presenting to primary care settings with inguinal hernia were male.[4] It found that the incidence rose from about 11/10 000 person-years in men aged 16–24 years to about 200/10 000 person-years in men aged 75 years or above.

AETIOLOGY/ RISK FACTORS Age and male sex are risk factors (see incidence/prevalence above). Chronic cough and manual labour involving heavy lifting are conventionally regarded as risk factors because they lead to high intra-abdominal pressure. Obesity has also been suggested to be a risk factor. However, we found no reliable data to quantify these risks.

PROGNOSIS We found few reliable data on untreated prognosis. Strangulation, intestinal obstruction, and infarction are the most important acute complications of untreated hernia and are potentially life threatening. National statistics from England found that 5% of primary inguinal hernia repairs were undertaken as emergencies (presumably because of acute complications) in 1998–1999.[2]

Inguinal hernia

Older age, longer duration of hernia, and longer duration of irreducibility are thought to be risk factors for acute complication,[5] although we found no reliable data to quantify these effects.

Please refer to clinicalevidence.com for full text and references.

Irritable bowel syndrome

Search date June 2005

Niek de Wit, Gregory Rubin, and Roger H Jones

What are the effects of treatments in people with irritable bowel syndrome?

LIKELY TO BE BENEFICIAL

Antidepressants (amitriptyline, clomipramine, desipramine, doxepin, mianserin, trimipramine, fluoxetine)

One systematic review found limited evidence from low to moderate quality RCTs that antidepressants (amitriptyline, clomipramine, desipramine, doxepin, mianserin, trimipramine) reduced symptoms of irritable bowel syndrome compared with placebo. A subsequent systematic review found no clear evidence of benefit for tricyclic antidepressants on abdominal pain or global symptom improvement compared with placebo. A third systematic review with less rigorous inclusion criteria found limited evidence that antidepressants (amitriptyline, desipramine, doxepin, fluoxetine, mianserin, trimipramine) improved global symptoms compared with control. It was not clear in some RCTs whether the effects on irritable bowel syndrome were independent of the effects on psychological symptoms.

Antispasmodics

One systematic review found that antispasmodics had a consistent beneficial effect on abdominal pain and global symptom assessment compared with placebo. However, another systematic review using less rigorous inclusion criteria comparing antispasmodics to placebo was unable to decide whether this group of drugs was beneficial. One RCT identified by a systematic review found that mebeverine was less effective for symptoms than alosetron (a $5HT_3$ receptor antagonist) in women with diarrhoea predominant irritable bowel syndrome, although there are concerns that alosetron may be associated with ischaemic colitis.

TRADE OFF BETWEEN BENEFITS AND HARMS

$5HT_4$ receptor agonists (tegaserod)

Two systematic reviews found that in women with constipation predominant irritable bowel syndrome, tegaserod improved symptoms compared with placebo. Both reviews found insufficient evidence about the effects of tegaserod in men. The first systematic review found that tegaserod increased diarrhoea compared with placebo. A warning has been issued that serious diarrhoea, sometimes requiring hospitalisation, can occur with tegaserod as an adverse event.

Alosetron

Two systematic reviews of the same RCTs found that alosetron (a $5HT_3$ receptor antagonist) improved symptoms in women with diarrhoea predominant irritable bowel syndrome compared with placebo. However, alosetron is associated with adverse effects, particularly constipation, and has been restricted in some countries because of concerns that it may be associated with ischaemic colitis. The systematic reviews provided insufficient evidence about the effects of alosetron in men. One RCT identified by a systematic review found that alosetron improved symptoms in women with diarrhoea predominant irritable bowel syndrome compared with mebeverine.

Irritable bowel syndrome

UNKNOWN EFFECTIVENESS

$5HT_3$ receptor antagonists other than alosetron

We found no RCTs examining $5HT_3$ receptor antagonists other than alosetron.

Fibre supplementation

One systematic review found limited evidence that fibre supplementation improved symptoms of irritable bowel syndrome and irritable bowel syndrome related constipation.

Loperamide *New*

Small, methodologically weak RCTs found limited evidence that loperamide decreased stool frequency compared with placebo, but found no effect on irritable bowel syndrome symptoms or pain compared with placebo.

DEFINITION Irritable bowel syndrome (IBS) is a chronic non-inflammatory condition characterised by abdominal pain, altered bowel habit (diarrhoea or constipation), and abdominal bloating, but with no identifiable structural or biochemical disorder. Symptom based criteria, such as the Manning criteria (see table 1Ⓣ),[1] the Rome I criteria (see table 2Ⓣ),[2] and the Rome II criteria (see table 3Ⓣ),[3] aid diagnosis but their main use is in defining populations in clinical trials. The Rome criteria also subcategorise IBS according to predominant symptoms (diarrhoea, constipation, or alternating between diarrhoea and constipation). In practice, the division between constipation predominant and diarrhoea predominant IBS may not be clear-cut in all people. Restriction of trial entry to a subcategory of IBS limits the generalisability of study results.

INCIDENCE/ PREVALENCE Estimates of incidence and prevalence vary depending on the diagnostic criteria used to define IBS. One cross-sectional postal survey (4476 people aged 20–69 years) in Teeside, UK, defined IBS as recurrent abdominal pain on more than six occasions during the previous year plus two or more of the Manning criteria (see table 1Ⓣ).[4] It estimated prevalence in the UK to be 16.7% (95% CI 15.4% to 18.0%) overall, with a prevalence of 22.8% (95% CI 20.8% to 24.8%) among women and 10.5% (95% CI 8.9% to 12.1%) among men.[4] A cross-sectional postal survey (4500 people aged > 17 years) in Australia found prevalences of IBS of 13.6% (95% CI 12.3% to 14.8%) using the Manning criteria (see table 1Ⓣ), 6.9% (95% CI 6.0% to 7.8%) using the Rome I criteria (see table 2Ⓣ), and 4.4% (95% CI 3.5% to 5.1%) using the Rome II criteria (see table 3Ⓣ).[5]

AETIOLOGY/ RISK FACTORS The pathophysiology of IBS is not certain but abnormal gastrointestinal motor function,[6-8] and enhanced visceral perception,[9-11] appear important. Other determinants include psychosocial factors such as a history of childhood abuse,[12] genetic predisposition,[13-15] and a history of enteric mucosal inflammation.[16,17] We found no reliable prospective data to measure these associations.

PROGNOSIS A retrospective study reviewed the medical records of people with IBS (112 people aged 20–64 years when diagnosed with IBS at the Mayo Clinic, USA, in 1961–1963). IBS was defined as the presence of abdominal pain associated with either disturbed defecation or abdominal distension and the absence of organic bowel disease.[18] Over a 32 year period, death rates were similar among people with IBS compared with age and gender matched controls. One postal survey (4432 adults aged 20–69 years) found that people with IBS are significantly more likely to have had a cholecystectomy than controls (OR 1.9, 95% CI 1.2 to 3.2).[4] A paper reporting on the same survey population (2238 women aged 20–69 years) found that women with IBS were significantly more likely to have had a hysterectomy than controls (OR 1.6, 95% CI 1.1 to 2.2).[19] We found no reliable estimates of the duration of IBS if left untreated.

Please refer to clinicalevidence.com for full text and references.

Stomach cancer

Search date August 2005

Charles Bailey

What are the effects of radical versus conservative surgical resection?

LIKELY TO BE BENEFICIAL

Subtotal gastrectomy for resectable distal tumours (as effective as total gastrectomy)

Two RCTs in people with primary tumours in the distal stomach found no significant difference in 5 year survival or postoperative mortality between total and subtotal gastrectomy.

UNKNOWN EFFECTIVENESS

Radical versus conservative lymphadenectomy

One systematic review found no significant difference in 5 year survival between radical and conservative lymphadenectomy. However, confounding factors may have affected the reliability of results, and we found conflicting data from subgroup analyses of prospective cohort studies.

LIKELY TO BE INEFFECTIVE OR HARMFUL

Removal of adjacent organs

One RCT found no significant difference between radical gastrectomy plus splenectomy and radical gastrectomy alone in 5 year survival rates or postoperative mortality. The RCT found that radical gastrectomy plus splenectomy increased the number of postoperative infections compared with radical gastrectomy alone. Retrospective analyses of observational studies and RCTs in people with stomach cancer found that removal of additional organs (spleen and distal pancreas) increased morbidity and mortality compared with no organ removal.

What are the effects of adjuvant chemotherapy?

LIKELY TO BE BENEFICIAL

Adjuvant chemoradiotherapy

One large RCT found that adjuvant chemoradiotherapy improved survival compared with surgery alone in people with resectable stomach adenocarcinoma.

UNKNOWN EFFECTIVENESS

Adjuvant chemotherapy

One large systematic review and two subsequent RCTs found that adjuvant chemotherapy increased survival compared with surgery alone in people with gastric adenocarcinoma. Three subsequent RCTs found no significant difference between adjuvant chemotherapy and surgery alone in 5 year survival. Subsequent RCTs found that adjuvant chemotherapy was poorly tolerated.

Stomach cancer

DEFINITION Stomach cancer is usually an adenocarcinoma arising in the stomach and includes tumours arising at or just below the gastro-oesophageal junction (type II and III junctional tumours). Tumours are staged according to degree of invasion and spread (see table 1)Ⓣ. Only non-metastatic stomach cancers are considered in this chapter.

INCIDENCE/ PREVALENCE The incidence of stomach cancer varies among countries and by gender (incidence per 100 000 population a year in Japanese men is about 80, Japanese women 30, British men 18, British women 10, white American men 11, white American women 7).[1] Incidence has declined dramatically in North America, Australia, and New Zealand since 1930, but the decline in Europe has been slower.[2] In the USA, stomach cancer remains relatively common among particular ethnic groups, especially Japanese–Americans and some Hispanic groups. The incidence of cancer of the proximal stomach and gastro-oesophageal junction is rising rapidly in many European populations and in North America.[3,4] The reasons for this are poorly understood.

AETIOLOGY/ RISK FACTORS Distal stomach cancer is strongly associated with lifelong infection with *Helicobacter pylori* and poor dietary intake of antioxidant vitamins (A, C, and E).[5,6] In Western Europe and North America, distal stomach cancer is associated with relative socioeconomic deprivation. Proximal stomach cancer is strongly associated with smoking (OR about 4),[7] and is probably associated with gastro-oesophageal reflux, obesity, high fat intake, and medium to high socioeconomic status.

PROGNOSIS Invasive stomach cancer (stages T2–T4) is fatal without surgery. Mean survival without treatment is less than 6 months from diagnosis.[8,9] Intramucosal or submucosal cancer (stage T1) may progress slowly to invasive cancer over several years.[10] In the USA, over 50% of people recently diagnosed with stomach cancer have regional lymph node metastasis or involvement of adjacent organs. The prognosis after macroscopically and microscopically complete resection (R0) is related strongly to disease stage, particularly penetration of the serosa (stage T3) and lymph node involvement. Five year survival rates range from over 90% in intramucosal cancer to about 20% in people with stage T3N2 disease (see table 1)Ⓣ. In Japan, the 5 year survival rate for people with advanced disease is reported to be about 50%, but the explanation for the difference remains unclear. Comparisons between Japanese and Western practice are confounded by factors such as age, fitness, and disease stage, as well as by tumour location, because many Western series include gastro-oesophageal junction adenocarcinoma, which is associated with a much lower survival rate after surgery.

Please refer to clinicalevidence.com for full text and references.

Chronic suppurative otitis media

Search date November 2004

Jose Acuin

What are the effects of treatments for chronic suppurative otitis media in adults?

LIKELY TO BE BENEFICIAL

Antibiotics (topical) plus corticosteroids (topical)

One systematic review found limited evidence from three RCTs that topical antibiotics plus topical steroids improved symptoms compared with placebo or topical steroids alone in adults with chronic suppurative otitis media (CSOM). One of the RCTs had weak methods and one was published only as an abstract. Three RCTs of adults with CSOM found no clear evidence of a difference in clinical response rate with topical antibiotics plus topical steroids compared with topical antibiotics alone.

UNKNOWN EFFECTIVENESS

Antibiotics (systemic)

RCTs provided insufficient evidence about the effects of systemic antibiotics compared with placebo, each other, or topical antiseptics in adults with chronic suppurative otitis media (CSOM). One systematic review found that systemic antibiotics were less effective than topical antibiotics in reducing otoscopic activity in people with CSOM. One RCT found no significant difference between topical ceftizoxime plus systemic ceftizoxime and systemic ceftizoxime alone.

Antibiotics (topical)

We found no RCTs with long term follow up. Two RCTs with weak methods provided limited evidence that topical quinolone antibiotics improved otorrhoea and middle ear inflammation at 1–3 weeks compared with placebo in adults with chronic suppurative otitis media (CSOM). Five RCTs found no clear evidence of clinically important differences among topical antibiotics in adults. Three RCTs in adults with CSOM found no clear evidence of a difference in clinical response rate with topical antibiotics plus topical steroids compared with topical antibiotics alone. One systematic review found that topical antibiotics were more effective than systemic antibiotics for reducing otoscopic features of CSOM. Two RCTs found no significant difference between systemic plus topical quinolone antibiotics and topical quinolone antibiotics alone, although a third RCT found that topical quinolone alone was more effective than oral plus topical non-quinolones. One small RCT identified by a systematic review provided insufficient evidence to compare topical antibiotics versus topical antiseptics. One RCT found no significant difference between preoperative topical antibiotics and no preoperative treatment in people undergoing tympanoplasty. Short term topical antibiotics have been associated with few adverse events in RCTs. Uncontrolled case studies have reported vestibular ototoxicity after topical non-quinolone antibiotics.

Antibiotics (topical plus systemic)

We found no systematic review or RCTs comparing topical plus systemic antibiotics versus placebo in adults with chronic suppurative otitis media. Two RCTs found no significant difference between systemic plus topical quinolone antibiotics and topical quinolone antibiotics alone, although a third RCT found ▶

that topical quinolone alone was more effective than oral plus topical non-quinolones. One RCT found no significant difference between topical ceftizoxime plus systemic ceftizoxime and systemic ceftizoxime alone.

Antiseptics (topical)

We found no systematic review or RCTs comparing topical antiseptics versus placebo or no treatment in adults with chronic suppurative otitis media. One small RCT identified by a systematic review provided insufficient evidence to compare topical antiseptics versus topical antibiotics or systemic antibiotics.

Corticosteroids (topical)

We found no systematic review or RCTs comparing topical corticosteroids versus placebo or no treatment in adults. One weak RCT identified by a systematic review found limited evidence that topical steroids plus topical antibiotics in adults with chronic suppurative otitis media improved symptoms compared with topical steroids alone.

Ear cleansing

We found no RCTs or observational studies of sufficient quality comparing ear cleansing versus no treatment in adults with chronic suppurative otitis media.

Tympanoplasty with or without mastoidectomy

We found no RCTs comparing tympanoplasty with or without mastoidectomy versus no surgery in adults with chronic suppurative otitis media without cholesteatoma.

What are the effects of treatments for chronic suppurative otitis media in children?

UNKNOWN EFFECTIVENESS

Antibiotics (systemic)

One small open label RCT in children with chronic suppurative otitis media (CSOM) having ear cleansing and debridement found limited evidence that intravenous mezlocillin or ceftazidime reduced persistent otorrhoea after 6 months compared with no antibiotic and found no significant difference between antibiotics. Two systematic reviews identified no RCTs comparing topical versus systemic antibiotics that were undertaken solely in children with CSOM. One systematic review identified no RCTs comparing systemic antibiotics versus topical antiseptics.

Antibiotics (topical)

We found no systematic review and no RCTs comparing topical antibiotics versus placebo or versus each other in children with chronic suppurative otitis media (CSOM). Two systematic reviews identified no RCTs comparing topical versus systemic antibiotics that were undertaken solely in children with CSOM. We found no RCTs comparing topical antibiotics versus topical antibiotics plus topical corticosteroids in children.

Antibiotics (topical) plus corticosteroids (topical)

We found no RCTs comparing topical antibiotics plus topical corticosteroids versus placebo or other treatments in children with chronic suppurative otitis media.

Chronic suppurative otitis media

Antiseptics (topical)

Two RCTs found no significant difference in otorrhoea between topical antiseptics (aluminium acetate or boric acid) and control in children with chronic suppurative otitis media. However, the RCT was too small to detect a clinically important effect. One systematic review identified no RCTs comparing topical antiseptics versus systemic antibiotics.

Corticosteroids (topical)

We found no systematic review or RCTs comparing topical corticosteroids versus placebo or no treatment in children with chronic suppurative otitis media.

Ear cleansing

One systematic review of two RCTs with weak methods provided insufficient evidence to compare a simple form of ear cleansing versus no ear cleansing in children with chronic suppurative otitis media. We found no observational studies of sufficient quality of ear cleansing.

Tympanoplasty with or without mastoidectomy

We found no systematic review or RCTs comparing tympanoplasty with or without mastoidectomy versus no surgery in children with chronic suppurative otitis media without cholesteatoma.

DEFINITION Chronic suppurative otitis media (CSOM) is persistent inflammation of the middle ear or mastoid cavity. Synonyms include "chronic otitis media (without effusion)", chronic mastoiditis, and chronic tympanomastoiditis. CSOM is characterised by recurrent or persistent ear discharge (otorrhoea) over 2–6 weeks through a perforation of the tympanic membrane. Typical findings also include thickened granular middle ear mucosa, mucosal polyps, and cholesteatoma within the middle ear. CSOM is differentiated from chronic otitis media with effusion, in which there is an intact tympanic membrane with fluid in the middle ear but no active infection. CSOM does not include chronic perforations of the eardrum that are dry, or only occasionally discharge, and have no signs of active infection.

INCIDENCE/ PREVALENCE The worldwide prevalence of chronic suppurative otitis media (CSOM) is 65–330 million people. Between 39–200 million (60%) suffer from clinically significant hearing impairment.[1] Otitis media was estimated to have caused 28 000 deaths and loss of over 2 million Disability Adjusted Life Years in 2000, 94% of which were in developing countries.[2] Most of these deaths were probably due to CSOM because acute otitis media is a self limiting infection.

AETIOLOGY/ RISK FACTORS Chronic suppurative otitis media (CSOM) is assumed to be a complication of acute otitis media, but the risk factors for CSOM are not clear. Frequent upper respiratory tract infections and poor socioeconomic conditions (overcrowded housing,[3] hygiene, and nutrition) may be related to the development of CSOM.[4,5] Improvement in housing, hygiene, and nutrition in Maori children was associated with a halving of the prevalence of CSOM between 1978 and 1987.[6] Also see acute otitis media.

PROGNOSIS Most children with chronic suppurative otitis media (CSOM) have mild to moderate hearing impairment (about 26–60 dB increase in hearing thresholds), based on surveys among children in Africa, Brazil,[7] India,[8] and Sierra Leone,[9] and among the general population in Thailand.[10] In many developing countries, CSOM represents the most frequent cause of moderate hearing loss (40–60 dB).[11] Persistent hearing loss during the first 2 years of life may increase learning disabilities and poor scholastic performance.[12] Spread of infection may lead to life threatening complications such as intracranial infections and acute mastoiditis.[13] The frequency of serious complications fell from 20% in 1938 to 2.5% in 1948 and is currently estimated to be about 0.24% in Thailand and 1.8% in Africa. This is believed to be associated with increased use of antibiotic treatment, tympanoplasty, and mastoidectomy.[14-16] Cholesteatoma is another serious complication that has been found in a variable proportion of people with chronic suppurative otitis media (range 0–60%).[17-20] In the West, the incidence of cholesteatoma is low; in Finland in 1993, the age standardised incidence of cholesteatoma was eight new cases per 100 000 population/year.[21]

Please refer to clinicalevidence.com for full text and references.

Ear wax

Search date November 2005

George Browning

What are the effects of methods to remove ear wax?

TRADE OFF BETWEEN BENEFITS AND HARMS

Ear syringing*

There is consensus that ear syringing is effective at removing wax, but we found no RCTs comparing ear syringing alone versus no treatment. Reported complications of ear syringing include pain, damage to the skin of the external canal with haemorrhage, otitis externa, perforation of the ear drum, and vertigo. One small unblinded RCT found limited evidence that water instilled in the ear 15 minutes prior to syringing reduced the volume of water needed to syringe the ear clear of wax compared with no treatment.

UNKNOWN EFFECTIVENESS

Manual removal (other than ear syringing)*

We found no systematic review or RCTs about mechanical methods of removing ear wax other than syringing, although most otologists consider microsuction to be a standard management to enable the tympanic membrane to be visualised.

Wax softeners alone

Two systematic reviews of poor quality RCTs provided inconclusive evidence on the effects of wax softeners alone for clearing wax. The reviews included one RCT which found limited evidence that a proprietary wax softening agent, sodium bicarbonate, or sterile water eardrops, all increased wax clearance compared with no treatment, but found no significant difference in wax clearance between the different eardrops. One systematic review of two small RCTs found limited evidence that one proprietary agent increased wax clearance compared with normal saline, but found no significant difference between another proprietary agent and normal saline. The reviews found no consistent evidence that any one type of wax softener was superior to any other.

Wax softeners prior to syringing

Two systematic reviews of poor quality RCTs and one subsequent RCT provided inconclusive evidence on the effects of wax softeners prior to syringing. One review included one small RCT with weak methods which found that a proprietary wax softening agent increased successful syringing compared with no treatment. One systematic review of two RCTs and one subsequent RCT found no significant difference in successful syringing between three different proprietary wax softening agents and saline. The reviews found no consistent evidence that any one type of wax softener was superior to any other.

*Although many practitioners consider these to be standard treatments, we found no RCTs of these interventions.

DEFINITION Ear wax is normal and becomes a problem only if it produces deafness, pain, or other ear related symptoms. Ear wax may also need to be removed if it prevents inspection of the ear drum. The term "impacted wax" (see glossary) is used in different ways, and can merely imply the coexistence of wax obscuring the ear drum with symptoms in that ear.[1]

INCIDENCE/ PREVALENCE We found four surveys of the prevalence of impacted wax.[2-5] The studies were carried out in a variety of populations and used a variety of definitions of impacted wax; prevalence ranged from 7–35%. It is unclear how these figures relate to prevalence in the general population.

AETIOLOGY/ RISK FACTORS Factors that prevent the normal extrusion of wax from the ear canal (e.g. wearing a hearing aid, using cotton buds to clean ears) increase the chance of ear wax accumulating.

PROGNOSIS Most ear wax emerges from the external canal spontaneously; one small RCT that included a no treatment group found that 32% of ears with impacted wax showed some degree of spontaneous resolution after 5 days (26.3% described as moderately clear; 5.3% described as completely clear).[1] Without impaction or adherence to the drum, there is likely to be minimal, if any, hearing loss.

Please refer to clinicalevidence.com for full text and references.

Menière's disease

Search date January 2005

Adrian James and Marc Thorp

What are the effects of treatments for acute attacks?

UNKNOWN EFFECTIVENESS

Anticholinergics

We found no systematic review or RCTs about the effects of anticholinergics for acute attacks of Menière's disease.

Benzodiazepines

We found no systematic review or RCTs about the effects of benzodiazepines for acute attacks of Menière's disease.

Betahistine

We found no systematic review or RCTs about the effects of betahistine for acute attacks of Menière's disease.

What are the effects of interventions to prevent attacks and delay disease progression?

UNKNOWN EFFECTIVENESS

Aminoglycosides

We found no systematic review or RCTs about the effects of systemic aminoglycosides in preventing attacks of Menière's disease on delaying disease progression.

Betahistine (for vertigo or tinnitus)

Seven RCTs provided insufficient evidence to compare betahistine versus placebo in terms of their effects on frequency and severity of attacks of vertigo, tinnitus, and aural fullness. Two small RCTs in people with definite or possible Menière's disease found no significant difference in tinnitus between betahistine and trimetazidine. One of these RCTs found that trimetazidine reduced the intensity of vertigo compared with betahistine, but the other RCT found no significant difference in vertigo intensity between trimetazidine and betahistine.

Dietary modification

We found no systematic review or RCTs about the effects of dietary modification in preventing attacks of Menière's disease on delaying disease progression.

Diuretics

One small crossover RCT provided insufficient evidence about the effects of triamterene plus hydrochlorothiazide on hearing, tinnitus or on the frequency of attacks of vertigo. We found no evidence on the effects of diuretics on disease progression.

Psychological support

We found no systematic review or RCTs about the effects of psychological support, such as reassurance, in preventing attacks of Menière's disease on delaying disease progression.

Trimetazidine

We found no RCTs comparing trimetazidine versus placebo to prevent attacks of Menière's disease. Two small RCTs in people with definite or possible Menière's disease found no significant difference between trimetazidine and betahistine in hearing or tinnitus. One of these RCTs found that trimetazidine reduced the intensity of vertigo compared with betahistine, but the other RCT found no significant difference in vertigo intensity between trimetazidine and betahistine. We found no evidence on the effects of trimetazidine on disease progression.

Vestibular rehabilitation

We found no systematic review or RCTs about the effects of vestibular rehabilitation in preventing attacks of Menière's disease on delaying disease progression.

UNLIKELY TO BE BENEFICIAL

Betahistine (for hearing loss)

Four RCTs in people with possible Menière's disease found no significant difference between betahistine and placebo in change in hearing assessed by pure tone audiograms. Two small RCTs in people with definite or possible Menière's disease found no significant difference in hearing between betahistine and trimetazidine.

DEFINITION Menière's disease is characterised by recurrent episodes of spontaneous rotational vertigo, sensorineural hearing loss, tinnitus, and a feeling of fullness or pressure in the ear. It may be unilateral or bilateral. Acute episodes can occur in clusters of about 6–11 a year, although remission may last several months.[1] The diagnosis is made clinically.[2] It is important to distinguish Menière's disease from other types of vertigo that might occur independently with hearing loss and tinnitus, and respond differently to treatment (e.g. benign positional vertigo, acute labyrinthitis). Strict diagnostic criteria help to identify the condition. In this chapter we applied the classification of the American Academy of Otolaryngology — Head and Neck Surgery to assess the diagnostic rigour used in RCTs (see table 1Ⓣ).[3-5]

INCIDENCE/ PREVALENCE Menière's disease is most common between 40–60 years of age, although younger people may be affected.[6,7] In Europe, the incidence is about 50–200/100 000 a year. A survey of general practitioner records of 27 365 people in the UK found an incidence of 43 affected people in a 1 year period (157/100 000).[8] Diagnostic criteria were not defined in this survey. A survey of over 8 million people in Sweden found an incidence of 46/100 000 a year with diagnosis strictly based on the triad of vertigo, hearing loss, and tinnitus.[9] From smaller studies, the incidence appears lower in Uganda[10] and higher in Japan (350/100 000, based on a national survey of hospital attendances during a single week).[7]

AETIOLOGY/ RISK FACTORS Menière's disease is associated with endolymphatic hydrops (raised endolymph pressure in the membranous labyrinth of the inner ear),[11] but a causal relationship remains unproved.[12] Specific disorders associated with hydrops (such as temporal bone fracture, syphilis, hypothyroidism, Cogan's syndrome, and Mondini dysplasia) can produce symptoms similar to those of Menière's disease.

PROGNOSIS Menière's disease is progressive but fluctuates unpredictably. It is difficult to distinguish natural resolution from the effects of treatment. Significant improvement in vertigo is usually seen in the placebo arm of RCTs.[13,14] Acute attacks of vertigo often increase in frequency during the first few years after presentation and then decrease in frequency in association with sustained deterioration in hearing.[6] In most people, vertiginous episodes eventually cease completely.[15] In one 20 year cohort study in 34 people, 28 (82%) people had at least moderate hearing loss (mean pure tone hearing loss > 50 dB) and 16 (47%) developed bilateral disease.[1] Symptoms other than hearing loss improve in 60–80% of people irrespective of treatment.[16]

Please refer to clinicalevidence.com for full text and references.

Middle ear pain and trauma during air travel

Search date April 2006

Arin Basu

Preventing middle ear pain during air travel

LIKELY TO BE BENEFICIAL

Nasal balloon inflation

One RCT found that 69% of adult air passengers receiving nasal balloon inflation during or after a flight had reduced barotitis following flight descent.

Oral pseudoephedrine in adults

One RCT in adult passengers with a history of ear pain during air travel found that oral pseudoephedrine decreased symptoms of barotrauma during air travel compared with placebo. Another RCT in adult passengers with a history of ear pain during air travel found that oral pseudoephedrine decreased ear pain and hearing loss compared with placebo. The results of both RCTs should be treated with caution as they assessed outcomes by post-flight questionnaire, which may lead to recall bias.

UNKNOWN EFFECTIVENESS

Oral pseudoephedrine in children

One small RCT in children up to the age of 6 years found no significant difference between oral pseudoephedrine and placebo in ear pain at take off or landing. It found that more children were drowsy on take off with oral pseudoephedrine compared with placebo.

Topical nasal decongestants

One small RCT in adults with a history of ear pain during air travel found no significant difference between oxymetazoline nasal spray and placebo in preventing symptoms of barotrauma, but may have been too small to detect a clinically important effect of decongestants. We found no RCTs comparing other topical nasal decongestants with placebo during air travel.

DEFINITION The effects of air travel on the middle ear, due to changes in air pressure, can include ear drum pain, vertigo, hearing loss, and ear drum perforation.

INCIDENCE/ PREVALENCE The prevalence of symptoms depends on the altitude, type of aircraft, and characteristics of the passengers. One point prevalence study found that, in commercial passengers, 20% of adult and 40% of child passengers had negative pressure in the middle ear after flight, and that 10% of adults and 22% of children had otoscopic evidence of damage to the ear drum.[1] We found no data on the incidence of perforation, which seems to be extremely rare in commercial passengers.

AETIOLOGY/ RISK FACTORS During aircraft descent, the pressure in the middle ear drops relative to that in the ear canal. A narrow, inflamed, or poorly functioning Eustachian tube impedes the necessary influx of air. As the pressure difference between the middle and outer ear increases, the ear drum is pulled inward.

PROGNOSIS In most people, symptoms resolve spontaneously. Experience in military aviation shows that most ear drum perforations will heal spontaneously.[2]

Please refer to clinicalevidence.com for full text and references.

Otitis externa

Search date March 2006

Daniel Hajioff

What are the effects of empirical treatment for otitis externa?

LIKELY TO BE BENEFICIAL

Topical aluminium acetate drops (as effective as topical antibiotics)

We found no systematic review or RCTs that compared topical aluminium acetate versus placebo. One RCT in people with acute diffuse otitis externa found no significant difference between aluminium acetate drops and topical polymyxin–neomycin–hydrocortisone drops in time to clinical cure or clinical cure rate at 4 weeks.

Topical antibacterials (with or without steroids)

One RCT found that methylprednisolone–neomycin drops improved symptoms and signs compared with placebo at 28 days. Two RCTs found no significant difference in cure rate between topical quinolones and other topical anti-infective agents. One RCT found that triamcinolone–neomycin drops improved resolution rates compared with hydrocortisone–neomycin–polymyxin B drops. Two RCTs found limited evidence that neomycin–dexamethasone–acetic acid spray improved clinical cure compared with topical anti-infective drops that did not contain acetic acid. We found no RCTs on the effects of topical anti-infective agents versus oral antibiotics. One RCT found limited evidence of no significant difference between topical antibacterial ointment plus oral co-trimoxazole and topical antibacterial ointment alone in symptom severity, symptom duration, and cure rate. One RCT in people with acute diffuse otitis externa found no significant difference between topical polymyxin–neomycin–hydrocortisone drops and aluminium acetate drops in time to clinical cure or cure rate at 4 weeks.

Topical steroids

One RCT in people with mild or moderate acute or chronic otitis externa found that topical budesonide improved symptoms and signs compared with placebo. We found no RCTs of topical steroids compared with topical anti-infective agents. One RCT found no significant difference in symptom scores between low potency steroid (topical hydrocortisone) and high potency steroid (topical hydrocortisone butyrate) after 1 week.

UNKNOWN EFFECTIVENESS

Oral antibiotics

We found no systematic review or RCTs of oral antibiotics compared with placebo or topical anti-infective agents.

Specialist aural toilet

We found no systematic review or RCTs that compared specialist aural toilet versus no aural toilet. One RCT in a secondary care setting found no significant difference between an ear wick plus anti-infective drops versus ribbon gauze impregnated with anti-infective ointment in resolution rates after 4 weeks.

Topical acetic acid (insufficient evidence to demonstrate effectiveness compared with placebo)

We found no systematic review or RCTs comparing topical acetic acid versus placebo. One RCT in adults with acute diffuse otitis externa found that acetic ▶

acid increased the duration of symptoms and risk of recurrence, and reduced overall cure rates compared with topical steroids plus antibiotics and topical acetic acid plus steroids.

Topical antifungals (with or without steroids)

We found no RCTs of topical antifungals (with or without steroids, alone or in combination with oral antibiotics) in people with otitis externa.

UNLIKELY TO BE BENEFICIAL

Oral antibiotics plus topical anti-infective agents (no better than topical anti-infective agents alone)

One RCT found limited evidence of no significant difference between oral co-trimoxazole plus topical anti-infective ointment and topical anti-infective ointment alone in symptom severity, symptom duration, and cure rate.

What are the effects of prophylactic treatments for otitis externa?

UNKNOWN EFFECTIVENESS

Topical acetic acid spray or drops

We found no RCT or systematic review of topical acetic acid as prophylaxis for otitis externa,

Topical steroids

We found no RCT or systematic review of topical steroids as prophylaxis for otitis externa.

Water exclusion

We found no RCTs or systematic review of water exclusion for prevention for otitis externa.

DEFINITION Otitis externa is inflammation, often with infection, of the external ear canal. This inflammation is usually generalised throughout the ear canal, so it is often referred to as "diffuse otitis externa". The present topic excludes localised inflammations such as furuncles. Otitis externa has acute (< 6 weeks), chronic (> 3 months), and necrotising (malignant) forms. Acute otitis externa may present as a single episode, or recur. It causes pain with aural discharge and associated hearing loss.[1] If the ear canal is visible, it appears red and inflamed. *Pseudomonas aeruginosa* and *Staphylococcus aureus* are the most frequent bacterial pathogens in otitis externa. Fungal overgrowth (e.g. with *Aspergillus niger*) is also quite common, especially after prolonged antibiotic treatment. Chronic otitis externa may result in canal stenosis with associated hearing loss, for which it may be difficult to fit hearing aids. Necrotising otitis externa is defined by destruction of the temporal bone, usually in people with diabetes or in people who are immunocompromised, and can be life threatening.[2] In this chapter, we look at the empirical treatment of acute and chronic otitis externa only.

INCIDENCE/ PREVALENCE Otitis externa is common in all parts of the world. The incidence is not known precisely, but 10% of people are thought to have been affected at some time.[3] The condition affects children but is more common in adults. It accounts for a large proportion of the workload of otolaryngology departments, but milder cases are often managed in primary care.[3]

AETIOLOGY/ RISK FACTORS Otitis externa may be associated with local or generalised eczema of the ear canal. It is more common in swimmers, in humid environments, in people with an absence of ear wax or narrow external ear canals, in hearing aid users, and after mechanical trauma.[4]

PROGNOSIS We found few reliable data. Many cases of otitis externa resolve spontaneously over several weeks or months. Acute episodes have a tendency to recur, although the risk of recurrence is unknown. Experience suggests that chronic inflammation affects a small proportion of people after a single episode of acute otitis externa, and may rarely lead to canal stenosis.[1]

Please refer to clinicalevidence.com for full text and references.

Otitis media with effusion

Search date March 2006

Ian Williamson

What are the effects of interventions to prevent otitis media with effusion?

UNKNOWN EFFECTIVENESS

Modifying risk factors to prevent otitis media with effusion

We found no RCTs on the effects of interventions aimed at modifying risk factors, such as passive smoking and bottle feeding, in preventing otitis media with effusion.

What are the effects of pharmacological, mechanical, and surgical interventions to treat otitis media with effusion?

LIKELY TO BE BENEFICIAL

Autoinflation (with purpose manufactured nasal balloon)

One systematic review found that autoinflation with a purpose manufactured nasal balloon improved effusion compared with no treatment after 2 weeks to 3 months. Some children may find autoinflation difficult.

TRADE OFF BETWEEN BENEFITS AND HARMS

Ventilation tubes alone

One systematic review found that ventilation tubes improved hearing at up to 2 years but not at 5 years compared with no ventilation tubes. The clinical significance of the hearing improvement seen (less than 10 decibels) was unclear. The review found that ventilation tubes did not significantly improve cognition, language comprehension, or expression compared with no ventilation tubes, although relatively insensitive outcomes may have been used. The review found no significant difference between ventilation tubes alone and ventilation tubes plus adenoidectomy in hearing at up to 12 months. Ventilation tubes were associated with an increased risk of tympanosclerosis at 1 year.

Ventilation tubes plus adenoidectomy

One systematic review found that ventilation tubes plus adenoidectomy improved hearing at 6 months compared with no treatment, although the difference between groups was reduced at 12 months. The review found no significant difference between the combined treatment and ventilation tubes alone in hearing at up to 12 months. Another review found that the combined treatment improved hearing more than adenoidectomy alone at up to 12 months, but it found no significant difference between treatments at 2–5 years. The clinical significance of the improvements seen was unclear. Ventilation tubes were associated with an increased risk of tympanosclerosis at 1 year.

UNKNOWN EFFECTIVENESS

Adenoidectomy alone

One systematic review found inconclusive evidence on the effects of adenoidectomy alone compared with no treatment.

Otitis media with effusion

Autoinflation (with devices other than purpose manufactured nasal balloon)

Two small RCTs found no significant difference in improvement in symptoms between autoinflation using a carnival blower or an anaesthetic mask and no treatment.

Corticosteroids (intranasal)

One small RCT found no significant difference between intranasal corticosteroids alone and placebo for resolution of effusion at 3 weeks. A second small RCT found limited evidence that intranasal corticosteroids plus antibiotics reduced effusions compared with antibiotics alone at 4–12 weeks.

UNLIKELY TO BE BENEFICIAL

Antibiotics (oral)

One systematic review found no significant difference between antibiotics and placebo in cure rate. Another systematic review found limited evidence from four RCTs that antibiotics plus oral corticosteroids improved resolution rates at 2 weeks compared with antibiotics alone. One small RCT in the review found limited evidence that antibiotics plus intranasal corticosteroids reduced effusion compared with antibiotics alone at 4–12 weeks. Adverse effects with antibiotics (mainly nausea, vomiting, and diarrhoea) were reported in 2–32% of children.

Mucolytics

One systematic review found no significant difference between 1–3 month courses of carbocisteine or carbocisteine lysine and placebo or no treatment in resolution of effusion. Three small RCTs of bromhexine versus placebo found inconclusive results.

LIKELY TO BE INEFFECTIVE OR HARMFUL

Antihistamines plus oral decongestants

One systematic review found no significant difference between antihistamines plus oral decongestants and placebo in clearance of effusion after 4 weeks. Adverse effects of antihistamines include hyperactivity, insomnia, drowsiness, behavioural change, blood pressure variability, and seizures. One RCT in healthy volunteers found that decongestant nose drops given for 3 weeks or more led to iatrogenic rhinitis.

Corticosteroids (oral)

One systematic review found no significant difference between 7–14 days of treatment with oral corticosteroids and placebo in clearance of effusion after 2 weeks. It found limited evidence that oral corticosteroids plus antibiotics improved resolution rates at 2 weeks compared with antibiotics alone. However, oral corticosteroids have been associated with growth retardation in children.

DEFINITION Otitis media with effusion (OME), or "glue ear", is serous or mucoid but not mucopurulent fluid in the middle ear. Children usually present with hearing impairment and speech problems. In contrast to those with acute otitis media (see acute otitis media), children with OME do not suffer from acute ear pain, fever, or malaise. Hearing impairment is usually mild and often identified when parents express concern regarding their child's behaviour, performance at school, or language development.

INCIDENCE/ PREVALENCE OME is commonly seen in paediatric practice and accounts for 25–35% of all cases of otitis media.[1] One study in the UK found that, at any time, 5% of children aged 5 years had persistent (at least 3 months) bilateral hearing impairment associated with OME.[2] The prevalence declines considerably beyond 6 years of age.[3] Studies in the USA and Europe have estimated that about 50–80% of children aged 4 years have been affected by OME at some time in the past.[3,4] One study in the USA estimated that, between the ages of 2 months and 2 years, 91.1% of young children will have one episode of middle ear effusion, and 52.2% will have bilateral involvement.[5] OME is the most common reason for referral for surgery in children in the UK.[6] The number of general practitioner consultations for OME increased from 15.2 per 1000 (2–10 year olds) per year to 16.7 per 1000 per year between 1991 and 2001.[7] Middle ear effusions also occur infrequently in adults after upper respiratory tract infection or after air travel, and may persist for weeks or months after an episode of acute otitis media.[8]

AETIOLOGY/ RISK FACTORS Contributory factors include upper respiratory tract infection and narrow upper respiratory airways.[8,9] Case control studies have identified risk factors, including age 6 years or younger, day care centre attendance, large number of siblings, low socioeconomic group, frequent upper respiratory tract infection, bottle feeding, and household smoking.[3,8] These factors may be associated with about twice the risk of developing OME.[9]

PROGNOSIS Data from one prospective study of children aged 2–4 years showed that 50% of OME cases resolved within 3 months and 95% within a year.[10] In 5% of preschool children, OME (identified by tympanometric screening) persisted for at least 1 year.[10,11] One cohort study of 3 year olds found that 65% of OME cases cleared spontaneously within 3 months.[11] Most children aged 6 years or older will not have further problems.[2] The disease is ultimately self limiting in most cases.[2,5,6] However, one large cohort study (534 children) found that middle ear disease increased reported hearing difficulty at 5 years of age (OR 1.44, 95% CI 1.18 to 1.76) and was associated with delayed language development in children up to 10 years of age.[12] Hearing impairment is the most common complication of OME. Most children with OME have fluctuating or persistent hearing deficits with mild to moderate degrees of hearing loss, averaging 27 decibels. The type of hearing impairment is usually conductive but it may be sensorineural, or both. The sensorineural type is usually permanent.[13] Tympanic membrane perforation, tympanosclerosis, otorrhoea, and cholesteatoma occur more frequently among children with OME than among those without OME.

Please refer to clinicalevidence.com for full text and references.

Seasonal allergic rhinitis

Search date September 2004

Aziz Sheikh, Sukhmeet Singh Panesar, and Sangeeta Dhami

What are the effects of treatments of seasonal allergic rhinitis?

BENEFICIAL

Oral antihistamines (acrivastine, azatadine, brompheniramine, cetirizine, levocetirizine, ebastine, fexofenadine, loratadine, desloratidine, rupatadine, and mizolastine)

RCTs found that fexofenadine and loratadine improved quality of life and rhinitis symptoms compared with placebo. RCTs found that other oral antihistamines (acrivastine, azatadine, brompheniramine, cetirizine, desloratidine, ebastine, levocetirizine, mizolastine, and rupatadine) improved rhinitis symptoms compared with placebo. Drowsiness, sedation, and somnolence were the most commonly reported adverse effects of oral antihistamines.

Oral pseudoephedrine plus oral antihistamines

We found no systematic review or RCTs evaluating the effect of oral decongestants on quality of life. RCTs found that pseudoephedrine plus oral antihistamines (fexofenadine, acrivastine, cetirizine, terfenadine, triprolidine, loratadine, or azatadine) improved overall symptoms of seasonal allergic rhinitis compared with pseudoephedrine, oral antihistamine, or placebo alone. The most common adverse effects reported with combination treatment were headache and insomnia.

LIKELY TO BE BENEFICIAL

Intranasal levocabastine

RCTs found that intranasal levocabastine improved symptoms of seasonal allergic rhinitis compared with placebo.

Oral leukotriene receptor antagonists

One systematic review and two RCTs found that an oral leukotriene receptor antagonist, montelukast, improved nasal symptoms and quality of life compared with placebo. One RCT found inconclusive evidence about the effects of pranlukast compared with placebo on symptoms.

Oral leukotriene receptor antagonists plus oral antihistamines

Three RCTs identified by a systematic review found that montelukast plus loratadine improved nasal symptoms and quality of life compared with placebo. However, it found no evidence that combined treatment was any more effective than loratadine or montelukast alone.

TRADE OFF BETWEEN BENEFITS AND HARMS

Oral astemizole

RCTs found that astemizole improved rhinitis symptoms compared with placebo, but astemizole has been associated with prolongation of the QTc interval, and may induce ventricular arrhythmias.

Oral terfenadine

RCTs found conflicting results about the effectiveness of terfenadine compared with placebo on rhinitis symptoms. Terfenadine is associated with risk of fatal cardiac toxicity if used in conjunction with macrolide antibiotics, oral antifungal agents, or grapefruit juice.

UNKNOWN EFFECTIVENESS

Intranasal azelastine

Four RCTs found conflicting results on the effectiveness of intranasal azelastine compared with placebo on symptoms of seasonal allergic rhinitis. Two small RCTs found no significant difference in nasal symptoms between intranasal antihistamines (azelastine, levocabastine) and oral antihistamines (cetirizine, terfenadine).

Intranasal ipratropium bromide

We found no systematic review or published RCTs.

Oral decongestants

We found no systematic review or RCTs evaluating the effect of oral decongestants on quality of life. We found no RCTs only comparing oral decongestants with placebo. RCTs found that pseudoephedrine plus oral antihistamines (fexofenadine, acrivastine, cetirizine, terfenadine, triprolidine, loratadine, desloratadine, or azatadine) improved overall symptoms of seasonal allergic rhinitis compared with pseudoephedrine, oral antihistamine, or placebo alone. The most common adverse effects reported with combination treatment were headache and insomnia.

DEFINITION Seasonal allergic rhinitis is a symptom complex that may affect several organ systems. Symptoms will typically consist of seasonal sneezing, nasal itching, nasal blockage, and watery nasal discharge.[1] Eye symptoms (red eyes, itchy eyes, and tearing) are common. Other symptoms may include peak seasonal coughing, wheezing, and shortness of breath, oral allergy syndrome (manifesting as an itchy swollen oropharynx on eating stoned fruits), and systemic symptoms such as tiredness, fever, a pressure sensation in the head, and itchiness. Confirming the presence of pollen hypersensitivity using objective allergy tests such as skin prick tests, detection of serum specific IgE, and nasal provocation challenge testing may improve diagnostic accuracy.

INCIDENCE/ PREVALENCE Seasonal allergic rhinitis is found throughout the world. Epidemiological evidence suggests that there is considerable geographical variation in its prevalence. Prevalence is highest in socioeconomically developed countries, where the condition may affect as much as 25% of the population.[2-4] Prevalence and severity are increasing. It is thought that improved living standards and reduced risk of childhood infections may lead to immune deviation of T helper cells in early life, which may increase susceptibility to seasonal allergic rhinitis (the so called "hygiene hypothesis").[5,6] Although people of all ages may be affected, the peak age of onset is adolescence.[7]

AETIOLOGY/ RISK FACTORS The symptoms of seasonal allergic rhinitis are caused by an IgE mediated type 1 hypersensitivity reaction to grass, tree, or weed pollen. Allergy to other seasonal aeroallergens such as fungal spores may also provoke symptoms. Typically, symptoms become worse during the relevant pollen season and in the open, when pollen exposure is increased. Risk factors include a personal or family history of atopy or other allergic disorders, male sex, birth order (increased risk being seen in first born), and small family size.[8,9]

Seasonal allergic rhinitis

PROGNOSIS Seasonal allergic rhinitis may impair quality of life, interfering with work, sleep, and recreational activities.[10] Other allergic problems such as asthma and eczema frequently coexist, adding to the impact of rhinitis.[11]

Please refer to clinicalevidence.com for full text and references.

Sinusitis (acute)

Search date August 2005

Kim Ah-See

What are the effects of treatments in people with clinically diagnosed acute sinusitis?

UNKNOWN EFFECTIVENESS

Antibiotics (amoxicillin, amoxicillin–clavulanate, doxycycline, cephalosporins, macrolides)

Three RCTs found no good evidence that amoxicillin, with or without clavulanate, reduced or cured symptoms compared with placebo in people with clinically diagnosed acute sinusitis, who had not had radiological or bacteriological confirmation of disease. Two RCTs found that amoxicillin, with or without clavulanate, increased diarrhoea compared with placebo. Two RCTs in people with clinically diagnosed acute sinusitis compared doxycycline versus placebo. One RCT in people receiving nose drops and steam inhalation found limited evidence of no significant difference between doxycycline and placebo in cure rates, while another smaller RCT found similar recovery rates between doxycycline and placebo but did not assess the significance of the difference between groups. One RCT in people with clinically diagnosed acute sinusitis found no significant difference in clinical cure rate between a 5 day and a 10 day course of a cephalosporin.

Antihistamines

We found no systematic review or RCTs examining the effects of antihistamines in people with clinically diagnosed acute sinusitis.

Decongestants (xylometazoline, phenylephrine, pseudoephedrine)

We found no systematic review or RCTs examining the effects of decongestants (xylometazoline, phenylephrine, pseudoephedrine) in people with clinically diagnosed acute sinusitis.

Topical steroids (intra-nasal)

We found no systematic review or RCTs examining the effects of topical (intra-nasal) steroids in people with clinically diagnosed acute sinusitis.

What are the effects of treatments in people with radiologically or bacteriologically confirmed acute sinusitis?

LIKELY TO BE BENEFICIAL

Cephalosporins or macrolides (fewer adverse effects than amoxicillin or amoxicillin–clavulanate)

We found no RCTs comparing cephalosporins or macrolides versus placebo. One systematic review and two subsequent RCTs in people with radiologically or bacteriologically confirmed acute sinusitis found no significant difference in clinical resolution between amoxicillin or amoxicillin–clavulanate and cephalosporins or macrolides. However, cephalosporins and macrolides caused fewer adverse effects than amoxicillin and amoxicillin–clavulanate. Three RCTs in people with radiologically or bacteriologically confirmed acute sinusitis compared a cephalosporin versus a macrolide. One RCT found no significant ▶

difference in clinical improvement or clinical cure between cefaclor and azithromycin; another RCT found no significant difference in cure rate between clarithromycin and cefuroxime; and a third RCT found limited evidence of no significant difference in cure rate between telithromycin and cefuroxime.

TRADE OFF BETWEEN BENEFITS AND HARMS

Amoxicillin or amoxicillin–clavulanate (more adverse effects than cephalosporins or macrolides)

One systematic review identified two RCTs in people with radiologically or bacteriologically confirmed acute maxillary sinusitis, which found that amoxicillin improved early clinical cure rate compared with placebo, but was associated with more frequent adverse effects, mainly gastrointestinal. One systematic review and two subsequent RCTs in people with radiologically or bacteriologically confirmed acute sinusitis found no significant difference in clinical resolution between amoxicillin or amoxicillin–clavulanate and cephalosporins or macrolides. However, amoxicillin and amoxicillin–clavulanate caused more adverse effects.

UNKNOWN EFFECTIVENESS

Antihistamines

We found no systematic review or RCTs examining the effects of antihistamines in people with radiologically or bacteriologically confirmed acute sinusitis.

Decongestants (xylometazoline, phenylephrine, pseudoephedrine)

We found no systematic review or RCTs examining the effects of decongestants (xylometazoline, phenylephrine, pseudoephedrine) in people with radiologically or bacteriologically confirmed acute sinusitis.

Different dosages of antibiotics (amoxicillin, amoxicillin–clavulanate, doxycycline, cephalosporins, macrolides)

One RCT in people with radiologically or bacteriologically confirmed acute sinusitis found no significant difference in clinical resolution rates or adverse events between two and three daily doses of cefaclor. One RCT in people with radiologically or bacteriologically confirmed acute sinusitis comparing an extended versus an immediate release formulation of clarithromycin found no significant difference between groups in clinical cure rates. We found no RCTs of other antibiotics comparing different dosage regimens.

Doxycycline *New*

One RCT provided insufficient evidence on the effects of doxycycline compared with placebo in people with radiologically or bacteriologically confirmed acute sinusitis. We found no RCTs in people with radiologically or bacteriologically confirmed acute sinusitis comparing doxycycline versus amoxicillin with or without clavulanate, macrolides, or cephalosporins.

Topical steroids (intra-nasal)

We found no systematic review or RCTs examining the effects of topical (intra-nasal) steroids in people with radiologically or bacteriologically confirmed acute sinusitis.

UNLIKELY TO BE BENEFICIAL

Long course antibiotic regimens (amoxicillin, amoxicillin–clavulanate, doxycycline, cephalosporins, macrolides) (no more effective than short course regimens, and more adverse effects)

RCTs in people with confirmed acute sinusitis found no significant difference in clinical resolution rates between 6–10 day courses and 3–5 day courses of azithromycin, telithromycin, or cefuroxime (a cephalosporin) up to 3 weeks after treatment. RCTs found similar rates of adverse effects and diarrhoea between longer and shorter courses of azithromycin and telithromycin. One RCT found that adverse effects, which were mainly gastrointestinal, were more frequent with a longer course of cefuroxime than with a shorter course of cefuroxime.

DEFINITION Acute sinusitis is defined pathologically, by transient inflammation of the mucosal lining of the paranasal sinuses lasting less than 4 weeks. Clinically, it is characterised by nasal congestion, rhinorrhoea, facial pain, hyposmia, sneezing, and, if more severe, additional malaise and fever. The diagnosis is usually made clinically (on the basis of history and examination, but without radiological or bacteriological investigation). Clinically diagnosed acute sinusitis is less likely to be caused by bacterial infection than is acute sinusitis confirmed by radiological or bacteriological investigation.[1] In this chapter, we have excluded studies in children, in people with symptoms for more than 4 weeks (chronic sinusitis), and in people with symptoms after facial trauma. We have made it clear in each section whether we are dealing with clinically diagnosed acute sinusitis or acute sinusitis with clinical symptoms that have also been confirmed by bacteriological or radiological investigation, because the effects of treatment may be different in these groups.

INCIDENCE/ PREVALENCE Each year in Europe, 1–5% of adults are diagnosed with acute sinusitis by their general practitioner.[2] Extrapolated to the British population, this is estimated to cause 6 million restricted working days a year.[3,4] Most people with acute sinusitis are assessed and treated in a primary care setting. The prevalence varies according to whether diagnosis is made on clinical grounds or on the basis of radiological or bacteriological investigation.

AETIOLOGY/ RISK FACTORS One systematic review (search date 1998) reported that about 50% of people with a clinical diagnosis of acute sinusitis have bacterial sinus infection.[1] The usual pathogens in acute bacterial sinusitis are *Streptococcus pneumoniae* and *Haemophilus influenzae*, with occasional infection with *Moraxella catarrhalis*. Preceding viral upper respiratory tract infection is often the trigger for acute bacterial sinusitis,[5] with about 0.5% of common colds becoming complicated by the development of acute sinusitis.[6]

PROGNOSIS One meta-analysis of RCTs found that up to two thirds of people with acute sinusitis had spontaneous resolution of symptoms without active treatment.[7] One non-systematic review reported that people with acute sinusitis are at risk of chronic sinusitis and irreversible damage to the normal mucociliary mucosal surface.[8] One further non-systematic review reported rare life-threatening complications such as orbital cellulitis and meningitis after acute sinusitis.[9] However, we found no reliable data to measure these risks.

Please refer to clinicalevidence.com for full text and references.

Tinnitus

Search date November 2005

Stephanie Cook, Julian Savage, Angus Waddell

What are the effects of treatments for chronic tinnitus?

TRADE OFF BETWEEN BENEFITS AND HARMS

Tricyclic antidepressants

One RCT identified by a systematic review in people with depression and chronic tinnitus found that tricyclic antidepressants (nortriptyline) improved global satisfaction and depression at 6 weeks compared with placebo, but found no significant difference in self reported tinnitus severity compared with placebo. One small subsequent RCT in people with tinnitus and no depression found that a greater proportion of people rated themselves as improved with tricyclic antidepressants (amitriptyline) compared with placebo at 6 weeks, but did not assess the significance of the difference between groups. Tricyclic antidepressants are associated with adverse effects such as dry mouth, blurred vision, and constipation.

UNKNOWN EFFECTIVENESS

Acupuncture

RCTs identified by a systematic review provided inconclusive evidence about the effects of acupuncture in people with chronic tinnitus.

Baclofen

One RCT identified by a systematic review found no significant difference between baclofen and placebo in tinnitus severity. The RCT may have lacked power to detect a clinically important effect.

Benzodiazepines (alprazolam)

One small RCT identified by a systematic review found limited evidence that alprazolam, a benzodiazepine, improved self reported tinnitus severity compared with placebo after 12 weeks, but did not assess the significance of the difference between groups. Benzodiazepines can have adverse effects that may outweigh potential benefits.

Cinnarizine

One small RCT identified by a systematic review found no significant difference between cinnarizine and placebo in tinnitus severity. The RCT may have lacked power to detect a clinically important effect.

Electromagnetic stimulation/ear canal magnets

Two small RCTs provided insufficient evidence to compare electromagnetic stimulation versus placebo. One RCT found similar effects between simple ear canal magnets and placebo on tinnitus symptoms after 4 weeks, but did not assess the significance of the difference between groups.

Ginkgo biloba

One RCT found no significant difference in Tinnitus Handicap Inventory scores between ginkgo biloba and placebo in people with chronic tinnitus.

◀ **Hearing aids** *New*

One small RCT in people having hearing aids fitted for hearing loss and who also had tinnitus, found no significant difference in tinnitus between hearing aid and waiting list control.

Hyperbaric oxygen

One small RCT in people who had idiopathic sudden sensorineural hearing loss over 6 months previously found no significant difference in tinnitus between hyperbaric oxygen and control.

Hypnosis

One RCT found no significant difference between hypnosis and counselling for symptom severity at 3 months.

Lamotrigine

One small crossover RCT found insufficient evidence on the effects of lamotrigine versus placebo.

Nicotinamide

One RCT identified by a systematic review found similar effects between nicotinamide and placebo in tinnitus severity at 30 days, but did not assess the significance of the difference between groups. The RCT may have lacked power to detect a clinically important effect.

Psychotherapy

One systematic review provided insufficient evidence to assess the effects of cognitive behavioural treatment, relaxation therapy, education, or biofeedback compared with other or no treatment in people with chronic tinnitus. One subsequent RCT found limited evidence that cognitive behavioural treatment improved tinnitus related disability compared with control.

Tinnitus masking devices

One small crossover RCT identified by a systematic review found similar effects between a masking device and placebo in tinnitus symptoms, but did not assess the significance of the difference between groups.

Tinnitus retraining therapy

We found no systematic review or RCTs of tinnitus retraining therapy in people with chronic tinnitus.

Zinc

One RCT identified by a systematic review found no significant difference between zinc and placebo in tinnitus severity at 8 weeks. The RCT may have lacked power to detect a clinically important effect.

LIKELY TO BE INEFFECTIVE OR HARMFUL

Carbamazepine

One RCT identified by a systematic review found similar effects between carbamazepine and placebo in tinnitus severity at 30 days, but did not assess the significance of the difference between groups. Treatment with carbamazepine was associated with an increased proportion of people reporting side effects including dizziness, nausea, and headaches. ▶

Tinnitus

DEFINITION Tinnitus is the perception of sound in the ear or head which does not arise from the external environment, from within the body (e.g. vascular sounds), or from auditory hallucinations related to mental illness. This review is concerned with tinnitus, where tinnitus is the only, or the predominant, symptom in an affected person.

INCIDENCE/ PREVALENCE Up to 18% of the general population in industrialised countries are mildly affected by chronic tinnitus, and 0.5% report tinnitus having a severe effect on their ability to lead a normal life.[1]

AETIOLOGY/ RISK FACTORS Tinnitus may occur as an isolated idiopathic symptom or in association with any type of hearing loss. Tinnitus may be a particular feature of presbycusis (age related hearing loss), noise induced hearing loss, Menière's disease (see Menière's disease), or the presence of an acoustic neuroma. In people with toxicity from aspirin or quinine, tinnitus can occur while hearing thresholds remain normal. Tinnitus is also associated with depression, although it may be unclear whether the tinnitus is a manifestation of the depressive illness or a factor contributing to its development.[2] Studies involving people with tinnitus due to Menière's disease, acoustic neuroma, chronic otitis media, head injury, barotraumas, or other clear pathology have been excluded from this review. This review is principally concerned with idiopathic tinnitus with or without degenerative sensorineural hearing loss.

PROGNOSIS Tinnitus may have an insidious onset, with a long delay before clinical presentation. It may persist for many years or decades, particularly when associated with a sensorineural hearing loss. Tinnitus may cause disruption of sleep patterns, an inability to concentrate, and depression.[3]

Please refer to clinicalevidence.com for full text and references.

Tonsillitis

Search date November 2005

William McKerrow

What are the effects of tonsillectomy in children and adults with severe tonsillitis?

TRADE OFF BETWEEN BENEFITS AND HARMS

Tonsillectomy versus watchful waiting with antibiotics in children

Two systematic reviews that included the same two RCTs in children found insufficient evidence to compare surgical versus non-surgical treatment. One subsequent RCT in less severely affected children found that surgery reduced the frequency of throat infection compared with medical treatment over 3 years. However, it suggested that the modest benefit may be outweighed by the morbidity associated with the surgery in populations with a low incidence of tonsillitis.

UNKNOWN EFFECTIVENESS

Tonsillectomy compared with antibiotics in adults

We found no systematic review or RCTs evaluating tonsillectomy in adults.

DEFINITION Tonsillitis is an infection of the parenchyma of the palatine tonsils. The definition of severe recurrent tonsillitis is arbitrary, but recent criteria have defined severe tonsillitis as five or more episodes of true tonsillitis a year, symptoms for at least a year, and episodes that are disabling and prevent normal functioning.[1] The definition does not include tonsillitis owing to infectious mononucleosis, which usually occurs as a single episode. However, acute tonsillitis in this situation may be followed by recurrent tonsillitis in some people. Tonsillitis may occur in isolation or as part of a generalised pharyngitis. The clinical distinction between tonsillitis and pharyngitis is unclear in the literature, and the condition is often referred to simply as "acute sore throat". A sore throat lasting for 24–48 hours as part of the prodrome of minor upper respiratory tract infection is excluded from this definition. Diagnosis of acute tonsillitis is primarily clinical, with the main interest being in whether the illness is viral or bacterial, this being of relevance if antibiotics are being considered. Studies have attempted to distinguish viral from bacterial sore throat on clinical grounds, but the results are conflicting, suggesting a lack of reliable diagnostic criteria. Investigations to assist with this distinction include throat swabs and serological tests, including the rapid antigen test and the antistreptolysin O titre. Rapid antigen testing is convenient and popular in North America but has doubtful sensitivity (61–95%), at least when measured against throat swab results, although specificity is higher (88–100%).[1] However, the inevitable delay in reporting of both swabs and the antistreptolysin O titre reduce their value in the routine clinical situation.

INCIDENCE/ PREVALENCE Recurrent sore throat has an incidence in general practice in the UK of 100 per 1000 population a year.[2] Acute tonsillitis is more common in childhood.

AETIOLOGY/ RISK FACTORS Common bacterial pathogens include beta haemolytic and other streptococci. Bacteria are cultured only from a minority of people with tonsillitis. The role of viruses is uncertain. In tonsillitis associated with infectious mononucleosis, the most common infective agent is the Epstein–Barr virus (present in 50% of children and 90% of adults with the condition). Cytomegalovirus infection may also result in the clinical picture of infectious mononucleosis, and the differential diagnosis also includes toxoplasmosis, HIV, hepatitis A, and rubella.[3]

Tonsillitis

PROGNOSIS We found no good data on the natural history of tonsillitis or recurrent sore throat in children or adults. People in RCTs randomised to medical treatment (courses of antibiotics as required) have shown a tendency towards improvement over time.[4,5] Recurrent severe tonsillitis results in considerable morbidity, including time lost from school or work. The most common complication of acute tonsillitis is peritonsillar abscess, but we found no good evidence on its incidence. Rheumatic fever and acute glomerulonephritis are recognised complications of acute tonsillitis associated with group A beta haemolytic streptococci. These diseases are rare in developed countries, but do occasionally occur. They are still a common problem in certain populations, notably Australian Aboriginals, and may be effectively prevented in closed communities by the use of penicillin. A recently updated systematic review found that antibiotics reduced the incidence of these diseases.[6] However, in the developed world, these diseases are so rare that routine aggressive antibiotic use is not justified. The review also found that antibiotics shorten the duration of illness by about 16 hours overall.[6]

Please refer to clinicalevidence.com for full text and references.

Obesity

Search date July 2005

David E Arterburn, David E DeLaet, and Daniel P Schauer

What are the effects of drug treatments in adults with obesity?

TRADE OFF BETWEEN BENEFITS AND HARMS

Diethylpropion

One systematic review found that, in people having lifestyle interventions, diethylpropion promoted modest weight loss compared with placebo in obese adults. The review provided insufficient evidence to compare diethylpropion versus other agents. We found two case reports describing pulmonary hypertension and psychosis with diethylpropion. We found insufficient evidence on weight regain and long term safety. A European Commission review concluded that a link between diethylpropion and heart and lung problems could not be excluded.

Mazindol

One systematic review found that, in people having lifestyle interventions, mazindol promoted modest weight loss compared with placebo in obese adults. The review provided insufficient evidence to compare mazindol versus other agents. We found one case report of pulmonary hypertension diagnosed 1 year after stopping treatment with mazindol. We found one case series of mazindol in people with stable cardiac disease, which reported cardiac events such as atrial fibrillation and syncope. We found insufficient evidence on weight regain and long term safety.

Orlistat

Two systematic reviews and five subsequent RCTs found that, in people on a low calorie diet, orlistat modestly increased weight loss at 6–12 months compared with placebo in obese adults, in both those who did and who did not have diabetes, hyperlipidaemia, and hypertension. Two RCTs found that orlistat was less effective than sibutramine in achieving weight loss. [Two other RCTs found a similar reduction in body mass index or weight from baseline with orlistat and sibutramine]. Adverse effects such as diarrhoea, flatulence, bloating, and abdominal pain occurred in a high proportion of people taking orlistat. We found insufficient evidence on the effects of orlistat on weight regain and long term safety.

Phentermine

One systematic review found that, in people having lifestyle interventions, phentermine promoted modest weight loss compared with placebo in obese adults. RCTs identified by the review provided insufficient evidence to compare phentermine versus other agents. We found insufficient evidence on weight regain and long term safety with phentermine. A European Commission review concluded that a link between phentermine and heart and lung problems could not be excluded.

Rimonabant *New*

One RCT provided limited evidence that rimonabant 5 mg and 20 mg daily in addition to a calorie restricted diet, increased weight loss at 1 year compared ▶

with placebo. It also found that rimonabant 20 mg daily increased the proportion of people who withdrew due to adverse effects (including nausea, vomiting, diarrhoea, headache, dizziness, and anxiety) compared with rimonabant 5 mg daily or placebo.

Sibutramine

One systematic review and three subsequent RCTs found that, in people having dietary interventions with or without exercise, sibutramine increased weight loss at 8 weeks, 6 months, and 1 year compared with placebo in obese adults, in both those who did and who did not have diabetes, hypertension, hyperlipidaemia, or binge eating disorder. RCTs in obese adults who had lost weight by taking sibutramine found limited evidence that sibutramine was more effective than placebo for weight maintenance. Other RCTs found that weight regain occurred when sibutramine was discontinued. Two RCTs found that sibutramine achieved greater weight loss than orlistat. Two other RCTs found a similar reduction in body mass index or weight from baseline with sibutramine and orlistat. We found insufficient evidence to compare sibutramine versus other drugs. Sibutramine was temporarily suspended from the market in Italy for use in obesity because of concerns about severe adverse reactions, including arrhythmias, hypertension, and two deaths resulting from cardiac arrest. Two RCTs found no significant difference in the incidence of valvular heart disease between sibutramine and placebo, although these trials may have lacked power to detect a clinically important difference.

UNKNOWN EFFECTIVENESS

Sibutramine plus orlistat

We found no RCTs comparing sibutramine plus orlistat versus placebo. One small RCT provided limited evidence that, in addition to a reduced calorie diet, sibutramine plus orlistat increased weight loss compared with orlistat alone at 6 months, but not compared with sibutramine alone. One RCT found no significant difference in weight loss maintenance between sibutramine plus orlistat and sibutramine plus placebo, but found that sibutramine plus orlistat increased gastrointestinal adverse events (soft stools, bowel movements, oily evacuation, and faecal urge).

What are the effects of bariatric surgery in adults with morbid obesity?

LIKELY TO BE BENEFICIAL

Bariatric surgery (more effective than non-surgical treatment for clinically important weight loss in morbidly obese adults; but operative complications common)

Two systematic reviews identified one prospective, multicentre cohort study, which found that bariatric surgery (vertical banded gastroplasty, gastric bypass, or gastric banding) increased weight loss compared with non-surgical treatment (low calorie diet or usual care) in morbidly obese adults. Long term follow up of the prospective cohort study found that the differences in weight loss between surgery and non-surgical treatments were sustained at 10 years. The study found that, on average, bariatric surgery for obesity resulted in 23.4% weight loss after 2 years (compared with a 0.1% weight gain in matched participants who did not have surgery) and sustained a 16.1% weight loss 10 years later. The 30 day risk of death from surgery varies with the type of bariatric procedure performed, and ranges from 0.25–1.9%. Operative and postoperative complications are common and vary with the type of bariatric procedure performed. The systematic reviews also identified two retrospective cohort studies, which found that bariatric surgery decreased mortality compared with non-surgical treatment in morbidly obese adults at 5–15 year follow up. The two retrospective cohort studies also reported postoperative complications including bleeding, thromboembolism, wound complications, deep infections, pulmonary complications, and digestive disorders. We found no RCTs or observational studies of sufficient quality comparing biliopancreatic diversion or sleeve gastrectomy versus non-surgical treatment.

Gastric banding

Two systematic reviews found that gastric banding is effective in promoting clinically important weight loss in morbidly obese adults. One small RCT found that gastric banding was less effective than gastric bypass in reducing weight at 18 months. Three RCTs found inconclusive results regarding weight loss with gastric banding compared with vertical banded gastroplasty. One small RCT identified by a systematic review found no significant difference in weight loss between open and laparoscopic gastric banding at 12 months. However, laparoscopic gastric banding was found to be associated with shorter hospital stays and fewer readmissions than was open gastric banding. There is a small risk of perioperative death with gastric banding, but postoperative complications are common and may require reoperation. There is insufficient evidence to draw conclusions about the relative benefits and harms of gastric banding compared with gastric bypass or vertical banded gastroplasty.

Gastric bypass

Two systematic reviews found that gastric bypass is effective in promoting clinically important weight loss in morbidly obese adults. One small RCT identified by a systematic review found limited evidence of greater weight loss with gastric bypass than with gastric banding. The systematic review also identified six RCTs, which compared gastric bypass versus vertical banded gastroplasty. Four of the RCTs found that gastric bypass increased weight loss at 1–3 years compared with vertical banded gastroplasty, but another two RCTs found no significant difference between the procedures. Two subsequent RCTs found that laparoscopic gastric bypass increased weight loss compared with laparoscopic vertical banded gastroplasty at 1 and 2 year follow up. One small RCT found no significant difference in weight loss between proximal and distal gastric bypass at 1 or 2 year follow up. Three RCTs, two identified by a systematic review, found no significant difference in weight loss between open and laparoscopic gastric bypass. However, laparoscopic gastric bypass reduced hospital stay compared with open gastric bypass. There is a small risk of perioperative death with gastric bypass, but postoperative complications are common and may require reoperation. There is insufficient evidence to draw conclusions about the relative benefits and harms of gastric bypass compared with gastric banding or vertical banded gastroplasty.

Vertical banded gastroplasty

Two systematic reviews found that vertical banded gastroplasty is effective in promoting clinically important weight loss in morbidly obese adults. Three RCTs found inconclusive results regarding weight loss with vertical banded gastroplasty compared with gastric banding. One systematic review also identified six RCTs, which compared gastric bypass versus vertical banded gastroplasty. Four of these RCTs found that vertical banded gastroplasty was less effective than gastric bypass in increasing weight loss at 1–3 years, but another two RCTs

Obesity

found no significant difference between the procedures. Two subsequent RCTs also found that laparoscopic vertical banded gastroplasty was less effective than laparoscopic gastric bypass for increasing weight loss at 1 and 2 year follow up. One small RCT identified by the systematic review found no significant difference in weight loss at 1 year or in hospital stay between open and laparoscopic vertical banded gastroplasty, but found that operating time was significantly longer with laparoscopic gastroplasty. There is a small risk of perioperative death with vertical banded gastroplasty, but postoperative complications are common and may require reoperation. There is insufficient evidence to draw conclusions about the relative benefits and harms of vertical banded gastroplasty compared with gastric banding or gastric bypass.

UNKNOWN EFFECTIVENESS

Biliopancreatic diversion (no studies comparing biliopancreatic diversion versus other bariatric techniques)

Two systematic reviews found no RCTs comparing biliopancreatic diversion versus other bariatric procedures.

Sleeve gastrectomy (no studies comparing sleeve gastrectomy versus other bariatric techniques) *New*

Two systematic reviews identified no RCTs comparing sleeve gastrectomy versus other bariatric procedures.

See glossary

DEFINITION Obesity is a chronic condition characterised by an excess of body fat. It is most often defined by the body mass index (BMI), a mathematical formula that is highly correlated with body fat. BMI is weight in kilograms divided by height in metres squared (kg/m^2). Worldwide, adults with BMIs between 25–30 kg/m^2 are categorised as overweight, and those with BMIs above 30 kg/m^2 are categorised as obese.[1,2] Nearly 5 million US adults used prescription weight loss medication between 1996 and 1998. A quarter of users were not overweight. Inappropriate use of prescription medication is more common among women, white people, and Hispanic people.[3] The National Institutes of Health in the USA has issued guidelines for obesity treatment, which indicate that all obese adults (BMI > 30 kg/m^2) and all adults with a BMI of 27 kg/m^2 or more and obesity associated chronic diseases are candidates for drug treatment.[1] Morbidly obese adults (BMI > 40 kg/m^2) and all adults with a BMI of 35 kg/m^2 or more and obesity associated chronic diseases are candidates for bariatric surgery.

INCIDENCE/ PREVALENCE Obesity has increased steadily in many countries since 1900. In the UK in 2002, it was estimated that 23% of men and 25% of women were obese.[4] In the past decade alone, the prevalence of obesity in the USA has increased from 22.9% between 1988 and 1994, to 32.2% in 2004.[5,6]

AETIOLOGY/ RISK FACTORS Obesity is the result of long term mismatches in energy balance, where daily energy intake exceeds daily energy expenditure.[7] Energy balance is modulated by a myriad of factors, including metabolic rate, appetite, diet, and physical activity.[8] Although these factors are influenced by genetic traits, the increase in obesity prevalence in the past few decades cannot be explained by changes in the human gene pool, and is more often attributed to environmental changes that promote excessive food intake and discourage physical activity.[8,9] Less commonly, obesity may also be induced by drugs (e.g. high dose glucocorticoids), or be secondary to a variety of neuroendocrine disorders such as Cushing's syndrome and polycystic ovary syndrome.[10]

PROGNOSIS Obesity is a risk factor for several chronic diseases, including hypertension, dyslipidaemia, diabetes, cardiovascular disease, sleep apnoea, osteoarthritis, and some cancers.[1] The relationship between increasing body weight and mortality is curvilinear, where mortality is highest among adults with very low body weight (BMI < 18.5 kg/m^2) and among adults with the highest body weight (BMI > 35 kg/m^2).[2] Obese adults have more annual admissions to hospitals, more outpatient visits, higher prescription drug costs, and worse health related quality of life than normal weight adults.[11,12] Less than 10% of overweight or obese adults aged 40–49 years revert to a normal body weight after 4 years.[13]

Please refer to clinicalevidence.com for full text and references.

Primary hypothyroidism

Search date January 2006

Birte Nygaard

What are the effects of treatments for clinical (overt) hypothyroidism?

BENEFICIAL

Levothyroxine (L-thyroxine)*

We found no systematic review or RCTs that compared levothyroxine versus placebo, although there is consensus that treatment is beneficial. A placebo controlled trial would be considered unethical. One systematic review found no good evidence of an improvement in outcomes with a combination of levothyroxine plus liothyronine compared with levothyroxine alone. Treating clinical (overt) hypothyroidism with thyroid hormone (levothyroxine) may induce hyperthyroidism and reduce bone mass in postmenopausal women and increase the risk of atrial fibrillation.

*No RCT evidence, but there is clinical consensus that levothyroxine is beneficial in clinical (overt) hypothyroidism. A placebo controlled trial would be considered unethical.

UNKNOWN EFFECTIVENESS

Levothyroxine (L-thyroxine) plus liothyronine

One systematic review found no good evidence of an improvement in outcomes with a combination of levothyroxine plus liothyronine compared with levothyroxine alone. Treating clinical (overt) hypothyroidism with thyroid hormone (levothyroxine) can induce hyperthyroidism and reduce bone mass in postmenopausal women and increase the risk of atrial fibrillation.

What are the effects of treatments for subclinical hypothyroidism?

UNKNOWN EFFECTIVENESS

Levothyroxine (L-thyroxine)

One small RCT in women with biochemically defined subclinical hypothyroidism found limited evidence that L-thyroxine improved overall symptoms compared with placebo after 1 year. However, another small RCT found no significant difference in health related quality of life scores between levothyroxine and placebo at 6 months. One small RCT found inconclusive results about the effect of levothyroxine versus placebo on cognitive function in people with subclinical hypothyroidism. One small RCT found that levothyroxine improved left ventricular function at 6 months compared with placebo. Treating subclinical hypothyroidism with thyroid hormone can induce hyperthyroidism and reduce bone mass in postmenopausal women and increase the risk of atrial fibrillation.

DEFINITION Hypothyroidism is characterised by low levels of blood thyroid hormone. **Clinical (overt) hypothyroidism** is diagnosed on the basis of characteristic clinical features consisting of mental slowing, depression, dementia, weight gain, constipation, dry skin, hair loss, cold intolerance, hoarse voice, irregular menstruation, infertility, muscle stiffness and pain, bradycardia, hypercholesterolaemia, combined with a raised blood level of thyroid stimulating hormone (TSH) (serum TSH levels > 12 mU/L), and a low serum thyroxine (T4) level ▶

(serum T4 < 60 nmol/L). **Subclinical hypothyroidism** is diagnosed when serum TSH is raised (serum TSH levels > 4 mU/L) but serum T_4 is normal and there are no symptoms or signs, or only minor symptoms or signs, of thyroid dysfunction. **Primary hypothyroidism** is seen after destruction of the thyroid gland because of autoimmunity (the most common cause), or medical intervention such as surgery, radioiodine, and radiation. **Secondary hypothyroidism** is seen after pituitary or hypothalamic damage, and results in insufficient production of TSH. Secondary hypothyroidism is not covered in this review. **Euthyroid sick syndrome** is diagnosed when tri-iodothyronine (T3) levels are low, serum T_4 is low, and TSH levels are normal or low. Euthyroid sick syndrome is not covered in this review.

INCIDENCE/ PREVALENCE Hypothyroidism is more common in women than in men (in the UK, female : male ratio of 6 : 1). One study (2779 people in the UK with a median age of 58 years) found that the incidence of clinical (overt) hypothyroidism was 40/10 000 women a year and 6/10 000 men a year. The prevalence was 9.3% in women and 1.3% in men.[1] In areas with high iodine intake, the incidence of hypothyroidism can be higher than in areas with normal or low iodine intake. In Denmark, where there is moderate iodine insufficiency, the overall incidence of hypothyroidism is 1.4/10 000 a year, increasing to 8/10 000 a year in people older than 70 years.[2] The incidence of subclinical hypothyroidism increases with age. Up to 10% of women over the age of 60 years have subclinical hypothyroidism (evaluated from data from the Netherlands and USA).[3,4]

AETIOLOGY/ RISK FACTORS Primary thyroid gland failure can occur as a result of chronic autoimmune thyroiditis, radioactive iodine treatment, or thyroidectomy. Other causes include drug adverse effects (e.g. amiodarone and lithium), transient hypothyroidism due to silent thyroiditis, subacute thyroiditis, or postpartum thyroiditis.

PROGNOSIS In people with subclinical hypothyroidism, the risk of developing clinical (overt) hypothyroidism is described in the UK Whickham Survey (25 years' follow up; for women: OR 8, 95% CI 3 to 20; for men: OR 44, 95% CI 19 to 104; if both a raised TSH and positive antithyroid antibodies were present; for women: OR 38, 95% CI 22 to 65; for men: OR 173, 95% CI 81 to 370). For women, the survey found an annual risk of 4.3% per year (if both raised serum TSH and antithyroid antibodies were present) and 2.6% per year (if raised serum TSH was present alone); the minimum number of people with raised TSH and antithyroid antibodies who would need treating to prevent this progression to clinical (overt) hypothyroidism in one person over 5 years is 5–8.[1] **Cardiovascular disease:** A large cross sectional study (25 862 people with serum TSH between 5.1 mU/L and 10.0 mU/L) found significantly higher mean total cholesterol concentrations in people who were hypothyroid compared with people who were euthyroid (5.8 mmol/L *v* 5.6 mmol/L).[3] Another study (124 elderly women with subclinical hypothyroidism, 931 women who were euthyroid) found a significantly increased risk of myocardial infarction in women with subclinical hypothyroidism (OR 2.3, 95% CI 1.3 to 4.0) and of aortic atherosclerosis (OR 1.7, 95% CI 1.1 to 2.6).[4] **Mental health:** Subclinical hypothyroidism is associated with depression.[5] People with subclinical hypothyroidism may have depression that is refractory to both antidepressant drugs and thyroid hormone alone. Memory impairment, hysteria, anxiety, somatic complaints, and depressive features without depression have been described in people with subclinical hypothyroidism.[6]

Please refer to clinicalevidence.com for full text and references.

Age related macular degeneration

Search date March 2005

Jennifer Arnold

What are the effects of interventions to prevent progression of age related macular degeneration?

LIKELY TO BE BENEFICIAL

Antioxidant vitamin and zinc supplementation

One systematic review found modest evidence from one large RCT that, in people with early to late age related macular degeneration, antioxidant vitamins plus zinc supplements reduced the risk of progression and vision loss over 6 years compared with placebo.

UNKNOWN EFFECTIVENESS

Laser to drusen

Two RCTs provided insufficient evidence to assess whether laser to drusen decreased incidence of late age related macular degeneration, choroidal neovascularisation, or geographic atrophy. The first RCT found that threshold laser treatment improved visual acuity after 2 years compared with no treatment, but not compared with subthreshold treatment. The second, larger RCT, found a similar improvement in visual acuity after 1 year but the difference was not significant. Subgroup analysis found improved visual acuity where laser treatment had reduced the number of drusen by 50% or more. The RCT also found that, in people with unilateral (but not bilateral) drusen, laser increased the short term incidence of choroidal neovascularisation compared with no treatment. Another RCT also found a higher rate of choroidal neovascularisation with laser in people with unilateral drusen.

What are the effects of treatments for exudative age related macular degeneration?

BENEFICIAL

Photodynamic treatment with verteporfin

Systematic reviews of two RCTs in people with age related macular degeneration found that photodynamic treatment with verteporfin reduced the risk of moderate or severe loss of visual acuity and of legal blindness after 1–2 years in people with vision better than 20/100 or 20/200 compared with placebo. Photodynamic treatment with verteporfin was associated with an initial loss of vision and photosensitive reactions in a small proportion of people.

TRADE OFF BETWEEN BENEFITS AND HARMS

Thermal laser photocoagulation

Four large RCTs found that, in people with well demarcated exudative age related macular degeneration, thermal laser photocoagulation reduced severe visual loss after 2–5 years compared with no treatment, but was frequently associated with an immediate and permanent reduction in visual acuity. Choroidal neovascularisation recurred within 3 years in about half of those treated. One small RCT provided insufficient evidence to compare thermal laser photocoagulation versus submacular surgery.

UNKNOWN EFFECTIVENESS

External beam radiation

One systematic review found no evidence that external beam radiotherapy compared with observation or sham or low dose radiotherapy is an effective treatment for subfoveal choroidal neovascularisation. Most trials found effects that favoured treatment, but there was inconsistency in results. We found insufficient evidence on long term safety, although the systematic review found no evidence of toxicity to the optic nerve or retina after 12–24 months.

LIKELY TO BE INEFFECTIVE OR HARMFUL

Interferon alfa-2a (subcutaneous)

One large RCT found that in people with age related macular degeneration, visual loss was higher with subcutaneous interferon alfa-2a (an anti-angiogenesis drug) after 1 year compared with placebo, although the difference was not significant. The RCT also found evidence of serious ocular and systemic adverse effects.

Submacular surgery

Two large RCTs found little or no improvement in vision from surgery in people with age related macular degeneration, with new choroidal neovascularisation, with or without haemorrhagic choroidal neovascularisation. Surgery carries an increased risk of retinal detachment and cataract formation.

DEFINITION Age related macular degeneration (AMD) has two clinical stages: **early AMD** marked by drusen and pigmentary change, and usually associated with normal vision; and **late or sight threatening AMD** associated with a decrease in central vision. Late stage AMD has two forms: **atrophic (or dry) AMD**, characterised by geographic atrophy; and **exudative (or wet) AMD**, characterised by choroidal neovascularisation, which eventually causes a disciform scar.

INCIDENCE/ PREVALENCE AMD is a common cause of blindness registration in industrialised countries. Atrophic AMD is more common than the more sight threatening exudative AMD, affecting about 85% of people with AMD.[1] Late (sight threatening) AMD is found in about 2% of all people aged over 50 years, and prevalence rises with age (0.7–1.4% of people aged 65–75 years; 11–19% of people aged > 85 years).[2-4]

AETIOLOGY/ RISK FACTORS Proposed hypotheses for the cause of atrophic and exudative AMD involve vascular factors and oxidative damage coupled with genetic predisposition.[5] Age is the strongest risk factor. Systemic risk factors include hypertension, smoking, and a family history of AMD.[5-7] Ocular risk factors for the development of exudative AMD include the presence of soft drusen, macular pigmentary change, CNV in the other eye, and previous cataract surgery.[8] Hypertension, diet (especially intake of antioxidant micronutrients), and oestrogen are suspected as causal agents for atrophic and exudative AMD, but the effects of these factors remain unproven.[5,9]

PROGNOSIS AMD impairs central vision, which is required for reading, driving, face recognition, and all fine visual tasks. **Atrophic AMD** progresses slowly over many years, and time to legal blindness is highly variable (usually about 5–10 years).[10,11] **Exudative AMD** is more often threatening to vision; 90% of people with severe visual loss owing to AMD have the exudative type. This condition usually manifests with a sudden worsening and distortion of central vision. One study estimated (based on data derived primarily from cohort studies) that the risk of developing exudative AMD in people with bilateral soft drusen was 1–5%

Age related macular degeneration

at 1 year and 13–18% at 3 years.[12] The observed 5 year rate in a population survey was 7%.[13] Most eyes (estimates vary from 60% to 90%) with exudative AMD progress to legal blindness and develop a central defect (scotoma) in the visual field.[14-17] Peripheral vision is preserved, allowing the person to be mobile and independent. The ability to read with visual aids depends on the size and density of the central scotoma and the degree to which the person retains sensitivity to contrast. Once exudative AMD has developed in one eye, the other eye is at high risk (cumulative estimated incidence: 10% at 1 year, 28% at 3 years, and 42% at 5 years).[18]

Please refer to clinicalevidence.com for full text and references.

Bacterial conjunctivitis

Search date January 2006

John Epling, John Smucny

What are the effects of antibiotics in adults and children with bacterial conjunctivitis?

BENEFICIAL

Antibiotics (topical) in people with non-gonococcal culture positive bacterial conjunctivitis

One systematic review and two additional RCTs found that topical antibiotics (polymyxin B sulphate–bacitracin, ciprofloxacin, ofloxacin, levofloxacin, moxifloxacin) increased rates of both clinical and microbiological cure at 2–10 days compared with placebo, but these differences were minor. One RCT found that a significant increase in clinical cure at 3–5 days with polymyxin B sulphate plus bacitracin compared with placebo was not sustained at 8–10 days. Four RCTs found no significant difference between different antibiotics in clinical or microbiological cure. One RCT found that fusidic acid increased clinical cure rate compared with chloramphenicol. One RCT found that topical netilmicin increased clinical cure rate compared with topical gentamicin. One RCT found that topical levofloxacin increased microbiological cure rate, but not clinical cure rate, compared with topical ofloxacin. The RCTs found minimal and infrequent side effects, with no significant differences between topical antibiotics and placebo. RCTs comparing different antibiotics versus each other found that some antibiotics caused higher rates of punctuate epithelial erosions, stinging, burning, and slight irritation than others.

UNKNOWN EFFECTIVENESS

Empirical treatment with topical antibiotics in people with suspected bacterial conjunctivitis

One systematic review found high clinical cure rates with both topical antibiotics and placebo in people with suspected bacterial conjunctivitis, with no significant difference between topical antibiotics and placebo in two out of three RCTs identified. The third RCT found that norfloxacin increased clinical cure compared with placebo at 5 days. In a subgroup of people with culture positive bacterial conjunctivitis, all three RCTs found that topical antibiotics increased microbiological cure rates compared with placebo. The review found similar rates of adverse events with topical antibiotics and placebo, apart from with fusidic acid, which increased adverse events compared with placebo. RCTs comparing different topical antibiotics versus each other found high rates of clinical or microbiological cure, with no significant difference in rates between groups. One RCT found no significant difference between topical polymyxin B sulphate–bacitracin ointment and oral cefixime for clinical or microbiological improvement or cure, but it may have been underpowered to detect a clinically important difference. Topical antibiotics are associated with burning, stinging, and bad taste.

DEFINITION Conjunctivitis is any inflammation of the conjunctiva, generally characterised by irritation, itching, foreign body sensation, and watering or discharge. Treatment is often based on clinical suspicion that the conjunctivitis is bacterial, without waiting for the results of microbiological investigations. In this topic, we have therefore distinguished the effects of empirical treatment ▶

Bacterial conjunctivitis

from effects of treatment in people with culture positive bacterial conjunctivitis. This review covers only non-gonococcal bacterial conjunctivitis. Bacterial conjunctivitis in contact lens wearers is of particular concern because of the risk of bacterial keratitis, an infection of the cornea accompanying acute or subacute corneal trauma, which is more difficult to treat than conjunctivitis and can threaten vision.[1,2]

INCIDENCE/ PREVALENCE We found no good evidence on the incidence or prevalence of bacterial conjunctivitis.

AETIOLOGY/ RISK FACTORS Conjunctivitis may be infectious (caused by bacteria or viruses) or allergic. In adults, bacterial conjunctivitis is less common than viral conjunctivitis, although estimates vary widely (viral conjunctivitis has been reported to account for 8–75% of acute conjunctivitis).[3-5] *Staphylococcus* species are the most common pathogens for bacterial conjunctivitis in adults, followed by *Streptococcus pneumoniae* and *Haemophilus influenzae*.[6,7] In children, bacterial conjunctivitis is more common than the viral form, and is mainly caused by *H influenzae*, *S pneumoniae*, and *Moraxella catarrhalis*.[8,9] Narrative reviews suggest that the causative agents of bacterial conjunctivitis and keratitis in contact lens wearers are more frequently gram negative bacteria (such as *Pseudomonas aeruginosa*), but may include all of the above aetiologies. *Acanthamoeba spp*. infections can be particularly difficult to diagnose and treat and are most common in contact lens wearers.[1,2]

DIAGNOSIS The traditional criteria differentiating bacterial from other types of conjunctivitis have been: a yellow–white mucopurulent discharge, a papillary reaction (small bumps with fibrovascular cores on the palpebral conjunctiva, appearing grossly as a fine velvety surface), and bilateral infection. A recent systematic review was unable to find any quality research basis for these criteria, but a follow-up study performed by the authors of the review found that glued eyes and the absence of itching were predictive of a bacterial cause. A history of conjunctivitis in the recent past argued against a bacterial aetiology.[10,11]

PROGNOSIS Most bacterial conjunctivitis is self limiting. One systematic review (search date 2004) found clinical cure or significant improvement with placebo within 2–5 days in 65% of people.[12] Some organisms cause corneal or systemic complications, or both. Otitis media may develop in 25% of children with *H influenzae* conjunctivitis,[13] and systemic meningitis may complicate primary meningococcal conjunctivitis in 18% of people.[14] Bacterial keratitis is estimated to occur in 10–30 per 100 000 contact lens wearers.[15]

Please refer to clinicalevidence.com for full text and references.

Cataract

Search date October 2005

David Allen

What are the effects of surgery for age related cataract without other ocular comorbidity?

BENEFICIAL

Manual extracapsular extraction (more effective than intracapsular extraction but less effective than phaco extracapsular extraction)

We found no RCTs comparing manual extracapsular extraction versus no extraction, although there is consensus that cataract extraction is preferable to no intervention. One RCT found that manual extracapsular extraction plus intraocular lens implant improved visual acuity and quality of life compared with intracapsular extraction plus aphakic glasses. The RCT also found a higher rate of complications with intracapsular extraction plus aphakic glasses than with a manual extracapsular extraction plus intraocular lens implant. One RCT identified by a systematic review found that manual extracapsular extraction plus rigid posterior chamber intraocular lens implant was less effective for improving vision at up to 1 year compared with phaco extracapsular extraction plus foldable posterior chamber intraocular lens implant. The RCT and a systematic review of observational studies found that a higher proportion of people had complications with manual extracapsular extraction than with phaco extracapsular extraction.

Phaco extracapsular extraction (improved visual acuity and fewer complications than manual extracapsular extraction)

We found no systematic review or RCTs comparing phaco extracapsular extraction versus no extraction, although there is consensus that cataract extraction is preferable to no intervention. One RCT found phaco extracapsular extraction improved visual acuity at 6 months and reduced falls at 12 months compared with waiting list control. One RCT identified by a systematic review found improved vision up to 1 year after phaco extracapsular extraction plus foldable posterior chamber intraocular lens implant compared with manual extracapsular extraction plus rigid posterior chamber intraocular lens implant. The RCT and a systematic review of observational studies found that a higher proportion of people had complications with manual extracapsular extraction than with phaco extracapsular extraction. We found no systematic review or RCTs comparing phaco extracapsular extraction versus intracapsular extraction.

LIKELY TO BE BENEFICIAL

Intracapsular extraction (more effective than no extraction*; less effective than manual extracapsular extraction and has more complications)

We found no systematic review or RCTs comparing intracapsular extraction versus no extraction, however, there is consensus that the clinical and quality of life benefits of modern cataract removal are such that an RCT that includes non-intervention would be unethical. One RCT found that manual extracapsular extraction plus intraocular lens implant improved visual acuity and quality of life compared with intracapsular extraction plus aphakic glasses. The RCT also found a higher rate of complications with intracapsular extraction plus aphakic glasses than with manual extracapsular extraction plus intraocular lens implant. We found no systematic review or RCTs comparing intracapsular extraction ▶

versus phaco extracapsular extraction. Such RCTs are unlikely to be performed as intracapsular extraction has been superseded by manual extracapsular extraction in the developed world.

*Based on consensus.

What are the effects of treatment for age related cataracts in people with glaucoma?

LIKELY TO BE BENEFICIAL

Concomitant cataract and glaucoma surgery (reduced intraocular pressure compared with cataract surgery alone)

Three RCTs identified by a systematic review found that concomitant cataract surgery (phaco or manual extracapsular extraction) and glaucoma surgery reduced intraocular pressure compared with cataract surgery alone in people with glaucoma. Another RCT identified by the review found a similar reduction in intraocular pressure with phaco extracapsular extraction plus glaucoma surgery and phaco extracapsular extraction alone. No significant differences were found in visual acuity changes between treatments. One systematic review found no RCTs comparing the effects of phaco extracapsular extraction versus manual extracapsular extraction in people having concomitant glaucoma surgery.

UNKNOWN EFFECTIVENESS

Cataract surgery (manual or phaco extracapsular extraction) alone

One systematic review found no RCTs on the effectiveness of cataract surgery alone (phaco extraction and manual extracapsular extraction) compared with no surgery in people with glaucoma. The review identified four RCTs comparing cataract surgery alone versus concomitant cataract and glaucoma surgery. Three of the RCTs found that cataract surgery alone was less effective at reducing intraocular pressure compared with concomitant cataract surgery and glaucoma surgery in people with glaucoma. Another RCT identified by the review found a similar reduction in intraocular pressure with phaco extracapsular extraction plus glaucoma surgery and with phaco extracapsular extraction alone. No significant differences were found in visual acuity changes between treatments.

Cataract surgery plus non-concomitant glaucoma surgery

One systematic review identified no RCTs comparing cataract surgery plus non-concomitant glaucoma surgery versus cataract surgery alone or concomitant cataract surgery and glaucoma surgery.

DEFINITION **Cataracts** are cloudy or opaque areas in the lens of the eye (which should usually be completely clear). This results in changes that can impair vision. **Age related (or senile) cataract** is defined as cataract occurring in people over 16 years of age in the absence of known mechanical, chemical, or radiation trauma. This chapter covers treatment for age related cataract. It does not cover cataract in people with diabetes mellitus or recurrent uveitis; these conditions can affect the surgical outcome. This chapter also addresses the treatment of age related cataract in people with glaucoma. Surgery for cataracts in people with glaucoma may affect glaucoma control, and the optimal strategy for treating these conditions when they co-exist is not clear. See also glaucoma.

INCIDENCE/ PREVALENCE Cataract accounts for over 40% of blindness worldwide, causing blindness in about 15.8 million people in 1990.[1] A cross-sectional study in a representative sample of an urban population in New South Wales, Australia in 1997

(3654 people aged 49–96 years) found that the prevalence of late cataract (of all types) in people aged 65–74 years was 21.6%, and in people aged 85 years and over was 67.3%.[2] This rate excluded those people who had already had cataract surgery. The incidence of non-age related cataract within this population is so small that this can be taken as the effective incidence of age related cataract. Glaucoma has an overall prevalence of about 2.0% rising to about 4.5% in people aged 70 years or over (the peak age for cataract surgery). The 5 year incidence of nuclear cataract in people aged over 50 years old and with open angle glaucoma was estimated to be 25% in 2006.[3]

AETIOLOGY/ RISK FACTORS Diet, smoking,[4] and exposure to ultraviolet light[5] are thought to be risk factors in the development of age related cataract. In addition, some people may have a genetic predisposition to development of age related cataract.[6]

PROGNOSIS Age related cataract progresses with age, but at an unpredictable rate. Cataract surgery is indicated when the chances of significant visual improvement outweigh the risks of a poor surgical outcome. It is not dependent on reaching a specific visual acuity standard. Cataract surgery may also be indicated where the presence of cataract makes it hard to treat or monitor concurrent retinal disease, such as diabetic retinopathy.

Please refer to clinicalevidence.com for full text and references.

Glaucoma

Search date January 2006

Rajiv Shah and Richard Wormald

What are the effects of treatments for established primary open angle glaucoma, ocular hypertension, or both?

LIKELY TO BE BENEFICIAL

Laser trabeculoplasty plus topical medical treatment (compared with no initial treatment or topical medical treatment alone)

RCTs in people with newly diagnosed primary open angle or pseudoexfoliation glaucoma found that laser trabeculoplasty plus topical medical treatment to lower intraocular pressure reduced progression of glaucoma compared with no initial treatment or compared with topical treatment alone at 6–7 years.

Topical medical treatment (in people with primary open angle glaucoma or ocular hypertension)

One systematic review found that, compared with placebo, topical medical treatment (primarily timolol and betaxolol) reduced the proportion of people who developed glaucoma (defined as visual field loss, deterioration of optic disc, or both in people with ocular hypertension). However, one large subsequent RCT in people with ocular hypertension found no significant difference between dorzolamide and placebo in the proportion of people who developed primary open angle glaucoma over 5 years. The review found limited evidence from one RCT that topical medical treatment also reduced progression of glaucoma at 6 years in people with primary open angle glaucoma. Analysis of longer term data in African American participants found similar beneficial effects of topical medical treatment. One RCT in people with primary open angle glaucoma found that, compared with topical medical treatment alone, initial laser trabeculoplasty followed by topical medical treatment reduced intraocular pressure and deterioration in optic disc appearance, and improved visual fields after a mean of 7 years. One systematic review found no significant difference in visual field loss at 2–5 years between topical medical treatment and surgical trabulectomy in people with primary open angle glaucoma but found that surgery increased the risk of developing cataracts and the need for cataract surgery. Results for loss in visual field acuity were inconclusive, with two RCTs finding no significant difference between groups but one larger RCT finding that participants treated medically had a lower risk of visual acuity loss than people treated surgically.

TRADE OFF BETWEEN BENEFITS AND HARMS

Surgical trabeculectomy

One systematic review found no significant difference in visual field loss at 2–5 years between surgical trabulectomy and topical medical treatment in people with primary open angle glaucoma and found that surgery increased the risk of developing cataracts and the need for cataract surgery. Results for loss in visual field and visual acuity were inconclusive. Two RCTs in people with newly diagnosed or advanced primary open angle glaucoma found that surgical trabeculectomy reduced intraocular pressure compared with laser trabeculoplasty. They found mixed effects for changes in visual acuity and visual field loss after 5–7 years. Surgical trabeculectomy has been reported to be associated with a reduction in central vision.

UNKNOWN EFFECTIVENESS

Laser trabeculoplasty (compared with surgical trabeculectomy)

Two RCTs found that laser trabeculoplasty was less effective than surgical trabeculectomy in reducing intraocular pressure, but found mixed effects for changes in visual acuity after 5–7 years.

What are the effects of lowering intraocular pressure in people with normal tension glaucoma?

LIKELY TO BE BENEFICIAL

Medical treatment

One systematic review of two RCTs in people with normal tension or primary open angle glaucoma found that topical medical treatment reduced the proportion of people with glaucoma progression at 5–6 years compared with placebo. Subgroup analysis found no significant difference in people with normal tension glaucoma, although fewer people having topical medical treatment had progression.

TRADE OFF BETWEEN BENEFITS AND HARMS

Surgical treatment

One RCT identified by a systematic review found that both surgical and topical medical treatment, either singly or combined, reduced progression of visual field loss after 5 years in people with people with normal tension glaucoma compared with no treatment, but found that surgery increased cataract formation after 8 years.

What are the effects of treatment for acute angle closure glaucoma?

LIKELY TO BE BENEFICIAL

Medical treatment*

We found no placebo controlled RCTs, but consensus suggests that medical treatments are effective for acute angle closure glaucoma. One small RCT in people with angle closure glaucoma receiving acetazolamide found that low dose pilocarpine, an intensive pilocarpine regimen, or pilocarpine ocular inserts all reduced intraocular pressures after 2 hours with no significant difference among groups. We found no RCTs of other medical treatments.

Surgical treatment*

We found no placebo controlled RCTs, but consensus suggests that surgical treatments are effective for acute angle closure glaucoma. One small RCT in people with uniocular acute angle closure glaucoma found no significant difference between surgical iridectomy and laser iridotomy in visual acuity or intraocular pressure after 3 years.

*No placebo controlled RCTs but strong consensus that treatments are effective.

DEFINITION Glaucoma is a group of diseases characterised by progressive optic neuropathy. It is usually bilateral but asymmetric and may occur at any intraocular pressure. All forms of glaucoma show optic nerve damage (cupping, pallor, or both) associated with peripheral visual field loss. **Primary open angle glaucoma** occurs in people with an open anterior chamber drainage angle and no secondary identifiable cause. Knowledge of the natural history of these conditions is incomplete, but it is thought that the problem starts with an intraocular pressure that is too high for the optic nerve. However, in a large proportion of people with glaucoma (about 40%) intraocular pressure is within the statistically defined normal range. The term ocular hypertension generally applies to eyes with an intraocular pressure greater than the statistical upper limit of normal (about 21 mm Hg). However, only a relatively small proportion of eyes with raised intraocular pressure have an optic nerve that is vulnerable to its effects (about 10%). However, because intraocular pressure is the main and only modifiable risk factor for the disease, studies on the effectiveness of reducing intraocular pressure often include people who have both ocular hypertension and primary open angle glaucoma. Previously, trialists were anxious about withholding active treatment in overt primary open angle glaucoma, and so many placebo or no treatment trials selected people just with ocular hypertension. Trials comparing treatments often include both people with primary open angle glaucoma and people with ocular hypertension, but in these the outcome is usually intraocular pressure alone. **Normal tension glaucoma** occurs in people with intraocular pressures that are consistently below the statistical upper limit of normal (21 mm Hg; 2 standard deviations above the population mean). **Acute angle closure glaucoma** is glaucoma resulting from a rapid and severe rise in intraocular pressure caused by physical obstruction of the anterior chamber drainage angle.

INCIDENCE/ PREVALENCE Glaucoma occurs in 1–2% of white people aged over 40 years, rising to 5% at 70 years. Primary open angle glaucoma accounts for two thirds of those affected, and normal tension glaucoma for about a quarter.[1,2] In black people glaucoma is more prevalent, presents at a younger age with higher intraocular pressures, is more difficult to control, and is the main irreversible cause of blindness in black populations of African origin.[1,3] Glaucoma related blindness is responsible for 8% of new blind registrations in the UK.[4]

AETIOLOGY/ RISK FACTORS The major risk factor for developing primary open angle glaucoma is raised intraocular pressure. In one RCT (90 people with intraocular pressure > 22 mm Hg, 1 other glaucoma risk factor, and normal visual fields, mean age 55–56 years), three baseline risk factors were identified to be independently associated with glaucomatous field loss.[5] These were higher intraocular pressure ($P = 0.047$, intraocular pressure per mm Hg), suspect discs ($P = 0.007$), and older age ($P = 0.034$, age per year).[6] Lesser risk factors include family history and ethnic origin. The relationship between systemic blood pressure and intraocular pressure may be an important determinant of blood flow to the optic nerve head and, as a consequence, may represent a risk factor for glaucoma.[6] Systemic hypotension, vasospasm (including Raynaud's disease and migraine), and a history of major blood loss have been reported as risk factors for normal tension glaucoma in hospital based studies.[7] Risk factors for acute angle closure glaucoma include family history, female sex, being long sighted, and cataract. One systematic review (search date 1999, 6 observational studies, 594 662 people with mydriasis) did not find any evidence supporting the theory that routine pupillary dilatation with short acting mydriatics was a risk factor for acute angle closure glaucoma.[8]

PROGNOSIS Advanced visual field loss is found in about 20% of people with primary open angle glaucoma at diagnosis,[9] and is an important prognostic factor for glaucoma related blindness.[10] Blindness owing to glaucoma results from gross loss of visual field or loss of central vision. Once early field defects have appeared, and where the intraocular pressure is greater than 30 mm Hg, untreated people may lose the remainder of the visual field in 3 years or less.[11] As the disease progresses, people with glaucoma have difficulty moving from a bright room to a darker room, and judging steps and kerbs. Progression of visual field loss is often slower in normal tension glaucoma. Acute angle glaucoma leads to rapid loss of vision, initially from corneal oedema and subsequently from ischaemic optic neuropathy.

Please refer to clinicalevidence.com for full text and references.

Ocular herpes simplex

Search date June 2006

Nigel H Barker

What are the effects of treatments in people with epithelial keratitis?

BENEFICIAL

Antiviral agents (topical)

One systematic review found that topical antivirals (idoxuridine or vidarabine) increased healing after 14 days compared with placebo, and that trifluridine or aciclovir increased healing compared with idoxuridine after 7 and 14 days. The review also found that antiviral treatment plus debridement increased healing after 7 days compared with antivirals alone. The review found no significant difference in healing at 14 days between antiviral treatment plus debridement and antiviral treatment alone. It also found no significant difference between topical antivirals (idoxuridine) and topical interferon in healing after 7 days, but found that topical interferon increased healing after 14 days. The review also found that adding topical interferon to a topical antiviral agent increased healing at 7 days compared with the antiviral agent alone. "Healing" was not always clearly defined.

Interferons (topical)

One systematic review found that topical interferons (alfa or beta) increased healing after 7 and 14 days compared with placebo. The review found no significant difference between a topical interferon beta and a topical nucleoside antiviral agent (idoxuridine) in healing after 7 days, but found that a topical interferon increased healing after 14 days. The review also found that topical interferon plus a topical antiviral agent increased healing compared with a topical antiviral agent alone after 7 days. "Healing" was not always clearly defined.

UNKNOWN EFFECTIVENESS

Debridement

One systematic review found no significant difference between physicochemical debridement and no treatment. The review also found that physicochemical debridement plus antiviral treatment improved healing at 7 days compared with either treatment alone. This difference remained significant at 14 days for combined treatment compared with physicochemical debridement alone. The review found no significant difference in healing at 7 or 14 days between physical debridement plus aciclovir compared with physical debridement plus idoxuridine.

What are the effects of treatments in people with stromal keratitis?

BENEFICIAL

Adding topical corticosteroids to topical antiviral treatment

One RCT in people receiving topical antiviral treatment found that adding topical corticosteroids reduced progression and shortened the duration of stromal keratitis compared with placebo.

UNLIKELY TO BE BENEFICIAL

Adding oral aciclovir to topical corticosteroids plus topical antiviral treatment

One RCT in people receiving topical corticosteroids plus topical antiviral treatment found no significant difference between oral aciclovir and placebo in rates of treatment failure at 16 weeks.

What are the effects of interventions to prevent recurrence of ocular herpes simplex?

BENEFICIAL

Long term (1 year) oral aciclovir

One large RCT in people with at least one previous episode of epithelial or stromal keratitis found that long term oral aciclovir reduced recurrence after 1 year compared with placebo.

UNLIKELY TO BE BENEFICIAL

Short term (3 weeks) oral aciclovir

One RCT in people with epithelial keratitis receiving a topical antiviral agent (trifluridine) found no significant difference between short term prophylaxis with oral aciclovir and placebo in the rate of stromal keratitis or iritis at 1 year.

What are the effects of interventions to prevent recurrence of ocular herpes simplex in people with corneal grafts?

UNKNOWN EFFECTIVENESS

Oral aciclovir

One small open label RCT found limited evidence that prophylactic use of oral aciclovir reduced recurrence and improved graft survival compared with placebo.

DEFINITION Ocular herpes simplex is usually caused by herpes simplex virus type 1 (HSV-1) but also occasionally by the type 2 virus (HSV-2). Ocular manifestations of HSV are varied and include blepharitis (inflammation of the eyelids), canalicular obstruction, conjunctivitis, corneal complications, iritis, and retinitis. Corneal complications are of two main types: **epithelial keratitis** is inflammation of the cells that form the surface layer of the cornea and **stromal keratitis** is inflammation of the middle layer (stroma) of the cornea. HSV infections are classified as neonatal, primary (HSV in a person with no previous viral exposure), and recurrent (previous viral exposure with humoral and cellular immunity present).

INCIDENCE/ PREVALENCE Infections with HSV are usually acquired in early life. A US study found antibodies against HSV-1 in about 50% of people with high socioeconomic status and 80% of people with low socioeconomic status by the age of 30 years. It quoted one report, which suggested that overcrowding may be a causal factor.[1] However, only about 20–25% of people with HSV antibodies had any history of clinical manifestations of ocular or cutaneous herpetic disease.[2] Ocular HSV is the most common cause of corneal blindness in high income countries and is the most common cause of unilateral corneal blindness in the world.[3] A 33 year study of the population of Rochester, Minnesota, found the annual incidence of new cases of ocular herpes simplex was 8.4/100 000 (95% CI 6.9/100 000 to 9.9/100 000) and the annual

Ocular herpes simplex

incidence of all episodes (new and recurrent) was 20.7/100 000 (95% CI 18.3/100 000 to 23.1/100 000).[4] The prevalence of ocular herpes was 149/100 000 population (95% CI 115/100 000 to 183/100 000). Twelve per cent of people had bilateral disease.[4]

AETIOLOGY/ RISK FACTORS Epithelial keratitis results from productive, lytic viral infection of the corneal epithelial cells. Stromal keratitis and iritis are thought to result from a combination of viral infection and compromised immune mechanisms. Observational evidence (346 people with ocular HSV in the placebo arm of an RCT) showed that a previous history of stromal keratitis was a risk factor for the recurrence of stromal keratitis (6/174 [4%] without previous stromal keratitis *v* 53/172 [32%] with previous stromal keratitis; RR 10.0, 95% CI 4.3 to 23.0; $P < 0.001$).[5] Age, sex, ethnicity, and previous history of non-ocular HSV disease were not associated with an increased risk of recurrence.[5]

PROGNOSIS HSV epithelial keratitis tends to resolve spontaneously within 1–2 weeks while stromal keratitis is more likely to result in corneal scarring and loss of vision. In a trial of 271 people treated with topical trifluorothymidine and randomly assigned to receive either oral aciclovir or placebo, the epithelial lesion had resolved completely or was at least less than 1 mm after 1 week of treatment with placebo in 89% of people and after 2 weeks in 99% of people.[6] Stromal keratitis or iritis occurs in about 25% of people after epithelial keratitis.[7] The effects of HSV stromal keratitis include scarring, tissue destruction, neovascularisation, glaucoma, and persistent epithelial defects. The rate of recurrence of ocular herpes for people with one episode is 10% at 1 year, 23% at 2 years, and 50% at 10 years.[8] The risk of recurrent ocular HSV infection (epithelial or stromal) also increases with the number of previous episodes reported (2 or 3 previous episodes: RR 1.41, 95% CI 0.82 to 2.42; 4 or more previous episodes: RR 2.09, 95% CI 1.24 to 3.50).[5] Of corneal grafts performed in Australia over a 10 year period, 5% were in people with visual disability or with actual or impending corneal perforation after stromal ocular herpes simplex. The recurrence of HSV in a corneal graft has a major effect on graft survival. The Australian Corneal Graft Registry found that, in corneal grafts performed for HSV keratitis, there was at least one HSV recurrence in 58% of corneal grafts that failed over a follow up period of 9 years.[9]

Please refer to clinicalevidence.com for full text and references.

Trachoma

Search date January 2006

Anthony W Solomon, Denise Mabey, and David CW Mabey

What are the effects of interventions to prevent scarring trachoma by reducing the prevalence of active trachoma?

LIKELY TO BE BENEFICIAL

Fly control using insecticide

A small pilot study for an RCT found that fly control using deltamethrin reduced the incidence of active trachoma after 3 months compared with no intervention. A larger RCT found that fly control using permethrin reduced the prevalence of active trachoma compared with no intervention. Although the RCTs found evidence of a short term benefit, it is unlikely that this intervention would be cost effective or acceptable (from an individual or an environmental point of view) if an attempt was made to implement it on a large scale. The purpose of this trial was to demonstrate that fly control interventions in general might be effective.

Promotion of face washing plus topical tetracycline (better than tetracycline alone)

One RCT found that promotion of face washing plus topical tetracycline reduced the prevalence of "severe trachoma" (a non-standard diagnosis) after 1 year compared with topical tetracycline alone. It found no significant difference in the prevalence of "any trachoma". However, the RCT may have lacked power to rule out a clinically important effect. Another RCT found that face washing (performed by a teacher) plus topical tetracycline reduced the proportion of children with trachoma after 3 months compared with no intervention.

UNKNOWN EFFECTIVENESS

Antibiotics

One systematic review found insufficient evidence comparing antibiotics with placebo or each other in people with active trachoma. The same review also found insufficient evidence comparing oral azithromycin versus topical tetracycline in active trachoma, and insufficient evidence comparing oral antibiotics other than azithromycin with topical antibiotics for active trachoma. Trials were heterogeneous and the review did not exclude clinically important effects.

Face washing alone

One RCT found no significant difference between face washing alone (performed by a teacher) and no intervention on the prevalence of trachoma in children after 3 months.

Fly control through the provision of pit latrines

One RCT found no significant difference between the provision of improved household pit latrines and no intervention (using existing facilities, mainly no or local latrine) on the prevalence of active trachoma.

Health education

One small RCT found limited evidence of a reduction in the incidence of active trachoma with health education compared with no intervention.

Trachoma

What are the effects of eye lid surgery for entropion and trichiasis?

LIKELY TO BE BENEFICIAL

Bilamellar tarsal rotation or tarsal advance and rotation (better than other types of eyelid surgery)

In people with major trichiasis, one RCT found limited evidence that bilamellar tarsal rotation increased operative success and reduced adverse effects after 2 weeks compared with eversion splinting, tarsal advance, or tarsal grooving. However, it found no significant difference between bilamellar tarsal rotation and tarsal advance and rotation in operative success after 2 weeks. A second RCT found that bilamellar tarsal rotation increased operative success after 25 months compared with tarsal advance and rotation. In both RCTs, one experienced surgeon performed most of the operations. In people with minor trichiasis, one of the RCTs found that tarsal rotation increased operative success after 25 months compared with cryoablation or electrolysis. One further RCT reporting combined results for major and minor trichiasis found no significant difference in recurrence between bilamellar tarsal rotation and tarsal advance and lid margin rotation after 3 months, although there were more minor complications (lid notching and pyogenic granuloma) with the bilamellar procedure. In this RCT, the operations were undertaken by less experienced surgeons under supervision.

DEFINITION **Active trachoma** is chronic inflammation of the conjunctiva caused by infection with *Chlamydia trachomatis*. The World Health Organization simplified trachoma grading scheme defines active trachoma as TF and/or TI, where TF (trachomatous inflammation — follicular) is the presence of five or more follicles in the central part of the upper tarsal conjunctiva each at least 0.5 mm in diameter, and TI (trachomatous inflammation — intense) is pronounced inflammatory thickening of the upper tarsal conjunctiva that obscures more than half of the normal deep vessels.[1] **Cicatricial trachoma** is caused by repeated infection by *C trachomatis*; it includes the presence of visible scars on the tarsal conjunctiva (trachomatous scarring), shortening and inversion of the upper eye lid (entropion), and malposition of the lashes so that they abrade the eye (trichiasis). Trachomatous scarring can be present without entropion/trichiasis but if entropion/trichiasis is present because of trachoma, there will be scarring. Trachoma blindness results from corneal opacification, which occurs due to the mechanical trauma wrought by entropion/trichiasis. **Diagnosis** of trachoma is by clinical examination, using the criteria set out in either the modified WHO grading system[2] or the WHO simplified grading system.[1] The simplified grading system is now the most commonly employed.

INCIDENCE/ PREVALENCE Trachoma is the world's leading cause of infectious blindness.[3] Globally, active trachoma affects an estimated 84 million people, most of them children. About 7.6 million people are blind or at risk of blindness as a consequence.[4] Trachoma is a disease of poverty, regardless of geographical region. Cicatricial trachoma is prevalent in large regions of Africa, the Middle East, Asia, and Aboriginal communities in Australia, and there are also small foci in Central and South America.[3] In areas where trachoma is constantly present at high prevalence, active disease is found in more than 50% of preschool children and may have a prevalence as high as 60–90%,[5] and as many as 75% of women and 50% of men over the age of 45 years may show signs of scarring disease.[6] The prevalence of active trachoma decreases with increasing age.[5] Although similar prevalences of active disease are observed in boys and girls, the later sequelae of trichiasis, entropion, and corneal opacification are usually more common in women than men.[5]

AETIOLOGY/ RISK FACTORS Active trachoma is associated with youth, poor access to water and sanitation, and close contact between people. Discharge from the eyes and nose may facilitate transmission of ocular *C trachomatis* infection.[7] Sharing a bedroom with someone who has active trachoma is a risk factor for infection.[8] The density of eye seeking flies in a community is held to be associated with active trachoma.[9,10] Flies important to trachoma transmission lay their eggs on human faeces lying exposed on the soil, suggesting that access to improved sanitation might help to control trachoma.[11,12]

PROGNOSIS Corneal damage from trachoma is caused by multiple processes. Scarring trachoma damages glandular structures and may cause an inadequate tear film; a dry eye may be more susceptible to damage from inturned lashes and superadded infection by other bacteria and fungi, leading to corneal opacification.

Please refer to clinicalevidence.com for full text and references.

Uveitis (acute anterior)

Search date February 2006

André Curi, Kimble Matos, and Carlos Pavesio

What are the effects of anti-inflammatory eye drops on acute anterior uveitis?

LIKELY TO BE BENEFICIAL

Corticosteroid eye drops*

Corticosteroid eye drops have been standard treatment for anterior uveitis since the early 1950s. However, we found insufficient evidence from RCTs about their effects in people with acute anterior uveitis. One small RCT found no significant difference between corticosteroid (betamethasone phosphate/clobetasone butyrate) eye drops and placebo in symptom severity after 14 or 21 days. Two RCTs found no significant difference between prednisolone and rimexolone in the anterior chamber cell count (a marker of disease severity). One RCT found that prednisolone increased the proportion of people with fewer than five anterior chamber cells per examination field after 28 days compared with loteprednol. The results of a second RCT comparing prednisolone with loteprednol were difficult to interpret. RCTs found that rimexolone and loteprednol were less likely than prednisolone to be associated with increased intraocular pressure, although differences were not significant. Three RCTs found no significant difference between corticosteroid and non-steroidal anti-inflammatory drug (NSAID) eye drops in clinical cure rate after 14 or 21 days.

*Based on consensus; RCTs unlikely to be conducted.

Non-steroidal anti-inflammatory drug (NSAID) eye drops (as effective as corticosteroids)

One RCT found no significant difference between non-steroidal anti-inflammatory drug (NSAID) eye drops and placebo eye drops in clinical cure rate after 21 days. Three RCTs found no significant difference between NSAID eye drops and corticosteroid eye drops in clinical cure rate after 14 or 21 days.

DEFINITION Anterior uveitis is inflammation of the uveal tract, and includes iritis and iridocyclitis. It can be classified according to its clinical course into acute or chronic anterior uveitis, or according to its clinical appearance into granulomatous or non-granulomatous anterior uveitis. **Acute anterior uveitis** is characterised by an extremely painful red eye, often associated with photophobia and occasionally with decreased visual acuity.[1] **Chronic anterior uveitis** is defined as inflammation lasting over 6 weeks. It is usually asymptomatic, but many people have mild symptoms during exacerbations.

INCIDENCE/ PREVALENCE Acute anterior uveitis is rare with an annual incidence of 12/100 000 population.[2] It is particularly common in Finland (annual incidence 22.6/100 000 population, prevalence 68.7/100 000 population), probably owing to genetic factors such as the high frequency of HLA-B27 in the Finnish population.[3] It is equally common in men and women, and more than 90% of cases occur in people older than 20 years of age.[3,4]

AETIOLOGY/ RISK FACTORS No cause is identified in 60–80% of people with acute anterior uveitis. Systemic disorders that may be associated with acute anterior uveitis include ankylosing spondylitis, Reiter's syndrome, Kawasaki's disease, infectious uveitis, Behçet's syndrome, inflammatory bowel disease, interstitial nephritis, sarcoidosis, Vogt-Koyanagi-Harada syndrome, and masquerade syndromes.[5] Acute anterior ▶

uveitis also occurs in association with HLA-B27 expression not linked to any systemic disease. Acute anterior uveitis may occur after surgery or as an adverse drug or hypersensitivity reaction.[3,4]

PROGNOSIS Acute anterior uveitis is often self limiting, but we found no evidence about how often it resolves spontaneously, in which people, or over what length of time. Complications include posterior synechiae, cataract, glaucoma, and chronic uveitis. In a study of 154 people (232 eyes) with acute anterior uveitis (119 people HLA-B27 positive), visual acuity was better than 20/60 in 209/232 eyes (90%), and 20/60 or worse in 23/232 eyes (10%), including worse than 20/200 (classified as legally blind) in 11/232 eyes (5%).[6]

Please refer to clinicalevidence.com for full text and references.

HIV infection

Search date June 2005

Martin Talbot

What are the effects of preventive interventions?

LIKELY TO BE BENEFICIAL

Early diagnosis and treatment of sexually transmitted diseases (in regions with emerging HIV epidemics)

Three RCTs found different results concerning the effect of early diagnosis and treatment of sexually transmitted infections on HIV incidence. One large community based RCT in a region with a relatively mature HIV epidemic and one smaller RCT in female sex workers found no significant difference between routine care and improved diagnosis and management of sexually transmitted infections in the incidence of HIV infection. One large community based RCT in a region with an emerging HIV epidemic found that improved diagnosis and management of sexually transmitted infections reduced the incidence of HIV over 2 years compared with routine care. Interventions to decrease HIV transmission by reducing sexually transmitted infections may be effective only in regions where the HIV epidemic is emerging, and infection is concentrated within a population where the incidence of sexually transmitted infections is high.

Postexposure prophylaxis in health care workers

One case control study found limited evidence that postexposure prophylaxis with zidovudine may reduce the risk of HIV infection over 6 months. RCTs in people with established HIV infection found that combinations of antiretroviral drugs are more effective than antiretroviral monotherapy for treating HIV, suggesting that the same may be true in a prophylactic setting. However, adverse effects of antiretroviral treatments are common, especially with combination treatment, and cause a significant proportion of people receiving postexposure prophylaxis to discontinue treatment after a short time.

UNKNOWN EFFECTIVENESS

Presumptive mass treatment of sexually transmitted infections

One RCT found no significant difference between presumptive mass antibiotic treatment of sexually transmitted infections and control in the incidence of HIV infection over 20 months. One RCT found no significant difference in HIV-1 infection at 2 years between monthly empirical antibiotics (azithromycin) and placebo as part of a package of HIV preventive services in initially HIV negative female sex workers.

What are the effects of different antiretroviral drug treatment regimens in HIV infection?

BENEFICIAL

Boosted protease inhibitor based regimens (at least as effective as standard protease based triple regimens at reducing viral load)

Two RCTs found that boosted protease inhibitor based regimens reduced viral load compared with standard protease inhibitor based triple regimens at 24–48 weeks. They found no significant difference between treatments in overall adverse events. One RCT found no significant difference between a boosted ▶

protease inhibitor based regimen and two different standard protease inhibitor based triple regimens in progression to an AIDS defining event or death, or in proportion of people with undetectable viraemia at 72 weeks. It found that more people taking ritonavir as part of the standard protease inhibitor triple regimen discontinued their assigned protease inhibitor treatment compared with people taking the boosted protease inhibitor regimen or the indinavir based standard protease inhibitor triple regimen. We found no RCTs comparing boosted protease inhibitor based regimens versus dual NRTI regimens, triple NRTI regimens, or NNRTI based triple regimens. One systematic review of observational studies found that protease inhibitor based regimens increased total cholesterol, triglycerides, and low density lipoprotein. Findings from other observational studies suggest that some NRTIs (notably stavudine) may play a role in the development of lipodystrophy.

Dual NRTI regimens (more effective than NRTI monotherapy, but less effective than protease inhibitor based or NNRTI based triple regimens)

It is well established that dual NRTI regimens are more effective than NRTI monotherapy. One systematic review found that dual NRTI regimens were less effective than protease inhibitor based triple regimens at reducing HIV viral load at up to 1 year. The review found reduced adverse events with dual NRTI regimens compared with protease inhibitor triple regimens. The systematic review found that dual NRTI regimens were less effective than protease inhibitor based triple regimens at reducing progression to AIDS and death at up to 1 year. We found no RCTs comparing dual NRTI treatment with boosted protease inhibitor based triple treatment. One systematic review found that dual NRTI regimens were less effective at viral suppression than NNRTI based triple regimens at up to 1 year and found similar rates of overall adverse events between treatments. One RCT found no significant difference between dual and triple NRTI regimens in viral load or adverse events. However, the triple NRTI regimen increased CD4 cell count at up to 48 weeks. One systematic review of observational studies found that protease inhibitor based regimens increased total cholesterol, triglycerides, and low density lipoprotein. Findings from other observational studies suggest that some NRTIs (notably stavudine) may play a role in the development of lipodystrophy.

NNRTI based triple regimens (increase viral suppression compared with dual NRTI regimens or protease inhibitor based triple regimens)

One systematic review found that NNRTI (efavirenz or nevirapine) based triple regimens increased viral suppression at up to 1 year compared with dual NRTI regimens and found no significant difference between treatments in overall adverse events. One systematic review found no significant difference between NNRTI based triple regimens and protease inhibitor based triple regimens in HIV progression and found that protease inhibitors increased overall adverse events but decreased rash. This systematic review and subsequent RCTs provided evidence that NNRTI based triple regimens increased virological response compared with protease inhibitor based triple regimens. One of the RCTs provided evidence that the relative efficacy of NNRTI and protease inhibitor based triple regimens may depend on which NRTIs are used. We found no RCTs comparing NNRTI based triple regimens versus boosted protease inhibitor based regimens or triple NRTI regimens. One systematic review of observational studies found that protease inhibitor based regimens increased total cholesterol, triglycerides, and low density lipoprotein. Findings from other observational studies suggest that some NRTIs (notably stavudine) may play a role in the development of lipodystrophy.

Protease inhibitor based triple regimens (more effective than dual NRTI regimens, less effective at achieving viral response than NNRTI based triple regimens)

One systematic review found that protease inhibitor based triple regimens reduced viral load at up to 1 year compared with dual NRTI regimens. The systematic review found that protease inhibitor based triple regimens reduced progression to AIDS and death at up to 1 year compared with dual NRTI regimens. The review found reduced adverse events with dual NRTI regimens compared with protease inhibitor based triple regimens. Two RCTs found that boosted protease inhibitor based regimens reduced viral load compared with standard protease inhibitor based triple regimens at 24–48 weeks and found no significant difference between treatments in overall adverse effects. One RCT found no significant difference between a boosted protease inhibitor based regimen and two different standard protease inhibitor based triple regimens in progression to an AIDS defining event or death, or in the proportion of people with undetectable viraemia at 72 weeks. It found that more people taking ritonavir as part of the standard protease inhibitor triple regimen discontinued their assigned protease inhibitor treatment compared with people taking the boosted protease inhibitor or indinavir. One systematic review found no significant difference between protease inhibitor based triple regimens and NNRTI based triple regimens in HIV progression and found that NNRTI based triple regimens decreased overall adverse events but increased rash compared with protease inhibitor based triple regimens. This systematic review and subsequent RCTs provided evidence that NNRTI based triple regimens increased virological response compared with protease inhibitor based triple regimens. One of the RCTs provided evidence that the relative efficacy of NNRTI and protease inhibitor based triple regimens may depend on which NRTIs are used. One systematic review of observational studies found that protease inhibitor based regimens increased total cholesterol, triglycerides, and low density lipoprotein. Findings from other observational studies suggest that some NRTIs (notably stavudine) may play a role in the development of lipodystrophy.

Triple NRTI regimens (similar viral suppression to dual NRTI regimens)

One RCT found no significant difference between dual and triple NRTI regimens in viral load but found that the triple NRTI regimen increased CD4 cell count at up to 48 weeks. This RCT found similar rates of grade 3 to 4 adverse events between treatments. One RCT found no significant difference between protease inhibitor based triple regimens and triple NRTI regimens in viral suppression, CD4 cell count, or rates of treatment withdrawal owing to adverse events at 48 weeks. We found no RCTs comparing triple NRTI regimens versus NNRTI based triple regimens or boosted protease inhibitor based regimens. One systematic review of observational studies found that protease inhibitor based regimens increased total cholesterol, triglycerides, and low density lipoprotein. Findings from other observational studies suggest that some NRTIs (notably stavudine) may play a role in the development of lipodystrophy.

UNKNOWN EFFECTIVENESS

Early versus delayed treatment

One systematic review found no significant difference between early and delayed zidovudine monotherapy in AIDS free survival or overall survival at median follow up of 50 months. The review did not report harms. We found no RCTs exploring this question with dual or triple drug regimens.

HIV infection

DEFINITION HIV infection refers to infection with the human immunodeficiency virus (HIV) type 1 or type 2. Clinically, this is characterised by a variable period (about 8–10 years on average) of asymptomatic infection, followed by repeated episodes of illness of varying and increasing severity as immune function deteriorates, resulting in acquired immune deficiency syndrome (AIDS). The type of illness varies by country, availability of specific treatments for HIV, and prophylaxis for opportunistic infections. Current treatments interrupt the life cycle of the virus without effecting a cure: mutations in the viral genome result in gradual resistance drift and increasing ineffectiveness of drug treatments.

INCIDENCE/ PREVALENCE Worldwide estimates suggest that by December 2004 about 39.4 million people were living with HIV. In 2004 alone there were estimated to be 4.9 million new cases of HIV and 3.1 million deaths from AIDS.[1] About 95% of HIV infections occur in the developing world.[1] By 1999, occupationally acquired HIV infection in health care workers had been documented in at least 102 definite and 217 possible cases, although this is likely to be an underestimate.[2]

AETIOLOGY/ RISK FACTORS The major risk factor for transmission of HIV is unprotected heterosexual or homosexual intercourse. Other risk factors include needlestick injury, sharing drug injecting equipment, and blood transfusion. An HIV infected woman may also transmit the virus to her baby transplacentally, during birth, or through breast milk. This has been reported in 15–30% of pregnant women with HIV infection. Mother to child transmission of HIV is dealt with in a separate chapter (HIV: mother to child transmission). Not everyone who is exposed to HIV will become infected, although risk increases if exposure is repeated, at high dose, or through blood. There is at least a two to fivefold greater risk of HIV infection among people with sexually transmitted diseases.[3]

PROGNOSIS Without treatment, about 50% of people infected with HIV will become ill and die from AIDS over about 10 years. A meta-analysis of 13 cohort studies from Europe and the USA looked at 12 574 treatment naive people starting HAART with a combination of at least three drugs.[4] A lower baseline CD4 cell count and higher baseline HIV-1 viral load were associated with an increased probability of progression to AIDS or death. Other independent predictors of poorer outcome were advanced age, infection through injection drug use, and a previous diagnosis of AIDS. The CD4 cell count at initiation was the dominant prognostic factor in people starting HAART. People with the most favourable prognostic factors (aged < 50 years old, not infected through injection drug use, viral load < 100 000 copies/mL, and CD4 count > 350 cells/mL on initiation of HAART) were estimated to have a 3.5% chance of progression to AIDS or death within 3 years. People with the most unfavourable prognostic factors (aged ≥ 50 years old, infected through injection drug use, viral load ≥ 100 000 copies/mL, and CD4 count < 50 cells/mL on initiation of HAART) had an estimated 50% chance of progression to AIDS or death within 3 years. Genetic factors have been shown to affect response to antiretroviral treatment, but were not considered in the meta-analysis.[4]

Please refer to clinicalevidence.com for full text and references.

HIV: mother to child transmission

Search date January 2006

Jimmy Volmink and Unati Mahlati

What are the effects of measures to reduce mother to child transmission of HIV?

BENEFICIAL

Antiretroviral drugs

One systematic review found that zidovudine reduced the incidence of HIV in infants compared with placebo. One RCT identified by the review found that longer courses of zidovudine given to mother and infant reduced the incidence of HIV in infants compared with shorter courses of zidovudine. One RCT found no advantage in giving nevirapine compared with placebo to mother and baby when transmission rates were already reduced by mothers receiving standard antiretroviral treatment. However, one RCT found that nevirapine given to the mother and her newborn baby reduced the risk of HIV transmission compared with zidovudine. One RCT found no significant difference between a single dose of nevirapine given to infants within 24 hours of birth and 6 weeks of zidovudine in the rate of HIV-1 infection at 12 weeks. One RCT found that zidovudine plus lamivudine given in the antenatal, intrapartum, and postpartum periods, or during the intrapartum and postpartum periods reduced the risk of transmission of HIV at 6 weeks compared with placebo. One RCT found no significant difference in newborn HIV infection rates between nevirapine monotherapy and zidovudine plus lamivudine given to the mother during labour and to the mother and baby after delivery. However, one RCT found that nevirapine plus zidovudine given twice daily to babies for 7 days after birth reduced HIV transmission at 6–8 weeks compared with a single dose of nevirapine given to babies immediately after birth. One RCT found that in mothers receiving intrapartum nevirapine, rates of HIV infection in their babies at 6–8 weeks were similar whether babies received a single dose of nevirapine at birth plus zidovudine for 7 days or single dose nevirapine alone. One RCT found that, in mothers and babies receiving zidovudine prophylaxis, adding nevirapine reduced HIV transmission at 6 months compared with adding placebo. It found no significant difference in HIV infection rates in babies at 6 months between the addition of a single dose of nevirapine given to mothers and babies compared with the addition of a single dose of nevirapine given to mothers only.

LIKELY TO BE BENEFICIAL

Avoiding breast feeding (provided there is access to clean water and health education)

One RCT in women with HIV who had access to clean water and health education found that, compared with breastfeeding, formula feeding reduced the incidence of HIV in infants at 24 months without increasing mortality.

Elective caesarean section

One RCT identified by two systematic reviews provided limited evidence that elective caesarean section reduced the incidence of HIV in infants at 18 months compared with vaginal delivery.

UNKNOWN EFFECTIVENESS

Immunotherapy

One RCT found no significant difference in HIV transmission to infants from mothers taking zidovudine and either HIV hyperimmune globulin or immunoglobulin without HIV antibody. However, the study might have been too small to detect a clinically important difference.

Vaginal microbicides

One systematic review of two RCTs with methodological weaknesses found no significant difference between vaginal cleansing with microbicides and no microbicides in the risk of HIV transmission.

LIKELY TO BE INEFFECTIVE OR HARMFUL

Vitamin supplements

One systematic review found that vitamin A supplements given to HIV positive pregnant women had no significant effect on the risk of transmission of HIV infection in their infants compared with placebo or no vitamin A supplements. One RCT found that multivitamins given to mothers during pregnancy and lactation had no significant effect on HIV infection in their infants compared with placebo.

DEFINITION Mother to child transmission of HIV infection is defined as transmission of HIV infection from an infected mother to her child during gestation, labour, or through breastfeeding in infancy. HIV-1 infection may be transmitted from mother to child,[1] although HIV-2 is rarely transmitted in this way.[2] Infected children usually have no symptoms or signs of HIV at birth, but develop them over subsequent months or years.[3]

INCIDENCE/ PREVALENCE A review of 13 cohort studies found that the risk of mother to child transmission of HIV without antiviral treatment is on average about 15–20% in Europe, 15–30% in the USA, and 25–35% in Africa.[4] The risk of transmission is estimated to be 15–30% during pregnancy, with an additional risk of about 10–20% postpartum through breastfeeding.[5] UNAIDS estimated that, at the end of 2005, 2.3 million children worldwide under the age of 15 years were living with HIV/AIDS. Of these, more than 80% were in sub-Saharan Africa.[6] An estimated 700 000 children under 15 years of age were newly infected with HIV in 2004 alone; more than 75% of them were in sub-Saharan Africa.[6]

AETIOLOGY/ RISK FACTORS Transmission of HIV to children is more likely if the mother has a high viral load.[1,7,8] Women with detectable viraemia (by p24 antigen or culture) have double the risk of transmitting HIV-1 to their infants compared with those who do not.[1] Prospective studies have also found that breastfeeding is a risk factor for mother to child transmission of HIV.[9,10] Other risk factors include sexually transmitted diseases, chorioamnionitis, prolonged rupture of membranes, vaginal mode of delivery, low $CD4^+$ count, advanced maternal HIV disease, obstetric events increasing bleeding (episiotomy, perineal laceration, and intrapartum haemorrhage), young maternal age, and history of stillbirth.[6,11-15]

PROGNOSIS About 25% of infants infected with HIV progress rapidly to AIDS or death in the first year. Some survive beyond 12 years of age.[3] One European study found a mortality of 15% in the first year of life and a mortality of 28% by the age of 5 years.[16] A recent study reported that, in children under 5 years of age in sub-Saharan Africa, HIV accounted for 2% of deaths in 1990 and almost 8% in

HIV: mother to child transmission

1999.[17] Five countries (Botswana, Namibia, Swaziland, Zambia, and Zimbabwe) had rates of HIV attributable mortality in excess of 30/1000 in children under the age of 5 years.

Please refer to clinicalevidence.com for full text and references.

HIV: prevention of opportunistic infections

Search date December 2004

John Ioannidis and Taryn Young

What are the effects of prophylaxis for P carinii *pneumonia (PCP) and toxoplasmosis?*

LIKELY TO BE BENEFICIAL

Atovaquone

We found no RCTs comparing atovaquone versus placebo. Atovaquone is usually used in people who are either intolerant of or fail to respond to trimethoprim–sulfamethoxazole. It would be considered unethical to perform a trial comparing atovaquone versus placebo. RCTs in people who are either intolerant of or fail to respond to trimethoprim–sulfamethoxazole found that atovaquone is as effective as dapsone or aerosolised pentamidine in preventing *Pneumocystis carinii* pneumonia (PCP).

Azithromycin (alone or plus rifabutin, compared with rifabutin alone, for PCP prevention)

One RCT found that azithromycin, either alone or in combination with rifabutin, reduced the risk of *Pneumocystis carinii* pneumonia (PCP) compared with rifabutin alone in people receiving standard PCP prophylaxis.

Trimethoprim–sulfamethoxazole for PCP

Systematic reviews found that trimethoprim–sulfamethoxazole reduced the incidence of *Pneumocystis carinii* pneumonia (PCP) compared with placebo or pentamidine. One systematic review and one subsequent RCT found no significant difference between high and low dose trimethoprim–sulfamethoxazole for PCP prophylaxis, although adverse effects were more common with the higher dose. Two systematic reviews found that trimethoprim–sulfamethoxazole reduced incidence of PCP compared with dapsone (with or without pyrimethamine), although only one of these reviews found that the reduction was statistically significant.

UNKNOWN EFFECTIVENESS

Trimethoprim–sulfamethoxazole for toxoplasmosis

One RCT found no significant difference between trimethoprim–sulfamethoxazole and placebo for preventing toxoplasmosis. One systematic review found no significant difference between trimethoprim–sulfamethoxazole and dapsone (with or without pyrimethamine) for preventing toxoplasmosis.

What are the effects of antituberculosis prophylaxis in people with HIV infection?

BENEFICIAL

Antituberculosis prophylaxis versus placebo

One systematic review found that in people who are HIV and tuberculin skin test positive, antituberculosis prophylaxis drugs reduced the frequency of tuberculosis compared with placebo over 1–3 years. However it found no significant difference between treatments in the risk of death from any cause. The review found no significant difference between antituberculosis prophylaxis drugs and ▶

HIV: prevention of opportunistic infections

placebo in the frequency of tuberculosis, or death from any cause in people who were HIV positive but tuberculin skin test negative. One RCT found that the benefit of prophylaxis diminished with time after treatment was stopped.

TRADE OFF BETWEEN BENEFITS AND HARMS

Isoniazid for 6–12 months (versus combination treatment for 2–3 months — longer treatment regimen, but similar benefits and fewer harms)

One systematic review found no significant difference in the risk of tuberculosis or death (any cause) between isoniazid monotherapy for 6–12 months and combination treatment (isoniazid plus rifampicin, rifampicin plus pyrazinamide, or isoniazid plus rifampicin plus pyrazinamide) for 2–3 months. The review found that adverse effects leading to treatment discontinuation were more common with combination treatment than with isoniazid monotherapy.

What are the effects of prophylaxis for disseminated **M avium** *complex (MAC) disease for people without previous MAC disease?*

LIKELY TO BE BENEFICIAL

Azithromycin

One RCT found that azithromycin reduced the incidence of *Mycobacterium avium* complex (MAC) compared with placebo. One RCT found that both azithromycin alone and azithromycin plus rifabutin reduced the incidence of MAC compared with rifabutin alone.

Clarithromycin

One RCT found that clarithromycin reduced the incidence of *Mycobacterium avium* complex (MAC) compared with placebo. One RCT found that both clarithromycin alone and clarithromycin plus rifabutin reduced the incidence of MAC compared with rifabutin alone.

TRADE OFF BETWEEN BENEFITS AND HARMS

Rifabutin plus macrolides

One RCT found that rifabutin plus clarithromycin reduced the incidence of *M avium* complex (MAC) compared with rifabutin alone. One RCT found that azithromycin plus rifabutin reduced the incidence of MAC compared with azithromycin alone or rifabutin alone. One systematic review and two subsequent RCTs found that toxicity, including uveitis, was more common with combination treatment than with clarithromycin or rifabutin alone.

What are the effects of prophylaxis for disseminated **M avium** *complex (MAC) disease for people with previous MAC disease?*

LIKELY TO BE BENEFICIAL

Clarithromycin, rifabutin, and ethambutol (more effective than clarithromycin plus clofazimine)

One RCT found that clarithromycin plus rifabutin plus ethambutol reduced *Mycobacterium avium* complex (MAC) relapse compared with clarithromycin plus clofazimine.

Ethambutol added to clarithromycin plus clofazimine

One RCT found that adding ethambutol to clarithromycin plus clofazimine reduced *Mycobacterium avium* complex (MAC) relapse compared with clarithromycin plus clofazimine.

UNKNOWN EFFECTIVENESS

Rifabutin added to clarithromycin plus ethambutol

One RCT found no significant difference in survival by adding rifabutin to clarithromycin plus ethambutol in people with previous *Mycobacterium avium* complex (MAC).

LIKELY TO BE INEFFECTIVE OR HARMFUL

Clofazimine added to clarithromycin and ethambutol (higher mortality than clofazimine plus ethambutol)

One RCT found that adding clarithromycin to clofazimine plus ethambutol increased mortality compared with clofazimine plus ethambutol.

What are the effects of prophylaxis for cytomegalovirus (CMV), herpes simplex virus (HSV), and varicella zoster virus (VZV)?

BENEFICIAL

Aciclovir

One systematic review found that aciclovir reduced herpes simplex virus (HSV) and varicella zoster virus (VZV) infection, and overall mortality, compared with placebo in people at different clinical stages of HIV infection. However, it found no significant difference between treatments in the incidence of cytomegalovirus (CMV) disease. One RCT found that valaciclovir reduced the incidence of CMV disease compared with aciclovir, but may be associated with increased mortality. One RCT found no significant difference between aciclovir and valaciclovir in anogenital HSV recurrence.

TRADE OFF BETWEEN BENEFITS AND HARMS

Oral ganciclovir (in people with severe CD4 depletion)

One RCT found that oral ganciclovir reduced the incidence of cytomegalovirus (CMV) in people with severe CD4 depletion compared with placebo. It found that 26% of people who took ganciclovir developed severe neutropenia. A second RCT found no significant difference in prevention of CMV between ganciclovir and placebo.

Valaciclovir

One RCT found that valaciclovir reduced genital and oral herpes simplex virus (HSV) recurrence compared with placebo at 6 months in people on HAART. One RCT found that valaciclovir reduced the incidence of cytomegalovirus disease compared with aciclovir, but may be associated with increased mortality. One RCT found no significant difference between aciclovir and valaciclovir in anogenital HSV recurrence. One RCT found that valaciclovir 500 mg twice daily reduced anogenital HSV recurrence compared with valaciclovir 1000 mg once daily.

HIV: prevention of opportunistic infections

UNKNOWN EFFECTIVENESS

Famciclovir (for recurrent HSV)

One small RCT found that famciclovir reduced the rate of viral shedding compared with placebo, but provided insufficient evidence on the effect of famciclovir on herpes simplex virus (HSV) recurrence.

What are the effects of prophylaxis for invasive fungal disease in people without previous fungal disease?

TRADE OFF BETWEEN BENEFITS AND HARMS

Fluconazole or itraconazole

RCTs in people with advanced HIV disease found that both fluconazole and itraconazole reduced the incidence of invasive fungal infections compared with placebo. One RCT found that fluconazole reduced the incidence of invasive fungal disease and mucocutaneous candidiasis compared with clotrimazole. One RCT found no difference between high and low dose fluconazole. Azoles have been associated with congenital problems and potentially serious interactions with other drugs.

What are the effects of prophylaxis for invasive fungal disease in people with previous invasive fungal disease?

LIKELY TO BE BENEFICIAL

Itraconazole (more effective than placebo for preventing *Penicillium marneffei* relapse)

Two RCTs found that itraconazole reduced the incidence of relapse of *Penicillium marneffei* infection and candidiasis compared with placebo.

LIKELY TO BE INEFFECTIVE OR HARMFUL

Itraconazole (less effective than fluconazole for preventing relapse of cryptococcal meningitis)

One RCT found that itraconazole increased the risk of relapse of cryptococcal meningitis compared with fluconazole. We found no RCTs on itraconazole for histoplasmosis.

What are the effects of discontinuing prophylaxis against opportunistic pathogens in people on highly active antiretroviral treatment (HAART)?

LIKELY TO BE BENEFICIAL

Discontinuing prophylaxis for MAC in people with CD4 > 100/mm^3

Two RCTs in people with CD4 counts over 100/mm^3 taking highly active antiretroviral treatment (HAART) found that discontinuation of prophylaxis for *Mycobacterium avium* complex (MAC) disease did not increase the incidence of MAC disease.

Discontinuing prophylaxis for PCP and toxoplasmosis in people with CD4 > 200/mm^3

One systematic review of two unblinded RCTs in people with CD4 counts over 200/mm^3 taking highly active antiretroviral treatment (HAART) found that discontinuation of prophylaxis did not increase the incidence of *Pneumocystis carinii* pneumonia (PCP). Two unblinded RCTs found that discontinuation of prophylaxis did not increase the incidence of toxoplasmosis in people with a satisfactory response to HAART.

UNKNOWN EFFECTIVENESS

Discontinuing prophylaxis for CMV in people with CD4 > 100/mm^3

We found insufficient evidence on the effects of discontinuation of maintenance treatment for cytomegalovirus (CMV) retinitis or other end organ disease in people with CD4 counts over 100/mm^3 taking highly active antiretroviral treatment (HAART).

DEFINITION Opportunistic infections are intercurrent infections that occur in people infected with HIV. Prophylaxis aims to avoid either the first occurrence of these infections (primary prophylaxis) or their recurrence (secondary prophylaxis, maintenance treatment). This review includes *Pneumocystis carinii* pneumonia (PCP), *Toxoplasma gondii* encephalitis, *Mycobacterium tuberculosis*, *Mycobacterium avium* complex (MAC) disease, cytomegalovirus (CMV) disease (most often retinitis), infections from other herpes viruses (herpes simplex virus [HSV] and varicella zoster virus [VZV]), and invasive fungal disease (*Cryptococcus neoformans, Histoplasma capsulatum*, and *Penicillium marneffei*).

INCIDENCE/ PREVALENCE The incidence of opportunistic infections is high in people with immune impairment. Data available before the introduction of highly active antiretroviral treatment (HAART) suggest that, with a CD4 < 250/mm^3, the 2 year probability of developing an opportunistic infection is 40% for PCP, 22% for CMV, 18% for MAC, 6% for toxoplasmosis, and 5% for cryptococcal meningitis.[1] The introduction of HAART has reduced the rate of opportunistic infections. One cohort study found that the introduction of HAART decreased the incidence of PCP by 94%, CMV by 82%, and MAC by 64%, as presenting AIDS events. HAART decreased the incidence of events subsequent to the diagnosis of AIDS by 84% for PCP, 82% for CMV, and 97% for MAC.[2]

AETIOLOGY/ RISK FACTORS Opportunistic infections are caused by a wide array of pathogens and result from immune system defects induced by HIV. The risk of developing opportunistic infections increases dramatically with progressive impairment of the immune system. Each opportunistic infection has a different threshold of immune impairment, beyond which the risk increases substantially.[1] Opportunistic pathogens may infect the immunocompromised host *de novo*, but usually they are simply reactivations of latent pathogens in such hosts.

PROGNOSIS Prognosis depends on the type of opportunistic infection. Even with treatment they may cause serious morbidity and mortality. Most deaths owing to HIV infection are caused by opportunistic infections.

Please refer to clinicalevidence.com for full text and references.

Pneumocystis pneumonia in people with HIV

Search date November 2005

Richard Bellamy

What are the effects of first line antipneumocystis treatments for Pneumocystis *pneumonia in people infected with HIV?*

BENEFICIAL

Atovaquone

We found no RCTs comparing atovaquone versus placebo or no treatment as the first line treatment for *Pneumocystis* pneumonia in people infected with HIV; such RCTs would be considered unethical. One RCT found that atovaquone and intravenous pentamidine were equally effective. One RCT found that atovaquone was less effective than trimethoprim–sulfamethoxazole (co-trimoxazole). Adverse effects requiring termination of treatment occurred less frequently with atovaquone than with trimethoprim–sulfamethoxazole or intravenous pentamidine.

Clindamycin–primaquine

We found no RCTs comparing clindamycin–primaquine versus placebo or no treatment as the first line treatment for *Pneumocystis* pneumonia in people infected with HIV; such RCTs would be considered unethical. RCTs found that clindamycin–primaquine was as effective as trimethoprim–sulfamethoxazole (co-trimoxazole) and trimethoprim–dapsone and found no significant difference between interventions in rates of serious adverse effects.

Pentamidine (aerosolised)

We found no RCTs comparing aerosolised pentamidine versus placebo or no treatment as first line treatment for *Pneumocystis* pneumonia in people infected with HIV; such RCTs would be considered unethical. One RCT found no significant difference in mortality or treatment failure between aerosolised and intravenous pentamidine. Two RCTs found no significant difference in mortality between aerosolised pentamidine and trimethoprim–sulfamethoxazole. They found lower rates of serious adverse effects with aerosolised pentamidine.

Pentamidine (intravenous)

We found no RCTs comparing intravenous pentamidine versus placebo or no treatment as first line treatment for *Pneumocystis* pneumonia in people infected with HIV; such RCTs would be considered unethical. One RCT found no significant difference between intravenous pentamidine and atovaquone, but atovaquone caused fewer adverse effects requiring termination of treatment. One RCT found no significant difference in mortality or treatment failure between intravenous and aerosolised pentamidine. Two RCTs found no significant difference in mortality, treatment failure, or adverse effects between intravenous pentamidine and trimethoprim–sulfamethoxazole (co-trimoxazole). However, a third RCT found that intravenous pentamidine increased mortality compared with trimethoprim–sulfamethoxazole.

Trimethoprim–dapsone

We found no RCTs comparing trimethoprim–dapsone versus placebo or no treatment as first line treatment for *Pneumocystis* pneumonia in people infected with HIV; such RCTs would be considered unethical. One RCT found that ►

trimethoprim–dapsone was as effective as clindamycin–primaquine. RCTs found that trimethoprim–dapsone was as effective as trimethoprim–sulfamethoxazole (co-trimoxazole), with similar rates of adverse effects.

Trimethoprim–sulfamethoxazole (co-trimoxazole)

We found no RCTs comparing trimethoprim–sulfamethoxazole (co-trimoxazole) versus placebo or no treatment as first line treatment for *Pneumocystis* pneumonia in people infected with HIV; such RCTs would be considered unethical. One RCT found that trimethoprim–sulfamethoxazole was more effective than atovaquone. RCTs have found that trimethoprim–sulfamethoxazole was as effective as clindamycin–primaquine and trimethoprim–dapsone, and aerosolised pentamidine. Two RCTs found no significant difference in mortality, treatment failure, or adverse effects between trimethoprim–sulfamethoxazole and intravenous pentamidine. However, a third RCT found that trimethoprim–sulfamethoxazole reduced mortality compared with intravenous pentamidine. RCTs have found that adverse events requiring termination of treatment were more frequent with trimethoprim–sulfamethoxazole than atovaquone or aerosolised pentamidine.

What are the effects of adjuvant corticosteroids in people receiving first line antipneumocystis treatments for Pneumocystis *pneumonia in people infected with HIV?*

BENEFICIAL

Adjuvant corticosteroids for moderate to severe *Pneumocystis* pneumonia

One systematic review found that adjuvant corticosteroids reduced mortality when used early in the treatment of moderate to severe *Pneumocystis* pneumonia (see definition).

UNKNOWN EFFECTIVENESS

Adjuvant corticosteroids for mild *Pneumocystis* pneumonia

We found insufficient evidence on the effects of adjuvant corticosteroids in the early treatment of mild *Pneumocystis* pneumonia in people infected with HIV (see definition).

What are the effects of treatments for Pneumocystis *pneumonia in people infected with HIV who have not responded to first line antipneumocystis treatment?*

UNKNOWN EFFECTIVENESS

Treatment after failure of first line treatment

We found no systematic review or RCTs comparing the effectiveness or adverse effects of different treatments after failure of first line treatment for *Pneumocystis* pneumonia in people infected with HIV. One systematic review of controlled studies, case series, and case reports suggested that clindamycin–primaquine may be more effective than alternative treatments in this situation.

DEFINITION *Pneumocystis* pneumonia (PCP) is caused by the opportunistic fungus *Pneumocystis jiroveci*. The infection occurs in people with impaired immune function. Most cases occur in people infected with HIV, in whom PCP is an AIDS defining illness. The pneumonia is generally classified as **mild** if PaO_2 is

Pneumocystis pneumonia in people with HIV

greater than 70 mm Hg on room air, if the alveolar–arterial oxygen gradient is less than 35 mm Hg, or both. It is generally classified as **moderate/severe** if PaO_2 is less than 70 mm Hg, if the alveolar–arterial oxygen gradient is greater than 35 mm Hg, or both. This chapter focuses on the treatment of PCP in adults infected with HIV. Prevention of PCP is covered under HIV: prevention of opportunistic infections.

INCIDENCE/ PREVALENCE PCP is the most common AIDS defining illness in developed nations.[1] It is probably also common throughout the developing world, although the prevalence is harder to assess here because of difficulties in making the diagnosis. Before the widespread use of prophylaxis it was estimated that up to 80% of people with AIDS would eventually develop PCP.[2] Widespread use of prophylaxis against PCP and of highly active antiretroviral treatment has dramatically reduced the incidence of this infection (see HIV: prevention of opportunistic infections).

AETIOLOGY/ RISK FACTORS Risk factors for PCP include HIV infection, primary immune deficiencies, prematurity, cancer, use of immune suppressants after organ transplantation, and prolonged use of high dose corticosteroids. HIV infection is now responsible for the vast majority of cases of PCP. Among adults with HIV infection, those with a CD4 count below 200 cells/mm^3 are at highest risk, and the median CD4 count at diagnosis of PCP is about 50 cells/mm^3.[3]

PROGNOSIS It is generally believed that without treatment PCP would almost certainly be fatal in a person with AIDS. For ethical reasons, no studies have examined short term prognosis without treatment. People with AIDS and PCP frequently have other serious opportunistic infections, which can adversely affect their prognosis.

Please refer to clinicalevidence.com for full text and references.

Tuberculosis in people with HIV

Search date July 2005

Richard Bellamy

What are the effects of first line treatments for tuberculosis in people infected with HIV?

BENEFICIAL

Conventional anti-tuberculous treatment*

There is consensus that conventional anti-tuberculous treatment (2 months of rifampicin, isoniazid, and pyrazinamide [plus ethambutol in areas where drug resistant tuberculosis is likely] followed by 4–7 months of rifampicin and isoniazid) is effective for the treatment of tuberculosis in people with HIV. We found insufficient evidence about the effects of conventional anti-tuberculous treatment compared with regimens containing rifabutin or quinolones. One RCT provided limited evidence that conventional anti-tuberculous treatment increased the proportion of people with negative sputum culture after 2 months of treatment compared with a thiacetazone containing regimen. The RCT found no significant difference in survival between treatments, and found fewer adverse effects with conventional anti-tuberculous treatment than with the thiacetazone containing regimen.

*Categorisation based on consensus.

UNKNOWN EFFECTIVENESS

Adjuvant highly active antiretroviral treatment (compared with delayed initiation of highly active antiretroviral treatment)

We found no RCTs comparing anti-tuberculous treatment plus adjuvant highly active antiretroviral treatment versus conventional anti-tuberculous treatment with delayed initiation of highly active antiretroviral treatment.

Anti-tuberculous treatment containing quinolones (compared with alternative regimens)

One RCT provided insufficient evidence about the effects of a quinolone (levofloxacin) containing regimen compared with conventional anti-tuberculous treatment. We found no RCTs comparing anti-tuberculous treatment containing quinolones versus regimens containing rifabutin or thiacetazone as the first line treatment for tuberculosis in people infected with HIV.

Anti-tuberculous treatment containing rifabutin (compared with alternative regimens)

One small RCT provided insufficient evidence about the effects of a rifabutin containing regimen compared with conventional anti-tuberculous treatment. We found no systematic review or RCTs comparing anti-tuberculous treatment containing rifabutin versus anti-tuberculous treatment containing thiacetazone or quinolones as the first line treatment for tuberculosis in people infected with HIV.

Directly observed therapy, short course (compared with unsupervised treatment)

We found no RCTs comparing directly observed therapy versus unsupervised treatment for tuberculosis in people with HIV.

Tuberculosis in people with HIV

Longer courses of anti-tuberculous treatment (compared with conventional short course treatment)

RCTs provided insufficient evidence about the effects of regimens longer than 6 months compared with conventional short course (6 months) anti-tuberculous treatment.

UNLIKELY TO BE BENEFICIAL

Adjuvant immunotherapy with *Mycobacterium vaccae*

RCTs found that anti-tuberculous treatment plus *Mycobacterium vaccae* immunisation achieved no additional benefits in survival or negative sputum *M tuberculosis* culture rates compared with anti-tuberculous treatment plus placebo immunisation.

LIKELY TO BE INEFFECTIVE OR HARMFUL

Anti-tuberculous treatment containing thiacetazone

One RCT provided limited evidence that a thiacetazone containing regimen decreased the proportion of people with negative sputum culture at 2 months compared with conventional anti-tuberculous treatment. It found no significant difference in survival between treatments, and found that the thiacetazone containing regimen was associated with a greater number of adverse effects, mostly skin rash. One observational study reported a high rate of fatal mucocutaneous reactions among HIV positive children receiving thiacetazone containing regimens. We found no systematic review or RCTs comparing anti-tuberculous treatment containing thiacetazone versus regimens containing rifabutin or quinolones as the first line treatment for tuberculosis in people infected with HIV. Many countries no longer use thiacetazone because of the high frequency of adverse events associated with this drug.

Anti-tuberculous treatment containing $\leq$ 3 months of rifampicin (compared with rifampicin for $\geq$ 5 months)

One systematic review of observational evidence found that anti-tuberculous regimens including rifampicin for at least 5 months reduced recurrence of tuberculosis compared with regimens containing rifampicin for 3 months or shorter.

What are the effects of second line treatments for tuberculosis in people infected with HIV?

UNKNOWN EFFECTIVENESS

Antimycobacterial treatment combinations (comparative benefits of different regimens unclear)

We found no RCTs comparing different regimens of anti-tuberculous treatment after failure of first line treatment for tuberculosis in people with HIV.

DEFINITION HIV infection kills more people than any other infectious disease.[1] Infection with *Mycobacterium tuberculosis* is among the most important HIV related opportunistic infections, in both the developed and the developing world. HIV infection compromises the host's immune defences and can lead to failure to control latent *M tuberculosis* infection with the subsequent development of active (i.e. symptomatic) tuberculosis. The HIV pandemic has been a major contributing factor in the spread of tuberculosis in many countries. Tuberculosis most commonly affects the lungs, but it can also affect many other organs such as lymph nodes, kidneys, liver, gastrointestinal tract, and the central nervous system. In a study of 132 HIV positive people with tuberculosis in San Francisco, 50 (38%) had solely pulmonary disease, 40 (30%) had solely extra-pulmonary disease, and 42 (32%) had both pulmonary and extra-pulmonary disease.[2] In Africa and South America, 40–80% of HIV positive people presenting with tuberculosis have pulmonary disease.[3] The specific symptoms of tuberculosis depend on the site of infection. Pulmonary disease characteristically presents with cough, haemoptysis, chest pain, and systemic symptoms such as weight loss and night sweats. This topic deals with the treatment of active tuberculosis (both pulmonary and extra-pulmonary) in people with HIV. Prevention of tuberculosis in people with HIV is covered in a separate chapter (see HIV: prevention of opportunistic infections).

INCIDENCE/ PREVALENCE About a third of the world's population has latent *M tuberculosis* infection.[4] Each year about 3 million cases of active tuberculosis occur in people who are HIV positive, resulting in one million deaths.[1] HIV infection has been a major factor in the increase in the number of cases of tuberculosis occurring worldwide.[5] Most people infected with HIV live in sub-Saharan Africa. In several countries of this region, over 40% of people who develop tuberculosis are infected with HIV.[5-8] Tuberculosis is the most frequent cause of death in people infected with HIV in Africa.[9]

AETIOLOGY/ RISK FACTORS Risk factors for tuberculosis include social factors such as poverty, overcrowding, and homelessness, and medical factors such as steroid treatment. In people co-infected with HIV and *M tuberculosis*, the annual risk of developing active tuberculosis is about 5–10%,[10,11] more than 10 times greater than for people infected with *M tuberculosis* who do not have HIV.

PROGNOSIS Without treatment, active tuberculosis would most likely be fatal in a person infected with HIV. For ethical reasons, no studies have examined the prognosis of active tuberculosis without treatment in people infected with HIV. In one study in the pre-highly active antiretroviral treatment era, the median survival of HIV infected people treated for tuberculosis was 16 months.[2] However, only 13/99 (13%) of the deaths were attributed to tuberculosis. The other common causes of death were *Pneumocystis carinii* pneumonia (24%), bacterial pneumonia (14%), wasting syndrome (9%), and Kaposi's sarcoma (9%).[2] Recurrence of tuberculosis after completion of treatment is more common among people with HIV than among HIV uninfected people. In one study in New York, 83/1530 (5.4%) people with HIV who completed tuberculosis treatment had a recurrence of disease compared with 21/1413 (1.5%) HIV uninfected people who completed tuberculosis treatment.[12] One cohort study in 326 South African mineworkers successfully treated for tuberculosis found a higher recurrence rate of tuberculosis in HIV positive people, with 16.0 cases per 100 person years of follow up compared with 6.4 cases per 100 person years of follow up among HIV negative people.[13]

Please refer to clinicalevidence.com for full text and references.

Amoebic dysentery

Search date July 2005

Leonila Dans and Elizabeth Martínez

What are the effects of drug treatments for amoebic dysentery in endemic areas?

LIKELY TO BE BENEFICIAL

Ornidazole

One RCT found that ornidazole reduced treatment failure rate compared with placebo. Nausea and vomiting were more common with ornidazole than with placebo. Two RCTs found similar treatment failure rates with ornidazole compared with tinidazole or secnidazole in children with amoebic dysentery.

Secnidazole*

We found no RCTs comparing secnidazole versus placebo. One RCT found similar treatment failure rates with secnidazole and ornidazole in children with amoebic dysentery.

Tinidazole*

We found no RCTs comparing tinidazole versus placebo. We found nine RCTs comparing tinidazole versus metronidazole, most of which found lower rates of treatment failure and adverse effects with tinidazole. One RCT found similar parasite clearance for tinidazole and ornidazole in children with amoebic dysentery. We found no RCTs comparing tinidazole versus secnidazole, emetine, or paromomycin.

UNKNOWN EFFECTIVENESS

Emetine

We found no RCTs evaluating emetine for the treatment of amoebic dysentery.

Paromomycin

We found no RCTs evaluating paromomycin for the treatment of amoebic dysentery.

UNLIKELY TO BE BENEFICIAL

Metronidazole*

We found no RCTs comparing metronidazole versus placebo. We found nine RCTs comparing metronidazole versus tinidazole, most of which found higher rates of treatment failure and adverse events with metronidazole.

*No placebo controlled RCTs. Categorisation based on consensus and evidence of similar effectiveness among these drugs.

DEFINITION Amoebic dysentery is caused by the protozoan parasite *Entamoeba histolytica*. Invasive intestinal parasitic infection can result in symptoms of fulminant dysentery, such as fever, chills, and bloody or mucous diarrhoea, abdominal discomfort, or diarrhoea containing blood or mucus. The dysentery can alternate, with periods of constipation or remission. This chapter focuses on amoebic dysentery only, and includes populations with both suspected and documented disease in endemic areas where levels of infection do not exhibit wide fluctuations through time.[1] The term "amoebic dysentery" encompasses people described as having symptomatic intestinal amoebiasis, amoebic colitis, amoebic diarrhoea, or invasive intestinal amoebiasis. Extraintestinal amoebiasis (e.g. amoebic liver abscess) and asymptomatic amoebiasis are not covered.

INCIDENCE/ PREVALENCE We found no accurate global prevalence data for *E histolytica* infection and amoebic dysentery. Estimates on the prevalence of *Entamoeba* infection range from 1–40% of the population in Central and South America, Africa, and Asia, and from 0.2–10.8% in endemic areas of developed countries such as the USA.[2-5] However, these estimates are difficult to interpret, mainly because infection can remain asymptomatic or go unreported,[6] and because many older reports do not distinguish *E histolytica* from the non-pathogenic, morphologically identical species *Entamoeba dispar*. Development and availability of more sophisticated methods (such as the enzyme-linked immunosorbent assay [ELISA] based test) to differentiate the two species might give a more accurate estimate of its global prevalence.[7] Infection with *E histolytica* is a common cause of acute diarrhoea in developing countries. One survey conducted in Egypt found that 38% of people with acute diarrhoea in an outpatient clinic had amoebic dysentery.[8]

AETIOLOGY/ RISK FACTORS Ingestion of cysts from food or water contaminated with faeces is the main route of *E histolytica* transmission. Low standards of hygiene and sanitation, particularly those related to crowding, tropical climate, contamination of food and water with faeces, and inadequate disposal of faeces, all account for the high rates of infection seen in developing countries.[9,10] It has been suggested that some animals, such as dogs, pigs, and monkeys, may act as reservoir hosts to the protozoa, but this has not been proven. In developed countries, risk factors include communal living, oral and anal sex, compromised immune system, and migration or travel from endemic areas.[9,11,12]

PROGNOSIS Amoebic dysentery may progress to amoeboma, fulminant colitis, toxic megacolon and colonic ulcers, and may lead to perforation.[13] Amoeboma may be mistaken for colonic carcinoma or pyogenic abscess. Amoebic dysentery may also result in chronic carriage and the chronic passing of amoebic cysts. Fulminant amoebic dysentery is reported to have 55–88% mortality.[14,15] It is estimated that more than 500 million people are infected with *E histolytica* worldwide.[10] Between 40 000 and 100 000 will die each year, placing this infection second to malaria in mortality caused by protozoan parasites.[16]

Please refer to clinicalevidence.com for full text and references.

Chickenpox

Search date March 2006

George Swingler

What are the effects of interventions to prevent chickenpox in healthy adults and children?

BENEFICIAL

Live attenuated vaccine in healthy children

Two RCTs identified by a systematic review found that live attenuated varicella vaccine reduced clinical chickenpox in healthy children compared with placebo, with no significant increase in adverse effects. One RCT of postexposure vaccination found no significant difference in the clinical incidence between live attenuated varicella vaccine and placebo. However, it found that the vaccine reduced severity of chickenpox.

UNKNOWN EFFECTIVENESS

Live attenuated vaccine in healthy adults

We found no systematic review or RCTs in healthy adults on the effects of live attenuated varicella vaccine.

What are the effects of interventions to prevent chickenpox in children exposed prenatally?

UNKNOWN EFFECTIVENESS

Aciclovir

We found no systematic review or RCTs on the effects of aciclovir in prenatally exposed children.

Zoster immune globulin in prenatally exposed children

We found no systematic review or RCTs on the effects of zoster immune globulin in prenatally exposed children.

What are the effects of interventions to prevent chickenpox in immunocompromised adults and children?

BENEFICIAL

High dose aciclovir (> 3200 mg/day) in people with HIV infection

One systematic review in people with HIV infection found that high dose aciclovir (≥ 3200 mg/day) reduced the risk of clinical chickenpox and reduced all cause mortality over 22 months' treatment compared with placebo.

UNKNOWN EFFECTIVENESS

Aciclovir in people with immunocompromise other than HIV

We found no systematic review or RCTs on the effects of aciclovir in people with immunocompromise other than HIV.

Live attenuated vaccine in immunocompromised people

We found no systematic review or RCTs in immunocompromised adults or children on the effects of live attenuated varicella vaccine.

Zoster immune globulin in immunocompromised adults

We found no systematic review or RCTs on the effects of zoster immune globulin in immunocompromised adults.

Zoster immune globulin versus varicella zoster immune globulin in immunocompromised children

One RCT in immunocompromised children exposed to a sibling with chickenpox found no significant difference in clinical chickenpox with zoster immune globulin compared with varicella zoster immune globulin at 12 weeks.

What are the effects of treatments for chickenpox in healthy adults and children?

LIKELY TO BE BENEFICIAL

Aciclovir (oral) in healthy people (given < 24 hours of onset of rash)

One systematic review in children found that oral aciclovir given less than 24 hours after onset of rash reduced the duration of fever. It found no significant difference in time to last new lesions. One RCT identified by a systematic review also found that early aciclovir reduced symptoms of chickenpox in adults.

UNKNOWN EFFECTIVENESS

Aciclovir (oral) in healthy people (given > 24 hours after onset of rash)

One systematic review in adults found that oral aciclovir given beyond 24 hours after onset of rash did not reduce the symptoms of chickenpox compared with placebo.

What are the effects of treatments for chickenpox in immunocompromised adults and children?

LIKELY TO BE BENEFICIAL

Aciclovir (intravenous) for treatment of chickenpox in children with malignancy

Two RCTs compared intravenous aciclovir versus placebo in children with cancer. One large RCT found that aciclovir reduced clinical deterioration. The other smaller RCT found no significant difference in clinical deterioration.

UNKNOWN EFFECTIVENESS

Aciclovir in immunocompromised adults

We found no systematic review or RCTs on the effects of aciclovir in immunocompromised adults.

DEFINITION Chickenpox is caused by primary infection with varicella zoster virus. In healthy people, it is usually a mild self limiting illness, characterised by low grade fever, malaise, and a generalised, itchy, vesicular rash.[1]

INCIDENCE/ PREVALENCE Chickenpox is extremely contagious. Over 90% of unvaccinated people become infected, but infection occurs at different ages in different parts of the world: over 80% of people have been infected by the age of 10 years in the USA, the UK, and Japan, and by the age of 30 years in India, South East Asia, and the West Indies.[2,3]

Chickenpox

AETIOLOGY/ RISK FACTORS Chickenpox is caused by exposure to varicella zoster virus.

PROGNOSIS **Infants and children:** In healthy children the illness is usually mild and self limiting. In the USA, mortality in infants and children (aged 1–14 years) with chickenpox is about 7/100 000 in infants and 1.4/100 000 in children.[4] In Australia, mortality from chickenpox is about 0.5–0.6/100 000 in children aged 1–11 years, and about 1.2/100 000 in infants.[5] Bacterial skin sepsis is the most common complication in children under 5 years of age, and acute cerebellar ataxia is the most common complication in older children; both cause hospital admission in 2–3/10 000 children.[1] **Adults:** Mortality in adults is higher, at about 31/100 000.[4] Varicella pneumonia is the most common complication, causing 20–30 hospital admissions/10 000 adults.[1] Activation of latent varicella zoster virus infection can cause herpes zoster, also known as shingles (see postherpetic neuralgia). **Cancer chemotherapy:** One case series (77 children with both cancer and chickenpox; 1 child received zoster immune globulin within 72 hours of exposure) found that more children receiving chemotherapy compared with those in remission developed progressive chickenpox with multiple organ involvement (19/60 [32%] of children receiving chemotherapy *v* 0/17 [0%] of children in remission) and more children died (4/60 [7%] of children receiving chemotherapy *v* 0/17 [0%] of children in remission).[6] **HIV infection:** One retrospective case series (45 children with AIDS; no treatment reported) found that 1/4 (25%) children with AIDS who acquired chickenpox in hospital developed pneumonia and 5% died.[7] In a retrospective cohort study (73 children with HIV and chickenpox; 83% with symptomatic HIV; 14 children received varicella zoster immune globulin, 9 within 48 hours of exposure), infection beyond 2 months occurred in 10 children (14%) and recurrent varicella zoster virus infections occurred in 38 children (55%). There was a strong association between an increasing number of recurrences and low CD4 cell counts.[8] Half of recurrent infections involved generalised rashes and the other half had zoster. **Newborns:** We found no cohort studies of untreated children with perinatal exposure to chickenpox. One cohort study (281 neonates receiving varicella zoster immune globulin because their mothers had developed a chickenpox rash during the month before or after delivery) found that 134 (48%) developed a chickenpox rash and 19 (14%) developed severe chickenpox.[9] Sixteen (84%) of the 19 cases of severe chickenpox occurred in neonates of mothers whose rash had started between 4 days before and 2 days after delivery.

Please refer to clinicalevidence.com for full text and references.

Congenital toxoplasmosis

Search date March 2004

Piero Olliaro

What are the effects on mother and baby of treating toxoplasmosis during pregnancy?

UNKNOWN EFFECTIVENESS

Antiparasitic drugs

Two systematic reviews studies in women who seroconverted during pregnancy found insufficient evidence on the effects of current antiparasitic treatment compared with no treatment on mother or baby.

See glossary

DEFINITION Toxoplasmosis is caused by the parasite *Toxoplasma gondii*. Infection is asymptomatic or unremarkable in immunocompetent individuals, but leads to a lifelong antibody response. During pregnancy, toxoplasmosis can be transmitted across the placenta and may cause intrauterine death, neonatal growth retardation, mental retardation, ocular defects, and blindness in later life. Congenital toxoplasmosis (confirmed infection of the fetus or newborn) can also present at birth: either as subclinical disease, which may evolve with neurological or ophthalmological disease later in life; or as a disease of varying severity, ranging from mild ocular damage to severe mental retardation.

INCIDENCE/ PREVALENCE Reported rates of toxoplasma seroprevalence vary among and within countries, as well as over time. The risk of primary infection is highest in young people, including young women during pregnancy. We found no cohort studies describing annual seroconversion rates in women of childbearing age nor incidence of primary infection. One systematic review (search date 1996) identified 15 studies that reported rates of seroconversion in non-immune pregnant women ranging from 2.4–16/1000 in Europe and from 2–6/1000 in the USA.[1] France began screening for congenital toxoplasmosis in 1978, and during the period 1980–1995 the seroconversion rate during pregnancy in non-immune women was 4–5/1000.[2]

AETIOLOGY/ RISK FACTORS Toxoplasma infection is usually acquired by ingesting either sporocysts (from unwashed fruit or vegetables contaminated by cat faeces) or tissue cysts (from raw or undercooked meat). The risk of contracting toxoplasma infection varies with eating habits, contact with cats and other pets, and occupational exposure.

PROGNOSIS One systematic review of studies conducted from 1983–1996 found no population based prospective studies of the natural history of toxoplasma infection during pregnancy.[1] One systematic review (search date 1997; 9 controlled, non-randomised studies) found that untreated toxoplasmosis acquired during pregnancy was associated with infection rates in children of between 10–100%.[3] We found two European studies that correlated gestation at time of maternal seroconversion with risk of transmission and severity of disease at birth.[4,5] Risk of transmission increased with gestational age at maternal seroconversion, reaching 70–90% when seroconversion occurred after 30 weeks' gestation. In contrast, the risk of the infant developing clinical disease was highest when maternal seroconversion occurred early in pregnancy. The highest risk of developing early signs of disease (including chorioretinitis and hydrocephaly) was about 10%, recorded when seroconversion occurred between 24 and 30 weeks' gestation.[5] Infants with congenital toxoplasmosis and generalised neurological abnormalities at birth develop ▶

mental retardation, growth retardation, blindness or visual defects, seizures, and spasticity. Children with subclinical infection at birth may have cognitive, motor, and visual deficits, which may go undiagnosed for many years. One case control study (845 school children in Brazil) found mental retardation and retinochoroiditis to be significantly associated with positive toxoplasma serology (population attributable risk 6–9%).[6]

Please refer to clinicalevidence.com for full text and references.

Dengue fever

Search date November 2005

Marissa Alejandria

What are the effects of supportive treatments for dengue haemorrhagic fever or dengue shock syndrome in children?

LIKELY TO BE BENEFICIAL

Crystalloids compared with colloids (evidence crystalloids as effective as colloids in moderately severe dengue shock syndrome; evidence insufficient in severe dengue shock syndrome)

Two RCTs found no significant difference in mortality, recurrence of shock, or requirement for further infusions between crystalloids and colloids for acute resuscitation in Vietnamese children with dengue shock syndrome, but they are likely to have been underpowered to detect a clinically important difference. A third large adequately powered RCT in Vietnamese children found that crystalloids (Ringers lactate) were as effective as colloids in the initial resuscitation of children with moderately severe dengue shock syndrome in terms of the requirement for rescue colloids. It did not compare crystalloids versus colloids in children with severe dengue shock syndrome.

Intravenous fluids*

We found no RCTs comparing intravenous fluids versus placebo or no treatment. It is widely accepted that immediate fluid replacement should be undertaken in a child who has dengue haemorrhagic fever or dengue shock syndrome; it would be considered unethical to test its role in a placebo controlled trial.

UNKNOWN EFFECTIVENESS

Adding carbazochrome sodium sulfonate (AC-17) to standard intravenous fluids

One RCT in Thai children with dengue haemorrhagic fever/dengue shock syndrome found no significant difference in the development of shock, pleural effusion, and duration of hospital stay between adding carbazochrome sodium sulfonate and adding placebo to standard intravenous fluids. Another RCT with weak methods in Indonesian children with grade II dengue haemorrhagic fever found limited evidence that adding carbazochrome sodium sulfonate to standard intravenous fluids decreased the occurrence of pleural effusion compared with standard intravenous fluids alone.

Adding corticosteroids to standard intravenous fluids

Two RCTs in Thai and Indonesian children with dengue shock syndrome found no significant difference in mortality between adding corticosteroids to standard fluid replacement and adding placebo to standard fluid replacement. One open label RCT with weak methods in Burmese children with dengue shock syndrome found limited evidence that adding hydrocortisone to intravenous fluids reduced mortality compared with intravenous fluids alone.

Adding intravenous immunoglobulin to standard intravenous fluids

We found no published RCTs on the effects of intravenous immunoglobulin in people with dengue haemorrhagic fever or dengue shock syndrome. One unpublished RCT in Filipino children with dengue shock syndrome found that adding intravenous immunoglobulin to standard intravenous fluids reduced mortality compared with adding placebo to standard intravenous fluids.

BMJ Clin Evid Concise 2006;16:311–313.

Dengue fever

*Although we found no direct evidence to support their use, widespread consensus holds that intravenous fluid replacement with crystalloids should be used universally in children with dengue haemorrhagic fever or dengue shock syndrome because these conditions lead to an acute increase in vascular permeability that leads to plasma leakage, resulting in increased haematocrit and decreased blood pressure. Placebo controlled trials would be considered unethical.

DEFINITION Dengue infection is a mosquito borne arboviral infection. The spectrum of dengue virus infection ranges from asymptomatic or undifferentiated febrile illness to dengue fever and dengue haemorrhagic fever or dengue shock syndrome. An important criterion to consider in the diagnosis of dengue infection is history of travel or residence in a dengue endemic area within 2 weeks of the onset of fever. **Dengue fever** is an acute febrile illness whose clinical presentation varies with age. Infants and young children may have an undifferentiated febrile disease with a maculopapular rash. Children aged 15 years or older and adults may have either a mild febrile illness or the classic incapacitating disease also called "breakbone fever" presenting with high fever of sudden onset and non-specific signs and symptoms of severe headache; pain behind the eyes; muscle, bone, or joint pains; nausea; vomiting; and rash. **Dengue haemorrhagic fever** is characterised by four criteria: acute onset of high fever; haemorrhagic manifestations evidenced by a positive tourniquet test, skin haemorrhages, mucosal and gastrointestinal tract bleeding; thrombocytopenia; and evidence of plasma leakage manifested by a rise or drop in haematocrit, fluid in the lungs or abdomen, or hypoproteinaemia. Dengue haemorrhagic fever is classified into four grades of severity (see table 1 Ⓣ).[1] Presence of thrombocytopenia and haemoconcentration differentiates dengue haemorrhagic fever grades I and II from dengue fever. Grades III and IV dengue haemorrhagic fever are considered **dengue shock syndrome**.[1] Plasma leakage is the major pathophysiological feature observed in dengue haemorrhagic fever.

INCIDENCE/ PREVALENCE Dengue fever and dengue haemorrhagic fever are public health problems worldwide, particularly in low-lying areas where *Aedes aegypti*, a domestic mosquito, is present. Cities near to the equator but high in the Andes are free of dengue because *Aedes* mosquitoes do not survive at high altitudes. Worldwide, an estimated 50–100 million cases of dengue fever and hundreds of thousands of dengue haemorrhagic fever occur yearly.[2] Endemic regions are the Americas, South East Asia, western Pacific, Africa, and the eastern Mediterranean. Major global demographic changes and their consequences (particularly increases in the density and geographic distribution of the vector with declining vector control; unreliable water supply systems; increasing non-biodegradable container and poor solid waste disposal; increased geographic range of virus transmission owing to increased air travel; and increased population density in urban areas) are responsible for the resurgence of dengue in the past century.[3,4] The World Health Organization estimates that global temperature rises of 1.0–3.5 °C can increase transmission by shortening the extrinsic incubation period of viruses within the mosquito, adding 20 000–30 000 more fatal cases annually.[5]

AETIOLOGY/ RISK FACTORS Dengue virus serotypes 1–4 (DEN 1, 2, 3, 4) belonging to the flavivirus genus are the aetiologic agents. These serotypes are closely related but antigenically distinct. *Ae aegypti*, the principal vector, transmits the virus to humans. Dengue haemorrhagic fever and dengue shock syndrome typically occur in children under the age of 15 years, although dengue fever primarily occurs in adults and older children. Important risk factors influencing who will develop dengue haemorrhagic fever or severe disease during epidemics include the virus strain and serotype, immune status of the host, age, and genetic predisposition. There is evidence that sequential infection or pre-existing antidengue antibodies increases the risk of dengue haemorrhagic fever through antibody dependent enhancement.[3,4,6-8]

PROGNOSIS Dengue fever is an incapacitating disease but prognosis is favourable in previously healthy adults, although dengue haemorrhagic fever and dengue shock syndrome are major causes of hospital admission and mortality in children. Dengue fever is generally self limiting, with less than 1% case fatality. The acute phase of the illness lasts for 2–7 days but the convalescent phase may be prolonged for weeks associated with fatigue and depression, especially in adults. Prognosis in dengue haemorrhagic fever and dengue shock syndrome depends on prevention or early recognition and treatment of shock. Case fatality ranges from 2.5% to 5.0%. Once shock sets in, fatality may be as high as 12–44%.[9] In centres with appropriate intensive supportive treatment, fatality can be less than 1%. There is no specific antiviral treatment. The standard treatment is to give intravenous fluids to expand plasma volume. People usually recover after prompt and adequate fluid and electrolyte supportive treatment. The optimal fluid regimen, however, remains the subject of debate. This is particularly important in dengue, where one of the management difficulties is to correct hypovolaemia rapidly without precipitating fluid overload.

Please refer to clinicalevidence.com for full text and references.

Diarrhoea in adults (acute)

Search date January 2006

Guy de Bruyn

What are the effects of treatments for acute diarrhoea in adults living in developed countries?

LIKELY TO BE BENEFICIAL

Antimotility agents

RCTs found that loperamide hydrochloride and loperamide oxide reduced the duration of diarrhoea and improved symptoms of acute diarrhoeal illness compared with placebo. One RCT found that diphenoxylate–atropine reduced rate of bowel actions compared with placebo but found no significant difference in median time to last stool. One RCT found that loperamide hydrochloride and loperamide oxide 2 mg increased constipation like periods compared with placebo. However, it found no significant difference in constipation like periods between loperamide oxide 1 mg and placebo.

Antisecretory agents

Two RCTs found that racecadotril (acetorphan) reduced the duration of diarrhoea compared with placebo. Three RCTs found no significant difference in reduction of duration of diarrhoea between racecadotril and loperamide.

TRADE OFF BETWEEN BENEFITS AND HARMS

Antibiotics (empirical use for mild to moderate diarrhoea)

RCTs found that antibiotics reduced the duration of diarrhoea and improved symptoms of acute diarrhoeal illness compared with placebo, and were more effective in eradicating pathogens from stools. One RCT found various self limiting adverse effects in people taking antibiotics, but these only led to discontinuation of treatment in people with rash. The RCT also found that bacterial resistance developed in about 20% of people with *Campylobacter* taking antibiotics (ciprofloxacin or trimethoprim–sulfamethoxazole).

UNKNOWN EFFECTIVENESS

Diet

One RCT found no significant difference in time to resolution of diarrhoea in people on a restricted compared with an unrestricted diet.

Oral rehydration solutions

We found no systematic review or RCTs evaluating the effects of oral rehydration solutions for acute diarrhoea in adults living in developed countries.

What are the effects of treatments for acute mild to moderate diarrhoea in adults from the developed world travelling to developing countries?

LIKELY TO BE BENEFICIAL

Antimotility agents

Two RCTs found that loperamide hydrochloride reduced the duration of diarrhoea compared with placebo. One of these RCTs also found that loperamide alone and trimethoprim–sulfamethoxazole alone were associated with similar durations of diarrhoea but that combination treatment with loperamide plus trimethoprim–sulfamethoxazole reduced the duration of diarrhoea compared with loperamide alone. Two RCTs found no significant difference in improvement of symptoms of acute diarrhoea between loperamide plus ciprofloxacin and ciprofloxacin alone.

Bismuth subsalicylate

RCTs found that bismuth subsalicylate reduced the duration of acute diarrhoea compared with placebo but was not as effective as loperamide. Bismuth subsalicylate is associated with frequent minor adverse effects such as black tongue or black stools.

TRADE OFF BETWEEN BENEFITS AND HARMS

Antibiotics (empirical use for mild–moderate diarrhoea)

One systematic review, one subsequent RCT, and one additional RCT found that antibiotics reduced the duration of diarrhoea compared with placebo. The systematic review performed a meta-analysis of five RCTs and reported that antibiotics increased adverse effects compared with placebo, but none of the adverse effects were judged to be serious.

Antisecretory agents

One RCT found that zaldaride maleate shortened the duration of diarrhoea compared with placebo. One RCT found that loperamide reduced the mean number of unformed stools at 48 hours compared with zaldaride maleate. Further development of zaldaride maleate has been halted due to concerns over cardiovascular symptoms related to higher doses.

UNKNOWN EFFECTIVENESS

Diet

One RCT found insufficient evidence to assess the effects of restricted compared with unrestricted diet.

Oral rehydration solutions

We found no systematic review or RCTs evaluating the effects of oral rehydration solutions on acute mild to moderate diarrhoea in adults from the developed world travelling to developing countries. One RCT found no significant difference in duration of diarrhoea or symptom control between loperamide plus oral rehydration solution and loperamide alone.

What are the effects of treatments for acute mild to moderate diarrhoea in adults living in developing countries?

LIKELY TO BE BENEFICIAL

Antimotility agents

Two RCTs found that lidamidine and loperamide improved symptoms of acute diarrhoea compared with placebo.

Antisecretory agents

One RCT found no significant difference in duration of illness between racecadotril (acetorphan) and loperamide. People taking racecadotril had fewer adverse effects than those taking loperamide, in particular fewer had rebound constipation.

Diarrhoea in adults (acute)

UNKNOWN EFFECTIVENESS

Antibiotics (empirical use)

Two RCTs with methodological weaknesses found no significant difference in symptoms of acute mild to moderate diarrhoea between antibiotics and placebo in adults living in developing countries.

Oral rehydration solutions

One RCT found no significant difference in stool output at 48 hours between citrate oral rehydration solution and bicarbonate oral rehydration solution.

What are the effects of treatments for acute severe diarrhoea in adults living in developing countries?

BENEFICIAL

Amino acid oral rehydration solution

RCTs found modest clinical benefit with amino acid oral rehydration solution compared with standard oral rehydration solution both in people with cholera and non-cholera diarrhoea.

Rice based oral rehydration solution

One systematic review found that rice based oral rehydration solution (ORS) reduced stool volume compared with standard ORS both in people with cholera and non-cholera diarrhoea. One additional RCT found that rice ORS reduced stool output compared with standard ORS.

Standard oral rehydration solution*

RCTs comparing oral rehydration versus no rehydration would be considered unethical. There is consensus that rehydration with standard oral rehydration solution is beneficial in people with severe diarrhoea.

UNKNOWN EFFECTIVENESS

Antibiotics (empirical use)

We found no systematic review or RCTs evaluating the effects of empirical use of antibiotics in treating severe diarrhoea in adults living in developing countries.

Antimotility agents

We found no systematic review or RCTs evaluating the effects of antimotility agents in treating severe diarrhoea in adults living in developing countries.

Antisecretory agents

One RCT found no significant difference in duration of diarrhoea between racecadotril (acetorphan) and placebo. One RCT found no difference between berberine sulphate, tetracycline, berberine plus tetracycline, and placebo in mean duration of diarrhoea among people with non-cholera diarrhoea. The RCT found that among people with cholera berberine plus tetracycline and tetracycline reduced the mean duration of diarrhoea compared with placebo. A second RCT found that berberine sulphate reduced mean stool volumes and increased the proportion of people who stopped having diarrhoea at 24 hours compared with no treatment in people with *Escherichia coli*. The RCT also found that berberine sulphate decreased mean stool volume at the second 8 hour period in people with cholera compared with no treatment. One RCT found similar results between chlorpromazine and placebo for duration of hospitalisation, fluid requirement, and volume loss in adults and children with severe diarrhoea. A second RCT found that chlorpromazine reduced the duration of diarrhoea compared with no treatment in adults with cholera.

Bicarbonate oral rehydration solution

Three RCTs found no significant difference in total stool output or duration of diarrhoea between bicarbonate oral rehydration solution and standard or chloride oral rehydration solution in people with cholera and non-cholera diarrhoea.

Intravenous rehydration (compared with nasogastric tube rehydration or oral rehydration solution alone)

One small RCT in adults with cholera and severe dehydration, who all received initial intravenous fluids, found no significant difference in the duration of diarrhoea or total stool volume between enteral rehydration through a nasogastric tube and intravenous rehydration. We found no systematic review or RCTs comparing oral rehydration solution alone versus intravenous rehydration.

Reduced osmolarity oral rehydration solution

Three RCTs found modest and inconsistent effects of reduced osmolarity oral rehydration solution (ORS) on stool volume and duration of diarrhoea compared with standard ORS in people with cholera diarrhoea. Reduced osmolarity ORS was associated with an increased risk of non-symptomatic hyponatraemia.

*Categorisation based on consensus. RCTs are unlikely to be conducted.

DEFINITION Diarrhoea is watery or liquid stools, usually with an increase in stool weight above 200 g daily and an increase in daily stool frequency. This chapter covers empirical treatment of suspected infectious diarrhoea in adults.

INCIDENCE/ PREVALENCE An estimated 4000 million cases of diarrhoea occurred worldwide in 1996, resulting in 2.5 million deaths.[1] In the USA, the estimated incidence for infectious intestinal disease is 0.44 episodes per person per year (1 episode per person every 2.3 years), resulting in about one consultation with a doctor per person every 28 years.[2] A recent community study in the UK reported an incidence of 19 cases per 100 person years, of which 3.3 cases per 100 person years resulted in consultation with a general practitioner.[3] Both estimates derive from population based studies, including both adults and children. The epidemiology of travellers' diarrhoea is not well understood. Incidence is higher in travellers visiting developing countries, but it varies widely by location and season of travel.[4] The incidence of diarrhoea in adults in developing countries is largely unknown owing to the lack of large scale surveillance studies in these countries.

AETIOLOGY/ RISK FACTORS The cause of diarrhoea depends on geographical location, standards of food hygiene, sanitation, water supply, and season. Commonly identified causes of sporadic diarrhoea in adults in developed countries include *Campylobacter*, *Salmonella*, *Shigella*, *Escherichia coli*, *Yersinia*, protozoa, and viruses (see table 1)Ⓣ.[5,6] No pathogens are identified in more than half of people with diarrhoea. In returning travellers, about 50% of episodes are caused by bacteria such as enterotoxigenic *E coli*, *Salmonella*, *Shigella*, *Campylobacter*, *Vibrio*, enteroadherent *E coli*, *Yersinia*, and *Aeromonas* (see table 1)Ⓣ.[5]

PROGNOSIS In developed countries, death from infectious diarrhoea is rare, although serious complications, including severe dehydration and renal failure, can occur and may necessitate admission to hospital. Elderly people and those in long term care have an increased risk of death.[7] In developing countries, diarrhoea

Diarrhoea in adults (acute)

is reported to cause more deaths in children under 5 years of age than any other condition.[1] Few studies have examined which factors predict poor outcome in adults.

Please refer to clinicalevidence.com for full text and references.

Hepatitis B (prevention)

Search date November 2005

Suzanne Norris and Abdul Mohsen

What are the effects of immunisation in countries with high endemicity?

BENEFICIAL

Selective immunisation of high risk individuals (evidence only for children born to HBsAg positive mothers)

One non-systematic review of mainly observational studies with both plasma derived and recombinant vaccine, and two RCTs of plasma derived hepatitis B immunisation all found that immunisation prevented chronic carrier state compared with placebo or no treatment in children born to HBsAg positive mothers. One RCT found minor adverse effects with immunisation; the other RCTs did not report on adverse effects. We found no good evidence in other high risk groups. One cluster RCT found that selective immunisation in high risk individuals was less effective than universal immunisation of infants in preventing chronic carrier state and acute hepatitis events.

Universal immunisation of infants (more effective than placebo or no treatment; limited evidence that it may be better than selective immunisation of high risk individuals)

One non-systematic review and four additional and subsequent RCTs found that universal immunisation of infants (using either recombinant or plasma derived vaccines) reduced acute hepatitis and development of a chronic carrier state compared with placebo. The longest RCT found that universal immunisation protected at 15 years. Observational data from mass vaccination programmes found that universal immunisation reduced the incidence of hepatocellular carcinoma, mortality secondary to hepatocellular carcinoma, mortality rate of fulminant hepatitis, hepatitis B carrier rate, prevalence of chronic carrier state, chronic liver disease, and cirrhosis. Three non-systematic reviews and one RCT found only minor adverse reactions after recombinant hepatitis B immunisation. One cluster RCT found that universal immunisation with plasma or recombinant vaccine reduced the development of chronic carrier state and acute hepatitis events compared with selective immunisation of high risk groups.

What are the effects of immunisation in countries with low endemicity?

LIKELY TO BE BENEFICIAL

Selective immunisation of high risk individuals

One systematic review found that, in countries with low endemicity, plasma derived hepatitis B immunisation prevented acute hepatitis B and development of chronic carrier state in healthcare workers at high risk of exposure to bodily fluids. One systematic review found no significant difference in the incidence of hepatitis B infection or mortality between vaccination and placebo in people on haemodialysis. Three RCTs found that plasma derived hepatitis B immunisation prevented acute hepatitis B in homosexual men. One small RCT found no significant difference in hepatitis B events in heterosexual partners of infected people. One observational study showed a high prevalence of hepatitis B carrier state and low immunisation uptake in young homosexuals, despite a national ▶

strategy to immunise high risk groups. Surveillance data from a national programme in Japan found that immunisation of neonates (with recombinant hepatitis B vaccine plus hepatitis B immunoglobulin) born to HBsAg positive mothers provided 95% protection against the development of a chronic carrier state. We found insufficient evidence to compare the effectiveness of selective immunisation in high risk individuals versus other strategies in countries with low endemicity.

Universal immunisation of adolescents

One observational study found that mass immunisation reduced the rate of reported acute hepatitis B viral infection. Another observational study suggested minor adverse effects after hepatitis B immunisation in this group. We found insufficient evidence to compare universal adolescent immunisation versus other immunisation strategies.

Universal immunisation of infants

One historical cohort study in a country with low endemicity found a reduction in the prevalence of hepatitis B chronic carrier state after universal immunisation. We found insufficient evidence to compare its effectiveness versus other strategies. Two cohort studies and surveillance data did not report any links between hepatitis B immunisation and serious adverse reactions.

UNKNOWN EFFECTIVENESS

Selective immunisation of people with known chronic liver disease not caused by hepatitis B

We found insufficient evidence to compare the effectiveness of selective immunisation versus no immunisation in people with known chronic liver disease not caused by hepatitis B. One RCT comparing several different doses of vaccine, and several observational studies found no serious adverse effects with selective immunisation in people with chronic liver disease caused by alcoholism or hepatitis C.

DEFINITION Hepatitis B is a viral infectious disease with an incubation period of 40–160 days. Acute hepatitis B infection is characterised by anorexia, vague abdominal discomfort, nausea and vomiting, jaundice, and occasional fever. Illness is associated with deranged liver function tests (especially raised alanine transaminases) and presence of serological markers of acute hepatitis B infection (e.g. hepatitis B surface antigen [HBsAg], antiHBc IgM).[1]

INCIDENCE/ PREVALENCE The incidence of acute hepatitis B and prevalence of its chronic carrier state varies widely across the globe. In areas with high endemicity (HBsAg prevalence ≥ 8%; e.g. South East Asia and Africa), more than half of the population becomes infected at some point in their lives.[2] In countries with low endemicity (HBsAg prevalence < 2%; e.g. North America, western Europe, Australia), most of the population do not become infected.[2] Nearly a third of the world population has been infected by hepatitis B at some point, and at least 350 million people (5–6% of the world population) are currently chronic carriers of hepatitis B infection.[3]

AETIOLOGY/ RISK FACTORS In countries with high endemicity, most infections occur during childhood from an infected mother to her baby (vertical transmission) or from one family member to another (horizontal transmission).[4] Horizontal transmission is thought to be an important route of hepatitis B infection during early childhood, and probably occurs mainly through unnoticed contact with blood from infected family members.[5] In countries with high endemicity, the proportion of chronic HBsAg carriage attributable to vertical transmission has been estimated at 5–50%.[6-8] The proportion of chronic HBsAg carriage attributable to horizontal transmission is not known, although one survey in China found that 27.2% of families had one or more HBsAg positive members.[8] In developed countries most hepatitis B infection occurs later, from sexual activity, injection drug use, or occupational exposure. Less frequent causes of infection include household contact, regular haemodialysis, transmission from a healthcare professional, and receipt of organs or blood products.[9] The vaccination policy of a country is a large determinant of the risk of developing hepatitis B. Since the development of plasma derived hepatitis B vaccine in the early 1980s, subsequently replaced by recombinant vaccine, many countries have adopted a policy of universal immunisation of all infants. On the basis of disease burden, the World Health Organization recommended that hepatitis B vaccine be incorporated into routine infant and childhood immunisation programmes in countries with high endemicity by 1995 and in all countries by 1997.[10] However, in many countries with low endemicity, universal immunisation policy remains controversial and has still not been adopted.[11] Some of these countries have adopted a policy of selective immunisation of high risk individuals. Others have adopted a universal adolescent immunisation policy.

PROGNOSIS Hepatitis B infection resolves after the acute infection in 90–95% of cases. In the remainder (5–10%) it may result in several serious sequelae. Massive hepatic necrosis occurs in 1% of people with acute viral hepatitis, leading to a serious and often fatal condition called acute fulminant hepatitis. Between 2% and 10% of those infected as adults become chronic carriers, indicated by HBsAg persistence for more than 6 months. Chronic carriage is more frequent in those infected as children, and reaches up to 90% in those infected during the perinatal period.[1] Between 20% and 25% of chronic carriers develop a progressive chronic liver disease. In about one quarter to one third of cases, this progresses to cirrhosis and hepatocellular carcinoma.[12] These complications usually arise in older adults and are major causes of mortality in populations with high hepatitis B endemicity.[4] Observational studies suggest that in these countries, almost 80% of chronic liver disease and cirrhosis is attributed to hepatitis B, and these complications lead to at least 1 million deaths every year worldwide.

Please refer to clinicalevidence.com for full text and references.

Hepatitis C (chronic)

Search date May 2005

Abdul Mohsen and Suzanne Norris

What are the effects of interventions in treatment naive people with chronic infection, but without liver decompensation?

BENEFICIAL

Interferon

One systematic review found that more treatment naive people had a sustained virological response with interferon compared with placebo or no treatment. It also found that more people with cirrhosis or advanced fibrosis who were treated with interferon had a sustained virological response compared with no treatment. The review also found that interferon improved liver histology compared with placebo or no treatment. One RCT found no significant difference between interferon and no treatment in the incidence of hepatocellular carcinoma in people with Child–Pugh A cirrhosis.

Interferon plus ribavirin

One systematic review and two subsequent RCTs found that interferon plus ribavirin increased the proportion of treatment naive people with a sustained virological response compared with interferon monotherapy.

Peginterferon

One systematic review and one subsequent RCT found that peginterferon (alfa-2a or alfa-2b) increased the proportion of treatment naive people with a sustained virological response compared with standard interferon monotherapy. A meta-analysis of three RCTs identified by the review found that peginterferon reduced liver fibrosis compared with standard interferon.

Peginterferon plus ribavirin

Four RCTs found that peginterferon plus ribavirin increased the proportion of treatment naive people with a sustained virological response compared with peginterferon alone or plus placebo, standard interferon plus ribavirin, or no treatment.

What are the effects of interventions in treating interferon non-responsive people with chronic infection, but without liver decompensation?

BENEFICIAL

Interferon alfa plus ribavirin

Two systematic reviews and one subsequent RCT found that a larger proportion of interferon non-responsive people had a sustained virological response with interferon plus ribavirin compared with interferon monotherapy.

LIKELY TO BE BENEFICIAL

Peginterferon plus ribavirin*

We found no systematic review or RCTs on the effects of peginterferon plus ribavirin in interferon non-responsive people. However, interferon plus ribavirin is effective in interferon non-responsive people and there is consensus that peginterferon plus ribavirin is also likely to be beneficial.

UNKNOWN EFFECTIVENESS

Interferon

One systematic review found no RCTs reporting the effects of retreatment with interferon on virological outcomes in people who had previously not responded to interferon.

Peginterferon

We found no systematic review or RCTs on the effects of peginterferon in interferon non-responsive people.

What are the effects of interventions in people with chronic infection, but without liver decompensation, who relapse after interferon treatment?

BENEFICIAL

Interferon alfa plus ribavirin

One systematic review found that a larger proportion of people had a sustained virological response with interferon alfa plus ribavirin compared with interferon alfa monotherapy.

LIKELY TO BE BENEFICIAL

Peginterferon plus ribavirin*

We found no systematic review or RCTs on the effects of peginterferon plus ribavirin in people who had relapsed after interferon treatment. However, interferon plus ribavirin is effective in people who have relapsed from treatment, and there is consensus that peginterferon plus ribavirin is also likely to be beneficial.

UNKNOWN EFFECTIVENESS

Interferon

We found one systematic review, which identified no RCTs comparing interferon with placebo or no treatment in people who had relapsed after interferon treatment.

Peginterferon

We found no systematic review or RCTs on the effects of peginterferon in people who have relapsed after treatment.

*No RCTs. Categorisation based on consensus.

DEFINITION Hepatitis C virus (HCV), identified in 1989, is a member of the flaviviridae family of spherical, enveloped, positive strand RNA viruses.[1,2] There are six different HCV genotypes. Genotype 1 is the most common and is also the most resistant to treatment.[3] Chronic HCV infection is defined as persistent, detectable serum HCV RNA for a period greater than 6 months with or without

Hepatitis C (chronic)

derangement in liver function tests. This is in contrast to acute HCV infection, where serum HCV RNA clears within 6 months. Prospective studies have shown that 60–85% of HCV infected persons will develop chronic infection.[2,4] This chapter will only deal with interventions used to treat chronic HCV infection without liver decompensation. The effect of treatment is measured by the presence or absence of detectable serum HCV RNA. The loss of detectable HCV RNA at the end of the treatment period is defined as the end of treatment virological response. The loss of detectable HCV RNA 24 weeks or more after the completion of treatment is termed the sustained virological response. Response to treatment is defined as the loss of detectable serum HCV RNA. Non-response is defined as a failure to clear serum HCV RNA during the treatment period. A relapse from treatment is defined as loss of serum HCV RNA during treatment, which reappears during the follow up period, typically within 24 weeks of a treatment episode.

INCIDENCE/ PREVALENCE HCV has emerged as a major viral pandemic over the past two decades, with about 3% of the world's population chronically infected.[5] HCV prevalence varies throughout the world, with the highest number of infections reported in Egypt (6–28%).[6] In the USA, an estimated four million people are positive for HCV antibodies, reflecting a prevalence rate of 2%, and about 35 000 new HCV infections are estimated to occur each year.[2] In Europe, the prevalence of HCV infection ranges from about 0.5–2.0%.[7] The true incidence of HCV is difficult to calculate accurately because this relates to the prevalence of risk factors for HCV transmission, in particular injection drug use.

AETIOLOGY/ RISK FACTORS HCV is mainly blood borne and transmission occurs primarily through exposure to infected blood. This exposure may occur because of the use of infected needles used for drug injection, blood transfusion or solid organ transplantation from infected donors in the absence of universal screening procedures, maternal (vertical) transmission, unsafe medical practices, and occupational exposure to infected blood.[8] As a result of HCV screening, the absolute risk of acquiring infection through blood components or products is now very small, at lower than 1/400 000 units of blood transfused.[9] HCV vertical transmission is uncommon, with a transmission rate of lower than 6%.[10] Poverty, high risk sexual behaviour, and having fewer than 12 years of education are linked to an increased risk of infection.[11] However, in some cases no risk factors can be identified.[12]

DIAGNOSIS Diagnosis of HCV infection is often the result of active screening because many people chronically infected with HCV remain asymptomatic, including a significant number of those who progress to cirrhosis. Therefore, routine screening of people in high risk groups is advised.

PROGNOSIS Diagnosis of HCV infection is often the result of active screening because many people chronically infected with HCV remain asymptomatic, including a significant number of those who progress to cirrhosis. The spectrum of liver disease and the rate of disease progression vary in people with chronic HCV infection. Complications of chronic HCV infection include cirrhosis, compensated and decompensated liver disease, and hepatocellular carcinoma. Studies suggest that one third of people with chronic HCV infection are "rapid progressors" (time from infection to cirrhosis < 20 years); one third "intermediate progressors" (time to cirrhosis 20–50 years); and one third "slow or non-progressors" (time to cirrhosis > 50 years).[13] Factors associated with disease progression include: older age at acquisition; male sex; coinfection with HIV, hepatitis B virus, or both; coexisting liver disease; and excessive alcohol consumption. In people who develop cirrhosis, the 5 year risk of decompensation is 15–20%, the 5 year risk of hepatocellular carcinoma is 10% and the annual risk of hepatocellular carcinoma is 1–5% a year.[14-16]

Please refer to clinicalevidence.com for full text and references.

Influenza

Search date April 2006

Tom Jefferson

What are the effects of vaccines to prevent influenza?

LIKELY TO BE BENEFICIAL

Vaccines in adults (prevention of cases) *New*

One systematic review found that both live and inactivated influenza vaccines reduced the number of influenza cases compared with placebo, and to a greater extent if their antigen content matched World Health Organization recommendations. It found that vaccines moderately reduced time off work but found no evidence on the effects of complications. Aerosol vaccines increased sore throats, coryza, and inactivated vaccines caused local tenderness.

Vaccines in children (prevention of symptoms and/or infection) *New*

One systematic review of RCTs and observational studies found that in older children (aged 2–16 years), vaccines reduced the number of cases of influenza and influenza-like illness. There were no data in children below the age of 2 years. However, there is insufficient evidence to assess the effects of vaccines on complications. The review also found that vaccines reduced the number of school absences. It found insufficient evidence to assess adverse effects.

UNKNOWN EFFECTIVENESS

Vaccines in the elderly (prevention of cases and complications)

One systematic review of cohort and case control studies found no significant difference between inactivated split vaccines and placebo or no intervention in influenza or influenza-like illness in elderly community residents. The review found that newer vaccines reduce the number of cases of influenza-like illness compared with no intervention. In closed communities such as nursing homes, inactivated vaccines reduced the number of cases of influenza-like illness, but not influenza, compared with no intervention. The studies were generally of poor quality, and adverse effects were difficult to quantify.

What are the effects of antiviral chemoprophylaxis of influenza?

LIKELY TO BE BENEFICIAL

Orally inhaled zanamivir (prevention of symptoms in influenza A and B) *New*

One systematic review found that orally inhaled zanamivir increased the prevention of symptoms of influenza, but not influenza-like illness, compared with placebo. Therefore the benefit of orally inhaled zanamivir is likely to be seen when influenza is diagnosed or its local circulation is known to be high. The review found no significant difference in infection between zanamivir and placebo. Two RCTs found that postexposure prophylaxis with zanamivir reduced the number of cases of symptomatic influenza in households and individuals, and reduced the duration of symptoms by at least 1.5 days compared with placebo.

Oral oseltamivir (prevention of symptoms in influenza A and B) *New*

One systematic review found that oseltamivir improved symptoms in cases of influenza, but not in influenza-like illness, compared with placebo and did not ▶

prevent infection. Two RCTs found that postexposure prophylaxis with oseltamivir reduced symptomatic influenza in households and contacts compared with placebo. A common adverse effect was nausea.

LIKELY TO BE INEFFECTIVE OR HARMFUL

Oral amantadine* *New*

One systematic review found that amantadine prevented symptoms of seasonal influenza and influenza-like illness compared with placebo in adults, but had no effects on infection or nasal shedding. There is consensus that amantadine should not be used for first line chemoprophylaxis because resistance to amantadine is high and it is only effective against influenza A. There was insufficient evidence to assess amantadine for the prophylaxis of influenza A in the elderly, pregnant women, or children. Adverse effects include insomnia, hallucinations, and agitation.

Oral rimantadine *New*

One systematic review found no significant difference between rimantadine and placebo in the prevention of symptoms or infection with influenza A. The review found no studies in children, the elderly, or pregnant women. The review found that rimantadine increased adverse effects compared with placebo.

What are the effects of antiviral medications to treat influenza?

LIKELY TO BE BENEFICIAL

Orally inhaled zanamivir for early treatment of influenza A or B (reduced duration of symptoms and incidence of complications)

One systematic review found that orally inhaled zanamivir reduced the duration of influenza symptoms in adults and children aged up to 12 years and decreased viral load and viral shedding in adults compared with placebo. It found limited evidence that zanamivir reduced complications in adults. Adverse effects were similar in people taking zanamivir and those taking placebo. There is insufficient evidence to assess orally inhaled zanamivir for treatment of influenza in the elderly.

Oral oseltamivir for early treatment of influenza A and B (reduced duration of symptoms and incidence of complications)

One systematic review found that oral oseltamivir reduced the duration of influenza symptoms in children aged up to 12 years and in adults compared with placebo. It also reduced the incidence of respiratory tract complications in adults with influenza but not influenza-like illness. In adults, it decreased viral load and viral shedding. In adults, adverse effects were similar in people taking oseltamivir and placebo. The review found that oseltamivir increased vomiting in children.

LIKELY TO BE INEFFECTIVE OR HARMFUL

Oral amantadine for early treatment of influenza A*

One systematic review found that oral amantadine reduced the duration of fever in adults by about 1 day compared with placebo, but had no effect on viral shedding from the nose. There is consensus that amantadine should not be used as first line treatment, because resistance to amantadine is high and it is only effective against influenza A. There is insufficient evidence to assess oral amantadine for the treatment of influenza A in children or the elderly. Adverse effects include insomnia, hallucinations, and agitation.

Oral rimantadine for early treatment of influenza A*

One systematic review found that oral rimantadine reduced the duration of fever by about 1 day compared with placebo, but had no effect on viral shedding from the nose. We found insufficient evidence to assess adverse effects in this setting. There is consensus that rimantadine should not be used as first line treatment, because resistance to amantadine is high and it is only effective against influenza A. There is also insufficient evidence to assess oral rimantadine for the treatment of influenza A in children or the elderly.

*Categorisation based on consensus.

DEFINITION Influenza is an acute respiratory illness caused by infection with influenza A and B viruses. The illness affects the upper and/or lower respiratory tract and is often accompanied by systemic signs and symptoms such as the abrupt onset of fever, chills, non-productive cough, myalgias, headache, nasal congestion, sore throat, and fatigue.[1] **Diagnosis:** Not all people infected with influenza viruses become symptomatic, and not everybody with the above symptoms will have influenza. This is because each year many different viral and bacterial circulating agents cause an illness called influenza-like illness with a clinical picture which is indistinguishable from influenza.[2-4] . Between 40% and 85% of infections with influenza result in clinical illness, depending on age and pre-existing immunity to the virus.[5] Although influenza is usually diagnosed clinically, genuine influenza infection can only be diagnosed with laboratory confirmation either by culture, serological responses, or by bedside testing. The rapid bedside diagnostic tests available on the market are mainly antigen detection immunoassays and (unlike laboratory tests such as culture or reverse transcription–polymerase chain reaction) can be carried out within 30 minutes. However, the results of these tests must be interpreted with caution. During times of low influenza viral circulation, the positive predictive value is low, leading to an increased proportion of false positive results. In times of high viral circulation, the negative predictive value is low, leading to an increased proportion of false negatives.[6] It is also impractical to test all potential influenza cases. If a good surveillance system is in place, with quick feedback, it is likely that the positive predictive value of clinical diagnosis alone (based on high fever and a cough) will be similar to that of the bedside test (79–87%).[6] **Population:** For the purpose of this review, we have included trials that assessed both influenza-like illness and influenza, which are clinically indistinguishable. Where appropriate, the applicability of data to influenza pandemic has been discussed.

INCIDENCE/ PREVALENCE **Seasonal influenza:** Circulation of seasonal influenza viruses can vary from year to year, season to season, and even setting to setting. In temperate areas, seasonal influenza activity typically peaks between late December and early March in the northern hemisphere and between May and September in the southern hemisphere. In tropical areas, there is no temporal peak in influenza activity through the year.[7] The annual incidence of influenza varies, and depends partly on the underlying level of population immunity to circulating influenza viruses.[1] One localised study in the USA found that serological conversion, with or without symptoms, occurred in 10–20% of people a year, with the highest infection rates in people aged under 20 years.[8] A systematic review of the incidence of influenza in people aged up to 19 years found that the average incidence was between 4.6% and 9.5%.[9] The proportion of people affected by circulating influenza is higher in institutions and in areas of overcrowding.[10] **Pandemic influenza:** The incidence of symptomatic influenza depends, among other factors, on the susceptibility of the host. Occasionally, a new type of influenza virus appears, generated either by direct mutation or by reassortment of the viral genome. Because immunity to this new virus is low, it is able to behave in an aggressive way, causing morbidity and mortality on a global scale, mainly because of the body's inability to prevent the creation of a high viral load, the cytopathic effect of the new virus, and the complications in target organs such as lungs and airways. Widespread epidemics are known as pandemics (from the Greek pan = all). In the 20th century, there were three pandemics caused by different influenza A viral subtypes (see aetiology), in 1918–9 (H1N1), 1957 (H2N2), and 1968 (H3N2). **Avian influenza:** Influenza infection may also appear as a zoonotic infection, with direct spread of the avian virus to humans. In April 2003, 87 people in the Netherlands were infected with avian virus H7N7. In most cases, the only symptom was conjunctivitis. However, a 57 year old vet dealing with veterinary public health interventions died of acute respiratory distress. An avian virus (H5N1) has been transmitted from bird to human (and perhaps occasionally from human to human) sporadically since 1997. Such transmission has frequently taken place in situations of poor hygiene and close proximity between birds and humans.[11]

AETIOLOGY/ RISK FACTORS

Viral classification: The influenza virus is composed of a protein envelope around an RNA core. On the surface of the envelope are two antigens: neuraminidase (N antigen) and haemagglutinin (H antigen). The influenza virus has a marked propensity to mutate its external antigenic composition to escape the host's immune defences. Given this extreme mutability, a classification of viral subtype A based on H and N typing has been introduced. **Transmission:** Influenza viruses are transmitted primarily from person to person through respiratory droplets disseminated during sneezing, coughing, and talking, and through contact with contaminated surfaces.[1,12] The incubation period of influenza is 1–4 days, and infected adults are usually contagious from the day before symptom onset until 5 days after symptom onset. **Pandemic influenza:** Pandemics are thought to originate mostly in southern China, where ducks (the animal reservoir and breeding ground for new strains), pigs (which are thought to be the biological intermediate host or "mixing vessel"), and humans live in very close proximity.[13] Pigs are considered to be plausible intermediate hosts because their respiratory epithelial cells have receptors for both avian (i.e. duck) and human viral haemagglutinins. Minor changes in viral antigenic configurations, known as "drift", cause local or more circumscribed epidemics.

PROGNOSIS

The signs and symptoms of uncomplicated influenza usually resolve within 1 week, although cough and fatigue may persist.[1] Complications include otitis media, bacterial sinusitis, secondary bacterial pneumonia, and, less commonly, viral pneumonia, respiratory failure, and exacerbations of underlying disease.[1,7] In the UK, 1.3% of people with influenza-like illness are hospitalised each year (95% CI 0.6% to 2.6%).[14] It is estimated that 300–400 deaths each year are attributable to influenza, rising to in excess of 29 000 during an epidemic.[14] The risk of hospitalisation is highest in people 65 years or older, in very young children, and in those with chronic medical conditions.[1,15,16] Over 90% of influenza related deaths during recent seasonal epidemics in the USA have been in people 65 years or older.[1] During influenza pandemics, morbidity and mortality may be high in younger age groups as well.[1] Severe illness is more common with influenza A infections than with influenza B infections.[1] For pandemic influenza, see incidence.

Please refer to clinicalevidence.com for full text and references.

Leprosy

Search date September 2004

Diana Lockwood

What are the effects of interventions to prevent leprosy?

BENEFICIAL

Bacillus Calmette Guerin vaccine

One RCT and three non-randomised or quasi-randomised trials found that Bacillus Calmette Guerin (BCG) alone reduced the incidence of leprosy at 13–16 years of follow up. The RCT also evaluated other vaccines and found that BCG alone was more effective than *Mycobacterium w*, but less effective than ICRC vaccine and BCG plus killed *M leprae*. The RCT found minimal adverse effects with BCG alone.

BCG plus killed *Mycobacterium leprae* vaccine

Two RCTs found that BCG plus killed *M leprae* reduced the incidence of leprosy compared with placebo at 5–9 years of follow up. One of the RCTs also evaluated other vaccines and found that BCG plus killed *M leprae* was more effective than BCG alone and *Mycobacterium w*, but less effective than ICRC vaccine. This RCT found minimal adverse effects with BCG plus killed *Mycobacterium leprae*.

LIKELY TO BE BENEFICIAL

ICRC vaccine

One RCT found that ICRC vaccine reduced the incidence of leprosy compared with placebo at 6–7 years follow up. The RCT also evaluated other vaccines and found that ICRC vaccine was more effective than BCG plus killed *M leprae*, BCG alone, and *Mycobacterium w*. The RCT found minimal adverse effects with ICRC vaccine.

UNLIKELY TO BE BENEFICIAL

***Mycobacterium w* vaccine**

One RCT found that *Mycobacterium w* reduced the incidence of leprosy compared with placebo at 6–7 years of follow up, although the reduction was marginal. The RCT also evaluated other vaccines and found that *Mycobacterium w* was less effective than ICRC vaccine, BCG plus killed *M leprae*, and BCG alone. The RCT found minimal adverse effects with *Mycobacterium w*.

What are the effects of treatments for leprosy?

BENEFICIAL

Multidrug treatment for multibacillary leprosy*

We found no reliable studies comparing multidrug treatment with rifampicin plus clofazimine plus dapsone versus placebo, no treatment, dapsone plus rifampicin, or dapsone alone in multibacillary leprosy. Consensus regarding multidrug treatment efficacy and rising dapsone resistance rates would make such studies unethical. Case series found that multidrug treatment improved skin lesions, increased nerve impairment, and was associated with a low relapse rate. The evidence on the incidence of adverse effects is poor.

Leprosy

Multidrug treatment for paucibacillary leprosy*

We found no reliable studies comparing multidrug treatment with rifampicin plus dapsone versus placebo, no treatment, or dapsone alone in paucibacillary leprosy. Consensus regarding multidrug treatment efficacy and rising dapsone resistance rates would make such studies unethical. Case series found that multidrug treatment improved skin lesions, increased nerve impairment, and was associated with a low relapse rate. We found poor evidence on the incidence of adverse effects.

Multiple dose compared with single dose treatment for single skin lesion leprosy (both achieve high cure rates but multiple dose is likely to achieve a higher rate)

One RCT found that multiple dose treatment with rifampicin monthly plus dapsone daily for 6 months achieved higher cure rates at 18 months than did single dose treatment with rifampicin plus minocycline plus ofloxacin. Some improvement occurred in 99% of people in both groups. Adverse effects were similar with both regimens.

*Categorisation based on observational evidence and consensus; RCTs unlikely to be conducted.

DEFINITION Leprosy is a chronic granulomatous disease caused by *Mycobacterium leprae*, primarily affecting the peripheral nerves and skin. The clinical picture depends on the individual's immune response to *M leprae*. At the tuberculoid end of the Ridley–Jopling scale, individuals have good cell mediated immunity and few skin lesions. At the lepromatous end of the scale, individuals have low reactivity for *M leprae*, causing uncontrolled bacterial spread and skin and mucosal infiltration. Peripheral nerve damage occurs across the spectrum. Nerve damage may occur before, during, or after treatment. Some people have no nerve damage, while others develop anaesthesia of the hands and feet, which puts them at risk of developing neuropathic injury. Weakness and paralysis of the small muscles of the hands, feet, and eyes puts patients at risk of developing deformity and contractures. Loss of the fingers and toes is due to repeated injury in a weak, anaesthetic limb. These visible deformities cause stigmatisation. Classification is based on clinical appearance and bacterial index of lesions. The World Health Organization field leprosy classification is based on the number of skin lesions: single lesion leprosy (1 lesion), paucibacillary leprosy (2–5 skin lesions), and multibacillary leprosy (> 5 skin lesions).[1]

INCIDENCE/ PREVALENCE Worldwide, about 720 000 new cases of leprosy are reported each year,[2] and about 2 million people have leprosy related disabilities. Six major endemic countries (India, Brazil, Myanmar, Madagascar, Nepal, and Mozambique) account for 88% of all new cases. Cohort studies show a peak of disease presentation between 10–20 years of age.[3] After puberty, there are twice as many cases in males as in females.

AETIOLOGY/ RISK FACTORS *M leprae* is discharged from the nasal mucosa of people with untreated lepromatous leprosy, and spreads, via the recipient's nasal mucosa, to infect their skin and nerves. It is a hardy organism and has been shown to survive outside human hosts in India for many months.[4] Risk factors for infection include household contact with a person with leprosy. We found no good evidence of an association with HIV infection, nutrition, or socioeconomic status.[5]

PROGNOSIS Complications of leprosy include nerve damage, immunological reactions, and bacillary infiltration. Without treatment, tuberculoid infection eventually resolves spontaneously. Most people with borderline tuberculoid and borderline lepromatous leprosy gradually develop lepromatous infection. Many people have peripheral nerve damage at the time of diagnosis, ranging from 15% in Bangladesh[6] to 55% in Ethiopia.[7] Immunological reactions can occur with or without antibiotic treatment. Further nerve damage occurs through immune mediated reactions (type 1 reactions) and neuritis. Erythema nodosum leprosum (type 2 reaction) is an immune complex mediated reaction causing fever, malaise, and neuritis, which occurs in 20% of people with lepromatous leprosy and 5% with borderline lepromatous leprosy.[8] Secondary impairments (wounds, contractures, and digit resorption) occur in 33–56% of people with established nerve damage.[9] We found no recent information on mortality.

Please refer to clinicalevidence.com for full text and references.

Malaria: prevention in travellers

Search date February 2006

Ashley M Croft

What are the effects of non-drug preventive interventions in adult travellers?

LIKELY TO BE BENEFICIAL

Insecticide treated clothing

Two RCTs in soldiers and refugee householders who were not receiving chemoprophylaxis found that permethrin treated fabric (clothing or sheets) reduced the incidence of malaria. However, one controlled trial in soldiers receiving chemoprophylaxis found no significant difference in the incidence of malaria between those wearing permethrin treated uniforms and control soldiers in the incidence of malaria, although the presence of background chemoprophylaxis may have masked the effect of permethrin treated uniforms.

Insecticide treated nets

We found no systematic review or RCTs in travellers. One systematic review in adult and child residents of malaria endemic settings found that insecticide treated nets reduced the number of mild episodes of malaria and reduced child mortality.

Topical (skin applied) insect repellents containing diethyltoluamide (DEET)*

We found no systematic review or RCTs on the effects of topical (skin applied) insect repellents to prevent malaria in travellers. One small crossover RCT found that DEET preparations protected against mosquito bites. Many years of clinical experience have led to the consensus that using the topical insect repellent diethyltoluamide (DEET) is likely to be beneficial in preventing malaria. DEET has been reported to cause systemic and skin adverse reactions, particularly with prolonged use.

UNKNOWN EFFECTIVENESS

Acoustic buzzers

We found no systematic review or RCTs on the effects of acoustic buzzers to prevent malaria in adults.

Aerosol insecticides

We found no systematic review or RCTs on the effects of aerosol insecticides to prevent malaria in travellers. One large questionnaire survey in travellers found insufficient evidence on the effects of aerosol insecticides in preventing malaria. Two community RCTs in residents of malaria endemic areas found that indoor spraying of aerosol insecticides reduced clinical malaria.

Air conditioning and electric fans

We found no systematic review or RCTs on the effects of air conditioning or electric fans to prevent malaria in travellers. One large questionnaire survey found that air conditioning reduced the incidence of malaria. One small observational study found that electric ceiling fans reduced total catches of culicine mosquitoes in indoor spaces. However, it found no significant difference in total catches of anopheline mosquitoes.

Biological control measures

We found no systematic review or RCTs on the effects of biological control measures to prevent malaria in travellers.

Full length and light coloured clothing

We found no systematic review or RCTs on the effects of full-length clothing or light coloured clothing to prevent malaria in travellers. One controlled trial in military personnel and one large questionnaire survey in travellers reported that wearing long trousers and long sleeved shirts reduced the incidence of malaria.

Mosquito coils and vaporising mats

We found one systematic review but no RCTs on the effects of coils to prevent malaria in travellers, and no RCTs on the effects of vaporising mats. One case control study of coils in travellers found no evidence of a protective effect against malaria.

Smoke

We found no systematic review or RCTs on the effects of smoke to prevent malaria. One controlled clinical trial found that smoke repelled mosquitoes during the evening.

What are the effects of drug prophylaxis in adult travellers?

LIKELY TO BE BENEFICIAL

Atovaquone–proguanil

One RCT in migrants with limited immunity found that atovaquone–proguanil reduced the proportion of people with malaria compared with placebo. One RCT found no significant difference between atovaquone–proguanil and chloroquine–proguanil in preventing malaria. One RCT comparing atovaquone–proguanil versus mefloquine found no cases of clinical malaria throughout the trial but found a higher rate of neuropsychiatric harm with mefloquine than with atovaquone–proguanil. One RCT found that atovaquone–proguanil reduced adverse effects compared with mefloquine and chloroquine–proguanil and had similar adverse effect rates compared with doxycycline. Another RCT found no significant difference in adverse events between atovaquone–proguanil and chloroquine–proguanil.

Chloroquine (in areas of chloroquine sensitivity)*

We found no systematic review or RCTs on the effects of chloroquine in travellers. One RCT in Austrian workers residing in Nigeria found no significant difference between chloroquine and sulfadoxine–pyrimethamine in the incidence of malaria after 6–22 months. *P falciparum* resistance to chloroquine is now established in most malaria endemic regions of the world. However, clinical experience has led to the consensus that chloroquine is effective for preventing malaria in people travelling to areas where no chloroquine resistance has developed.

Doxycycline

One RCT in soldiers and one RCT in migrants with limited immunity found that doxycycline reduced the risk of malaria compared with placebo. The RCT in soldiers found a similarly low incidence of malaria with doxycyline and mefloquine. One of the RCTs found that doxycycline was associated with nausea and vomiting, diarrhoea, cough, headache, and unspecified dermatological symptoms over 13 weeks. We found no evidence on long term safety. One RCT

Malaria: prevention in travellers

found that doxycycline had fewer adverse effects than mefloquine or chloroquine–proguanil and had similar adverse effect rates compared with atovaquone–proguanil.

TRADE OFF BETWEEN BENEFITS AND HARMS

Chloroquine–proguanil

One RCT found no significant difference between chloroquine–proguanil and chloroquine plus pyrimethamine–sulfadoxine in the incidence of *P falciparum* malaria. One RCT found no significant difference between chloroquine–proguanil and proguanil alone in the incidence of *P falciparum* malaria. One RCT found no significant difference between chloroquine–proguanil and atovaquone–proguanil in preventing malaria. RCTs comparing adverse effects of chloroquine–proguanil versus atovaquone–proguanil found different results. One RCT found that chloroquine–proguanil increased adverse effects compared with three other common antimalaria drug regimens (doxycycline, mefloquine, and atovaquone–proguanil). Another RCT found no significant difference in adverse events between chloroquine–proguanil and atovaquone–proguanil.

Mefloquine

One systematic review of one RCT in soldiers found that mefloquine reduced cases of malaria compared with placebo and found that mefloquine had a protective efficacy of 100%. Three RCTs in non-military travellers found that mefloquine increased neuropsychiatric adverse effects compared with placebo or alternative chemoprophylaxis.

UNKNOWN EFFECTIVENESS

Pyrimethamine–dapsone

We found no RCTs in travellers. One RCT in Thai soldiers found insufficient evidence to compare pyrimethamine–dapsone versus proguanil–dapsone. We found limited observational evidence that pyrimethamine–dapsone may cause agranulocytosis.

Pyrimethamine–sulfadoxine

We found no RCTs of pyrimethamine–sulfadoxine alone. One RCT found no significant difference between chloroquine–proguanil and chloroquine plus pyrimethamine–sulfadoxine in the incidence of *P falciparum* malaria. One retrospective observational study suggested that pyrimethamine–sulfadoxine was associated with severe cutaneous reactions.

LIKELY TO BE INEFFECTIVE OR HARMFUL

Amodiaquine

We found no RCTs on the effects of amodiaquine in preventing malaria in travellers. We found limited observational evidence that amodiaquine may cause neutropenia, liver damage, and hepatitis. Because of concern over adverse events, amodiaquine use is restricted to the treatment of malaria rather than prevention of malaria in the developed world.

Primaquine *New*

One RCT found that primaquine had a protective efficacy of 94% for *P falciparum* and 85% for *P vivax* malaria in non-immune soldiers. It found that primaquine was associated with severe epigastric pain, abdominal pain, or vomiting in some people. Primaquine can cause potentially lethal acute intravascular haemolysis in people with glucose-6-phosphate dehydrogenase (G6PD) deficiency, and methaemoglobinaemia in people with normal G6PD activity. The small risk of severe haemolysis outweighs the possible benefit from using primaquine to prevent malaria.

What are the effects of antimalaria vaccines in travellers?

UNKNOWN EFFECTIVENESS

Vaccines

We found no RCTs in travellers. One systematic review of antimalaria vaccines in residents of malaria endemic areas found that the SPf66 vaccine reduced first attacks of malaria compared with placebo.

What are the effects of antimalaria interventions in child travellers?

LIKELY TO BE BENEFICIAL

Chloroquine (in areas of chloroquine sensitivity)*

Decades of experience of using chloroquine to prevent malaria, in areas where there is no parasite resistance to the drug, have led to the consensus that it is effective in this setting. We found insufficient evidence about the effects of other antimalaria drugs in preventing malaria in child travellers.

TRADE OFF BETWEEN BENEFITS AND HARMS

Topical (skin applied) insect repellents containing diethyltoluamide (DEET)*

We found no RCTs on the effects of diethyltoluamide (DEET) in preventing malaria in child travellers. However, many years of clinical experience have led to the consensus that using the topical insect repellent diethyltoluamide (DEET) is likely to beneficial in preventing malaria. Case reports in young children found serious adverse effects with DEET.

What are the effects of antimalaria interventions in pregnant travellers?

LIKELY TO BE BENEFICIAL

Chloroquine (in areas of chloroquine sensitivity)*

One systematic review identified no RCTs on the effects of antimalaria drugs in pregnant travellers. It found that, in pregnant residents of malaria endemic settings, antimalaria drugs reduced malaria and episodes of fever compared with no prophylaxis. It found no significant difference in perinatal deaths or preterm births. We found insufficient evidence on the safety of chloroquine, doxycycline and mefloquine in pregnancy. Decades of experience of using chloroquine to prevent malaria, in areas where there is no parasite resistance to the drug, have led to the consensus that it is effective in this setting.

UNKNOWN EFFECTIVENESS

Insecticide treated clothing

We found no RCTs in pregnant travellers of the effects of insecticide treated clothing.

Malaria: prevention in travellers

Insecticide treated nets

We found no RCTs on the effects of insecticide treated nets in preventing malaria in pregnant travellers. One RCT of pregnant residents of a malaria endemic area found insufficient evidence on the effects of permethrin treated nets in preventing malaria.

Topical (skin applied) insect repellents

We found no RCTs in pregnant travellers. It is unclear which topical (skin applied) insect repellents are safe in pregnancy.

What are the effects of antimalaria interventions in airline pilots?

UNKNOWN EFFECTIVENESS

Antimalaria drugs

We found one small RCT reporting on the adverse events of atovaquone-proguanil in non-travelling volunteers, under aircraft cabin pressure conditions. It found no significant difference in adverse events between atovaquone-proguanil and placebo.

*Categorisation based on consensus opinion.

DEFINITION Malaria is an acute parasitic disease of the tropics and subtropics, caused by the invasion and destruction of red blood cells by one or more of four species of the genus *Plasmodium: P falciparum*, *P vivax*, *P ovale*, and *P malariae*.[1] The clinical presentation of malaria varies according to the infecting species, and to the genetics, immune status, and age of the infected person.[2] The most severe form of human malaria is caused by *P falciparum*, in which variable clinical features include spiking fevers, chills, headache, muscular aching and weakness, vomiting, cough, diarrhoea, and abdominal pain; other symptoms related to organ failure may supervene, such as acute renal failure, generalised convulsions, and circulatory collapse, followed by coma and death.[3,4] *P falciparum* accounts for more than 50% of malaria infections in most East Asian countries, over 90% in sub-Saharan Africa, and almost 100% in Hispaniola.[5] Travellers are defined here as visitors from a malaria free area to a malaria endemic area, who stay in the endemic area for less than 1 year.

INCIDENCE/ PREVALENCE Malaria is the most dangerous parasitic disease of humans, infecting about 5% of the world's population, and causing about one million deaths each year.[6] The disease is strongly resurgent, owing to the effects of war, climate change, large scale population movements, increased breeding opportunities for vector mosquitoes, rapidly spreading drug and insecticide resistance, and neglect of public health infrastructure.[1,7] Malaria is currently endemic in more than 100 countries, which are visited by more than 125 million international travellers each year.[4] Cases of malaria acquired by international travellers from industrialised countries probably number 25 000 annually; of these, about 10 000 are reported and 150 are fatal.[8]

AETIOLOGY/ RISK FACTORS Humans acquire malaria from sporozoites transmitted by the bite of infected female anopheline mosquitoes.[9] Of about 3200 mosquito species so far described, some 430 belong to the genus *Anopheles*, and of these about 70 anopheline species are known to transmit malaria, with about 40 species considered important vectors.[10] When foraging, blood thirsty female mosquitoes fly upwind searching for the scent trail of an attractive host.[11] Female anophelines are attracted to their human hosts over a range of 7–20 m, through a variety of stimuli including exhaled carbon dioxide, lactic acid, other host odours, warmth, and moisture.[12] Larger people tend to be bitten by mosquitoes more than smaller individuals, and adults are bitten more often than infants and children.[12,13] Women get significantly more mosquito bites in trials than men.[14] Children secrete lower levels of chemical attractants than adults and therefore usually receive fewer mosquito bites.[15] Malaria transmission does not usually occur at temperatures below 16 °C or above 35 °C, or at altitudes greater than 3000 m above sea level at the equator (lower elevations in cooler climates), because sporozoite development in the mosquito cannot take place.[16] The optimal conditions for transmission are a humidity of over 60% and an ambient temperature of 25–30 °C.[17] Most of the important vectors of malaria breed in small temporary collections of fresh surface water exposed to sunlight and with little predation, and in sites such as residual pools in drying river beds.[18] Although rainfall provides breeding sites for mosquitoes, excessive rainfall may wash away mosquito larvae and pupae.[19] Conversely, prolonged droughts may be associated with increased malaria transmission if they reduce the size and flow rates of large rivers sufficiently to produce suitable *Anopheles* breeding sites.[20] Anopheline mosquitoes vary in their preferred feeding and resting locations, although most bite in the evening and at night.[21] The *Anopheles* mosquito will feed by day only if unusually hungry.[22] *Anopheles* adults usually fly not more than 2–3 km from their breeding sites, although a flight range of up to 7 km has been observed.[23] One cross sectional study of about 7000 children under the age of 10 years found that, during months of peak transmission, living within 3 km of an *Anopheles* breeding site significantly increased the risk of malaria compared with living 8–10 km away (RR 21.00, 95% CI 2.87 to 153.00).[24] Exceptionally, strong winds may carry *Anopheles* up to 30 km or more.[12] In travellers, malaria risk is related to destination, activity, and duration of travel. A retrospective cohort study (5898 confirmed cases) conducted in Italian travellers between 1989 and 1997 found that the malaria incidence was 1.5/1000 for travel to Africa, 0.11/1000 for travel to Asia, and 0.04/1000 for travel to Central and South America.[25] A survey of approximately 170 000 Swedish travellers found that the prevalence of malaria was lowest among travellers to Central America and the Caribbean (0.01/1000), and higher among travellers to East, Central, and West Africa (prevalence among travellers to East Africa 2.4/1000, Central Africa 3.6/1000, and West Africa 3.0/1000).[26] A survey of 2131 German travellers to sub-Saharan Africa found that solo travellers were at almost a ninefold greater risk of infection than those on package tours.[27] A case control study (46 cases, 557 controls) reported that a visit to the tropics for longer than 21 days doubled the malaria risk compared with visits lasting 21 days or less.[28]

PROGNOSIS Malaria can develop after just one anopheline mosquito bite.[29] Human malaria has a usual incubation period that ranges from 10–14 days (*P falciparum*, *P vivax*, and *P ovale*) to about 28 days (*P malariae*).[30] Certain strains of *P vivax* and *P ovale* can have a much longer incubation period, of 6–18 months.[20] Some 90% of malaria attacks in travellers occur at home.[31] About 36% of cases that develop after returning home do so more than 2 months after the traveller's return.[32] People returning from an endemic area with any fever pattern should be considered to have malaria until proved otherwise.[4,6,22,29,33] Once malaria infection occurs, older travellers are at greater risk of poor clinical outcomes and death. In US travellers between 1966 and 1987, the case fatality rate was 0.4% for people aged 0–19 years, 2.2% for ages 20–39 years, 5.8% for ages 40–69 years, and 30.3% for those aged 70–79 years.[34] Complications and death from malaria are mainly because of inappropriate treatment or because of delayed initiation of treatment.[35] If malaria is diagnosed and treated promptly, about 88% of previously healthy travellers will recover completely.[36]

Please refer to clinicalevidence.com for full text and references.

Malaria: severe, life threatening

Search date December 2005

Aika Omari and Paul Garner

What are the effects of antimalarial treatments for complicated falciparum malaria in non-pregnant people?

LIKELY TO BE BENEFICIAL

High initial dose quinine (reduced parasite and fever clearance times, but no difference in mortality)

One systematic review of four small RCTs in adults and children found no significant difference in mortality between quinine regimens with high initial quinine dose and those with no loading dose. The systematic review found that high initial dose quinine reduced parasite and fever clearance times compared with no loading dose. One small RCT included in the review found that high initial dose quinine increased transient partial hearing loss compared with no loading dose. Another small RCT in the review found no significant difference between high initial dose and no loading dose of quinine in neurological sequelae.

Intramuscular artemether (as effective as quinine)

Two systematic reviews and five subsequent RCTs found no significant difference in death rates between intramuscular artemether and quinine in people with severe malaria. One of the reviews found no significant difference in the speed of coma recovery, fever clearance time, or neurological sequelae between intramuscular artemether and quinine. The second review found no significant difference in neurological sequelae at recovery between intramuscular artemether and quinine.

Quinine*

International consensus recommends quinine for the treatment of severe falciparum malaria. Placebo or no treatment controlled trials would be considered unethical.

Rectal artemisinin and its derivatives

One small RCT found no significant difference in mortality, fever and parasite clearance times, and coma recovery time between rectal artemether and quinine in children with cerebral malaria. One systematic review of small RCTs found no significant difference in mortality and coma recovery time between rectal artemisinin and quinine in people with severe malaria. One small RCT found no significant difference in mortality between rectal artesunate and quinine in people with moderately severe malaria. It found that artesunate reduced fever and parasite clearance times compared with quinine in children, but found no significant difference in these outcomes in adults. One small RCT found no significant difference in mortality and coma recovery time between rectal dihydroartemisinin and quinine in people with severe malaria, but found that dihydroartemisinin reduced parasite clearance time.

UNKNOWN EFFECTIVENESS

Intramuscular arteether versus quinine

One systematic review of small RCTs in children with malaria found no significant difference between intramuscular arteether and quinine in mortality, time to ▶

regain consciousness, parasite clearance time, fever clearance time, and parasite clearance on days 7 and 28. However, the review lacked power to detect clinically important differences.

Intramuscular versus intravenous quinine

One RCT in children found no significant difference between intramuscular and intravenous quinine in recovery times or death. However, the study may have lacked power to detect clinically important differences between treatments.

Intravenous artesunate versus quinine

Two small RCTs found no significant difference in mortality between intravenous artesunate and quinine, but they may have lacked power to detect a clinically important difference.

What are the effects of adjunctive treatment for complicated falciparum malaria in non-pregnant people?

UNKNOWN EFFECTIVENESS

Desferrioxamine mesylate

One systematic review found limited evidence that desferrioxamine mesylate reduced the risk of persistent seizures in children with cerebral malaria compared with placebo.

Exchange blood transfusion

One systematic review found no suitable RCTs. A systematic review of case control studies found no significant difference in mortality between exchange transfusion plus antimalarial drugs and antimalarial drugs alone.

Initial blood transfusion

One systematic review found no significant difference in mortality between initial and expectant blood transfusion among clinically stable children (no respiratory distress or cardiac failure) with malarial anaemia, but found that adverse events were more common with initial blood transfusion. The review found no significant difference between transfusion and no transfusion for the combined outcome of death or severe adverse events. Transmission of hepatitis B or HIV was not reported. We found no RCTs examining the effects of transfusion in adults with malaria.

LIKELY TO BE INEFFECTIVE OR HARMFUL

Dexamethasone

One systematic review found no significant difference in mortality between dexamethasone and placebo, but found that gastrointestinal bleeding and seizures were more common with dexamethasone.

Phenobarbitone *New*

One systematic review found that phenobarbitone reduced convulsions compared with placebo or no anticonvulsants, but may have increased mortality.

*Based on consensus. RCTs would be considered unethical.

DEFINITION Malaria is caused by protozoan infection of red blood cells with *Plasmodium falciparum* and comprises a variety of syndromes. This review deals with clinically complicated malaria (i.e. malaria that presents with life threatening conditions, including coma, severe anaemia, renal failure, respiratory distress

Malaria: severe, life threatening

syndrome, hypoglycaemia, shock, spontaneous haemorrhage, and convulsions). The diagnosis of cerebral malaria should be considered where there is encephalopathy in the presence of malaria parasites. A strict definition of cerebral malaria requires the presence of unrousable coma and no other cause of encephalopathy (e.g. hypoglycaemia, sedative drugs), in the presence of *P falciparum* infection.[1] This review does not currently cover the treatment of malaria in pregnancy.

INCIDENCE/ PREVALENCE Malaria is a major health problem in the tropics, with 300–500 million clinical cases occurring annually and an estimated 1.1–2.7 million deaths each year as a result of severe malaria.[2] Over 90% of deaths occur in children under 5 years of age, mainly from cerebral malaria and anaemia.[2] In areas where the rate of malaria transmission is stable (endemic), those most at risk of acquiring severe malaria are children under 5 years old, because adults and older children have partial immunity, which offers some protection. In areas where the rate of malaria transmission is unstable (non-endemic), severe malaria affects both adults and children. Non-immune travellers and migrants are also at risk of developing severe malaria.

AETIOLOGY/ RISK FACTORS Malaria is transmitted by the bite of infected female anopheline mosquitoes. Certain genes are associated with resistance to severe malaria. The human leukocyte antigens HLA-Bw53 and HLA-DRB1*1302 protect against severe malaria. However, associations of HLA antigens with severe malaria are limited to specific populations.[3,4] Haemoglobin S[3] and haemoglobin C[5] are also protective against severe malaria. Genes such as the tumour necrosis factor gene have also been associated with increased susceptibility to severe malaria (see aetiology under malaria: prevention in travellers).[6]

PROGNOSIS In children under 5 years of age with cerebral malaria, the estimated case fatality of treated malaria is 19%, although reported hospital case fatality may be as high as 40%.[1,7] Neurological sequelae persisting for more than 6 months occur in more than 2% of survivors, and include ataxia, hemiplegia, speech disorders, behavioural disorders, epilepsy, and blindness. Severe malarial anaemia has a case fatality rate higher than 13%.[7] In adults, the mortality of cerebral malaria is 20%; this rises to 50% in pregnancy, and neurological sequelae occur in about 3% of survivors.[8]

Please refer to clinicalevidence.com for full text and references.

Malaria: uncomplicated, caused by *Plasmodium falciparum*

Search date September 2006

David Taylor-Robinson, Katharine Jones, and Paul Garner

Are artemisinin combination treatments more effective than non-artemisinin combinations treatments in people living in endemic areas (excluding South East Asia)?

LIKELY TO BE BENEFICIAL

Artemether–lumefantrine (6 doses) (more effective than amodiaquine plus sulfadoxine–pyrimethamine)

One RCT included in a systematic review found that artemether–lumefantrine (6 doses) significantly reduced parasitological failure but not clinical failure at day 28 compared with amodiaquine plus sulfadoxine–pyrimethamine.

Artesunate (3 days) plus amodiaquine (more effective than amodiaquine plus sulfadoxine–pyrimethamine)

Two RCTs found that artesunate plus amodiaquine reduced treatment failure rate (excluding new infections) at 28 days compared with amodiaquine plus sulfadoxine–pyrimethamine, in children with uncomplicated malaria. The first RCT found no significant difference in the need for rescue therapy between artesunate plus amodiaquine and amodiaquine plus sulfadoxine–pyrimethamine, which suggested that the risk of new infection was greater with artesunate plus amodiaquine. It also found that artesunate plus amodiaquine reduced time to fever resolution.

UNKNOWN EFFECTIVENESS

Artesunate (3 days) plus sulfadoxine–pyrimethamine (no proven benefit compared with amiodaquine plus sulfadoxine–pyrimethamine)

One RCT found that artesunate plus sulfadoxine–pyrimethamine increased clinical and parasitological treatment failure compared with amodiaquine plus sulfadoxine–pyrimethamine, although these differences were no longer significant when new infections were excluded. A second RCT found no significant difference between artesunate plus sulfadoxine–pyrimethamine and amodiaquine plus sulfadoxine–pyrimethamine in adequate clinical and parasitological response after 28 days. It found that artesunate plus sulfadoxine–pyrimethamine increased new infection rate compared with amodiaquine plus sulfadoxine–pyrimethamine.

Which artemisinin combination treatment is most effective in people living in endemic areas?

LIKELY TO BE BENEFICIAL

Artemether–lumefantrine (6 doses) (more effective than a 4 dose regimen)

One RCT found that artemether–lumefantrine (6 doses) increased parasitological cure rates at 28 days compared with artemether–lumefantrine (4 doses).

Malaria: uncomplicated, caused by *Plasmodium falciparum*

Artemether–lumefantrine (6 doses) (more effective than artesunate plus amodiaquine)

One RCT included in a systematic review found that artemether–lumefantrine (6 doses) significantly reduced parasitological but not clinical failure at day 28 compared with artesunate plus amodiaquine.

UNKNOWN EFFECTIVENESS

Artemether–lumefantrine (6 doses) versus artesunate plus sulfadoxine–pyrimethamine

We found no RCTs comparing artemether–lumefantrine (6 doses) versus artesunate plus sulfadoxine–pyrimethamine.

Artesunate plus amodiaquine versus artesunate plus sulfadoxine–pyrimethamine (relative benefits unclear)

One RCT found no significant difference in adequate clinical and parasitological response rate between artesunate plus amodiaquine and artesunate plus sulfadoxine–pyrimethamine after 28 days. A second RCT found that artesunate plus amodiaquine significantly reduced adequate clinical and parasitological response rate compared with artesunate plus sulfadoxine–pyrimethamine after 28 days.

UNLIKELY TO BE BENEFICIAL

Artemether–lumefantrine (6 doses) (less effective than artesunate (3 days) plus mefloquine)

One systematic review found that artemether–lumefantrine increased treatment failures compared with artesunate (3 days) plus mefloquine at 42 days. Two RCTs identified by the review found no difference in treatment failure at 28 days. One subsequent RCT found no difference in between artemether–lumefantrine and artesunate plus mefloquine in cure rate at day 42. A second subsequent RCT found no difference between treatments in adequate clinical and parasitological response at 42 days. However, if new infections were included, then artemether–lumefrantrine increased parasitological failure at day 48.

DEFINITION Malaria is a parasite transmitted by *Anopheles* mosquitoes. There are four types of human malaria, namely *falciparum, vivax, ovale*, and *malariae*. The *falciparum* type is the most important cause of illness and death and *Plasmodium falciparum*, the responsible organism, is known to develop resistance to antimalarial drugs.[1] This chapter covers treatments only for *falciparum* malaria and a population of adults and children living in endemic malarial areas, who, by definition, are exposed (seasonally or all year round) to malaria. It does not cover treatment of malaria in non-immune travellers, pregnant women, and people infected with HIV. Repeated episodes of *falciparum* malaria result in temporary and incomplete immunity. Therefore, adults living in areas where malaria is common are often found to be "semi-immune", presenting with asymptomatic or chronic forms of malaria, with clinical episodes that are attenuated by their immunity. **Severe malaria** is defined as a form of symptomatic malaria with signs of vital organ disturbance (World Health Organization 2000).[1] Any person with symptomatic malaria who does not develop any such signs is defined as having **uncomplicated malaria**. This chapter assesses the effectiveness of antimalarial drugs only in people with uncomplicated malaria. Table 1 provides an overview of the number of RCTs for each treatment and the comparison included in this chapter.

INCIDENCE/ PREVALENCE Malaria is a major health problem in the tropics, with 300–500 million new clinical cases annually, most of them cases of uncomplicated malaria. An estimated 1.1–2.7 million deaths occur annually as a result of severe *falciparum* malaria.[1]

AETIOLOGY/ RISK FACTORS The malaria parasite is transmitted by infected *Anopheles* mosquitoes. Risk factors for developing the disease include exposure to infected mosquitoes (living in an endemic area; housing that allows mosquitoes to enter and absence of mosquito nets; and living in an area where *Anopheles* mosquitoes can thrive). Risk factors in relation to severity of the illness relate to host immunity, determined mainly by exposure to the parasite, and therefore varying with level of transmission in the area and the age of the host. Malaria is uncommon in the first 6 months of life (fetal haemoglobin is protective); it is, however, common in children over 6 months of age. In areas of intense transmission infection is attenuated by host immunity in older age groups, but with less intense transmission morbidity and mortality can be high in adults as well.

PROGNOSIS Uncomplicated malaria may progress to severe malaria, become chronic, or resolve with effective treatment or the development of improved immunity. The outcome is therefore dependent on host immunity and prompt access to effective treatment. In the absence of effective treatment, people with no or low immunity are at increased risk of developing severe malaria (see Malaria: severe, life threatening) resulting in high morbidity and mortality.

Please refer to clinicalevidence.com for full text and references.

Meningococcal disease

Search date May 2004

Jailson B Correia and C A Hart

What are the effects of interventions to prevent meningococcal disease in contacts and carriers?

LIKELY TO BE BENEFICIAL

Antibiotics for throat carriage (reduce carriage, but unknown effect on risk of disease)

RCTs found that antibiotics reduced throat carriage of meningococcus compared with placebo. We found no RCTs or observational evidence examining whether eradicating throat carriage of meningococcus reduces the risk of meningococcal disease.

Prophylactic antibiotics (sulfadiazine) in contacts*

We found no RCTs on the effects of prophylactic antibiotics on the incidence of meningococcal disease among contacts. One observational study found limited evidence that prophylactic sulfadiazine reduced the risk of meningococcal disease over 8 weeks compared with no prophylaxis. We found no evidence regarding which contacts should be treated.

What are the effects of interventions to treat suspected cases of meningococcal disease before admission to hospital?

UNKNOWN EFFECTIVENESS

Pre-admission parenteral penicillin in suspected cases*

We found no RCTs on the effects of pre-admission parenteral penicillin in suspected meningococcal disease in people of all ages. We found inconclusive evidence from observational studies on the benefit of pre-admission antibiotics. However, it is unlikely that RCTs on pre-admission antibiotics will be performed because of the unpredictably rapid course of disease in some people and the likely risks involved in delaying treatment, combined with a low risk of causing harm.

What are the effects of treatments for meningococcal meningitis on admission in children?

LIKELY TO BE BENEFICIAL

Adding corticosteroids (reduced severe hearing loss in bacterial meningitis of any cause, but no difference in mortality and unknown effectiveness in meningococcal meningitis)

We found no RCTs on adding corticosteroids specifically in children with meningococcal meningitis. One systematic review found no significant difference between adding corticosteroids and adding placebo in mortality in children with bacterial meningitis of any aetiology or in people of all ages with meningococcal meningitis. The review found that, compared with adding placebo, corticosteroids reduced severe hearing loss in children with bacterial meningitis of any aetiology, but it did not specifically assess the effect in children with meningococcal meningitis. The review found no significant difference between ▶

adding corticosteroids and adding placebo for short term or long term neurological sequelae in people of all ages with bacterial meningitis of any aetiology, but it did not separately assess the effect in children with meningococcal meningitis. Interpreting the results of available evidence on the use of corticosteroids in children with meningococcal meningitis demands caution, as age- and pathogen-specific evidence is scarce. In regions where the conjugate vaccine has been introduced, the incidence of *Haemophilus influenzae* type b (Hib) has fallen dramatically and the applicability of evidence from trials performed prior to this change in epidemiology is questionable. However, decisions on initial treatment such as adding corticosteroids almost always precede knowledge of the specific aetiology.

What are the effects of treatments for meningococcal meningitis on admission in adults?

LIKELY TO BE BENEFICIAL

Adding corticosteroids (reduced mortality in bacterial meningitis of any cause, but unknown effectiveness in meningococcal meningitis)

We found no RCTs on adding corticosteroids specifically in adults with meningococcal meningitis. One systematic review found that, compared with adding placebo, adding corticosteroids reduced mortality in adults with bacterial meningitis of any aetiology. Subgroup analysis for meningococcal meningitis found no significant difference in mortality with adding corticosteroids compared with adding placebo. The review found that, compared with adding placebo, adding corticosteroids reduced neurological sequelae in people with bacterial meningitis of any aetiology, but the difference did not quite reach significance. Subgroup analysis for meningococcal meningitis found no significant difference in neurological sequelae with adding corticosteroids compared with adding placebo. None of the RCTs included in the systematic review were powered to detect a significant effect of corticosteroid treatment in the subgroup of people with meningococcal meningitis, probably due to the lower rates of mortality and sequelae in this group. However, decisions on initial treatment with adding corticosteroids almost always precede knowledge of the specific aetiology.

What are the effects of treatments for meningococcal septicaemia in children?

UNKNOWN EFFECTIVENESS

Adding corticosteroids

We found no RCTs on the use of adding corticosteroids specifically in children with meningococcal septicaemia. Two RCTs found no significant difference in mortality between adding corticosteroids and adding placebo in children with severe sepsis and septic shock of any bacterial aetiology. It is questionable whether evidence from RCTs on severe sepsis and septic shock of any aetiology can be applied to children with meningococcal septicaemia.

Meningococcal disease

What are the effects of treatments for meningococcal septicaemia in adults?

UNKNOWN EFFECTIVENESS

Adding corticosteroids

We found no RCTs on adding corticosteroids specifically in adults with meningococcal septicaemia. One systematic review in adults with severe sepsis or septic shock of any aetiology found no significant difference in overall mortality at 28 days by adding corticosteroids to antibiotics or by adding high dose, short course corticosteroids compared with adding placebo, but that adding low dose, longer duration corticosteroids at doses of 300 mg or less of hydrocortisone or equivalent for 5 or more days reduced all cause mortality at 28 days compared with adding placebo. It is questionable whether evidence from RCTs on severe sepsis and septic shock of any aetiology can be applied to adults with meningococcal septicaemia.

*Based on consensus or observational evidence. RCTs unlikely to be conducted.

See glossary

DEFINITION Meningococcal disease is any clinical condition caused by *Neisseria meningitidis* (the meningococcus) groups A, B, C, W135, or other serogroups. These conditions include purulent conjunctivitis, septic arthritis, meningitis, and septicaemia with or without meningitis. In this chapter we cover meningococcal meningitis and meningococcal septicaemia with or without meningitis.

INCIDENCE/ PREVALENCE Meningococcal disease is sporadic in temperate countries, and is most commonly caused by group B or C meningococci. The annual incidence in Europe varies from fewer than 1 case/100 000 people in France, up to 4–5 cases/100 000 people in the UK and Spain, and in the USA it is 0.6–1.5 cases/100 000 people.[1,2] Occasional outbreaks occur among close family contacts, secondary school pupils, military recruits, and students living in halls of residence. Sub-Saharan Africa has regular epidemics in countries lying in the expanded "meningitis belt", reaching 500 cases/100 000 people during epidemics, which are usually due to serogroup A, although recent outbreaks of serogroup W135 cause concern.[3-5] In sub-Saharan Africa, over 90% of cases present with meningitis alone.[3]

AETIOLOGY/ RISK FACTORS The meningococcus colonises and infects healthy people, and is transmitted by close contact, probably by exchange of upper respiratory tract secretions Ⓣ.[6-14] The risk of transmission is greatest during the first week of contact.[9] Risk factors include crowding and exposure to cigarette smoke.[15] In the UK, children younger than 2 years have the highest incidence of meningococcal disease, with a second peak between ages 15–24 years. There is currently an increased incidence of meningococcal disease among university students, especially among those in their first term and living in catered accommodation,[16] although we found no accurate numerical estimate of risk from close contact in, for example, halls of residence. Close contacts of an index case have a much higher risk of infection than do people in the general population.[9,12,13] The risk of epidemic spread is higher with groups A and C meningococci than with group B meningococci.[6-8,10] It is not known what makes a meningococcus virulent. Certain clones tend to predominate at different times and in different groups. Carriage of meningococcus in the throat has been reported in 10–15% of people; recent acquisition of a virulent meningococcus is more likely to be associated with invasive disease.

Meningococcal disease

PROGNOSIS Mortality is highest in infants and adolescents, and is related to disease presentation and availability of therapeutic resources. In developed countries, case fatality rates have been around 19–25% for septicaemia, 10–12% for meningitis plus septicaemia, and less than 1% in meningitis alone, but an overall reduction in mortality was observed in recent years in people admitted to paediatric intensive care units.[17-21]

Please refer to clinicalevidence.com for full text and references.

MRSA (treatment)

Search date July 2005

Tim Weller

What are the effects of treatment for MRSA infections at any body site?

TRADE OFF BETWEEN BENEFITS AND HARMS

Linezolid (compared with glycopeptides) New

RCTs found no significant difference between linezolid compared with vancomycin or teicoplanin for MRSA infection of any body site. One meta-analysis of two RCTs found that linezolid plus aztreonam was more effective than vancomycin plus aztreonam for survival and cure for nosocomial pneumonia. However, a subgroup analysis of one RCT found no significant difference between linezolid alone and vancomycin alone. RCTs found mixed results of linezolid compared with vancomycin for MRSA skin and soft tissue infections; however, vancomycin was not found to be better than linezolid for any outcomes.

Teicoplanin, vancomycin (glycopeptides) (compared with linezolid, quinupristin–dalfopristin, or trimethoprim–sulfamethoxazole) New

RCTs found no significant difference between vancomycin or teicoplanin compared with linezolid for MRSA infection of any body site. One meta-analysis of two RCTs found that vancomycin plus aztreonam was less effective than linezolid plus aztreonam for survival and cure for nosocomial pneumonia. However, a subgroup analysis of one RCT found no significant difference between vancomycin alone and linezolid alone. RCTs found mixed results of vancomycin compared with linezolid for MRSA skin and soft tissue infections; however, vancomycin was not found to be better than linezolid for any outcomes. One RCT found no significant difference between vancomycin compared with quinupristin–dalfopristin for cure of MRSA nosocomial pneumonia. One RCT found that vancomycin and trimethoprim–sulfamethoxazole were equally as effective in the clinical cure of MRSA infection in injecting drug users.

UNKNOWN EFFECTIVENESS

Azithromycin, clarithromycin, erythromycin (macrolides) New

We found no systematic review or RCTs of macrolides (azithromycin, clarithromycin, erythromycin) in people with MRSA infection.

Ciprofloxacin, levofloxacin, moxifloxacin (quinolones) New

We found no systematic review or RCTs of quinolones (ciprofloxacin, levofloxacin, moxifloxacin) in people with MRSA infection.

Clindamycin New

We found no systematic review or RCTs of clindamycin in people with MRSA infection.

Daptomycin New

We found no systematic review or RCTs of daptomycin in people with MRSA infection.

Doxycycline, minocycline, oxytetracycline (tetracyclines) New

We found no systematic review or RCTs of tetracyclines (minocycline, doxycycline, and oxytetracycline) in people with MRSA infection.

Fusidic acid *New*

We found no systematic review or RCTs of fusidic acid (sodium fusidate) in people with MRSA infection.

Quinupristin–dalfopristin *New*

One RCT provided insufficient evidence to assess quinupristin–dalfopristin compared with vancomycin for cure of MRSA nosocomial pneumonia.

Rifampicin *New*

We found no systematic review or RCTs of rifampicin in people with MRSA infection.

Trimethoprim *New*

We found no systematic review or RCTs of trimethoprim alone in people with MRSA infection.

Trimethoprim–sulfamethoxazole (compared with vancomycin) *New*

One RCT found that trimethoprim–sulfamethoxazole and vancomycin were equally as effective in the clinical cure of MRSA infection in injecting drug users.

What are the effects of treatment for MRSA nasal or extra-nasal colonisation?

LIKELY TO BE BENEFICIAL

Mupirocin nasal ointment *New*

One RCT found that mupirocin nasal ointment improved eradication of MRSA from all body sites at 30 and 90 days compare with placebo. However, another RCT found no significant difference at 26 days. One RCT found that mupirocin nasal ointment or topical fusidic acid plus oral trimethoprim–sulfamethoxazole were equally as effective in the eradication of MRSA from nasal sites; however, adverse effects should be more frequent with oral antibiotics. One RCT identified by a systematic review found that mupirocin was more effective than tea tree preparations for eradication of MRSA nasal colonisation, but found no significant difference for extra-nasal sites. Another smaller, methodologically weaker RCT identified by the review, found no significant difference between the treatments.

UNKNOWN EFFECTIVENESS

Antiseptic body washes *New*

We found no systematic review or RCTs of antiseptic body washes in people with nasal or extra-nasal MRSA colonisation.

Chlorhexidine–neomycin nasal cream *New*

We found no systematic review or RCTs of chlorhexidine–neomycin nasal cream in people with nasal or extra-nasal MRSA colonisation.

Mupirocin nasal ointment for 5 days (compared with > 5 days) *New*

We found no systematic review or RCTs that compared mupirocin nasal ointment for 5 days with mupirocin nasal ointment for regimens longer than 5 days.

Systemic antimicrobials *New*

We found no good evidence that compared systemic antimicrobials versus placebo for nasal or extra-nasal colonisation. One RCT found no significant

MRSA (treatment)

difference between trimethoprim–sulfamethoxazole plus rifampicin compared with rifampicin plus novobiocin for eradication of MRSA from all colonised body sites.

UNLIKELY TO BE BENEFICIAL

Tea tree preparations *New*

We found no systematic review or RCTs comparing tea tree preparations versus placebo. One RCT identified by a systematic review found that tea tree preparations were less effective than mupirocin for eradication of MRSA nasal colonisation, but found no significant difference for extra-nasal sites. Another smaller, methodologically weaker RCT identified by the review, found no significant difference between the treatments.

DEFINITION Methicillin resistant *Staphylococcus aureus* (MRSA) is an organism resistant to methicillin by means of the *mecA* gene. This confers resistance to all beta lactam antibiotics, including flucloxacillin, oxacillin, cephalosporins, and carbapenems. Antimicrobial resistance is defined as the failure of the antimicrobial to reach a concentration in the infected tissue high enough to inhibit the growth of the infecting organism. MRSA presents in the same way as susceptible *S aureus*. It can be part of the normal flora (colonisation) or it can cause infection. The phenomena of colonisation and infection should be treated as separate entities. **MRSA colonisation:** Growth of MRSA from a body fluid or swab from any body site. The most common site of colonisation is the anterior nares but MRSA can also be found in other areas such as the axillae, abnormal skin (e.g. eczema), urine, and throat. There should be no signs or symptoms of infection. The colonised site may act as a reservoir of MRSA, which then causes infection at another site or can be passed on to others. Although the colonised patient (or staff member) does not need treatment, a course of decolonisation treatment may be given in order to eradicate carriage and prevent future infections or transmission.[1] **MRSA infection:** Growth of MRSA from a sterile body site (e.g. blood culture or cerebrospinal fluid) or growth of MRSA from a non-sterile body site (e.g. wound, urine, or sputum) in the presence of symptoms or signs of infection. MRSA infections are also accompanied by fever and signs of inflammation, including skin/soft tissue, wound, bone and joint, nosocomial pneumonia, endocarditis, and prosthetic material. MRSA is becoming an increasingly important issue as a community acquired infection in people who have not been recently admitted to hospital or had medical problems. However, the investigation of treatments strategies for community compared with nosocomial MRSA is ongoing, and will not be covered here.

INCIDENCE/ PREVALENCE The incidence of MRSA varies from country to country.[2] The UK, Ireland, and southern Europe (e.g. Spain, Italy, and Greece) have a high incidence when compared with northern Europe and Scandinavia. The most objective measure of incidence is the percentage of *S aureus* found in blood cultures that are resistant to methicillin. This currently stands at about 40% in the UK.[3]

AETIOLOGY/ RISK FACTORS Risk factors for MRSA colonisation include: prolonged stay in hospital, severe underlying disease, prior antibiotics, exposure to colonised people, and admission to a high risk unit (critical care, renal unit, etc).

PROGNOSIS The virulence of MRSA has been found to be equal to that of methicillin susceptible *S aureus* in animal models and case people the overall morbidity and mortality of people with MRSA is found to be higher if this is not taken into account. A meta-analysis of 31 cohort studies found that mortality associated with MRSA bacteraemia was significantly higher than that of methicillin susceptible *S aureus* bacteraemia (mean mortality not reported; OR 1.93, 95% CI 1.54 to 2.42).[4]

Please refer to clinicalevidence.com for full text and references.

Postherpetic neuralgia

Search date December 2005

David Wareham

What are the effects of interventions during an acute attack of herpes zoster aimed at preventing postherpetic neuralgia?

LIKELY TO BE BENEFICIAL

Oral antiviral agents (aciclovir, famciclovir, valaciclovir, netivudine)

One systematic review found limited evidence from RCTs that aciclovir given for 7–10 days reduced pain at 1–3 months compared with placebo. However, the RCTs found no significant difference in pain between aciclovir and placebo at 6 months. One systematic review of one large RCT found that famciclovir reduced mean pain duration after acute herpes zoster compared with placebo. One RCT found that valaciclovir reduced the prevalence of postherpetic neuralgia at 6 months compared with aciclovir. One RCT found that more people taking aciclovir than netivudine had complete resolution of postherpetic neuralgia at 6 months. One RCT found no significant difference between valaciclovir and famciclovir in the resolution of postherpetic neuralgia. One RCT found no significant difference in pain between oral aciclovir and topical idoxuridine at 1 month after rash healing. One systematic review found insufficient evidence from two RCTs about the effects of corticosteroids plus antiviral agents.

UNKNOWN EFFECTIVENESS

Dressings *New*

We found no systematic review or RCTs examining the effects of dressings during an acute attack of herpes zoster for the prevention of postherpetic neuralgia.

Topical antiviral agents (idoxuridine) for pain at 6 months

One systematic review of heterogeneous poor quality RCTs found no significant difference in pain between topical idoxuridine and placebo at 6 months. One RCT identified by the review found no significant difference in pain between topical idoxuridine and oral aciclovir 1 month after rash healing.

Tricyclic antidepressants (amitriptyline)

One RCT with weak methods provided insufficient evidence on the effects of amitriptyline in preventing postherpetic neuralgia.

LIKELY TO BE INEFFECTIVE OR HARMFUL

Corticosteroids

Systematic reviews found insufficient evidence from RCTs about the effects of corticosteroids alone or in combination with antiviral agents on postherpetic neuralgia. There is concern that corticosteroids may cause dissemination of herpes zoster.

What are the effects of interventions to relieve established postherpetic neuralgia after the rash has healed?

BENEFICIAL

Gabapentin

One systematic review of two RCTs found that gabapentin reduced pain at 7–8 weeks compared with placebo in people with postherpetic neuralgia.

Tricyclic antidepressants

One systematic review of four small crossover RCTs found that tricyclic antidepressants increased pain relief in postherpetic neuralgia after 3–8 weeks compared with placebo.

UNKNOWN EFFECTIVENESS

Oral opioids (oxycodone, morphine, methadone, tramadol)

We found no RCTs examining effects of morphine or methadone in people with postherpetic neuralgia. One small crossover RCT found limited evidence that oral oxycodone reduced pain compared with placebo, but was associated with more adverse effects. One systematic review of one small RCT found limited evidence that tramadol reduced pain compared with clomipramine with or without levomepromazine after 6 weeks. One subsequent RCT found limited evidence that tramadol reduced pain after 6 weeks compared with placebo.

Topical anaesthesia

We found insufficient evidence from three RCTs about the effects of lidocaine (lignocaine) in people with postherpetic neuralgia.

Topical counterirritants (capsaicin)

One systematic review of two RCTs found limited evidence that the topical counterirritant capsaicin improved pain relief in postherpetic neuralgia compared with placebo. One subsequent RCT found no significant difference in pain between capsaicin and placebo at 6 months. Capsaicin may cause painful skin reactions (including burning, stinging, and erythema).

LIKELY TO BE INEFFECTIVE OR HARMFUL

Dextromethorphan

One systematic review of one small crossover RCT and one subsequent RCT found no evidence that dextromethorphan was more effective than placebo or lorazepam after 3–6 weeks and found that dextromethorphan was associated with sedation and ataxia at high doses.

DEFINITION Postherpetic neuralgia is pain that sometimes follows resolution of acute herpes zoster and healing of the zoster rash. It can be severe, accompanied by itching, and follows the distribution of the original infection. Herpes zoster is caused by activation of latent varicella zoster virus (human herpes virus 3) in people who have been rendered partially immune by a previous attack of chickenpox. Herpes zoster infects the sensory ganglia and their areas of innervation. It is characterised by pain along the distribution of the affected nerve, and crops of clustered vesicles over the area.

INCIDENCE/ PREVALENCE In a UK general practice survey of 3600–3800 people, the annual incidence of herpes zoster was 3.4/1000.[1] Incidence varied with age. Herpes zoster was relatively uncommon in people under the age of 50 years (< 2/1000 a year), but rose to 5–7/1000 a year in people aged 50–79 years, and 11/1000 in people aged 80 years or older. A population based study in the Netherlands reported a similar incidence (3.4/1000 a year) and a similar increase of incidence with age (3–10/1000 a year in people over 50 years).[2] Prevalence of postherpetic neuralgia depends on when it is measured after acute infection. There is no agreed time point for diagnosis.

AETIOLOGY/ RISK FACTORS The main risk factor for postherpetic neuralgia is increasing age. In a UK general practice study (involving 3600–3800 people, 321 cases of acute herpes zoster) there was little risk in those under the age of 50 years, but postherpetic neuralgia developed in over 20% of people who had had acute herpes zoster aged 60–65 years and in 34% of those aged over 80 years.[1] No other risk factor has been found to predict consistently which people with herpes zoster will experience continued pain. In a general practice study in Iceland (421 people followed for up to 7 years after an initial episode of herpes zoster), the risk of postherpetic neuralgia was 1.8% (95% CI 0.6% to 4.2%) for people under 60 years of age and the pain was mild in all cases.[3] The risk of severe pain after 3 months in people aged over 60 years was 1.7% (95% CI 0% to 6.2%).

PROGNOSIS About 2% of people with acute herpes zoster in the UK general practice survey had pain for more than 5 years.[1] Prevalence of pain falls as time elapses after the initial episode. Among 183 people aged over 60 years in the placebo arm of a UK trial, the prevalence of pain was 61% at 1 month, 24% at 3 months, and 13% at 6 months after acute infection.[4] In a more recent RCT, the prevalence of postherpetic pain in the placebo arm at 6 months was 35% in 72 people over 60 years of age.[5]

Please refer to clinicalevidence.com for full text and references.

Tuberculosis

Search date July 2005

Lilia Ziganshina and Paul Garner

What are the effects of interventions to prevent tuberculosis in people without HIV infection at high risk of developing tuberculosis?

TRADE OFF BETWEEN BENEFITS AND HARMS

Isoniazid

One systematic review, in people without HIV infection at high risk of tuberculosis, found that isoniazid prophylaxis for 6–12 months reduced the risk of active tuberculosis or extrapulmonary tuberculosis compared with placebo. It also found that a short 6 month course was as effective as a 12 month course. One large RCT found that treatment with isoniazid increased the risk of hepatotoxicity compared with placebo.

Rifampicin plus isoniazid New

One RCT found that, in people with latent tuberculosis infection, rifampicin plus isoniazid for 3 months and isoniazid alone for 6–12 months led to similar reductions in rates of active tuberculosis over 1–3 years. Rates of adverse effects requiring withdrawal (hepatotoxicity, rash, gastrointestinal intolerance) were similar between groups.

What are the effects of different drug regimens in people with newly diagnosed pulmonary tuberculosis without HIV infection?

BENEFICIAL

Shorter course chemotherapy (6 month regimen as good as longer courses)

Two RCTs found no significant difference in relapse rates between 6 month and longer course chemotherapy regimens.

LIKELY TO BE BENEFICIAL

Adding pyrazinamide in chemotherapy regimens for ≥ 6 months

Three RCTs found that chemotherapy regimens containing pyrazinamide improved sputum clearance in the first 2 months compared with other regimens, but found limited evidence about effects on relapse rates.

Adding rifampicin to isoniazid (more effective than isoniazid alone)

One large RCT found that a 6 month regimen of rifampicin plus isoniazid reduced relapse rate compared with isoniazid alone.

UNKNOWN EFFECTIVENESS

Intermittent chemotherapy for ≥ 6 months

Two RCTs, one identified by a systematic review, in people with newly diagnosed tuberculosis found no significant difference in cure rates between daily and two or three times weekly short course chemotherapy regimens. However, the RCTs may have lacked power to detect a clinically important difference. ▶

Tuberculosis

Regimens containing quinolones

One systematic review found that ciprofloxacin was less effective in reducing relapse rates than standard first line drugs (ethambutol, rifampicin, pyrazinamide) in people with tuberculosis with or without HIV. Other quinolones have not been adequately evaluated.

UNLIKELY TO BE BENEFICIAL

Ethambutol in place of rifampicin in continuation phase *New*

One multicentre RCT comparing 8 months' chemotherapy regimens found that ethambutol plus isoniazid in the continuation phase was less effective than rifampicin plus isoniazid in reducing bacteriological failures and relapse rates at 12 months.

LIKELY TO BE INEFFECTIVE OR HARMFUL

Chemotherapy for less than 6 months

One systematic review found limited evidence that 3 month chemotherapy regimens were less effective in reducing relapse rates than 12 month regimens.

What are the effects of different drug regimens in people with multidrug resistant tuberculosis without HIV infection?

UNKNOWN EFFECTIVENESS

Comparative benefits of different regimens in multidrug resistant tuberculosis

We found no systematic review and no RCTs comparing different drug regimens for multidrug resistant tuberculosis.

What are the effects of low level laser therapy in people with tuberculosis without HIV infection?

UNKNOWN EFFECTIVENESS

Low level laser therapy

One systematic review provided insufficient evidence to assess effects of low level laser therapy in people with tuberculosis.

Which interventions improve adherence to treatment in people with tuberculosis without HIV infection?

LIKELY TO BE BENEFICIAL

Cash incentives

One systematic review found that cash incentives improved attendance among people living in deprived circumstances compared with usual care. One subsequent RCT found that cash incentives improved treatment completion in intravenous drug users. A second subsequent RCT found no significant difference in treatment completion between immediate and deferred cash incentives. A third subsequent RCT found no significant difference in treatment completion between cash payment and non-cash payment (fast food or grocery coupon, phone cards, or bus tokens).

Defaulter actions

One systematic review found that intensive action (repeated home visits and reminder letters) improved completion of treatment compared with routine action (single reminder letter and home visit) for defaulters.

Health education by a nurse

One RCT found that health education by a nurse improved treatment completion compared with an educational leaflet alone. One RCT in drug users found no significant effect of 5–10 minutes of health education by a clinic nurse compared with no targeted health education on attendance rates for scheduled follow up.

UNKNOWN EFFECTIVENESS

Community health advisors

One RCT found that consultation with peer health advisors recruited from the community significantly increased the rate of attendance for treatment compared with no consultation.

Direct observation treatment versus self administered treatment

One systematic review provided insufficient evidence to compare direct observation of treatment versus self treatment for improving cure rates in people with tuberculosis.

Health education by a doctor or peer educator

One RCT found no significant difference in treatment completion between consultation by the clinic doctor and the education leaflet alone. One RCT found no significant difference in completion rates between adherence coaching by peer educators plus usual care, self esteem counselling by college students plus usual care, and usual care alone.

Prompts to adhere to treatment

One systematic review identified no RCTs about the effects of prompts on adherence to treatment in people with tuberculosis.

Sanctions for non-adherence

One systematic review identified no RCTs on the effect of sanctions in people with tuberculosis.

Staff training

Two RCTs provided insufficient evidence to assess the effects of staff training on adherence to treatment.

Support mechanisms for directly observed treatment *New*

RCTs found no significant difference in non-compliance direction observation at different sites (participant chosen *v* designated) or direct observation and direct observation done by different people (health professionals *v* family members).

Which interventions improve reattendance for Mantoux test reading in people who have had tuberculosis?

UNKNOWN EFFECTIVENESS

Prompts and contracts to improve reattendance for Mantoux test reading

One RCT in healthy people found that telephone prompts to return for Mantoux test reading slightly increased the number of people who reattended compared

Tuberculosis

with no prompts, but the difference was not significant. One RCT found that healthy people were more likely to reattend for Mantoux test reading after providing either a verbal or written commitment compared with no such commitment.

DEFINITION Tuberculosis is caused by *Mycobacterium tuberculosis* and can affect many organs. Specific symptoms relate to site of infection and are generally accompanied by fever, sweats, and weight loss.

INCIDENCE/ PREVALENCE The *Mycobacterium tuberculosis* organism kills more people than any other infectious agent. The number of cases of tuberculosis was stable or falling in five of six World Health Organization (WHO) regions in 2004, but growing at 0.6% per year globally.[1] Incidence is rising in Africa where the tuberculosis epidemic is still driven by the spread of the human immunodeficiency virus (HIV). According to WHO data, there were 8.9 million new cases of tuberculosis worldwide in 2004 (140/100 000 population), of which 3.9 million (62/100 000) were smear positive and 741 000 were in adults infected with HIV. There were 14.6 million prevalent cases (229/100 000), of which 6.1 million were smear positive (95/100 000). More than 80% of all people newly diagnosed with tuberculosis in 2004 were in the African, South-East Asia and Western Pacific regions.[1] About a third of the world's population have latent tuberculosis (see aetiology).[2]

AETIOLOGY/ RISK FACTORS **Aetiology:** The chief route of infection is by inhalation of airborne bacteria released by people with active respiratory tuberculosis by cough, sneeze, or speech. Inhaled mycobacteria reach the lung and grow slowly over several weeks. The immune system of most healthy exposed people (80–90%) kills the bacteria and they are removed from the body with only a positive skin test left as a marker of exposure. In a small proportion of people infected, a defensive barrier is built round the infection but the tuberculosis bacteria are not killed and lie dormant.[2] This is known as latent tuberculosis, where the person is asymptomatic and is not infectious. In the rest of those infected, active tuberculosis develops immediately. **Risk factors:** Social factors include poverty, overcrowding, homelessness, and inadequate health services. Medical factors include HIV and immunosuppression.

PROGNOSIS Prognosis varies widely and depends on treatment.[3] An estimated 1.7 million people (27/100 000) died from tuberculosis in 2004, including those co-infected with HIV (248 000).[1]

Please refer to clinicalevidence.com for full text and references.

End stage renal disease

Search date March 2005

Yoshio N Hall and Glenn M Chertow

What are the effects of different doses and osmotic agents for peritoneal dialysis?

LIKELY TO BE BENEFICIAL

Icodextrin (reduces volume overload compared with 1.36% or 2.27% dextrose solutions)

Three RCTs in people receiving continuous ambulatory peritoneal dialysis found that 7.5% icodextrin solution for the long dwell increased ultrafiltration (fluid loss) compared with 1.36% or 2.27% dextrose solutions. Two of the RCTs found that 7.5% icodextrin reduced extracellular water or total body water compared with 1.36% or 2.27% dextrose solutions. One of the RCTs found that 7.5% icodextrin reduced left ventricular mass compared with 1.36% dextrose solution. However, one of the RCTs found no significant difference between 7.5% icodextrin solution and 3.86% dextrose solution in mean ultrafiltration during the long dwell.

UNLIKELY TO BE BENEFICIAL

Increased dose dialysis (no more effective than standard dose dialysis in reducing mortality)

One RCT found no significant difference in mortality between standard dose and increased dose peritoneal dialysis.

What are the effects of different doses and membrane fluxes for haemodialysis?

UNLIKELY TO BE BENEFICIAL

High membrane flux haemodialysis (no more effective than low membrane flux haemodialysis in reducing mortality)

One RCT found no significant difference in all cause mortality between high membrane flux and low membrane flux (with standard or increased dose haemodialysis).

Increased dose haemodialysis (no more effective than standard dose haemodialysis in reducing mortality)

One RCT found no significant difference in all cause mortality between standard dose haemodialysis and increased dose haemodialysis (at high or low membrane flux).

What are the effects of interventions aimed at preventing secondary complications?

BENEFICIAL

Sevelamer (reduces progression of coronary artery and aortic calcification compared with calcium salts)

One RCT found that sevelamer reduced the progression of coronary artery and aortic calcification compared with calcium salts at 52 weeks. One crossover RCT ▶

End stage renal disease

found no difference in reduction of serum phosphorus between sevelamer and calcium acetate. The two RCTs found that sevelamer reduced serum low density lipoprotein cholesterol levels and the incidence of hypercalcaemia compared with calcium salts. We found no RCTs comparing sevelamer versus aluminium or lanthanum carbonate.

LIKELY TO BE BENEFICIAL

Erythropoietin or darbepoetin

One RCT found no significant difference between darbepoetin alfa and recombinant human erythropoietin in maintenance of haemoglobin levels at 25–32 weeks. There is consensus based on observational studies that erythropoietin is effective for the treatment of anaemia in people with end stage renal disease.

DEFINITION End stage renal disease (ESRD) is defined as irreversible decline in a person's own kidney function, which is severe enough to be fatal in the absence of dialysis or transplantation. ESRD is included under stage 5 of the National Kidney Foundation Kidney Disease Outcomes Quality Initiative classification of chronic kidney disease (CKD), where it refers to individuals with an estimated glomerular filtration rate below 15 mL per minute per 1.73 m^2 body surface area, or those requiring dialysis irrespective of glomerular filtration rate.[1] The reduction or absence of kidney function leads to a host of maladaptive changes including fluid retention (extracellular volume overload), anaemia, disturbances of bone and mineral metabolism, dyslipidaemia, and protein energy malnutrition. This chapter deals with ESRD in adults only. **Fluid retention** in people with ESRD contributes significantly to the hypertension, ventricular dysfunction, and excess cardiovascular events observed in this population. **Anaemia** associated with CKD is normocytic and normochromic, and most commonly attributed to reduced erythropoietin synthesis by the affected kidneys. Additional factors such as iron deficiency from frequent phlebotomy, blood retention in the dialyser and tubing, and gastrointestinal bleeding; severe secondary hyperparathyroidism; acute and chronic inflammatory conditions (e.g. infection); and shortened red blood cell survival also contribute to the anaemia. **Disturbances of bone and mineral metabolism**, such as hyperparathyroidism, hyperphosphataemia, and hypo- or hypercalcaemia, are common in people with CKD.[1] If untreated, these disturbances can cause pain, pruritus, anaemia, bone loss, and increased fracture risk, and can contribute to hypertension and cardiovascular disease.[2] **Dyslipidaemia** in people with CKD is characterised by high levels of very low density lipoprotein, low levels of high density lipoprotein, and elevated levels of modified low density lipoprotein, and is associated with increased cardiovascular risk.

INCIDENCE/ PREVALENCE The incidence and prevalence of ESRD continues to grow worldwide. According to data collected from 120 countries with dialysis programmes, at the end of 2001, about 1 479 000 people were receiving renal replacement therapy (RRT).[3] Among these individuals, 1 015 000 (69%) received haemodialysis and 126 000 (9%) received peritoneal dialysis, although an additional 338 000 (23%) were living with a kidney transplant.[3] Precise estimates of ESRD incidence and prevalence remain elusive, because international databases of renal registries exclude individuals with ESRD who do not receive RRT.[4] International comparisons of RRT pose similar challenges owing to differences in health care systems, government funding, acceptance of treatment, demographics, and access to care. Worldwide, the highest incidence and prevalence rates are reported from the USA, Taiwan, and Japan. Prevalence data from several countries are listed below, although this list is not exhaustive. According to the United States Renal Data System 2004 annual report, there were 100 359 new cases of ESRD in 2002, equivalent to an annual incidence of 333 cases per million population.[5] The prevalence of

ESRD in the USA in 2002 was 456 010 (1446 cases/million population). Similarly, according to reports published by the Japanese Society for Dialysis Therapy, 255 people per million population started dialysis in 2002. In 2002, there were 1801 people per million population in Japan receiving dialysis, the highest reported prevalence for industrialised nations.[6,7] According to Taiwanese government reports, the prevalence of ESRD was 1352 cases per million population and the incidence of ESRD was 355 cases per million population in 2000.[8] In comparison, based on data pooled from the European Renal Association–European Dialysis and Transplant Association Registry and UK Renal Registry, the incidence of RRT in 2002 ranged from 76 cases per million population in Iceland to 170 cases per million population in Belgium. The prevalence of RRT in 2002 ranged from about 438 cases per million population in Iceland to 1080 cases per million population in Spain. In 2003, the Australia and New Zealand Dialysis and Transplant Registry reported an annual incidence of ESRD of 98 people per million population in Australia and 112 people per million population in New Zealand. The prevalence of ESRD in 2003 was 685 people per million population for Australia and 715 people per million population for New Zealand.[4,9-12]

AETIOLOGY/ RISK FACTORS The amount of daily proteinuria remains one of the strongest predictors of progression to ESRD.[13-15] Hypertension is a strong independent risk for progression to ESRD, particularly in people with proteinuria.[15,16] Age is also a predictor for ESRD: people over 65 years of age have a four to five-fold increase in risk of ESRD compared with people under 65 years of age.[17] Additional risk factors for developing ESRD include a history of chronic renal insufficiency, diabetes mellitus, heroin abuse, tobacco or analgesic use, black race, lower socioeconomic status, obesity, hyperuricaemia, and a family history of kidney disease.[18-26]

PROGNOSIS The overall prognosis of untreated ESRD remains poor. Most people with ESRD eventually die from complications of cardiovascular disease, infection, or, if dialysis is not provided, progressive uraemia (hyperkalaemia, acidosis, malnutrition).[1,5,9,27] Precise mortality estimates, however, are unavailable because international renal registries omit individuals with ESRD who do not receive RRT.[4] Among people receiving RRT, cardiovascular disease is the leading cause of mortality, and accounts for over 40% of deaths in this population.[1,5,9] Extracellular volume overload and hypertension, common among people with CKD, are known predictors of left ventricular hypertrophy and cardiovascular mortality in this population.[28] Even after adjustment for age, gender, race or ethnicity, and the presence of diabetes, annual cardiovascular mortality remains roughly an order of magnitude higher in people with ESRD compared with the general population, particularly among younger individuals.[1,10]

Please refer to clinicalevidence.com for full text and references.

Kidney stones

Search date April 2005

Robyn Webber, David Tolley, James Lingeman

What are the effects of treatments for stone removal in people with asymptomatic kidney stones?

UNKNOWN EFFECTIVENESS

Extracorporeal shockwave lithotripsy (ESWL) in people with asymptomatic renal or ureteric stones

One RCT found no significant difference in stone free rate at about 1 year between prophylactic extracorporeal shockwave lithotripsy (ESWL) and expectant management for people with asymptomatic renal stones less than 15 mm in diameter. However, it found limited evidence that more people required invasive procedures after conservative management. We found no systematic review or RCTs on ESWL in people with larger renal stones or with ureteric stones. We also found no RCTs comparing ESWL versus percutaneous nephrolithotomy or ureteroscopy in people with asymptomatic kidney stones.

Percutaneous nephrolithotomy (PCNL) in people with asymptomatic renal or ureteric stones

We found no systematic review or RCTs on percutaneous nephrolithotomy in people with asymptomatic renal or ureteric stones.

Ureteroscopy in people with asymptomatic renal or ureteric stones

We found no systematic review or RCTs on ureteroscopy in people with asymptomatic renal or ureteric stones.

What are the effects of treatments for the removal of symptomatic renal stones?

LIKELY TO BE BENEFICIAL

Extracorporeal shockwave lithotripsy (ESWL) in people with renal stones less than 20 mm

One RCT found that extracorporeal shockwave lithotripsy was less effective in increasing the stone free rate at 3 months and increased the rate of treatment failure in people with symptomatic renal stones less than 30 mm in diameter compared with percutaneous nephrolithotomy. It found no significant difference in complication rate between extracorporeal shockwave lithotripsy and percutaneous nephrolithotomy, although complications were more frequent with percutaneous nephrolithotomy. We found no systematic review or RCTs comparing extracorporeal shockwave lithotripsy versus ureteroscopy or open nephrolithotomy in people with renal stones. There is consensus that extracorporeal shockwave lithotripsy is the first line treatment in people with renal stones less than 20mm in diameter as it is a less invasive intervention than percutaneous nephrolithotomy.

Percutaneous nephrolithotomy (PCNL) in people with renal stones

One RCT found that percutaneous nephrolithotomy increased the stone free rate at 3 months and reduced the rate of treatment failure in people with symptomatic renal stones less than 30 mm in diameter compared with extracorporeal shockwave lithotripsy. It found no significant difference in complication rates between percutaneous nephrolithotomy and extracorporeal shockwave lithotripsy, although complications were more frequent with percutaneous nephrolithotomy. We found no RCTs comparing percutaneous nephrolithotomy versus expectant management, ureteroscopy, or open nephrolithotomy in people with renal stones.

UNKNOWN EFFECTIVENESS

Open nephrolithotomy in people with renal stones

We found no systematic review or RCTs on open nephrolithotomy in people with renal stones.

Ureteroscopy in people with renal stones

We found no systematic review or RCTs on ureteroscopy in people with renal stones.

What are the effects of treatments for the removal of symptomatic ureteric stones?

LIKELY TO BE BENEFICIAL

Extracorporeal shockwave lithotripsy (ESWL) in people with mid- and distal ureteric stones

Three RCTs found that overall stone free rates were lower and the time needed to become stone free longer in people with mid- and distal ureteric stones with extracorporeal shockwave lithotripsy compared with ureteroscopy. However, one RCT found no significant difference in stone free rates between treatments in people with distal ureteric stones of less than 15 mm. One RCT found a lower rate of treatment failure with extracorporeal shockwave lithotripsy compared with ureteroscopy. Three of the RCTs found a lower rate of severe complications with extracorporeal shockwave lithotripsy compared with ureteroscopy.

TRADE OFF BETWEEN BENEFITS AND HARMS

Ureteroscopy in people with mid- and distal ureteric stones

Three RCTs found that ureteroscopy increased overall stone free rate and decreased the time needed to become stone free in people with mid- and distal ureteric stones compared with extracorporeal shockwave lithotripsy. However, one RCT found no significant difference in stone free rates between treatments in people with distal ureteric stones of less than 15 mm. One RCT found a higher rate of treatment failure with ureteroscopy compared with extracorporeal shockwave lithotripsy. Three RCTs found a higher complication rate with ureteroscopy compared with extracorporeal shockwave lithotripsy.

UNKNOWN EFFECTIVENESS

Extracorporeal shockwave lithotripsy (ESWL) in people with proximal ureteric stones

We found no systematic review or RCTs comparing extracorporeal shockwave lithotripsy versus ureteroscopy in people with proximal ureteric stones or comparing extracorporeal shockwave lithotripsy with conservative treatment or ureterolithotomy (open or laparoscopic) in people with ureteric stones.

Kidney stones

Ureterolithotomy (open or laparoscopic) in people with ureteric stones

We found no systematic review or RCTs on ureterolithotomy (open or laparoscopic) in people with ureteric stones.

Ureteroscopy in people with proximal ureteric stones

We found no systematic review or RCTs comparing ureteroscopy versus extracorporeal shockwave lithotripsy in people with proximal ureteric stones or comparing ureteroscopy versus conservative treatment, extracorporeal shockwave lithotripsy, or ureterolithotomy (open or laparoscopic) in people with ureteric stones.

DEFINITION **Nephrolithiasis** is the presence of stones within the kidney; **urolithiasis** is a more general term for stones anywhere within the urinary tract. Urolithiasis is usually categorised according to the anatomical location of the stones (i.e. renal calyces, renal pelvis, ureteric, bladder, and urethra). Ureteric urolithiasis is described further by stating in which portion (proximal, middle, or distal) the stone is situated. This chapter assesses the effects of treatments only for the removal of asymptomatic or symptomatic renal and ureteric stones. It excludes pregnant women, in whom some forms of diagnostic procedures and treatments for stone removal are contraindicated, and people with significant comorbidities (including severe cardiovascular and respiratory conditions) who may be at increased risk when having general anaesthesia.

INCIDENCE/ PREVALENCE The peak incidence for stone disease occurs at the ages of 20–40 years, although stones are seen in all age groups.[2] There is a male to female ratio of 3 : 1. Calcium oxalate stones, the most common variety, have a recurrence rate of 10% at 1 year, 35% at 5 years, and 50% at 5 years after the first episode of kidney stone disease in North America.

AETIOLOGY/ RISK FACTORS Kidney stones develop when crystals separate from the urine and aggregate within the kidney papillae, the renal pelvis, or the ureter. The most common type of stone contains varying amounts of calcium and oxalate, whereas "struvite" stones contain a mixture of magnesium, ammonium, and phosphate. Struvite stones are associated almost exclusively with infection with urease producing organisms, whilst calcium oxalate stones have several aetiologies. Rarer stones include those formed from uric acid, cysteine, and xanthine, although this list is not exhaustive. In many otherwise healthy people the aetiology is uncertain.[3] However, incidence is higher in people with hyperparathyroidism and people with disorders including small bowel dysfunction, urinary tract infection (in particular caused by urease producing organisms) and structural/anatomical abnormalities of the kidney and ureter (including obstruction of the pelviureteric junction, hydronephrotic renal pelvis or calyces, calyceal diverticulum, horseshoe kidney, ureterocele, vesicoureteral reflux, ureteric stricture, or medullary sponge kidney). Other conditions associated with the development of renal stones include gout (especially leading to uric acid calculi) and chronic metabolic acidosis (typically resulting in stones composed of calcium phosphate). Women with a history of surgical menopause are also at higher risk because of increased bone resorption, and urinary excretion of calcium. Drugs, including some decongestants, diuretics, and anticonvulsants are also associated with an increased risk of stone formation.

DIAGNOSIS Diagnosis is usually based on clinical history, supported by investigations with diagnostic imaging. A third of all kidney stones become clinically evident; typically causing pain, often severe in nature; renal angle tenderness; haematuria; or digestive symptoms (e.g. nausea, vomiting, or diarrhoea).[1] The onset of pain is usually sudden, typically felt in the loin, and radiating to the groin, and genitalia (scrotum or labia). People are typically restless, finding the pain excruciating and describing it as the worst pain ever experienced. The aetiology and chemical composition of a stone may have some bearing on its diagnosis, management, and particularly on prevention of recurrence. Although the choices for surgical management in general remain the same for all types of stone disease, the recognition of a specific cause, such as recurrent infection with a urease producing organism for struvite stones, or cysteinuria for cysteine stones, will inform further management. **Differential diagnosis:** Bleeding within the urinary tract may present with identical symptoms to kidney stones, particularly if there are blood clots present within the renal pelvis or ureter. Several other conditions may also mimic a renal colic and need to be considered for differential diagnosis. These include urinary tract infection (and indeed the two conditions may coexist), analgesic abuse (either renal damage from excessive ingestion of analgesics, or in people with a history of opiate abuse, who may feign a renal colic in an attempt to obtain opiate analgesia). Rarely, people with sickle cell disease may also present with severe abdominal pain, which needs to be distinguished from a renal colic.

PROGNOSIS Most kidney stones pass within 48 hours with expectant treatment (including adequate fluid intake and analgesia). Others may take longer to pass and the observation period can be extended to 3–4 weeks where appropriate. Ureteric stones less than 5 mm in diameter will pass spontaneously in about 90% of people, compared with 50% of ureteric stones between 5 mm and 10 mm.[4] Expectant (conservative) management is considered on a case to case basis, and only in people with stones which are asymptomatic or very small (although stone size may not correlate with symptom severity), or both, and in people with significant comorbidities (including severe cardiovascular and respiratory conditions, who may be at increased risk when having general anaesthesia), in whom the risks of treatment may outweigh the likely benefits. Stones may migrate regardless of treatment or after treatment for their removal, and may or may not present clinically once in the ureter. Stones blocking the urine flow may lead to hydronephrosis and renal atrophy. They may also result in life threatening complications including urinary infection, perinephric abscess, or urosepsis. Infection may also occur after invasive procedures for stone removal. Some of these complications may cause kidney damage and compromised renal function.[5] Eventually, 10–20% of all kidney stones need treatment.

Please refer to clinicalevidence.com for full text and references.

Renal failure (acute)

Search date April 2005

John Kellum, Martine Leblanc, and Ramesh Venkataraman

What are the effects of interventions to prevent acute renal failure in people at high risk?

BENEFICIAL

Low osmolality contrast media (reduced nephrotoxicity compared with standard media in people with underlying renal failure)

One systematic review found that low osmolality contrast media reduced nephrotoxicity in people with underlying renal failure needing contrast investigation compared with standard osmolality contrast media.

LIKELY TO BE BENEFICIAL

Fluids

One RCT of people having elective cardiac catheterisation found that intravenous sodium chloride hydration reduced acute renal failure compared with unrestricted oral fluids 48 hours after catheterisation. One RCT found that hydration with 0.9% sodium chloride infusion reduced contrast nephropathy compared with 0.45% sodium chloride. This effect was greater in women, people with diabetes, and people who received more than 250 mL of contrast. One RCT found inconclusive evidence on the effects of inpatient hydration regimens compared with outpatient hydration regimens.

Lipid formulations of amphotericin B (may cause less nephrotoxicity than standard formulations)

We found no RCTs. Lipid formulations of amphotericin B seem to cause less nephrotoxicity compared with standard formulations, but direct comparisons of long term safety are lacking.

***N*-Acetylcysteine**

Systematic reviews have found that *N*-acetylcysteine plus hydration reduced contrast nephropathy compared with hydration alone in people at high risk of contrast nephropathy who were undergoing contrast nephrography. One further small RCT found that double dose *N*-acetylcysteine may be more effective in preventing contrast nephropathy than single dose *N*-acetylcysteine, especially in people who receive high volumes of non-ionic, low osmolality contrast agent.

Non-ionic iso-osmolar contrast media (better than non-ionic low osmolar contrast agent)

One RCT found that non-ionic iso-osmolar contrast medium (iodixanol) reduced contrast media induced nephropathy compared with low osmolar non-ionic contrast medium (iohexol) in people with diabetes.

Single dose aminoglycosides (as effective as multiple doses for treating infection, but with reduced nephrotoxicity)

One systematic review and one additional RCT compared single and multiple doses of aminoglycosides and found different results for nephrotoxicity. The systematic review, in people with fever and neutropenia receiving antibiotic treatment including aminoglycosides, found no significant difference in cure rates or nephrotoxicity between once daily compared with three times daily administration of the aminoglycoside. However, the RCT found that single doses ▶

of aminoglycosides reduced nephrotoxicity compared with multiple doses in people with fever and receiving antibiotic treatment including an aminoglycoside.

UNKNOWN EFFECTIVENESS

Sodium bicarbonate based fluids (limited evidence better than sodium chloride for the prevention of contrast nephropathy)

One single centre RCT in people with stable serum creatinine found limited evidence that the administration of sodium bicarbonate solution before and after contrast exposure was more effective in preventing contrast induced nephropathy compared with the administration of sodium chloride.

UNLIKELY TO BE BENEFICIAL

Fenoldopam

Five RCTs examined the role of fenoldopam in preventing acute renal failure. Although four small, poor quality RCTs suggested that fenoldopam may improve renal perfusion and creatinine clearance compared with conventional care, the fifth and largest RCT, which focused on clinical outcomes in people having invasive cardiovascular procedures, found no evidence that it is more effective than conventional care for preventing acute renal failure. Fenoldopam may induce hypotension.

Mannitol

Small RCTs in people with traumatic rhabdomyolysis, or in people who had had coronary artery bypass, vascular, or biliary tract surgery, found that mannitol plus hydration did not reduce acute renal failure compared with hydration alone. One RCT found that mannitol increased the risk of acute renal failure compared with 0.45% sodium chloride infusion, but the difference was not significant.

Prophylactic renal replacement therapy (haemofiltration/dialysis)

One single centre RCT in people with baseline chronic renal dysfunction undergoing coronary interventions with contrast found better in-hospital and 1 year survival with low dose haemofiltration compared with saline hydration alone. However, a number of limitations to this study were identified. Haemofiltration is invasive, expensive, and can lead to important clinical complications such as hypotension.

Theophylline or aminophylline

One systematic review found that theophylline/aminophylline attenuated the degree of increase in serum creatinine after radiocontrast administration compared with control. However, no patient centred outcomes were affected. In many RCTs included in the review, the hydration status of people was unclear. One included RCT found that in people with adequate intravenous hydration who required radiocontrast investigations, theophylline did not prevent radiocontrast induced nephropathy compared with placebo. One RCT found no significant reduction in renal impairment after elective coronary artery bypass surgery with theophylline compared with hydration alone, but may have been underpowered to detect a clinically important difference.

LIKELY TO BE INEFFECTIVE OR HARMFUL

Calcium channel blockers (for early allograft dysfunction)

One RCT found no significant difference between isradipine and placebo in preventing early allograft dysfunction in people receiving cadaveric or living renal

Renal failure (acute)

transplant. One systematic review limited to people with cadaveric renal transplant found limited evidence from heterogeneous RCTs that calcium channel blockers given in the perioperative period reduced post-transplant acute tubular necrosis, although it found no significant effect on graft loss, need for haemodialysis, or mortality. We found no RCTs assessing the effects of calcium channel blockers in preventing other forms of acute renal failure. Calcium channel blockers are associated with hypotension and bradycardia.

Dopamine

Two systematic reviews and one subsequent RCT found no significant difference between dopamine and placebo in the development of acute renal failure, the need for dialysis, or death. Dopamine is associated with serious adverse effects, such as extravasation necrosis, gangrene, and conduction abnormalities.

Loop diuretics

One systematic review and one subsequent RCT found that adding loop diuretics to fluids was not effective and may be harmful in preventing acute renal failure compared with fluids alone in people at high risk of acute renal failure.

Natriuretic peptides

One large RCT found no significant difference between natriuretic peptides and placebo in the prevention of acute renal failure induced by contrast media. Subgroup analysis in another large RCT in people with early acute renal failure found that atrial natriuretic peptide reduced dialysis free survival in non-oliguric people compared with placebo. One small RCT in people with postcardiac surgical heart failure requiring inotropic and vasoactive support found limited evidence that prolonged infusion of human recombinant atrial natriuretic peptide reduced the proportion of people requiring dialysis (before or at day 21) and the composite outcome of dialysis or death (before or at day 21) compared with placebo.

What are the effects of treatments for critically ill people with acute renal failure?

LIKELY TO BE BENEFICIAL

High dose continuous renal replacement therapy (reduced mortality compared with low dose)

One RCT found that high dose continuous renal replacement therapy (haemofiltration) reduced mortality compared with low dose continuous therapy. A small prospective study found that intensive (daily) intermittent haemodialysis reduced mortality in people with acute renal failure compared with conventional alternate day haemodialysis. A subsequent small three arm RCT found no significant difference in survival at 28 days between early, low dose haemofiltration; early, high dose haemofiltration; and late, low dose haemofiltration.

UNKNOWN EFFECTIVENESS

Continuous infusion of loop diuretics (compared with bolus injection)

We found no RCTs comparing continuous infusion versus bolus injection of loop diuretics in critically ill people with acute renal failure.

Continuous renal replacement therapy (compared with intermittent renal replacement therapy)

One systematic review found no significant difference between continuous and intermittent renal replacement therapy in mortality, renal death, or dialysis dependence in critically ill adults with acute renal failure.

Intravenous albumin supplementation plus loop diuretics

We found no RCTs on the effects of intravenous albumin supplementation plus loop diuretics in people with acute renal failure.

Synthetic dialysis membranes (compared with cellulose based membranes)

Two systematic reviews provided inconclusive evidence of the effects of synthetic membranes on mortality in critically ill people with acute renal failure compared with cellulose based membranes.

UNLIKELY TO BE BENEFICIAL

Loop diuretics

One large and two small RCTs in people with oliguric renal failure found no significant difference between loop diuretics and placebo on renal recovery, the number of days spent on dialysis, or mortality. Loop diuretics have been associated with ototoxicity and may lead to volume depletion.

LIKELY TO BE INEFFECTIVE OR HARMFUL

Dopamine

One systematic review found no significant difference in mortality or need for dialysis between dopamine and placebo. One additional RCT found that low dose dopamine did not reduce renal dysfunction compared with placebo. Dopamine has been associated with important adverse effects, including extravasation necrosis, gangrene, and conduction abnormalities.

Natriuretic peptides

RCTs found no significant difference between atrial natriuretic peptide, ularitide (urodilatin), and placebo in dialysis free survival in oliguric and non-oliguric people with acute renal failure. One of the RCTs found that atrial natriuretic peptide may reduce survival in non-oliguric people.

DEFINITION Acute renal failure is characterised by abrupt and sustained decline in glomerular filtration rate,[1] which leads to accumulation of urea and other chemicals in the blood. Most studies define it biochemically as a serum creatinine of 2–3 mg/dL (200–250 μmol/L), an elevation of more than 0.5 mg/dL (45 μmol/L) over a baseline creatinine below 2 mg/dL, or a twofold increase of baseline creatinine. A recent international, interdisciplinary, consensus panel has classified acute renal failure according to a change from baseline serum creatinine or urine output. The three level classification begins with "Risk", defined by either a 50% increase in serum creatinine or a urine output of less than 0.5 mL/kg/hour for at least 6 hours, and concludes with "Failure", defined by a threefold increase in serum creatinine or a urine output of less than 0.3 mL/kg/hour for 24 hours.[2] Acute renal failure is usually additionally classified according to the location of the predominant primary pathology (prerenal, intrarenal, and postrenal failure). Critically ill people are clinically unstable and at imminent risk of death, which usually implies that they need to be in, or have been admitted to, the intensive care unit.

INCIDENCE/ PREVALENCE Two prospective observational studies (2576 people) found that established acute renal failure affected nearly 5% of people in hospital and as many as 15% of critically ill people, depending on the definitions used.[3,4]

Renal failure (acute)

AETIOLOGY/ RISK FACTORS **General risk factors:** Risk factors for acute renal failure that are consistent across multiple causes include age; hypovolaemia; hypotension; sepsis; pre-existing renal, hepatic, or cardiac dysfunction; diabetes mellitus; and exposure to nephrotoxins (e.g. aminoglycosides, amphotericin, immunosuppressive agents, non-steroidal anti-inflammatory drugs, angiotensin converting enzyme inhibitors, iv contrast media) (see table 1) Ⓣ.[4-8] **Risk factors/aetiology in critically ill people:** Isolated episodes of acute renal failure are rarely seen in critically ill people, but are usually part of multiple organ dysfunction syndromes. Acute renal failure requiring dialysis is rarely seen in isolation (< 5% of people). The kidneys are often the first organs to fail.[9] In the perioperative setting, acute renal failure risk factors include prolonged aortic clamping, emergency rather than elective surgery, and use of higher volumes (> 100 mL) of intravenous contrast media. One study (3695 people) using multiple logistic regression identified the following independent risk factors: baseline creatinine clearance below 47 mL/minute (OR 1.20, 95% CI 1.12 to 1.30), diabetes (OR 5.5, 95% CI 1.4 to 21.0), and a marginal effect for doses of contrast media above 100 mL (OR 1.01, 95% CI 1.00 to 1.01). Mortality of people with acute renal failure requiring dialysis was 36% while in hospital.[5] Prerenal acute renal failure is caused by reduced blood flow to the kidney from renal artery disease, systemic hypotension, or maldistribution of blood flow. Intrarenal acute renal failure is caused by parenchymal injury (acute tubular necrosis, interstitial nephritis, embolic disease, glomerulonephritis, vasculitis, or small vessel disease). Postrenal acute renal failure is caused by urinary tract obstruction. Observational studies (in several hundred people from Europe, North America, and West Africa with acute renal failure) found a prerenal cause in 40–80%, an intrarenal cause in 10–50%, and a postrenal cause in the remaining 10%.[7,8,10-13] Prerenal acute renal failure is the most common type of acute renal failure in people who are critically ill.[7,14] Intrarenal acute renal failure in this context is usually part of multisystem failure, and most frequently because of acute tubular necrosis resulting from ischaemic or nephrotoxic injury, or both.[15,16]

PROGNOSIS One retrospective study (1347 people with acute renal failure) found that mortality was less than 15% in people with isolated acute renal failure.[17] One recent prospective study (> 700 people) found that, in people with acute renal failure, overall mortality and the need for dialysis were higher in an intensive care unit (ICU) than in a non-ICU setting, despite no significant difference between the groups in mean maximal serum creatinine (need for dialysis: 71% in ICU *v* 18% in non-ICU; $P < 0.001$; mortality: 72% in ICU *v* 32% in non-ICU; $P = 0.001$).[18] One large study (> 17 000 people admitted to Austrian ICUs) found that acute renal failure was associated with a greater than fourfold increase in mortality.[19] Even after controlling for underlying severity of illness, mortality was still significantly higher in people with acute renal failure (62.8% *v* 38.5%), suggesting that acute renal failure is independently responsible for increased mortality, even if dialysis is used. However, the exact mechanism that leads to increased risk of death is uncertain.

Please refer to clinicalevidence.com for full text and references.

Benign prostatic hyperplasia

Search date May 2005

Robyn Webber

What are the effects of medical treatments?

BENEFICIAL

5 alpha-reductase inhibitors

One systematic review and three subsequent RCTs found that 5 alpha-reductase inhibitors improved symptoms and reduced complications compared with placebo. RCTs found that the 5 alpha-reductase inhibitor finasteride was less effective at improving symptoms than alpha-blockers. One systematic review found no significant difference in symptoms between finasteride and saw palmetto plant extracts. We found no RCTs comparing 5 alpha-reductase inhibitors versus other herbal treatments or versus surgical treatments.

Alpha-blockers

Systematic reviews and RCTs found that alpha-blockers improved symptoms compared with placebo. The reviews found that different alpha-blockers have similar effects. RCTs found that alpha-blockers improved symptoms compared with the 5 alpha-reductase inhibitor finasteride. One RCT found that the alpha-blocker terazosin was less effective than transurethral microwave thermotherapy in improving symptoms over 18 months. One RCT found no significant difference between tamsulosin and saw palmetto plant extracts in symptoms or maximum urinary flow rate after 1 year. We found no RCTs comparing alpha-blockers versus other herbal treatments.

What are the effects of surgical treatments?

BENEFICIAL

Transurethral microwave thermotherapy

Three RCTs found that transurethral microwave thermotherapy reduced symptoms compared with sham treatment. One systematic review found limited evidence that transurethral microwave thermotherapy was less effective in improving symptoms and peak urinary flow at 6 to 12 months compared with transurethral resection. It found that transurethral microwave thermotherapy reduced the need for transfusion, retreatment for strictures and reduced retrograde ejaculation compared with transurethral resection. However, men undergoing TURP had a lower rate of retreatment for benign prostatic hyperplasia. One RCT found that transurethral microwave thermotherapy improved symptoms over 18 months compared with the alpha-blocker terazosin.

Transurethral resection versus no surgery

RCTs found that transurethral resection improved symptoms more than watchful waiting, and did not increase the risk of erectile dysfunction or incontinence.

UNKNOWN EFFECTIVENESS

Transurethral resection versus less invasive surgical techniques

One systematic review found no significant difference in symptoms between transurethral resection and transurethral incision. One systematic review found no clear evidence of a difference in symptoms between transurethral resection and visual laser ablation or contact laser ablation. One systematic review and ▶

BMJ Clin Evid Concise 2006;16:371–373.

Benign prostatic hyperplasia

three subsequent RCTs found similar improvements in symptoms between transurethral resection and electrical vaporisation. One systematic review found limited evidence that transurethral microwave thermotherapy was less effective in improving symptoms and peak urinary flow at 6–12 months compared with transurethral resection. It found that transurethral microwave thermotherapy reduced the need for transfusion retreatment of strictures, and reduced retrograde ejaculation compared with transurethral resection. However, men undergoing transurethral resection had a lower rate of retreatment for benign prostatic hyperplasia.

Transurethral resection versus transurethral needle ablation

One RCT found that transurethral resection reduced symptoms compared with transurethral needle ablation after 1 year, although transurethral needle ablation caused fewer adverse effects.

What are the effects of herbal treatments?

LIKELY TO BE BENEFICIAL

Beta-sitosterol plant extract

One systematic review found that beta-sitosterol plant extract improved lower urinary tract symptoms compared with placebo in the short term. We found no RCTs comparing beta-sitosterol plant extract versus other treatments.

Saw palmetto plant extracts

One systematic review found that saw palmetto plant extracts improved symptoms compared with placebo. It found no significant difference in symptoms between saw palmetto plant extracts and the alpha-blocker tamsulosin or the 5 alpha-reductase inhibitor finasteride. One RCT found no significant difference in symptoms between tamsulosin and tamsulosin plus saw palmetto plant extracts.

UNKNOWN EFFECTIVENESS

Pygeum africanum

One systematic review found limited evidence that *Pygeum africanum* increased peak urinary flow and reduced residual urine volume at 4–16 weeks compared with placebo. We found no RCTs comparing *Pygeum africanum* versus other treatments.

Rye grass pollen extract

One systematic review found limited evidence that rye grass pollen extract increased self rated improvement and reduced nocturia at 12–24 weeks compared with placebo. However, the review identified only two small RCTs, from which we were unable to draw reliable conclusions. We found no RCTs comparing rye grass pollen extract versus other treatments.

DEFINITION Benign prostatic hyperplasia is defined histologically. Clinically, it is characterised by lower urinary tract symptoms (urinary frequency, urgency, a weak and intermittent stream, needing to strain, a sense of incomplete emptying, and nocturia) and can lead to complications, including acute urinary retention.

INCIDENCE/ PREVALENCE Estimates of the prevalence of symptomatic benign prostatic hyperplasia range from 10–30% for men in their early 70s, depending on how benign prostatic hyperplasia is defined.[1]

AETIOLOGY/ RISK FACTORS The mechanisms by which benign prostatic hyperplasia causes symptoms and complications are unclear, although bladder outlet obstruction is an important factor.[2] The best documented risk factors are increasing age and normal testicular function.[3]

PROGNOSIS Community and practice based studies suggest that men with lower urinary tract symptoms can expect slow progression of symptoms.[4,5] However, symptoms can wax and wane without treatment. In men with symptoms of benign prostatic hyperplasia, rates of acute urinary retention range from 1–2% a year.[5-7]

Please refer to clinicalevidence.com for full text and references.

Chronic prostatitis

Search date July 2005

Bradley A Erickson, Thomas L Jang, Christina Ching, and Anthony J Schaeffer

What are the effects of treatments for chronic bacterial prostatitis?

LIKELY TO BE BENEFICIAL

Alpha-blockers

We found no systematic review or RCTs comparing alpha-blockers versus placebo or no treatment in men with chronic bacterial prostatitis. We found limited evidence from one RCT suggesting that adding alpha-blockers to antimicrobials improved symptoms and reduced recurrence compared with antimicrobials alone.

Oral antimicrobial drugs

We found no systematic review or RCTs comparing oral antimicrobial drugs versus placebo or no antimicrobial treatment in men with chronic bacterial prostatitis. Two RCTs found no significant difference between ciprofloxacin and other quinolones (levofloxacin or lomefloxacin) in rates of clinical success or bacteriological cure at 6 months. In the two RCTs, the clinical success rate ranged between 73–89% and the bacteriological cure rate ranged between 63–77% depending on the antimicrobial used.

UNKNOWN EFFECTIVENESS

Local injection of antimicrobials

We found no systematic review or RCTs comparing local injection of antimicrobials versus placebo or no treatment in men with chronic bacterial prostatitis. One small RCT found that anal submucosal injection of amikacin improved symptom scores and bacterial eradication rates at 3 months compared with intramuscular amikacin.

Non-steroidal anti-inflammatory drugs

We found no systematic review or RCTs on the effects of non-steroidal anti-inflammatory drugs in men with chronic bacterial prostatitis.

Radical prostatectomy

We found no systematic review or RCTs on the effects of radical prostatectomy in men with chronic bacterial prostatitis.

Transurethral resection

We found no systematic review or RCTs on the effects of transurethral resection in men with chronic bacterial prostatitis.

What are the effects of treatments for chronic abacterial prostatitis (CP/CPPS)?

LIKELY TO BE BENEFICIAL

Alpha-blockers

Two small RCTs identified by a systematic review and four small subsequent RCTs found limited evidence that alpha-blockers improved quality of life and symptoms compared with placebo in men with chronic abacterial prostatitis (CP/CPPS). The RCTs may have been too small to detect other clinically important differences. We found no systematic review or RCTs comparing alpha-blockers versus each other.

UNKNOWN EFFECTIVENESS

5 alpha reductase inhibitors

One RCT identified by a systematic review and one subsequent RCT provided insufficient evidence about the effects of 5 alpha reductase inhibitors compared with placebo in men with chronic abacterial prostatitis (CP/CPPS).

Allopurinol

One RCT identified by a systematic review provided insufficient evidence about the effects of allopurinol compared with placebo in men with chronic abacterial prostatitis (CP/CPPS).

Biofeedback

We found no systematic review or RCTs on the effects of biofeedback in men with chronic abacterial prostatitis (CP/CPPS).

Non-steroidal anti-inflammatory drugs

We found no systematic review or RCTs on the effects of non-steroidal anti-inflammatory drugs in men with chronic abacterial prostatitis (CP/CPPS).

Oral antimicrobial drugs

Two RCTs found no significant difference in improvement in National Institutes of Health–Chronic Prostatitis Symptom Index (NIH-CPSI) scores between oral antimicrobial drugs and control after 6 weeks of treatment in men with chronic abacterial prostatitis (CP/CPPS). There is currently little evidence to support the role of antimicrobial therapy for the treatment of CP/CPPS.

Pentosan polysulfate

One RCT identified by a systematic review and one subsequent RCT provided insufficient evidence about the effects of pentosan polysulfate compared with placebo or no treatment in men with chronic abacterial prostatitis (CP/CPPS).

Prostatic massage

We found no systematic review or RCTs on the effects of prostatic massage in men with chronic abacterial prostatitis (CP/CPPS).

Sitz baths

We found no systematic review or RCTs on the effects of Sitz baths in men with chronic abacterial prostatitis (CP/CPPS).

Transurethral microwave thermotherapy

One systematic review found limited evidence from one small RCT suggesting that transurethral microwave thermotherapy improved quality of life at 3 months and symptoms over 21 months compared with sham treatment. However, we were unable to draw reliable conclusions from this one small study.

DEFINITION **Chronic bacterial prostatitis** is characterised by a positive culture of expressed prostatic secretions. It may cause symptoms such as suprapubic, lower back, or perineal pain, or mild urgency, frequency, and dysuria, and may be associated with recurrent urinary tract infections. However, it may also be asymptomatic between acute episodes/exacerbations. **Chronic abacterial prostatitis**, or chronic pelvic pain syndrome (CP/CPPS), is characterised by

Chronic prostatitis

pelvic or perineal pain in the absence of pathogenic bacteria in expressed prostatic secretions. It is often associated with irritative and obstructive voiding symptoms including urgency, frequency, hesitancy, and poor interrupted flow. Symptoms can also include pain in the suprapubic region, lower back, penis, testes, or scrotum, and painful ejaculation. CP/CPPS may be inflammatory (white cells present in prostatic secretions) or non-inflammatory (white cells absent in prostatic secretions).[1] A classification system for the prostatitis syndromes has been developed by the National Institutes of Health (NIH).[2]

INCIDENCE/ PREVALENCE One community based study in the USA (cohort of 2115 men aged 40–79 years old) estimated that 9% of men have a diagnosis of prostatitis at any one time.[3] Another observational study found that, in men presenting with genitourinary symptoms, 8% of them presenting to urologists and 1% of them presenting to primary care physicians were diagnosed as having chronic prostatitis.[4] Most cases of chronic prostatitis are abacterial. Chronic bacterial prostatitis, although easy to diagnose, is rare.

AETIOLOGY/ RISK FACTORS Organisms commonly implicated in bacterial prostatitis include *Escherichia coli*, other Gram negative enterobacteriaceae, occasionally *Pseudomonas* species, and rarely Gram positive enterococci. Risk factors for bacterial prostatitis include urethral catheterization or instrumentation, condom drainage, dysfunctional voiding (high pressure urination), and unprotected anal intercourse. The cause of abacterial prostatitis (CP/CPPS) is unclear, although it has been suggested that it may be caused by undocumented infections with *Chlamydia trachomatis*,[5] *Ureaplasma urealyticum*,[6] *Mycoplasma hominis*,[7] and *Trichomonas vaginalis*.[8] Viruses,[9,10] *Candida* (in immunosuppressed people),[11] and parasites[12] have also rarely been implicated. Non-infectious factors might also be involved, including inflammation,[13] autoimmunity,[14] hormonal imbalances,[15] pelvic floor tension myalgia,[16] intraprostatic urinary reflux,[17] and psychological disturbances.[18] In one case control study (463 men with CP/CPPS, 121 asymptomatic age matched controls), when compared to controls, men with CP/CPPS reported a significantly higher lifetime prevalence of non-specific urethritis (12% *v* 4%; $P = 0.008$), cardiovascular disease (11% *v* 2%; $P = 0.004$), neurological disease (41% *v* 14%; $P < 0.001$), psychiatric conditions (29% *v* 11%; $P < 0.001$), and haematopoietic, lymphatic, or infectious disease (41% *v* 20%; $P < 0.001$).[19] Further studies are necessary to determine whether these factors play a role in the pathogenesis of CP/CPPS.[19]

PROGNOSIS The natural history of untreated chronic bacterial and abacterial prostatitis (CP/CPPS) remains ill-defined. Chronic bacterial prostatitis may cause recurrent urinary tract infections in men whereas CP/CPPS does not.[20] Several investigators have reported an association between chronic bacterial prostatitis, CP/CPPS, and infertility.[21] One study found that CP/CPPS had an impact on quality of life similar to that from angina, Crohn's disease, or a previous myocardial infarction.[22]

Please refer to clinicalevidence.com for full text and references.

Erectile dysfunction

Search date August 2005

Prathap Tharyan and Ganesh Gopalakrishanan

What are the effects of treatments in men with erectile dysfunction?

BENEFICIAL

Alprostadil (intracavernosal)

Two RCTs found intracavernosal alprostadil improved erections compared with placebo. Three RCTs found intracavernosal alprostadil to be more effective than intraurethral alprostadil in improving erections and the chances of successful intercourse. Three RCTs found that alprostadil improved erections compared with intracavernosal papaverine injections. Two RCTs found alprostadil to be as effective as a mixture of papaverine plus phentolamine (bimix) in improving erections. Two RCTs found that alprostadil was less effective than a mix of alprostadil plus papaverine plus phentolamine (trimix) in producing erections in men who failed to get erections with bimix. One small RCT found no significant difference between sildenafil and intracavernosal alprostadil injections and that both were effective in improving erections and successful sexual intercourse. One small RCT found limited evidence that vacuum devices were as effective as intracavernosal alprostadil injections for rigidity but less effective for orgasm or rates of overall satisfaction. Penile pain over the injection site was the most common adverse effect with alprostadil and was seen in up to 40% of men.

Alprostadil (intraurethral)

One systematic review and one RCT (in men who had previously responded to alprostadil) found that intraurethral alprostadil (prostaglandin E1) improved erections and the chances of successful sexual intercourse compared with placebo. Three RCTs found that intraurethral alprostadil was less effective than intracavernosal alprostadil in improving erections and the chances of successful intercourse. Penile pain was the most common adverse effect and was seen in a third of men.

Apomorphine

Three RCTs found that sublingual apomorphine increased successful erections and the chances of successful intercourse compared with placebo. Nausea, dizziness, headache, and drowsiness were the most common adverse events. These adverse events were less common with continued use.

Sildenafil

One systematic review and 23 subsequent RCTs found that sildenafil improved erections and increased rates of successful intercourse compared with placebo. One small RCT found that sildenafil and intracavernosal alprostadil both increased erections sufficient for successful intercourse over 4–9 months (average 6 months) of treatment with no significant difference between treatments. Adverse effects of sildenafil were mild to moderate including headache, flushing, and dyspepsia, and were reported in up to a quarter of men. Sildenafil is contraindicated in men receiving nitrates concurrently, in whom deaths have been reported.

Tadalafil

One systematic review and three subsequent RCTs found that tadalafil improved erections and successful sexual intercourse compared with placebo and this ▶

advantage persisted up to 36 hours. Men in two crossover RCTs expressed a preference for tadalafil over sildenafil. In men with diabetes taking antihypertensives, tadalafil 20 mg was associated with a better response than tadalafil 10 mg or placebo. Mild to moderate adverse effects included headache, muscle pain, back ache, dyspepsia, and flushing, and were seen in a third of men. Tadalafil is contraindicated in people receiving nitrates due to the risk of potentially life threatening hypotension.

Vardenafil

One systematic review and one subsequent RCT found that vardenafil improved erections and increased rates of successful intercourse compared with placebo. Adverse effects were mild to moderate including headache, flushing, and dyspepsia and were reported in up to a third of men. Vardenafil is contraindicated in people receiving nitrates due to the risk of potentially life threatening hypotension. We found no direct comparisons of vardenafil with sildenafil or tadalafil.

LIKELY TO BE BENEFICIAL

Ginseng

One small RCT found limited evidence that Korean red ginseng increased successful erections, sexual desire, and successful intercourse compared with placebo. Adverse effects were not reported.

Penile prosthesis*

We found no systematic review or RCTs of penile prostheses in men with erectile dysfunction. Anecdotal evidence suggests that patient satisfaction may be high, but we found no studies of adequate quality to assess this. However, there is consensus belief that penile prostheses are likely to be beneficial. Mechanical failure and infections are the most serious complications of penile prosthesis implantation. Use of penile prostheses is usually considered only after less invasive treatments have failed.

Psychosexual counselling

One small RCT found no significant difference in the chances of successful intercourse between psychosexual counselling and waiting list control, whereas another found psychosexual counselling improved sexual functioning and satisfaction compared with a waiting list control. This RCT also found that interpersonal therapy aimed at improving social skills, with or without additional psychosexual counselling, improved sexual functioning and sexual satisfaction compared with psychosexual counselling alone. All RCTs were conducted in men with psychological erectile dysfunction. Harms were inadequately described.

Vacuum devices

Vacuum devices have not been adequately assessed in RCTs. One small RCT found limited evidence that vacuum devices were as effective as intracavernosal alprostadil (prostaglandin E1) injections for rigidity but not for orgasm. One RCT found that a combination of a vacuum device and psychosexual therapy was no more effective than psychosexual counselling alone, although more people having combined treatment were assessed as improved. The RCT may have been too small to detect a clinically important difference between groups. Some men found the vacuum device produced insufficiently rigid erections and blocked ejaculations.

Yohimbine

One systematic review found that yohimbine improved self reported sexual function and penile rigidity at 2–10 weeks compared with placebo. One subsequent RCT did not find yohimbine to be beneficial but it may have been too small to detect clinically important benefits. Transient adverse effects were reported in up to a third of men.

TRADE OFF BETWEEN BENEFITS AND HARMS

Alprostadil (topical)

Two RCTs found that alprostadil (prostaglandin E1) gel applied on the tip of the penis improved erections and the rates of successful intercourse compared with placebo. About a third of men reported penile pain and erythema.

Papaverine

One small RCT found limited evidence that intracavernosal papaverine injections were less effective than intracavernosal injections of a combination of papaverine plus phentolamine (bimix) in improving erections sufficient for intercourse. Three RCTs found that intracavernosal papaverine was less effective than intracavernosal alprostadil injections in improving erections. Transient burning pain in the penis was reported by up to 25% of men. On long term use, bruising, prolonged erections, fibrosis of the corpora cavernosa, and fibrous penile nodules were reported in up to one in 10 men in one study.

Papaverine plus phentolamine (bimix)

One small RCT found that a mixture of papaverine plus phentolamine (bimix) injected into the penis increased the proportion of men with erections sufficient for intercourse compared with normal saline injections. Another small RCT found limited evidence that bimix was more effective than intracavernosal papaverine injections in improving erections sufficient for intercourse. Two RCTs found bimix to be as effective as alprostadil injections in improving erections. Adverse effects included mild transient pain and bruises at injection site. One prospective cohort study found that painless fibrous penile nodules and mild to moderate alteration in liver function developed in up to half of the men after 12 months, and bruising, prolonged erections, and fibrosis of the corpora cavernosa in less than one in 10 men.

Papaverine plus phentolamine plus alprostadil (trimix)

Two RCTs found that a mix of alprostadil plus papaverine plus phentolamine (trimix) was more effective than intracavernosal alprostadil in producing erections in men who failed to get erections with bimix. Penile pain was less commonly reported after trimix than after intracavernosal alprostadil.

UNKNOWN EFFECTIVENESS

Cognitive behavioural therapy

We found no relevant systematic review or RCTs assessing cognitive behavioural therapy in men with erectile dysfunction. Anecdotal evidence suggests that this may be an effective treatment but we found no studies of adequate quality.

*Categorisation based on consensus; RCTs unlikely to be conducted.

DEFINITION Erectile dysfunction is defined as the persistent inability to obtain or maintain sufficient rigidity of the penis to allow satisfactory sexual performance. The term erectile dysfunction has largely replaced the term "impotence". For the purposes of this review we included only men with normal testosterone and

Erectile dysfunction

gonadotrophin levels, who could gain an erection while asleep. We also included men with comorbid conditions such as cardiovascular disorders, prostate cancer, diabetes, and spinal cord injury. We excluded men with drug induced sexual dysfunction. Because the cause of erectile dysfunction in men with cardiovascular disease is unclear (the disease or treatment drugs), we included them.

INCIDENCE/ PREVALENCE Cross-sectional epidemiological studies from around the world[1-4] reveal that 30–50% of men aged 40–70 years report some degree of erectile dysfunction. About 150 million men worldwide are unable to achieve and maintain an erection adequate for satisfactory sexual intercourse.[1] Age is the variable most strongly associated with erectile dysfunction; between the ages of 40 to 70 years, the incidence of moderate erectile dysfunction doubles from 17% to 34%, whereas that of severe erectile dysfunction triples from 5% to 15%.[4]

AETIOLOGY/ RISK FACTORS About 80% of cases are believed to have an organic cause, the rest being psychogenic in origin. Most cases of erectile dysfunction are believed to be multifactorial and secondary to disease, stress, trauma (such as spinal cord injury, pelvic and prostate surgery), or drug adverse effects that interfere with the coordinated psychological, neurological, endocrine, vascular, and muscular factors necessary for normal erections. Risk factors include increasing age, smoking, and obesity. The prevalence of erectile dysfunction also increases in people with diabetes mellitus, hypertension, heart disease, anxiety, and depression.[5]

PROGNOSIS We found no good evidence on prognosis in untreated organic erectile dysfunction.

Please refer to clinicalevidence.com for full text and references.

Prostate cancer (early)

Search date February 2006

Melissa L James

What are the effects of treatments for early prostate cancer?

TRADE OFF BETWEEN BENEFITS AND HARMS

Radical prostatectomy

One large RCT found that radical prostatectomy reduced death from prostate cancer, overall mortality, and metastases at 8.2 years compared with watchful waiting. One small RCT found limited evidence of no significant difference in overall mortality between radical prostatectomy and watchful waiting in men with clinically detected disease after a median follow up of 23 years. One RCT found that more men managed by radical prostatectomy than watchful waiting had erectile dysfunction and urinary leakage, but found no significant difference in quality of life between groups at 12 months or more after surgery. We found no RCTs of sufficient quality comparing the benefits of radical prostatectomy versus external beam radiation therapy. One systemic review found lower rates of erectile function after nerve sparing radical prostatectomy compared with external beam radiation therapy at 12 months. Radical prostatectomy carries the risks of major surgery and of increased sexual and urinary dysfunction.

Watchful waiting

One large RCT found that watchful waiting was less effective than radical prostatectomy at reducing death from prostate cancer, overall mortality, and metastases at 8.2 years. One small RCT found limited evidence of no significant difference in overall mortality between watchful waiting and radical prostatectomy in men with clinically detected disease after median follow up of 23 years. One RCT found that fewer men managed by watchful waiting than by radical prostatectomy had erectile dysfunction and urinary leakage, but found no significant difference in quality of life between groups at 12 months or more after surgery. We found no RCTs comparing watchful waiting versus external beam radiation therapy. One RCT provided limited evidence that watchful waiting was less effective than immediate oestrogen hormone therapy at reducing prostate cancer mortality, but found no significant difference in overall mortality.

UNKNOWN EFFECTIVENESS

Adding hormone therapy to external beam radiation therapy (to increase overall survival)

Two RCTs found that neoadjuvant hormone therapy plus external beam radiation therapy (EBRT) (with or without concurrent and adjuvant hormone therapy) improved prostate specific antigen levels, rates of residual disease, and biochemical free survival at between 12 months and 5 years compared with EBRT alone. One RCT found that neoadjuvant, concurrent, and adjuvant hormone therapy plus EBRT improved rates of overall mortality, deaths from prostate cancer, survival free from salvage androgen suppression, and prostate specific antigen failure at a median of 4.52 years. One RCT found no significant difference in rates of biochemical freedom from disease between different combinations of hormone therapy plus EBRT.

Brachytherapy

We found no RCTs comparing the beneficial effects of brachytherapy with other interventions in men with early prostate cancer.

Prostate cancer (early)

External beam radiation therapy

We found no RCTs comparing external beam radiation therapy (EBRT) versus watchful waiting. We found no RCTs of sufficient quality comparing the benefits of EBRT versus radical prostatectomy. One systemic review found higher rates of erectile function after EBRT compared with nerve sparing radical prostatectomy at 12 months. One RCT, which included one fifth of men with T3 disease, found no significant difference in overall survival at 5 years between conformal EBRT and conventional EBRT, but found increased rectal toxicity at longer term follow up with conformal treatment (with dose escalation) compared with conventional treatment. One RCT, which included a large proportion of men with T3–T4 disease, found that conventional EBRT increased anal toxicity during and immediately after treatment compared with conformal EBRT, but found no significant difference at 2 years, whereas another RCT, which included men with T3–T4 disease, found that conventional EBRT increased proctitis at 2 years compared with conformal EBRT. We found no RCTs comparing conformal EBRT versus intensity modulated EBRT.

Hormone therapy plus brachytherapy

We found no RCTs assessing the effects of adjuvant hormone therapy plus brachytherapy on length or quality of life in men with clinically localised prostate cancer.

Hormone therapy plus standard care

RCTs in men with stage T1 and T2 disease, which also included men with T3–T4 disease, found that hormone therapy plus standard care reduced objective disease progression compared with placebo plus standard care at a median follow up of between 2.6 and 5.3 years, but found no significant difference between groups in overall survival rates. Hormone therapy plus standard care was associated with increased adverse effects such as gynaecomastia and breast pain compared with placebo plus standard care.

Immediate hormone therapy for asymptomatic disease

We found no RCTs assessing the effects of immediate hormone therapy on mortality or quality of life in men with asymptomatic, clinically localised prostate cancer.

Immediate hormone therapy for symptomatic disease

One RCT provided limited evidence that immediate oestrogen therapy decreased prostate cancer mortality, but not overall mortality, compared with watchful waiting.

UNLIKELY TO BE BENEFICIAL

Adding neoadjuvant hormone therapy to surgery plus adjuvant hormonal therapy

One RCT, which included one quarter of men with stage C disease, found no significant difference in overall survival, clinical relapse free survival, or prostate specific antigen relapse free survival rates at 5 years between men who did and those who did not have neoadjuvant hormone therapy before they had surgery and adjuvant hormone therapy.

Neoadjuvant hormone therapy plus surgery

Four RCTs found no significant difference in rates of biochemical disease recurrence at up to 6 years between neoadjuvant hormone therapy plus surgery compared with surgery alone. However, in one of these RCTs only half of the men had stage T1–T2 disease, and another RCT included men with stage T3 disease. One RCT found limited evidence that neoadjuvant hormone therapy plus surgery increased adverse effects and surgical difficulty compared with surgery alone.

DEFINITION Prostatic cancer is staged according to two systems: the tumour, node, metastasis (TNM) classification system (where scores of T0, T1, T2, T3, T4, N0; M0 apply to non-metastatic prostate cancer) and the American Urologic Staging system (where stages A, B, C apply to non-metastatic prostate cancer) (see table 1 Ⓣ) Non-metastatic prostate cancer can be divided into clinically localised disease and advanced disease. Clinically localised disease (T0, T1, T2) is prostate cancer thought to still be confined to the prostate gland by clinical examination. Locally advanced disease (T3 and T4) is prostate cancer which has spread beyond the capsule of, but is still connected to, the prostate gland. Metastatic disease is prostate cancer which has spread outside the prostate gland with no remaining connection. This chapter focuses on clinically localised disease that has not extended beyond the prostate capsule (TNM classification system T0, T1, T2, and American Urologic Staging system stages A and B).

INCIDENCE/ PREVALENCE Prostate cancer is the sixth most common cancer in the world and the third most common cancer in men. In 2000, an estimated 513 000 new cases of prostate cancer were diagnosed and about 250 000 deaths were attributed to prostate cancers worldwide. The estimated number of new cases of prostate cancer in the United States in 2005 was 232 090.[1] Prostate cancer is uncommon under the age of 50 years. About 85% of men with prostate cancer are diagnosed after the age of 65 years. Autopsy studies suggest that the prevalence of subclinical prostate cancer is high at all ages: 30% for men aged 30–39 years, 50% for men aged 50–59 years, and more than 75% for men older than 85 years. Incidence varies widely by ethnic group and around the world.

AETIOLOGY/ RISK FACTORS Risk factors for prostate cancer include increasing age, family history of prostate cancer, black ethnic group, and possibly higher dietary consumption of fat and meat, low intake of lycopene (from tomato products), low intake of fruit, and high dietary calcium. In the USA, black men have about a 60% higher incidence than white men.[3] The prostate cancer incidence for black men living in the USA is about 90/100 000 in men aged less than 65 years and about 1300/100 000 in men aged 65–74 years. For white men, incidence is about 44/100 000 in men aged less than 65 years and 900/100 000 in men aged 65–74 years.[3]

PROGNOSIS The chance that men with well to moderately differentiated, palpable, clinically localised prostate cancer will remain free of symptomatic progression is 70% at 5 years and 40% at 10 years.[4] The risk of symptomatic disease progression is higher in men with poorly differentiated prostate cancer.[5] One retrospective analysis of a large surgical series in men with clinically localised prostate cancer found that the median time from the increase in prostate specific antigen (PSA) concentration to the development of metastatic disease was 8 years.[6] PSA doubling time and Gleason score were predictive of the probability and time to development of metastatic disease. Once men developed metastatic disease, the median actuarial time to death was less than 5 years.[6] Morbidity from local or regional disease progression includes haematuria, bladder obstruction, and lower extremity oedema. The age adjusted prostate cancer specific mortality in the USA for all men aged 65 years and older has decreased by about 15% (244 deaths/100 000 to 207 deaths/100 000) from 1991–1997. The reasons for this are unclear, although inaccurate death certification, PSA screening, and earlier, more intensive treatment, including radical prostatectomy, radiotherapy, and androgen suppression, have been suggested. However, regions of the USA and Canada where PSA testing and early treatment are more common have similar prostate cancer mortality to regions with lower rates of both testing and early treatment.[7] Similarly, countries with low rates of PSA testing and treatment, such as the UK, have similar age adjusted prostate cancer mortality to countries with high rates of testing and treatment, such as the USA.[8]

Please refer to clinicalevidence.com for full text and references.

Testicular cancer: seminoma

Search date April 2005

Richard Neal, Nicholas Stuart, and Clare Wilkinson

What are the effects of treatments in men with stage 1 seminoma (confined to testis) who have undergone orchidectomy?

BENEFICIAL

Adjuvant irradiation of 20 Gy in 10 fractions to para-aortic area compared with 30 Gy in 15 fractions to para-aortic area and iliac nodes (similarly effective but less toxicity)

One large RCT identified by a systematic review found that both para-aortic strip irradiation and ipsilateral iliac lymph node irradiation were similarly effective in reducing relapse rates over 3 years in men who had undergone orchidectomy for stage 1 seminoma, but that para-aortic irradiation was associated with less nausea, vomiting, and leucopenia. Another large RCT identified by the review also found no significant difference in relapse rates over a mean of 37 months between irradiation of 20 Gy in 10 fractions and irradiation of 30 Gy in 15 fractions, and found that 20 Gy irradiation was associated with less lethargy and an earlier return to work at 4 weeks than was 30 Gy; the difference in adverse effects was no longer significant at 12 weeks. The RCT also found that six men receiving 30 Gy irradiation developed secondary malignancies over 61 months.

TRADE OFF BETWEEN BENEFITS AND HARMS

Adjuvant chemotherapy (reduced risk of relapse compared with surveillance, increased immediate toxicity and possible long term fertility problems and development of secondary malignancies)*

We found no RCTs comparing adjuvant chemotherapy versus surveillance in men who had undergone orchidectomy for stage 1 seminoma. Observational evidence suggests that adjuvant chemotherapy reduces the risk of relapse compared with surveillance but that it is associated with immediate adverse effects (sickness, diarrhoea, indigestion), and possible long term risks of reduced fertility and development of secondary malignancies. One recently completed RCT, published only in abstract form, found that a single cycle of adjuvant carboplatin and adjuvant radiotherapy were similarly effective in increasing relapse free survival. This was supported by more limited evidence from a cohort study, which found that adjuvant chemotherapy and adjuvant radiotherapy were associated with similar relapse rates and a similar rate of immediate adverse effects, although carboplatin was associated with less nausea and an earlier return to work than radiotherapy.

Adjuvant radiotherapy (reduced risk of relapse compared with surveillance, increased immediate toxicity and possible long term fertility problems and development of secondary malignancies)*

We found no RCTs comparing adjuvant radiotherapy versus surveillance or adjuvant chemotherapy in men who have undergone orchidectomy for stage 1 seminoma. Seminoma is a radio-sensitive tumour, and the current standard treatment for stage 1 seminoma is orchidectomy followed by infradiaphragmatic lymph node irradiation. Observational evidence suggests that, although some patients relapse and need salvage chemotherapy, final cure rates with orchidectomy plus radiotherapy approach 100%. Observational evidence also suggests that adjuvant radiotherapy reduces the risk of relapse compared with ▶

surveillance, but that it is associated with immediate adverse effects (sickness, diarrhoea, indigestion) and with possible long term risks of reduced fertility and development of secondary malignancies. One recently completed RCT, published only in abstract form, found that adjuvant radiotherapy and a single cycle of adjuvant carboplatin were similarly effective in increasing relapse free survival. This was supported by more limited evidence from a cohort study, which found that adjuvant radiotherapy and adjuvant chemotherapy were associated with similar relapse rates and a similar rate of immediate adverse effects, although radiotherapy was associated with more nausea and a later return to work than carboplatin.

Surveillance (avoids toxicity associated with adjuvant radiotherapy or chemotherapy, increased risk of relapse)*

We found no RCTs comparing surveillance versus adjuvant radiotherapy or chemotherapy in men who had undergone orchidectomy for stage 1 seminoma. An RCT assessing survival is unlikely to be conducted; it would be difficult to detect differences in mortality between groups because of the excellent prognosis and small differences in long term outcomes between orchidectomy alone and orchidectomy plus radiotherapy or chemotherapy. Seminoma is a radiosensitive tumour, and the standard treatment for stage 1 seminoma is orchidectomy followed by infradiaphragmatic lymph node irradiation. Observational evidence suggests that surveillance avoids the adverse effects associated with adjuvant radiotherapy or chemotherapy but it may increase the risk of delayed relapse. Therefore, it requires follow up for as long as 10 years.

UNKNOWN EFFECTIVENESS

Comparative effects of different drug combinations for adjuvant chemotherapy

One systematic review identified no RCTs or observational studies of sufficient quality comparing different drug combinations in men who had undergone orchidectomy for good prognosis stage 1 seminoma.

Comparative effects of different number of cycles of adjuvant chemotherapy

One systematic review identified no RCTs comparing different number of cycles of chemotherapy in men who had undergone orchidectomy for stage 1 seminoma. One prospective cohort study comparing one versus two cycles of carboplatin found that 9% of men receiving one cycle and 0% receiving two cycles relapsed over 2 years and that relapse free survival in both groups was 91%.

What are the effects of treatments in men with good prognosis non-stage 1 seminoma who have undergone orchidectomy?

LIKELY TO BE BENEFICIAL

Chemotherapy using etoposide plus cisplatin with or without bleomycin (increased relapse free survival compared with other combined regimens)

One RCT identified by a systematic review found that etoposide plus cisplatin increased relapse free survival over a mean 2 years compared with etoposide plus carboplatin, but found no significant difference in overall survival. Another RCT identified by the review found that adding bleomycin to two drug regimens containing etoposide reduced relapse rates and mortality over 3–4 years. A third RCT identified by the review found no significant difference in relapse free or overall survival over a mean 5 years between a two drug regimen containing etoposide plus cisplatin and a five drug regimen containing cisplatin plus vinblastine plus bleomycin plus cyclophosphamide plus dactinomycin, and found that the two drug regimen reduced toxicity.

Chemotherapy using vinblastine plus cisplatin plus bleomycin (reduced relapse rates and mortality compared with two drug regimen of vinblastine plus cisplatin)

One RCT found that that adding bleomycin to two drug regimens containing vinblastine plus cisplatin reduced relapse rates and mortality over 3–4 years.

Radiotherapy (30–36 Gy in 15–18 fractions)

We found no RCTs comparing radiotherapy versus chemotherapy or assessing different radiotherapy regimens in men who had undergone orchidectomy for good prognosis non-stage 1 seminoma. Consensus and current practice supports the use of radiotherapy at 30–36 Gy in 15–18 fractions but we found no RCT evidence to confirm that this in the optimum dose. Although one RCT found that lower doses of irradiation were as effective as 30–36 Gy in people with stage 1 seminoma, this evidence does not necessarily apply to people with non-stage 1 seminoma.

Three cycles of chemotherapy compared with four cycles (no significant difference in survival; reduced toxicity)

Two RCTs found no significant difference in overall survival with three cycles of combination chemotherapy compared with four cycles, and a third RCT found that three cycles increased survival compared with four. The RCTs also found that three cycles may reduce toxicity compared with four. All of the RCTs were conducted in men with both seminomas and non-seminomas, but it is likely that the results are generalisable to men with good prognosis non-stage 1 seminoma.

TRADE OFF BETWEEN BENEFITS AND HARMS

Radiotherapy versus chemotherapy (less toxicity with radiotherapy compared with chemotherapy; higher risk of relapse)*

We found no RCTs comparing radiotherapy versus chemotherapy or assessing different radiotherapy regimens in men who had undergone orchidectomy for good prognosis non-stage 1 seminoma. Observational evidence suggests that the immediate toxicity of radiotherapy is less than that of chemotherapy but that the risk of relapse after radiotherapy is higher with larger volume disease (>2 cm disease, stage IIB). Therefore, radiotherapy is often preferred for small volume disease (stage IIA) and chemotherapy for larger volume disease (stage IIB).

UNKNOWN EFFECTIVENESS

Adding higher compared with lower doses of cisplatin or vinblastine to a two drug chemotherapy regimen

One RCT found that adding higher dose cisplatin to vinblastine plus bleomycin increased response rates at 1 year compared with adding lower dose cisplatin. However, another RCT found no significant difference in response rates at 1 year between adding higher dose vinblastine to cisplatin plus bleomycin and adding lower dose vinblastine.

Testicular cancer: seminoma

UNLIKELY TO BE BENEFICIAL

Chemotherapy using single agent carboplatin (may be less effective than combined chemotherapy in increasing relapse free survival)

One RCT found no significant difference in relapse free or overall survival at 3 years between single agent carboplatin and etoposide plus cisplatin but it may have been underpowered to detect a clinically important difference. Another RCT published only in abstract form identified by a systematic review found that single agent carboplatin was less effective than combined chemotherapy with etoposide plus cisplatin plus ifosfamide in increasing relapse free survival over a median 52 months, but it found no significant difference in overall survival.

What are the effects of maintenance chemotherapy in men who are in remission after orchidectomy and chemotherapy for good prognosis non-stage 1 seminoma?

UNLIKELY TO BE BENEFICIAL

Maintenance chemotherapy

Two RCTs found that, in men who had complete remission after initial chemotherapy, maintenance chemotherapy using vinblastine did not reduce relapse over 1–5 years. The RCTs were conducted in men with both seminomas and non-seminomas, but it is likely that the results are generalisable to men with good prognosis non-stage 1 seminoma.

What are the effects of treatments in men with intermediate prognosis seminomas who have undergone orchidectomy?

UNKNOWN EFFECTIVENESS

Chemotherapy

One systematic review identified no RCTs of chemotherapy in men with intermediate prognosis seminomas. Intermediate prognosis tumours represent only 10% of seminomas, and no seminomas are classified as worse than this category.

*No RCTs. Based on observational evidence and consensus.

DEFINITION Although testicular symptoms are common, testicular cancer is relatively rare. Solid swellings affecting the body of the testis have a high probability (>50%) of being due to cancer. The most common presenting symptoms of cancer are a painless lump or swelling (>85%). About 10% of patients present with acute pain and 20–30% experience a heavy dragging feeling or general ache. These symptoms may lead the cancer to be initially wrongly diagnosed as epididymitis or acute testicular torsion. A small percentage present with symptoms of metastatic disease and infertility. Testicular cancers are divided into seminomas, which make up about half of all testicular tumours and which occur in older patients; and non-seminomatous tumours, comprising teratomas, mixed tumours, and other cell types, which tend to occur in younger patients. Several staging systems for testicular cancer have been developed (see table 1)Ⓣ. The most commonly used system in current practice is the International Germ Cell Consensus Classification, which classifies testicular tumours as good prognosis, intermediate prognosis, or poor prognosis.[1] Because 90% of seminomas are classified as good prognosis, this system is less useful for seminomas, so we have further divided good prognosis seminoma into stage 1 (confined to testis) and non-stage 1 (with nodal but no non-visceral metastases), based on the Royal Marsden and TNM staging systems.

INCIDENCE/ PREVALENCE There are about 1400 new cases of testicular cancer (seminona, teratoma, or mixed seminoma/teratoma) in the UK annually, with the peak incidence in men aged 25–35 years.[2] It comprises 1% of all cancers in men and is the most common tumour in young men. Incidence varies markedly with geography; a study among 10 cancer registries in Northern Europe identified a 10-fold variation, with the highest incidence rate in Denmark (7.8 per 100 000) and lowest in Lithuania (0.9 per 100 000).[3]

AETIOLOGY/ RISK FACTORS There appear to be both individual and environmental risk factors for testicular cancer.[2] Having a close relative who has had testicular cancer increases the risk of getting the disease. Inherited genetic factors may play a role in up to one in five cancers. Men are more at risk of developing cancer if they have a history of developmental abnormality (e.g. maldescent, gonadal dysgenesis), previous cancer in the opposite testis, HIV infection and/or AIDS, torsion, trauma (although this may be coincidental), and in Klinefelter's syndrome.[2] The wide geographical variation and changes over time in incidence rates imply that there are likely to be important environmental factors because the individual risk factors described above do not explain global disease patterns.[3]

PROGNOSIS Testicular tumours generally have a good prognosis. The International Germ Cell Consensus Classification (see table 1)Ⓣ classifies 90% of all seminomas as "good prognosis". These include those confined to the testis (stage 1 of the Royal Marsden or TNM system) as well as tumours with nodal but no non-pulmonary visceral metastases. The remaining 10% of seminomas, including those with non-pulmonary visceral metastases, are classified as "intermediate prognosis". No seminomas are classified as "poor prognosis". Untreated disease will progress over time, leading to large local tumours and distant spread. The first site of spread is the lymphatic system, particularly the pelvic and para-aortic lymph nodes. Haematological spread leading to lung, liver and brain metastases is less common in seminomas; 75% of men present with stage 1 disease. From the perspective of the International Germ Cell Cancer Collaborative Group prognostic classification, 90% of seminomas present as "good prognosis" with a 5 year survival of 86%, and 10% present as "intermediate prognosis" with a 5 year survival of 73%.[1] Seminoma is a radio-sensitive tumour, and the standard treatment for stage I seminoma is orchidectomy followed by infradiaphragmatic lymph node irradiation.[4] Observational evidence suggests that, with this approach, cure rates are nearly 100%.

Please refer to clinicalevidence.com for full text and references.

Varicocele

Search date September 2005

Chandra Shekhar Biyani, Jon Cartledge, and Günter Janetschek

What are the effects of treatments in men with varicocele?

UNKNOWN EFFECTIVENESS

Embolisation

We found no systematic review or RCTs comparing embolisation with no treatment or sclerotherapy. Three RCTs provided insufficient evidence on the effects of embolisation for improving fertility in men with varicocele compared with ligation techniques. We found no evidence examining the effects of embolisation on pain or discomfort caused by varicocele.

Expectant management

One systematic review of poor quality, heterogeneous RCTs in couples with male factor subfertility found no consistent evidence of difference in pregnancy rate between expectant management and surgical ligation or sclerotherapy. The review found no RCTs comparing expectant management with embolisation. We found no systematic review or RCTs examining the effects of expectant management on pain or discomfort caused by varicocele.

Sclerotherapy

One RCT found no significant difference in pregnancy rate between sclerotherapy and no treatment. We found no systematic review examining the effects of sclerotherapy on pain or discomfort caused by varicocele.

Surgical ligation

One systematic review and additional RCTs provided insufficient evidence on the effects of different surgical ligation techniques in pregnancy rate compared with no treatment, embolisation, or each other. We found no RCTs comparing surgical ligation with sclerotherapy. We found no systematic review or RCTs examining the effects of ligation on pain or discomfort caused by varicocele.

DEFINITION Varicocele is a dilation of the pampiniform plexus of the spermatic cord. Severity is commonly graded as follows: **grade 0**, only demonstrable by technical investigation; **grade 1**, palpable or visible only on Valsalva manoeuvre (straining); **grade 2**, palpable but not visible when standing upright at room temperature; and **grade 3**, visible when standing upright at room temperature. Varicocele is unilateral and left sided in at least 85% of cases. In most of the remaining cases, the condition is bilateral. Unilateral right sided varicocele is rare. Many men who have a varicocele have no symptoms. Symptoms may include testicular ache or discomfort and distress about cosmetic appearance. The condition is widely believed to be associated with male factor infertility, which is the most common reason for referral for treatment. However, evidence for a causal relationship is sparse.[1]

INCIDENCE/ PREVALENCE We found few data on the prevalence of varicocele. Anecdotally, it has been estimated that about 10–15% of men and adolescent boys in the general population have varicocele.[1] One multicentre study found that, in couples with subfertility, the prevalence of varicocele in male partners was about 12%.[2] In men with abnormal semen analysis, the prevalence of varicocele was about 25%.

AETIOLOGY/ RISK FACTORS We found no reliable data on epidemiological risk factors for varicocele, such as a family history or environmental exposures. Anatomically, varicoceles are ▶

caused by dysfunction of the valves in the spermatic vein, which allows pooling of blood in the pampiniform plexus. This is more likely to occur in the left spermatic vein than in the right because of normal anatomical asymmetry.

PROGNOSIS Varicocele is believed to be associated with subfertility, although reliable evidence is sparse. The natural history of varicocele is unclear.

Please refer to clinicalevidence.com for full text and references.

Anorexia nervosa

Search date December 2004

Janet Treasure and Ulrike Schmidt

What are the effects of treatments in anorexia nervosa?

UNKNOWN EFFECTIVENESS

Cyproheptadine

Two RCTs in inpatient settings provided insufficient evidence to assess cyproheptadine in people with anorexia nervosa.

Inpatient versus outpatient treatment setting

One small RCT found no significant difference between outpatient treatment and inpatient treatment in weight gain or Morgan Russell scale global scores at 1, 2, and 5 years in women with anorexia nervosa who did not need emergency intervention.

Psychotherapy

Small RCTs provided insufficient evidence to compare psychotherapy versus treatment as usual, dietary counselling, or each other.

Selective serotonin reuptake inhibitors

Three small RCTs, primarily in people also receiving psychotherapy, provided insufficient evidence about the effects of selective serotonin reuptake inhibitors compared with placebo or no treatment in people with anorexia nervosa. Two of the RCTs had high withdrawal rates.

Zinc

One small RCT provided insufficient evidence to assess zinc in people with anorexia nervosa.

LIKELY TO BE INEFFECTIVE OR HARMFUL

Anxiolytic drugs

We found no systematic review or RCTs. The QT interval may be prolonged in people with anorexia nervosa, and many neuroleptic drugs (haloperidol, pimozide, sertindole, thioridazine, chlorpromazine, and others) also increase the QT interval. Prolongation of the QT interval may be associated with increased risk of ventricular tachycardia, torsades de pointes, and sudden death.

Tricyclic antidepressants

Two small RCTs, one in people also receiving psychotherapy, provided insufficient evidence to assess the effects of amitriptyline on weight gain. One of the RCTs found that amitriptyline was associated with more adverse effects, such as drowsiness, dry mouth, and blurred vision. The QT interval may be prolonged in people with anorexia nervosa, and tricyclic antidepressants (amitriptyline, protriptyline, nortriptyline, doxepin, and maprotiline) also increase the QT interval. Prolongation of the QT interval may be associated with increased risk of ventricular tachycardia, torsades de pointes, and sudden death.

What are the effects of interventions to prevent or treat complications of anorexia nervosa?

UNKNOWN EFFECTIVENESS

Oestrogen treatment

We found no systematic review or RCTs on the effects of oestrogen treatment on fracture rates in women with anorexia nervosa. Two small RCTs found no significant difference between oestrogen and placebo or no treatment in bone mineral density in women with anorexia nervosa.

DEFINITION Anorexia nervosa is characterised by a refusal to maintain weight at or above a minimally normal weight (< 85% of expected weight for age and height, or body mass index < 17.5 kg/m^2), or a failure to show the expected weight gain during growth. In association with this, there is often an intense fear of gaining weight, preoccupation with weight, denial of the current low weight and its adverse impact on health, and amenorrhoea. Two subtypes of anorexia nervosa, binge–purge and restricting, have been defined.[1]

INCIDENCE/ PREVALENCE A mean incidence of anorexia nervosa in the general population of 19/100 000 a year in females and 2/100 000 a year in males has been estimated from 12 cumulative studies published between 1950 and 1992, primarily in the USA (49%) and the Netherlands (22%).[2] The highest rate was in female teenagers (age 13–19 years), where there were 50.8 cases/ 100 000 a year. A large cohort study undertaken in 1985 screened 4291 Swedish school children, aged 16 years, by weighing and subsequent interview, and found the prevalence of anorexia nervosa (defined using DSM-III and DSM-III-R criteria) to be 7/1000 for girls and 1/1000 for boys.[3] Little is known of the incidence or prevalence in Asia, South America, or Africa.

AETIOLOGY/ RISK FACTORS Anorexia nervosa has been related to family, biological, social, and cultural factors. Studies have found that anorexia nervosa is associated with a family history of anorexia nervosa (adjusted HR 11.4, 95% CI 1.1 to 89.0), bulimia nervosa (adjusted HR 3.5, 95% CI 1.1 to 14.0),[4] depression, generalised anxiety disorder, obsessive compulsive disorder, or obsessive compulsive personality disorder (adjusted RR 3.6, 95% CI 1.6 to 8.0).[5] A twin study suggested that anorexia nervosa may be related to genetic factors but it was unable to estimate reliably the contribution of non-shared environmental factors.[6] Specific aspects of childhood temperament thought to be related include perfectionism, negative self evaluation, and extreme compliance.[7] Perinatal factors include prematurity, particularly if the baby was small for gestational age (prematurity: OR 3.2, 95% CI 1.6 to 6.2; prematurity and small for gestational age: OR 5.7, 95% CI 1.1 to 28.7).[8]

PROGNOSIS One prospective study followed up 51 people with teenage onset anorexia nervosa, about half of whom received no or minimal treatment (< 8 sessions).[9] After 10 years, 14/51 people (27%) had a persistent eating disorder, three (6%) had ongoing anorexia nervosa, and six (12%) had experienced a period of bulimia nervosa. People with anorexia nervosa were significantly more likely to have an affective disorder than controls matched for sex, age, and school (lifetime risk of affective disorder 96% in people with anorexia *v* 23% in controls; ARI 73%, 95% CI 60% to 85%). Obsessive compulsive disorder was, similarly, significantly more likely to be present in people with anorexia nervosa compared with controls (30% *v* 10%; ARI 20%, 95% CI 10% to 41%). However, in 35% of people with obsessive compulsive disorder and anorexia nervosa, obsessive compulsive disorder preceded the anorexia. About half of all participants continued to have poor psychosocial functioning at 10 years (assessed using the Morgan Russell scale and Global Assessment of Functioning Scale).[9] A summary of treatment studies (68 studies published between 1953 and 1989, 3104 people, length of follow up 1–33 years) found that 43% of people recover completely (range 7–86%), 36% improve (range 1–69%), 20% develop a chronic eating disorder (range 0–43%), and 5% die from anorexia nervosa (range 0–21%).[10] Favourable prognostic factors include an early age at onset and a short interval between onset of symptoms and the beginning of treatment. Unfavourable prognostic factors include vomiting, bulimia, profound weight loss, chronicity, and a history of premorbid developmental or clinical abnormalities. The all cause standardised mortality ratio of eating disorders (anorexia nervosa and bulimia nervosa) has been estimated at 538, about three times higher than that of other psychiatric illnesses.[11] In studies published between 1970 and 1996, the average annual mortality was 0.59% a year in females in 10 eating disorder populations (1322 people), with a minimum follow up of 6 years.[12] The mortality was higher for people with lower weight and with older age at presentation. Young women with anorexia nervosa are at an increased risk of fractures later in life.[13]

Please refer to clinicalevidence.com for full text and references.

Bipolar disorder

Search date November 2004

John Geddes and David Briess

What are the effects of treatments in mania?

BENEFICIAL

Lithium

One RCT in people with bipolar type I disorder experiencing a manic episode identified by a systematic review found that lithium increased the proportion of people who responded after 3–4 weeks compared with placebo. One systematic review found that lithium increased the proportion of people who had remission of manic symptoms at 3 weeks compared with chlorpromazine. It found no significant difference in symptoms at 3–6 weeks between lithium and haloperidol, carbamazepine, or clonazepam. Another systematic review found no significant difference between lithium and valproate. One RCT identified by the systematic review found that lithium was less effective than risperidone in reducing manic symptoms at 4 weeks. RCTs found no significant difference in symptoms at 4 weeks between lithium and olanzapine or lamotrigine. Another RCT identified by a systematic review found that lithium plus olanzapine increased the proportion of people who responded at 3–6 weeks compared with placebo. Lithium can cause a range of adverse effects, including gastrointestinal disturbances, fine tremor, renal impairment, polydipsia, leucocytosis, weight gain, oedema, and hypothyroidism. The RCTs provided insufficient evidence about how the adverse effects of lithium compared with those of other antipsychotic drugs.

Olanzapine

One systematic review and one subsequent RCT in people with bipolar type I disorder found that olanzapine increased the proportion of people who responded at 3–6 weeks compared with placebo, both as monotherapy and in combination with lithium or valproate. One RCT found no significant difference in symptoms at 28 days between olanzapine and lithium. One systematic review and one subsequent RCT found that olanzapine was more effective in reducing symptoms than valproate, but found no significant difference in response or remission. They found that olanzapine increased sedation, dry mouth, and weight gain compared with valproate, but caused less nausea and nervousness. One RCT found no significant difference between haloperidol and olanzapine in remission or relapse at 6 weeks, or in time to remission. The acceptability of olanzapine may be limited by weight gain.

Valproate

One systematic review in people with bipolar type I disorder experiencing a manic episode found that valproate increased the proportion of people who responded over 3 weeks compared with placebo but caused more dizziness. It found no significant difference in response rates at 1–6 weeks between valproate and lithium, haloperidol, or carbamazepine. It found that valproate was associated with fewer extrapyramidal adverse effects and less sedation than haloperidol. The review and one subsequent RCT found that valproate was less effective in reducing manic symptoms than olanzapine, but found no significant difference in response or remission. They found that valproate increased nausea and nervousness compared with olanzapine, but reduced ▶

sedation, dry mouth, and weight gain. One RCT identified by a systematic review found that valproate plus olanzapine increased the proportion of people who responded at 3–6 weeks compared with placebo.

LIKELY TO BE BENEFICIAL

Carbamazepine

One RCT found that extended release carbamazepine increased the response rate at 21 days compared with placebo, but it also increased adverse effects. RCTs in people with bipolar type I disorder experiencing a manic episode identified by a systematic review found no significant difference in manic symptoms at 4–6 weeks between carbamazepine and lithium or valproate. The review provided insufficient evidence to assess the adverse effects of carbamazepine.

Clonazepam

One small RCT found that clonazepam reduced manic symptoms, but not psychotic symptoms, at 5 days compared with placebo. One systematic review found no significant difference in symptoms at 3–6 weeks between lithium and clonazepam.

Haloperidol

We found no RCTs comparing haloperidol versus placebo in people with mania. RCTs in people with bipolar type I disorder experiencing a manic episode identified by a systematic review found no significant difference in manic symptoms at 1–3 weeks between haloperidol and lithium or valproate, although haloperidol was associated with more extrapyramidal adverse effects and sedation than valproate. One RCT found no significant difference between haloperidol and olanzapine in remission or relapse at 6 weeks, or in time to remission.

Risperidone

We found no RCTs comparing risperidone alone versus placebo. One RCT in people with mania taking lithium, valproate, or carbamazepine found no significant difference in symptoms between adding risperidone and placebo, and found that adding risperidone increased extrapyramidal adverse effects. Another RCT in people with bipolar type I disorder experiencing a manic episode found that risperidone reduced manic symptoms at 4 weeks compared with lithium.

Ziprasidone

One RCT found that ziprasidone increased the proportion of people who responded at 3 weeks compared with placebo, but also increased adverse effects such as sedation, dizziness, and akathisia.

UNKNOWN EFFECTIVENESS

Chlorpromazine

One very small RCT in people with mania found limited evidence that chlorpromazine may improve manic symptoms over 7 weeks more than placebo or imipramine. One systematic review found that fewer people had remission of symptoms at 3 weeks with chlorpromazine than with lithium. The review and RCT provided insufficient evidence to assess the adverse effects of chlorpromazine.

Gabapentin

One RCT in people with bipolar type I disorder experiencing a manic or mixed episode already taking lithium or valproate found that adding gabapentin was less effective in reducing manic symptoms over 10 months than placebo. Gabapentin was associated with somnolence, dizziness, diarrhoea, and memory loss.

Lamotrigine

We found no RCTs comparing lamotrigine versus placebo in people with mania. One RCT in people with bipolar type I disorder experiencing a manic episode identified by a systematic review found no significant difference in manic symptoms at 4 weeks between lamotrigine and lithium. The review provided insufficient evidence to assess the adverse effects of lamotrigine.

Quetiapine

One RCT in adolescents found limited evidence that quetiapine increased the proportion of people who responded at 6 weeks compared with placebo, but caused sedation.

Topiramate

One RCT identified by a systematic review found no significant difference between topiramate and placebo in symptoms at 3 weeks.

What are the effects of treatments in bipolar depression?

LIKELY TO BE BENEFICIAL

Antidepressants

One systematic review found that antidepressants (fluoxetine, paroxetine, imipramine, tranylcypromine, and deprenyl) significantly increased treatment response at 4–10 weeks compared with placebo. The review found that serotonin specific reuptake inhibitors increased clinical response at 4–10 weeks compared with tricyclic antidepressants. The analysis may have been too small to detect a clinically important difference. Antidepressants are associated with manic switching. The review suggested that tricyclic antidepressants may be more likely to induce mania than selective serotonin reuptake inhibitors.

Lamotrigine

One RCT in people with bipolar type I disorder experiencing a depressive episode identified by a systematic review found that lamotrigine 200 mg increased the proportion of people who responded over 7 weeks compared with placebo. Lamotrigine 200 mg increased the proportion of people with headache compared with placebo.

UNKNOWN EFFECTIVENESS

Carbamazepine

One systematic review identified no RCTs of sufficient quality to assess carbamazepine in people with bipolar depression.

Lithium

One systematic review identified no RCTs of sufficient quality to assess lithium in people with bipolar depression.

Bipolar disorder

Psychological treatments

We found no systematic review or RCTs of psychological treatments in people with bipolar depression.

Topiramate

One systematic review identified no RCTs of topiramate in people with bipolar depression. One subsequent RCT in people taking lithium or valproate found no significant difference in symptoms at 8 weeks between adding topiramate and adding bupropion. The RCT found that a third of people taking topiramate and a fifth of people taking bupropion withdrew because of adverse effects, including anxiety, increase or decrease in appetite, blurred vision, backache, headache, and nausea.

Valproate

We found no systematic review or RCTs of valproate in people with bipolar depression.

What are the effects of interventions to prevent relapse of mania or bipolar depression?

BENEFICIAL

Lithium

Systematic reviews and three subsequent RCTs found that lithium reduced relapse over 2 years compared with placebo. They found no significant difference in relapse between lithium and valproate, carbamazepine, or lamotrigine. RCTs found that more people had adverse effects, including diarrhoea, somnolence, and tremor, with lithium than with placebo, and that lithium may increase hypothyroidism. They found that lithium caused more polyuria, thirst, and diarrhoea than valproate but less sedation and infection. The review and subsequent RCT found that lithium was associated with more adverse effects than carbamazepine. Three subsequent RCTs found that lithium caused more diarrhoea and tremor than lamotrigine.

LIKELY TO BE BENEFICIAL

Carbamazepine

One small RCT identified by a systematic review found no significant difference between carbamazepine and placebo in effectiveness, but is likely to have been too small to detect a clinically important difference. One systematic review and one subsequent RCT found no significant difference between carbamazepine and lithium in the proportion of people who relapsed over 1–3 years. The review and subsequent RCT found that carbamazepine was associated with fewer adverse effects than lithium.

Cognitive therapy

Two RCTs identified by a systematic review found that cognitive therapy reduced relapse over 6–12 months compared with usual care. Another RCT found no significant difference between cognitive therapy and usual care in the proportion of people who relapsed over 6 months, although it is likely to have been underpowered to detect a clinically important difference between treatments. The RCTs provided insufficient evidence to assess the adverse effects of cognitive therapy.

Education to recognise symptoms of relapse

One RCT identified by a systematic review found limited evidence that an educational programme to recognise symptoms of relapse reduced manic relapse over 18 months, but it may have increased depressive episodes. A second RCT identified by the review found that group psychoeducation for 14 weeks reduced recurrence at 2 years compared with control in people taking standard drug treatments. A subsequent RCT, which may have included a subset of participants included in the second RCT identified by the review, found that group psychoeducation for 20 weeks reduced recurrence and hospitalisation at 2 years compared with control in highly compliant people taking standard drug treatments.

Family focused psychoeducation

One RCT found that 21 sessions of family focused psychoeducation reduced relapse up to 2 years compared with two family sessions plus crisis management. Another RCT found that family focused psychoeducation may reduce relapse compared with individual focused therapy. The RCTs gave no information on adverse effects.

Lamotrigine

Four RCTs found that lamotrigine reduced relapse compared with placebo. RCTs found no significant difference between lamotrigine and lithium in the proportion of people who relapsed, and found that lithium caused more diarrhoea than lamotrigine, but fewer headaches.

Valproate

One RCT identified by a systematic review found that valproate reduced relapse over 12 months compared with placebo, but increased tremor, weight gain, and alopecia. One systematic review found no significant difference between lithium and valproate in relapse over 12 months. The review found that valproate caused more sedation and infection than lithium but less polyuria, thirst, and diarrhoea.

UNKNOWN EFFECTIVENESS

Antidepressant drugs

One systematic review provided insufficient evidence to assess antidepressants in preventing relapse of bipolar disorder.

DEFINITION Bipolar disorder (bipolar affective disorder, manic depressive disorder) is characterised by marked mood swings between mania (mood elevation) and bipolar depression that cause significant personal distress or social dysfunction, and are not caused by drugs or known physical disorders. **Bipolar type I disorder** is diagnosed when episodes of depression are interspersed with mania or mixed episodes. **Bipolar type II disorder** is diagnosed when depression is interspersed with less severe episodes of elevated mood that do not lead to dysfunction or disability (hypomania). Bipolar disorder has been subdivided in several further ways (see table 1) Ⓣ.[1]

INCIDENCE/ PREVALENCE One 1996 cross-national community based study (38 000 people) found lifetime prevalence rates of bipolar disorder ranging from 0.3% in Taiwan to 1.5% in New Zealand.[2] It found that men and women were at similar risk, and that the age at first onset ranged from 19–29 years (average of 6 years earlier than first onset of major depression).

AETIOLOGY/ RISK FACTORS The cause of bipolar disorder is uncertain, although family and twin studies suggest a genetic basis.[3] The lifetime risk of bipolar disorder is increased in first

Bipolar disorder

degree relatives of a person with bipolar disorder (40–70% for a monozygotic twin; 5–10% for other first degree relatives). If the first episode of mania occurs in an older adult, it may be secondary mania due to underlying medical or substance induced factors.[4]

PROGNOSIS Bipolar disorder is a recurring illness and one of the leading causes of worldwide disability, especially in the 15–44 year age group.[3] One 4 year inception cohort study (173 people treated for a first episode of mania or mixed affective disorder) found that 93% of people no longer met criteria for mania at 2 years (median time to recover from a syndrome 4.6 weeks), but that only 36% had recovered to premorbid function.[4] It found that 40% of people had a recurrent manic (20%) or depressive (20%) episode within 2 years of recovering from the first episode. A meta-analysis, comparing observed versus expected rates of suicide in an age and sex matched sample of the general population, found that the lifetime prevalence of suicide was about 2%, or 15 times greater than expected, in people with bipolar disorder.[5]

Please refer to clinicalevidence.com for full text and references.

Bulimia nervosa

Search date June 2005

Phillipa J Hay and Josue Bacaltchuk

What are the effects of treatments for bulimia nervosa in adults?

LIKELY TO BE BENEFICIAL

Cognitive behavioural therapy for bulimia nervosa

One RCT identified by a systematic review found that cognitive behavioural therapy for bulimia nervosa (CBT-BN) improved the clinical effects of bulimia compared with waiting list control or no treatment. One RCT found no significant difference in remission rate or symptoms between CBT plus exposure response prevention and CBT-BN. Two RCTs found no significant difference in remission of binge vomiting between guided self help CBT and CBT-BN after about 1 year. One systematic review identified two RCTs, which found that significantly more people abstained from both binge eating and purging after CBT-BN compared with interpersonal psychotherapy at the end of treatment, but not at 1 year if follow up. One RCT found no significant difference between hypnobehavioural therapy and CBT-BN for bulimia behavioural symptoms but the two groups were not balanced at baseline. One RCT found no clinically important difference in binge frequency between motivational enhancement therapy and CBT-BN. Two RCTs found no significant difference in remission or symptoms between CBT-BN and fluoxetine. Two RCTs comparing tricyclic antidepressants versus CBT-BN found mixed results. One found that CBT-BN improved remission compared with imipramine, and the other found no significant difference in remission rate between CBT-BN and desipramine. Two RCTs found no significant difference in remission rates or symptoms between CBT-BN and CBT-BN plus tricyclic antidepressants. Two RCTs found no significant difference in remission rates or symptoms between CBT-BN and CBT-BN plus fluoxetine.

Combination treatment (antidepressants plus cognitive behavioural therapy as effective as either treatment alone)

Two RCTs found no significant difference in remission rates or symptoms between cognitive behavioural therapy for bulimia nervosa (CBT-BN) plus tricyclic antidepressants and CBT-BN or tricyclic antidepressants alone. One RCT identified by a systematic review found no significant difference in remission rates or symptoms between CBT-BN plus fluoxetine and CBT-BN or fluoxetine alone. One RCT found no significant difference in remission rates between unguided self help CBT plus fluoxetine and unguided self help CBT alone or fluoxetine alone.

Monoamine oxidase inhibitors

RCTs identified by a systematic review, found that monoamine oxidase inhibitors improved remission rates compared with placebo, but found no significant difference in improvement in bulimic symptoms or depression scores.

Selective serotonin reuptake inhibitors (evidence limited to fluoxetine)

Three RCTs identified by a systematic review found that fluoxetine 60 mg daily increased the number of people with clinical improvement but not remission compared with placebo. Two RCTs found no significant difference in remission or symptoms between cognitive behavioural therapy for bulimia nervosa and fluoxetine. We found no RCTs of other selective serotonin reuptake inhibitors ▶

(fluvoxamine, paroxetine, sertraline, or citalopram). One RCT found no significant difference in remission between fluoxetine and pure self help cognitive behavioural therapy or between fluoxetine and combination treatment.

Tricyclic antidepressants

One systematic review found that tricyclic antidepressants (desipramine and imipramine) improved bulimic symptoms and reduced binge eating compared with placebo. Two RCTs comparing tricyclic antidepressants versus cognitive behavioural therapy for bulimia nervosa (CBT-BN) found mixed results. One RCT found that imipramine was not as effective at improving remission compared with CBT-BN, and the other found no significant difference in remission rate between desipramine and CBT-BN. Both of these RCTs found no significant difference between the tricyclic antidepressant alone and the combination treatment.

UNKNOWN EFFECTIVENESS

Cognitive behavioural therapy plus exposure response prevention enhancement

One RCT found no significant difference in vomiting frequency between cognitive behavioural therapy (CBT) plus exposure response prevention and being on a waiting list, although it found that exposure response prevention improved depression scores compared with being on a waiting list. One RCT identified by a systematic review found no significant difference in remission rate or symptoms between CBT plus exposure response prevention and CBT for bulimia nervosa.

Cognitive orientation therapy

We found no RCTs of cognitive orientation therapy in people with bulimia nervosa.

Dialectical behavioural therapy

We found limited evidence from one small RCT that dialectical behavioural therapy increased cessation of binge eating or purging and improved bulimic symptoms compared with being on a waiting list. It found no significant difference in depression scores between dialectical behavioural therapy and being on a waiting list.

Guided self help cognitive behavioural therapy

One RCT found no significant difference in behavioural symptoms between face to face or telephone guided self help cognitive behavioural therapy and being on a waiting list. Two RCTs found no significant difference in remission of binge vomiting between guided self help cognitive behavioural therapy and cognitive behavioural therapy for bulimia nervosa after about 1 year.

Hypnobehavioural therapy

One RCT found limited evidence that hypnobehavioural therapy improved abstinence from bingeing and purging in the short term compared with being on a waiting list. The same RCT found no significant difference between hypnobehavioural therapy and cognitive behavioural therapy for bulimia behavioural symptoms but the two groups were not balanced at baseline.

Interpersonal psychotherapy (as effective as cognitive behavioural therapy for bulimia nervosa)

We found no RCTs comparing interpersonal psychotherapy versus no treatment, placebo, or waiting list control. One systematic review identified two RCTs, which found that significantly fewer people abstained from both binge eating and purging with interpersonal psychotherapy compared with cognitive behavioural therapy for bulimia nervosa at the end of treatment. However, there was no difference between treatments at 1 year follow up.

Mirtazapine

We found no RCTs.

Motivational enhancement therapy

We found no RCTs comparing motivational enhancement therapy versus no treatment, placebo, or being on a waiting list. One RCT found no clinically important difference in binge frequency between motivational enhancement therapy and cognitive behavioural therapy for bulimia nervosa for 4 weeks.

Nefazodone

We found no RCTs.

Pure or unguided self help cognitive behavioural therapy

Two RCTs found no significant difference in remission or reduction in binge purge frequency between pure or unguided self help cognitive behavioural therapy (CBT) and being on a waiting list. One RCT found no significant difference in remission between unguided self help CBT and fluoxetine alone or unguided self help CBT plus fluoxetine.

Reboxetine

We found no RCTs.

Venlafaxine

We found no RCTs.

What are the effects of discontinuing treatment in people with remission?

UNLIKELY TO BE BENEFICIAL

Discontinuing fluoxetine

One RCT has found that continuing fluoxetine 60 mg daily is more effective than placebo for maintaining a reduction in vomiting frequency in people who have responded well to an initial 8 week course of fluoxetine.

DEFINITION Bulimia nervosa is an intense preoccupation with body weight and shape, with regular episodes of uncontrolled overeating of large amounts of food (binge eating) associated with use of extreme methods to counteract the feared effects of overeating. If a person also meets the diagnostic criteria for anorexia nervosa, then the diagnosis of anorexia nervosa takes precedence.[1] Bulimia nervosa can be difficult to identify because of extreme secrecy about binge eating and purgative behaviour. Weight may be normal but there is often a history of anorexia nervosa or restrictive dieting. Some people alternate between anorexia nervosa and bulimia nervosa. Some RCTs included people with subthreshold bulimia nervosa or a related eating disorder, for example, binge eating disorder. Where possible, only results relevant to bulimia nervosa are reported in this chapter.

INCIDENCE/ PREVALENCE In community based studies, the prevalence of bulimia nervosa is between 0.5% and 1.0% in young women, with an even social class distribution.[2-6] About 90% of people diagnosed with bulimia nervosa are women. The numbers presenting with bulimia nervosa in industrialised countries increased

Bulimia nervosa

during the decade that followed its recognition in the late 1970s and "a cohort effect" is reported in community surveys,[2,7,8] implying an increase in incidence. The prevalence of eating disorders such as bulimia nervosa is lower in non-industrialised populations,[9] and varies across ethnic groups. African-American women have a lower rate of restrictive dieting than white American women, but they have a similar rate of recurrent binge eating.[10]

AETIOLOGY/ RISK FACTORS Young women from the developed world who restrict their dietary intake are at greatest risk of developing bulimia nervosa and other eating disorders. One community based case control study compared 102 people with bulimia nervosa versus 204 healthy controls and found higher rates of the following in people with the eating disorder: obesity, mood disorder, sexual and physical abuse, parental obesity, substance misuse, low self esteem, perfectionism, disturbed family dynamics, parental weight/shape concern, and early menarche.[11] Compared with a control group of 102 women who had other psychiatric disorders, women with bulimia nervosa had higher rates of parental problems and obesity.

PROGNOSIS A 10 year follow up study (50 people with bulimia nervosa from a placebo controlled trial of mianserin treatment) found that 52% receiving placebo had fully recovered, and only 9% continued to experience full symptoms of bulimia nervosa.[12] A larger study (222 people from a trial of antidepressants and structured, intensive group psychotherapy) found that, after a mean follow up of 11.5 years, 11% still met criteria for bulimia nervosa, whereas 70% were in full or partial remission.[13] Short term studies found similar results: about 50% of people made a full recovery, 30% made a partial recovery, and 20% continued to be symptomatic.[14] There are few consistent predictors of longer term outcome. Good prognosis has been associated with shorter illness duration, a younger age of onset, higher social class, and a family history of alcohol abuse.[12] Poor prognosis has been associated with a history of substance misuse,[15] premorbid and paternal obesity,[16] and, in some studies, personality disorder.[17-20] One study (102 women) of the natural course of bulimia nervosa found that 31% and 15% still had the disorder at 15 months and 5 years, respectively.[21] Only 28% received treatment during the follow up period. In an evaluation of the response to cognitive behavioural therapy, early progress (by session 6) best predicted outcome.[22] A subsequent systematic review of the outcome literature found no consistent evidence to support early intervention and a better prognosis.[23] A more recent systematic review evaluating the cost effectiveness of treatments and prognostic indicators found only four consistent pretreatment predictors of poorer outcome for treatment of bulimia nervosa: features of borderline personality disorder, concurrent substance misuse, low motivation for change, and a history of obesity.[24]

Please refer to clinicalevidence.com for full text and references.

Deliberate self harm (and attempted suicide)

Search date October 2005

G Mustafa Soomro

What are the effects of treatments for deliberate self harm in adolescents and adults?

UNKNOWN EFFECTIVENESS

Cognitive therapy

One RCT of 120 adults who had recently deliberately self harmed found that cognitive therapy in addition to usual care reduced repetition of suicide attempts, severity of depression, and hopelessness compared with usual care alone after 18 months. A separate RCT found no significant difference in repeat self harm rates at 1 year between manual assisted cognitive therapy and usual treatment (problem solving approaches, dynamic psychotherapy, short term counselling, or referral to a general practitioner or a voluntary group).

Continuity of care

One systematic review identified one RCT, which found limited evidence that follow up after hospital treatment with the same therapist may increase repetition of deliberate self harm compared with follow up with a different therapist over 3 months. However, the difference between groups may be explained by a higher level of risk factors for repetition in the group receiving follow up with the same therapist.

Dialectical behavioural therapy

One systematic review including one RCT found limited and equivocal evidence that dialectical behavioural therapy may reduce the proportion of people who repeat deliberate self harm over 12 months compared with usual care.

Emergency card

One RCT identified by a systematic review provided insufficient evidence to assess the efficacy of emergency card intervention compared with usual care.

Flupentixol depot injection

One systematic review including one small RCT found that flupentixol depot injection reduced the proportion of people who repeated deliberate self harm over 6 months compared with placebo. However, we were unable to draw reliable conclusions from this small study. Typical antipsychotics such as flupentixol are associated with a wide range of adverse effects.

Hospital admission

One systematic review found no significant difference between hospital admission and immediate discharge in the proportion of people who repeated deliberate self harm over 16 weeks.

Mianserin

One systematic review provided insufficient evidence to assess the effects of mianserin on deliberate self harm behaviour.

Deliberate self harm (and attempted suicide)

Nurse led case management

One RCT found no significant difference between nurse led case management and usual care in the proportion of people who were admitted to emergency departments for episodes of deliberate self harm over 12 months.

Oral antipsychotics

We found no RCTs of sufficient quality that examined the effects of oral antipsychotics on deliberate self harm behaviour.

Paroxetine

One systematic review, which included one RCT in people receiving concurrent psychotherapy who had previously deliberately self harmed, found no significant difference between paroxetine and placebo in the proportion of people who repeated self harm over 12 months. It found that paroxetine increased diarrhoea and tremor compared with placebo. Paroxetine, like other selective serotonin re-uptake inhibitors, has been linked to suicidal ideation. In clinical trials in children and adolescents with depression it showed higher rates of suicide related events. Abrupt withdrawal of selective serotonin re-uptake inhibitors should be avoided. Withdrawal adverse effects include headache, nausea, paraesthesia, dizziness, and anxiety. Extrapyramidal reactions (including orofacial dystonias) and withdrawal syndrome have been reported more commonly with paroxetine than with other selective serotonin re-uptake inhibitors.

Problem solving therapy

One systematic review of RCTs found no significant difference between problem solving therapy and usual care in the proportion of people who repeated deliberate self harm over 6–12 months. A second systematic review found that problem solving therapy reduced symptoms of depression, anxiety, and hopelessness, and improved problems compared with usual care.

Psychodynamic interpersonal therapy

One RCT found that brief psychodynamic interpersonal therapy for 4 weeks reduced repetition of deliberate self harm, depression, and suicidal ideation over 6 months compared with usual care. However, we were unable to draw reliable conclusions from this single RCT.

Telephone contact

One RCT found no significant difference between telephone contact at 4 and 8 months and usual care in repetition of deliberate self harm, global functioning, and suicidal ideation over 12 months.

UNLIKELY TO BE BENEFICIAL

General practice based guidelines

One large cluster randomised trial comparing the use of general practitioner guidelines for management of deliberate self harm versus usual care found no significant difference in the proportion of people who repeated deliberate self harm over 12 months or in the time to repetition of self harm.

Intensive outpatient follow up plus outreach

One systematic review found no significant difference in the proportion of people who repeated deliberate self harm over 4–12 months between intensive outpatient follow up plus outreach and usual care.

Deliberate self harm (and attempted suicide)

DEFINITION Deliberate self harm is an acute non-fatal act of self harm carried out deliberately in the form of an acute episode of behaviour by an individual with variable motivation.[1] The intention to end life may be absent or present to a variable degree. Other terms used to describe this phenomenon are "attempted suicide" and "parasuicide". For the purpose of this chapter the term deliberate self harm will be used throughout. Common methods of deliberate self harm include self cutting and self poisoning, such as overdosing on medicines. Some acts of deliberate self harm are characterised by high suicidal intent, meticulous planning (including precautions against being found out), and severe lethality of the method used. Other acts of deliberate self harm are characterised by no or low intention of suicide, lack of planning and concealing of the act, and low lethality of the method used. The related term of "suicide" is defined as an act with a fatal outcome that is deliberately initiated and performed by the person with the knowledge or expectation of its fatal outcome.[1] This review focuses on the literature with recent deliberate self harm (in people aged ≥ 15 years) as the main presenting problem and main selection criterion for the RCTs. It excludes RCTs in which deliberate self harm is an outcome in studies of others disorders, such as depression or borderline personality disorder, rather than the primary presenting problem. Deliberate self harm is not defined in the *Diagnostic and statistical manual of mental disorders* (DSM IV)[2] or the *International classification of mental and behavioural disorders* (ICD-10).[3]

INCIDENCE/ PREVALENCE Based on data from 16 European countries between 1989 and 1992, the lifetime prevalence of deliberate self harm in people treated in hospital and other medical facilities, including general practice settings, is estimated at about 3% for women and 2% for men.[4] Over the last 50 years there has been a rise in the incidence of deliberate self harm in the UK.[4] A reasonable current estimate is about 400/100 000 population a year.[5] In two community studies in the USA, 3–5% of responders said that they had made an attempt at deliberate self harm at some time.[6] Self poisoning using organophosphates is particularly common in developing countries.[7] A large hospital (catering for 900 000 people) in Sri Lanka reported 2559 adult hospital admissions and 41% occupancy of medical intensive care beds for deliberate self harm with organophosphates over 2 years.[8] An international survey using representative community samples of adults (aged 18–64 years) reported lifetime prevalence of self reported deliberate self harm of 3.82% in Canada, 5.93% in Puerto Rico, 4.95% in France, 3.44% in West Germany, 0.72% in Lebanon, 0.75% in Taiwan, 3.2% in Korea, and 4.43% in New Zealand.[6]

AETIOLOGY/ RISK FACTORS Familial, biological, and psychosocial factors may contribute to deliberate self harm. Evidence for genetic factors includes a higher risk of familial suicide and greater concordance in monozygotic than dizygotic twins for deliberate self harm.[9] Evidence for biological factors includes reduced cerebrospinal fluid 5-hydroxyindoleacetic acid levels and a blunted prolactin response to the fenfluramine challenge test, indicating a reduction in the function of serotonin in the central nervous system.[10] People who deliberately self harm also show traits of impulsiveness and aggression, inflexible and impulsive cognitive style, and impaired decision making and problem solving.[11] Deliberate self harm is more likely to occur in women, young adults, and people who are single or divorced, of low education level, unemployed, disabled, or suffering from a psychiatric disorder,[12] particularly depression,[13] substance misuse,[14] borderline and antisocial personality disorders,[15] severe anxiety disorders,[16] and physical illness.[17]

PROGNOSIS Suicide is highest during the first year after deliberate self harm.[18] One systematic review found median rates of repetition of 16% (interquartile range [IQR] 12% to 25%) within the first year, 21% (IQR 12% to 30%) within 1–4 years, and 23% (IQR 11% to 32%) within 4 years or longer. It found median mortality from suicide after deliberate self harm of 1.8% (IQR 0.8% to 2.6%)

Deliberate self harm (and attempted suicide)

within the first year, 3.0% (IQR 2.0% to 4.4%) within 1–4 years, 3.4% (IQR 2.5% to 6.0%) within 5–10 years, and 6.7% (IQR 5.0% to 11.0%) within 9 years or longer.[18] Repetition of deliberate self harm is more likely in people aged 25–49 years who are unemployed, divorced, from lower social class, or who suffer from substance misuse, depression, hopelessness, powerlessness, personality disorders, have unstable living conditions or live alone, have a criminal record, previous psychiatric treatment, a history of stressful traumatic life events, or a history of coming from a broken home or of family violence.[12] Factors associated with risk of suicide after deliberate self harm are being aged over 45 years, male sex, being unemployed, retired, separated, divorced, or widowed, living alone, having poor physical health, psychiatric disorder (particularly depression, alcoholism, schizophrenia, and sociopathic personality disorder), high suicidal intent in current episode including leaving a written note, violent method used in current episode, and history of previous deliberate self harm.[19]

Please refer to clinicalevidence.com for full text and references.

Dementia

Search date February 2006

James Warner, Rob Butler, and Balaji Wuntakal

What are the effects of treatments on cognitive symptoms of dementia?

BENEFICIAL

Donepezil

Two systematic reviews and one subsequent RCT found that, compared with placebo, donepezil improved cognitive function and global clinical state at up to 2 years in people with mild to severe Alzheimer's disease, and donepezil improved cognitive function but not global state in people with vascular dementia at 24 weeks. One large RCT identified by a review found that donepezil delayed the median time to "clinically evident functional decline" by 5 months compared with placebo. One open label RCT in people with mild to moderate Alzheimer's disease found no significant difference in cognitive function at 12 weeks between donepezil and rivastigmine, although fewer people taking donepezil withdrew from the trial. One RCT in people with Alzheimer's disease found no significant difference between donepezil and galantamine in cognitive function or adverse effects at 1 year. We found no RCTs of donepezil in people with Lewy body dementia.

Galantamine

RCTs found that galantamine improved cognitive function and global clinical state over 6 months compared with placebo in people with Alzheimer's disease or vascular dementia. One RCT in people with Alzheimer's disease found no significant difference between donepezil and galantamine in cognitive function or adverse effects at 1 year. We found no RCTs of galantamine in people with Lewy body dementia.

LIKELY TO BE BENEFICIAL

Ginkgo biloba

RCTs found limited evidence that ginkgo biloba improved cognitive function at up to 52 weeks compared with placebo in people with Alzheimer's disease or vascular dementia. Preparations of ginkgo biloba available without prescription differ in terms of purity and concentrations of active ingredients compared with the high purity extract (EGb 761) used in most RCTs. We found no RCTs of ginkgo biloba in people with Lewy body dementia.

Memantine

RCTs identified by a systematic review found that memantine improved cognition and global impression in people with mild to moderate Alzheimer's disease, and improved cognition and activities of daily living in people with moderate to severe Alzheimer's disease after 24–28 weeks. Two RCTs found that memantine improved cognitive function after 28 weeks in people with mild to moderate vascular dementia, but had no effect on global state. We found no RCTs of memantine in people with Lewy body dementia.

TRADE OFF BETWEEN BENEFITS AND HARMS

Rivastigmine

One systematic review found that rivastigmine improved cognitive function and clinical global state in people with Alzheimer's disease. Two RCTs found that, ▶

Dementia

compared with placebo, rivastigmine improved cognitive and global functioning in people with Lewy body dementia or dementia due to Parkinson's disease. Adverse effects such as nausea, vomiting, and anorexia were common with rivastigmine treatment. One open label RCT in people with mild to moderate Alzheimer's disease found no significant difference in cognitive function at 12 weeks between rivastigmine and donepezil, although more people taking rivastigmine withdrew from the trial. We found no RCTs of rivastigmine in people with vascular dementia.

Tacrine

Two systematic reviews found limited evidence that tacrine improved cognitive function and global state at 3–36 weeks compared with placebo in people with Alzheimer's disease, but adverse effects, including nausea, vomiting, diarrhoea, anorexia, and abdominal pain, were common. We found no RCTs of tacrine in people with Lewy body or vascular dementia.

UNKNOWN EFFECTIVENESS

Music therapy

One RCT found that music based exercise improved cognition after 3 months compared with one to one conversation with a therapist. Poor studies identified by two systematic reviews provided insufficient evidence to assess the effects of music therapy in people with dementia.

Non-steroidal anti-inflammatory drugs

One RCT in people with Alzheimer's disease found no significant difference in cognitive function after 25 weeks' treatment with diclofenac plus misoprostol compared with placebo. Another RCT in people with Alzheimer's disease found that indometacin improved cognitive function versus placebo after 6 months in people with Alzheimer's disease. A third RCT found no significant difference between naproxen or rofecoxib and placebo in cognitive function at 1 year. The use of non-steroidal anti-inflammatory drugs (NSAIDS) has been linked to an increased risk of heart failure and stroke. Rofecoxib has been withdrawn from the market worldwide. We found no RCTs of NSAIDS in people with Lewy body dementia.

Omega 3 (fish oil)

We found no systematic review or RCTs of Omega 3 in people with dementia.

Physostigmine

One small RCT in people with Alzheimer's disease found limited evidence that slow release physostigmine improved cognitive function over 12 weeks compared with placebo, but adverse effects, including nausea, vomiting, diarrhoea, dizziness, and stomach pain, were common. We found no RCTs of physostigmine in people with Lewy body or vascular dementia.

Reminiscence therapy

One systematic review found that reminiscence therapy improved cognition but had no effect on behavioural measures. The included studies used diverse outcome measures and were often small.

Selegiline

One systematic review found that, in people with mild to moderate Alzheimer's disease, selegiline for 2–4 months improved cognitive function compared with placebo. It found no significant difference in global clinical state or in activities of daily living. There is limited evidence from a few RCTs that outcomes beyond 4 months are not improved by selegiline. We found no RCTs of selegiline in people with Lewy body or vascular dementia.

Statins

We found no systematic review or RCTs of statins in people with dementia.

UNLIKELY TO BE BENEFICIAL

Oestrogen

One systematic review found insufficient evidence that oestrogen with or without progestogen improved cognitive symptoms in postmenopausal women with dementia. However, there is concern that oestrogen treatment may increase the risk of developing breast cancer and cardiovascular events. The review found no RCTs of oestrogen in people with Lewy body or vascular dementia

What are the effects of treatments on behavioural and psychological symptoms of dementia?

LIKELY TO BE BENEFICIAL

Carbamazepine

One RCT found that carbamazepine reduced agitation and aggression over 6 weeks compared with placebo in people with various types of dementia and behavioural and psychological symptoms. We found no RCTs of carbamazepine in people with Lewy body dementia.

TRADE OFF BETWEEN BENEFITS AND HARMS

Haloperidol

One systematic review in people with various types of dementia plus behavioural and psychological symptoms found no significant difference in agitation between haloperidol and placebo at 6–16 weeks. However, it found that haloperidol may reduce aggression at 3–13 weeks. It found that haloperidol increased the frequency and severity of extrapyramidal symptoms compared with placebo. Another systematic review in people with various types of dementia plus behavioural and psychological symptoms found limited evidence that haloperidol and risperidone were similarly effective in reducing agitation over 12 weeks, but found that haloperidol caused more frequent and more severe extrapyramidal symptoms. Two small RCTs found insufficient evidence on the effects of trazodone on global state or behaviour compared with haloperidol after 9–16 weeks. Behavioural problems may resolve spontaneously, and further research is required to determine whether newer atypical antipsychotics have a better ratio of benefits to harms than older antipsychotics, particularly in people with Lewy body dementia.

Olanzapine

One systematic review in people with various types of dementia plus behavioural and psychological symptoms of dementia found modest evidence for efficacy. Olanzapine has been associated with an increased risk of stroke, and is not considered safe in people with psychosis associated with dementia.

Risperidone

RCTs identified by two systematic reviews found that, in people with vascular dementia, Alzheimer's disease, and mixed dementia, risperidone improved behavioural and psychological symptoms compared with placebo over 12

Dementia

weeks. One review found limited evidence that risperidone and haloperidol were similarly effective in reducing agitation over 12 weeks, but that risperidone caused fewer and less severe extrapyramidal symptoms. Risperidone has been associated with an increased risk of mortality and cerebrovascular events, including stroke and transient ischaemic attacks. Risperidone has not been shown to be safe in people with psychosis associated with dementia.

UNKNOWN EFFECTIVENESS

Benzodiazepines

One systematic review found limited evidence that intramuscular lorazepam reduces agitation at 2 hours.

Donepezil

Two systematic reviews of four RCTs found conflicting effects of donepezil on behavioural symptoms in people with moderate to severe Alzheimer's disease.

Galantamine

RCTs provided inconclusive evidence about the effects of galantamine compared with placebo on behavioural and psychiatric symptoms in people with mild to moderate Alzheimer's disease.

Quetiapine

One RCT found no significant effects of quetiapine on the behavioural and psychological symptoms of dementia.

Rivastigmine

We found one systematic review and one subsequent RCT, which found no significant effects of rivastigmine on the behavioural and psychological symptoms of dementia compared with placebo.

Sodium valproate/valproic acid

One systematic review found limited evidence that sodium valproate/valproic acid had no effect on agitation, aggression, and hostility after 6 weeks compared with placebo in people with dementia plus behavioural and psychological problems.

Trazodone

One systematic review found insufficient evidence on the effects of trazodone on global state and behaviour compared with placebo after 6–16 weeks. Two small RCTs found insufficient evidence on the effects of trazodone on global state or behaviour compared with haloperidol after 9–16 weeks. One small RCT reported that adverse effects were less common with trazodone than with haloperidol.

DEFINITION **Dementia** is characterised by chronic, global, non-reversible impairment in cerebral function. It usually results in loss of memory (initially of recent events), loss of executive function (such as the ability to make decisions or sequence complex tasks), and changes in personality. **Alzheimer's disease** is a type of dementia characterised by an insidious onset and slow deterioration, and involves impairments in speech, motor, personality, and executive function. It should be diagnosed after other systemic, psychiatric, and neurological causes of dementia have been excluded clinically and by laboratory investigation. **Vascular dementia** is often due to multiple infarcts or generalised small vessel disease. It often presents with a stepwise deterioration in cognitive function with or without language and motor dysfunction. It usually occurs in the presence of vascular risk factors (diabetes, hypertension, arteriosclerosis, and smoking). Characteristically, it has a more sudden onset and stepwise progression than Alzheimer's disease. **Lewy body dementia** is a type of dementia that involves insidious impairment of executive function with Parkinsonism, visual hallucinations, fluctuating cognitive abilities, and increased risk of falls or autonomic failure.[1,2] Careful clinical examination of people with mild to moderate dementia, and the use of established diagnostic criteria, accurately identify 70–90% of causes confirmed at post mortem.[3,4] In all types of dementia, people will experience problems with cognitive functioning and are likely to experience behavioural and psychological symptoms of dementia. Where possible, we have divided outcomes into cognitive or behavioural/psychological, although there is often considerable crossover between these outcomes, both clinically and in research.

INCIDENCE/ PREVALENCE About 6% of people aged over 65 years and 30% of people aged over 90 years have some form of dementia.[5] Dementia is rare before the age of 60 years. Alzheimer's disease and vascular dementia (including mixed dementia) are each estimated to account for 35–50% of dementia, and Lewy body dementia is estimated to account for up to 20% of dementia in the elderly, varying with geographical, cultural, and racial factors.[1,5-9] There are numerous other causes of dementia, all of which are relatively rare, including frontotemporal dementia, alcohol related dementia, Huntington's disease, normal pressure hydrocephalus, HIV infection, syphilis, subdural haematoma, and some cerebral tumours.

AETIOLOGY/ RISK FACTORS **Alzheimer's disease:** The cause of Alzheimer's disease is unclear. A key pathological process is deposition of abnormal amyloid in the central nervous system.[10] Most people with the relatively rare condition of early onset Alzheimer's disease (before age 60 years) exhibit an autosomal dominant inheritance owing to mutations in presenilin or amyloid precursor protein genes. Several gene mutations (on *APP*, *PS-1*, and *PS-2* genes) have been identified. Later onset dementia is sometimes clustered in families, but specific gene mutations have not been identified. Head injury, Down's syndrome, and lower premorbid intellect may be risk factors for Alzheimer's disease. **Vascular dementia:** Vascular dementia is related to cardiovascular risk factors, such as smoking, arteriosclerosis, hypertension, and diabetes. **Lewy body dementia:** The cause of Lewy body dementia is unknown. Brain acetylcholine activity is reduced in many forms of dementia, and the level of reduction correlates with cognitive impairment. Many treatments for Alzheimer's disease enhance cholinergic activity.[1,6]

PROGNOSIS **Alzheimer's disease:** Alzheimer's disease usually has an insidious onset with progressive reduction in cerebral function. Diagnosis is difficult in the early stages. Median life expectancy after diagnosis is 5–6 years.[11] **Vascular dementia:** We found no reliable data on prognosis. **Lewy body dementia:** People with Lewy body dementia have an average life expectancy of about 6 years after diagnosis.[5] Behavioural problems, depression, and psychotic symptoms are common in all types of dementia.[12,13] Eventually, most people with dementia find it difficult to perform simple tasks without help.

Please refer to clinicalevidence.com for full text and references.

Mental health

Depression in adults

Search date September 2004

Rob Butler, Stuart Carney, Andrea Cipriani, John Geddes, Simon Hatcher, Jonathan Price, and Michael Von Korff

What are the effects of treatments in mild to moderate or severe depression?

BENEFICIAL

Cognitive therapy (in mild to moderate depression)

One systematic review in younger and older adults found that cognitive therapy improved symptoms compared with no treatment. Three systematic reviews in younger and older adults with mild to moderate depression found that psychological therapies (mainly interpersonal psychotherapy and cognitive therapy) increased the proportion of people who were in remission over 10–34 weeks compared with control (usual care, usual care plus pill placebo, or supportive therapy). These reviews did not report results for cognitive therapy alone compared with control. One systematic review found no significant difference between cognitive therapy and interpersonal therapy, though found that cognitive therapy was more successful than combined interpersonal therapy, brief psychodynamic therapy or supportive therapy. One systematic review found no significant difference in remission rates or improvement of depressive symptoms between short term psychodynamic psychotherapy and cognitive therapy. One systematic review of poor quality RCTs in people aged 55 years or over with mild to moderate depression found no significant difference in symptoms between psychological treatments (such as cognitive therapy or cognitive behavioural therapy) and no treatment.

Electroconvulsive therapy (in severe depression)

One systematic review in people with moderate to severe depressive disorder, many of whom were inpatients, found that electroconvulsive therapy improved symptoms over 1–6 weeks' treatment compared with simulated electroconvulsive therapy or antidepressant drugs. The review found that bilateral electroconvulsive therapy improved symptoms compared with unilateral electroconvulsive therapy and that high dose electroconvulsive therapy was more effective than low dose. The degree of reported short term cognitive impairment seemed to be inversely related to treatment efficacy. Another systematic review provided insufficient evidence to assess electroconvulsive therapy in older adults. Because electroconvulsive therapy may be unacceptable to some people and, because it is a short term treatment, there is consensus that it should normally be reserved for people who cannot tolerate or have not responded to antidepressant drug treatment, although it may be useful when a rapid response is required.

Interpersonal psychotherapy (in mild to moderate depression)

Two systematic reviews in adults with mild to moderate depression found that psychological therapies (mainly interpersonal psychotherapy and cognitive therapy) increased the proportion of people who were in remission over 10–34 weeks compared with control (usual care, usual care plus pill placebo, or supportive therapy). These reviews did not report results for interpersonal therapy alone compared with control. One RCT identified by a third review found that interpersonal therapy increased response rates compared with usual care, ▶

though the review found no difference between cognitive therapy and interpersonal therapy. One RCT found that group interpersonal psychotherapy improved depressive symptoms compared with no treatment in depressed adults in Uganda. One systematic review in older adults found no significant difference between interpersonal therapy, psychodynamic psychotherapy or no treatment.

Monoamine oxidase inhibitors versus other prescription antidepressant drugs

Three systematic reviews found no significant difference in outcomes with different kinds of antidepressant drug (tricyclic antidepressants, selective serotonin reuptake inhibitors, or monoamine oxidase inhibitors). One systematic review found that monoamine oxidase inhibitors were less effective than tricyclic antidepressants in people with severe depressive disorders. However, the review found that monoamine oxidase inhibitors may be more effective in atypical depressive disorders with biological features such as increased sleep and increased appetite.

Prescription antidepressant drugs (tricyclic antidepressants [including low dose tricyclic antidepressants], selective serotonin reuptake inhibitors, monoamine oxidase inhibitors, reboxetine, or venlafaxine) improved symptoms compared with placebo in mild to moderate and severe depression

Systematic reviews and subsequent RCTs in people aged 18 years or over in primary and secondary care found that prescription antidepressant drugs (tricyclic antidepressants [including low dose tricyclic antidepressants], selective serotonin reuptake inhibitors, monoamine oxidase inhibitors, or venlafaxine) were effective for treatment of all grades of depressive disorders compared with placebo. However, the most robust available evidence of efficacy of treatment with antidepressant drugs is in the pharmacological management of moderate and severe depression. One systematic review and two subsequent RCTs in people aged 55 years or over with all grades of depressive disorder found that tricyclic antidepressants, selective serotonin reuptake inhibitors, or monoamine oxidase inhibitors reduced the proportion of people who failed to recover over 26–49 days compared with placebo. The reviews gave little information on severe adverse effects of antidepressant drugs compared with placebo. There is evidence of publication bias in trials of selective serotonin reuptake inhibitors. Current evidence indicates no clear relationship between selective serotonin reuptake inhibitors and increased risk for suicide in adults, but selective serotonin reuptake inhibitors and tricyclic antidepressants may induce or worsen suicidal ideation and behaviour during the early phases of treatment. This may be because of increased agitation and activation. In children and adolescents selective serotonin reuptake inhibitors generally increase adverse events compared with placebo, and the safety of these drugs is currently under review by regulatory authorities in several countries.

Selective serotonin reuptake inhibitors and related drugs versus other prescription antidepressant drugs

Three systematic reviews found no significant difference in outcomes with different kinds of antidepressant drug (tricyclic antidepressants, selective serotonin reuptake inhibitors, or monoamine oxidase inhibitors), although one systematic review found that selective serotonin reuptake inhibitors were less effective than venlafaxine in increasing the proportion of people who responded. RCTs in people with major depression found similar response rates at 6 weeks between fluoxetine and reboxetine, but found that reboxetine may be slightly more effective in improving social functioning. One RCT found that mirtazapine was significantly more effective than sertraline during the first 2 weeks of treatment, though this benefit did not last beyond 2 weeks. Another RCT found no significant difference between paroxetine and mirtazapine after 24 weeks. One systematic review found that selective serotonin reuptake inhibitors were associated with fewer adverse effects than TCAs, but the difference was small. Two systematic reviews, one retrospective cohort study, and two case control studies found contradictory evidence about the risk of suicide in adults treated with selective serotonin reuptake inhibitors. One of the systematic reviews and the case control studies reported no significant difference in risk of suicide between selective serotonin reuptake inhibitors and TCAs. One RCT and observational data suggested that abrupt withdrawal of selective serotonin reuptake inhibitors was associated with symptoms including dizziness and rhinitis, and that these symptoms are more likely with drugs with a short half life, such as paroxetine. There is evidence of publication bias in trials of selective serotonin reuptake inhibitors. Current evidence indicates no clear relationship between selective serotonin reuptake inhibitors and increased risk for suicide in adults, but selective serotonin reuptake inhibitors and TCAs may induce or worsen suicidal ideation and behaviour during the early phases of treatment. This may be because of increased agitation and activation. In children and adolescents selective serotonin reuptake inhibitors generally increase adverse events compared with placebo, and the safety of these drugs is currently under review by regulatory authorities in several countries.

Tricyclic antidepressants versus other prescription antidepressant drugs

Three systematic reviews found no significant difference in outcomes with different kinds of antidepressant drug (tricyclic antidepressants, selective serotonin reuptake inhibitors, or monoamine oxidase inhibitors). One systematic review and one subsequent RCT found no significant difference between tricyclic antidepressants and venlafaxine in the proportion of people who responded over 1–12 months. Another systematic review suggested that tricyclic antidepressants were more effective than monoamine oxidase inhibitors in people with severe depressive disorders, but may be less effective in atypical depressive disorders with biological features such as increased sleep and increased appetite. A third systematic review found that tricyclic antidepressants were associated with higher rates of adverse effects than selective serotonin reuptake inhibitors, but the difference was small. One systematic review and two case control studies found no significant difference in risk of suicide between selective serotonin reuptake inhibitors and tricyclic antidepressants. Two RCTs, primarily in people with severe depression, found no significant difference in symptoms at 4 weeks between desipramine or imipramine and reboxetine, but results were sensitive to outcome scales used. One systematic review found no significant difference between milnacipran and imipramine in people with major depressive disorder, though found an overall higher incidence of adverse events in the imipramine group. One systematic review found no significant difference between low dosage tricyclic antidepressants and standard dosage tricyclic antidepressants in the proportion of responders at 6–8 weeks. One systematic review found that combined antidepressants (primarily tricyclic antidepressants) with benzodiazepines increased response rate within 1 week versus antidepressants alone, though this difference was not significant at 6 weeks.

Venlafaxine versus other prescription antidepressant drugs

One systematic review and one RCT found no significant difference between venlafaxine and tricyclic antidepressants in the proportion of people who responded over 1–12 months. The review found that venlafaxine increased the proportion of people who responded compared with selective serotonin reuptake inhibitors, although one subsequent RCT found no significant difference in numbers of responders between extended release venlafaxine and escitalopram. One RCT found no significant difference between venlafaxine and mirtazapine in proportion of responders, but found that both treatments improved depressive symptoms from baseline.

LIKELY TO BE BENEFICIAL

Combining prescription antidepressant drugs and psychological treatments (in mild to moderate and severe depression)

Two systematic reviews found that a combination of pharmacotherapy and psychotherapy improved depressive symptoms compared with either treatment alone. One subsequent RCT of poor quality found no significant difference in response rate between combination therapy with sertraline and interpersonal therapy and sertraline alone. A second subsequent RCT found no significant difference between short term psychodynamic psychotherapy plus antidepressants and antidepressants alone, though subgroup analysis found that combination therapy was more effective in people with depression and a personality disorder.

Non-directive counselling (in mild to moderate depression)

One systematic review in people aged 18 years or over with recent onset psychological problems, including depression, found that brief, non-directive counselling in primary care reduced symptom scores in the short term (< 6 months) in people with mild to moderate depression compared with usual care. However, it found no significant difference in scores in the long term (> 6 months). One RCT found that eight sessions of counselling significantly improved symptoms of anxiety and depression compared with no treatment.

Reboxetine versus other antidepressant drugs (in mild to moderate or severe depression)

Two RCTs, primarily in people with severe depression, found no significant difference in symptoms at 4 weeks between reboxetine and desipramine or imipramine, but results were sensitive to outcome scales used. RCTs in people with major depression found similar response rates at 6 weeks between reboxetine and fluoxetine, and found that reboxetine may slightly improve social functioning.

St John's Wort (more effective than placebo, as effective as other antidepressants in mild to moderate depression)

One systematic review found that, in people with depressive disorders, St John's Wort (*Hypericum perforatum*) improved depressive symptoms over 4–12 weeks compared with placebo. The review found no significant difference between St John's Wort and tricyclic antidepressants or selective serotonin reuptake inhibitors. The results of the RCTs should be interpreted with caution as many did not use standardised preparations of St John's Wort and doses of antidepressants varied. Questions have been raised regarding the methodological quality of available studies, which have examined heterogenous patient populations and inconsistently used standardised symptom rating instruments. St John's Wort is likely to interact with many more drugs than has been previously reported.

UNKNOWN EFFECTIVENESS

Befriending (in mild to moderate depression)

One small RCT provided insufficient evidence to assess befriending in people with mild to moderate depression.

Depression in adults

Exercise (in mild to moderate depression)

One systematic review in younger and older adults found limited evidence from poor RCTs that exercise may improve symptoms compared with no treatment, and may be as effective as cognitive therapy. One poor RCT in older adults identified by the review found limited evidence that exercise may be as effective as antidepressant drugs in improving symptoms and may reduce relapse over 10 months.

Problem solving therapy (in mild to moderate depression)

One systematic review in younger and older adults with mild to moderate depression in primary care found that psychological therapies (including problem solving therapy) improved outcomes compared with usual care. The review did not report results of problem solving therapy alone in people with moderate depression. It found no significant difference between problem solving therapy and usual care in symptoms at 6–11 weeks in people with mild depression or dysthymia. One large subsequent RCT found that problem solving therapy increased the proportion of people who were not depressed at 6 months compared with usual care. However, it found no significant difference at 1 year. Another smaller RCT found no significant difference in symptoms at 8 or 26 weeks between problem solving therapy and usual care for people presenting to general practitioners with emotional disorders, most of whom were depressed. RCTs found insufficient evidence to assess the relative efficacy of drug and non-drug treatment in severe depression.

What are the effects of interventions in treatment resistant depression?

UNKNOWN EFFECTIVENESS

Lithium augmentation

RCTs provided insufficient evidence to assess augmentation of prescription antidepressant drug treatment with lithium in younger and older adults with treatment resistant depression.

Pindolol augmentation

RCTs provided insufficient evidence to assess augmentation of prescription antidepressant drug treatment with pindolol in younger and older adults with treatment resistant depression.

Which interventions reduce relapse rates?

BENEFICIAL

Continuing prescription antidepressant drugs (reduced risk of relapse after recovery in people with mild to moderate depression)

One systematic review found that continuing prescription antidepressant drug treatment after recovery reduced the proportion of people who experienced a relapse over 1–3 years compared with placebo. The effect of continuing antidepressants was independent of the underlying risk of relapse, the duration of treatment before randomisation, or the duration of previous antidepressant treatment. Five subsequent RCTs also found that continuing antidepressant treatment reduced absolute risk of recurrence by up to one half compared with treatment discontinuation. Two RCTs in people aged over 60 years found that continued treatment with dosulepin (dothiepin) or citalopram after recovery reduced the risk of relapse over 1–2 years compared with placebo, but may increase the risk of ischaemic heart disease. One RCT found no benefit of continuing treatment with sertraline compared with placebo for a further 2 years in preventing relapse.

UNKNOWN EFFECTIVENESS

Cognitive therapy (weak evidence that may reduce relapse over 1–2 years after stopping treatment in people with mild to moderate depression compared with antidepressant drugs)

One systematic review in younger and older adults with mild to moderate depression found limited evidence by combining relapse rates across different RCTs that cognitive therapy reduced the risk of relapse over 1–2 years after stopping treatment compared with antidepressant drugs. Four subsequent RCTs found limited evidence that cognitive therapy reduced relapse rates up to a year post remission. We found no systematic review or RCTs specifically in older adults.

Relapse prevention programme (improved symptoms over 1 year after recovery in people with mild to moderate depression but no significant difference in relapse rates)

One RCT identified by a systematic review found that, in people who had recovered after 8 weeks of antidepressant treatment, a relapse prevention programme improved depressive symptoms over 1 year compared with usual care. However, there were no significant differences in relapse rates.

What are the effects of interventions to improve delivery of treatments?

LIKELY TO BE BENEFICIAL

Care pathways (in mild to moderate depression)

Two systematic reviews and eight subsequent RCTs found that care pathways improved the effectiveness of treatment for depression (antidepressant drugs or cognitive behavioural therapy) compared with usual care in people aged over 18 years with mild to moderate depression. These pathways included collaborative working between primary care clinicians and psychiatrists, intensive patient education, case management, and telephone support. The RCTs also found that clinical practice guidelines and educational strategies without other organisational processes improved neither detection nor outcome of depression compared with usual care. It was not possible to determine from the results which components of care pathways were most effective. One RCT in depressed elderly people found that initial care by a community mental health team did not improve depressive symptoms compared with usual general practitioner care. Another RCT found that management of depressed elderly people by a community nurse improved symptoms of depression and increased recovery after 3 months compared with usual general practitioner care. One RCT in people aged over 60 years with major depression, dysthymic depression, or both, treated in a variety of primary care clinics found that collaborative care was more effective than usual care in reducing depressive symptoms. One RCT found no significant effect of treatment recommendations on symptoms of depression in older depressed people compared with usual physician care. However, diagnosis of depression and prescription of antidepressants was greater in the intervention group.

Depression in adults

DEFINITION Depressive disorders are characterised by persistent low mood, loss of interest and enjoyment, and reduced energy. They often impair day to day functioning. Most of the RCTs assessed in this review classify depression using the Diagnostic and Statistical Manual of Mental Disorders (DSM-IV)[1] or the International Classification of Mental and Behavioural Disorders (ICD-10).[2] DSM-IV divides depression into major depressive disorder or dysthymic disorder. **Major depressive disorder** is characterised by one or more major depressive episodes (i.e. at least 2 weeks of depressed mood or loss of interest accompanied by at least 4 additional symptoms of depression). **Dysthymic disorder** is characterised by at least 2 years of depressed mood for more days than not, accompanied by additional symptoms that do not reach the criteria for major depressive disorder.[1] ICD-10 divides depression into mild to moderate or severe depressive episodes.[2] Mild to moderate depression is characterised by depressive symptoms and some functional impairment. Severe depression is characterised by additional agitation or psychomotor retardation with marked somatic symptoms.[2] **Treatment resistant depression** is defined as an absence of clinical response to treatment with a tricyclic antidepressant at a minimum dose of 150 mg daily of imipramine (or equivalent drug) for 4–6 weeks.[3] In this review, we use both DSM-IV and ICD-10 classifications, but treatments are considered to have been assessed in severe depression if the RCT included inpatients. **Older adults:** Older adults are generally defined as people aged 65 years or older. However, some of the RCTs of older people in this review included people aged 55 years or over. The presentation of depression in older adults may be atypical: low mood may be masked and anxiety or memory impairment may be the principal presenting symptoms. Dementia should be considered in the differential diagnosis of depression in older adults.[4] This review does not cover intervention in women with postnatal depression (see postnatal depression) or seasonal affective disorder.

INCIDENCE/ PREVALENCE Depressive disorders are common, with a prevalence of major depression between 5% and 10% of people seen in primary care settings.[5] Two to three times as many people may have depressive symptoms but do not meet DSM-IV criteria for major depression. Women are affected twice as often as men. Depressive disorders are the fourth most important cause of disability worldwide and they are expected to become the second most important cause by 2020.[6,7] **Older adults:** Between 10% and 15% of older people have depressive symptoms, although major depression is relatively rare in older adults.[8]

AETIOLOGY/ RISK FACTORS The causes of depression are uncertain but are thought to include both childhood events and current psychosocial adversity. Recent studies suggest that genetic factors may also be important, indicating that several chromosomal regions may be involved. Phenotypes, however, do not seem to exhibit classic Mendelian inheritance. Psychiatric research has also focused on the role that psychosocial factors, such as social context and personality dimensions, play in depression. Many theories emphasise the importance of temperament (differences in the adaptive systems), which can increase vulnerability to mood disturbances. Impairment in social relationships, gender, socioeconomic status, and dysfunctional cognition may also play a role. It seems that integrative models, which take into account the interaction of biological and social variables, offer the most reliable way to approach the complex aetiology of depression.

PROGNOSIS About half of people suffering a first episode of major depressive disorder experience further symptoms in the next 10 years.[9] **Older adults:** One systematic review (search date 1996, 12 prospective cohort studies, 1268 people, mean age 60 years) found that the prognosis may be especially poor in elderly people with a chronic or relapsing course of depression.[10] Another systematic review (search date 1999, 23 prospective cohort studies in people aged ≥ 65 years, including 5 identified by the first review) found that depression in older people was associated with increased mortality (15 studies; pooled OR 1.73, 95% CI 1.53 to 1.95).[11]

Please refer to clinicalevidence.com for full text and references.

Generalised anxiety disorder

Search date February 2006

Christopher Gale

What are the effects of treatments for generalised anxiety disorder?

BENEFICIAL

Cognitive behavioural therapy

Two systematic reviews and four subsequent RCTs found that cognitive behavioural therapy (using a combination of interventions, such as exposure, relaxation, and cognitive restructuring) improved anxiety and depression over 4–12 weeks compared with waiting list control, anxiety management alone, relaxation alone, or non-directive psychotherapy. Two subsequent RCTs found no significant difference in symptoms at 13 weeks and 6 months between cognitive therapy and applied relaxation. One subsequent RCT found no significant difference in anxiety and depression at 24 months between cognitive therapy (with a behavioural component), cognitive therapy (without a behavioural component), and applied relaxation with visualisation.

LIKELY TO BE BENEFICIAL

Antidepressants (imipramine, opipramol, paroxetine, sertraline, escitalopram and venlafaxine)

One systematic review found that antidepressants (imipramine, paroxetine, and venlafaxine) improved symptoms over 4–28 weeks compared with placebo. RCTs found that escitalopram improved anxiety outcomes compared with placebo at 8 weeks. One RCT found that opipramol, paroxetine, or sertraline improved symptoms compared with placebo. One subsequent RCT found no significant difference in response rates between venlafaxine and placebo at 24 weeks, although a second subsequent RCT found that venlafaxine increased remission. RCTs found no significant difference in effect among these antidepressants or between antidepressants and benzodiazepines or buspirone. RCTs and observational studies found that antidepressants are associated with sedation, dizziness, nausea, falls, and sexual dysfunction. One RCT found that escitalopram increased rates of sexual dysfunction compared with paroxetine. One RCT found no significant difference in Hamilton Anxiety Scale or number of responses between kava and opopramol at 8 weeks.

Applied relaxation

We found no RCTs comparing applied relaxation versus placebo or no treatment. Two RCTs found no significant difference in symptoms at 13 weeks and 6 months between applied relaxation and cognitive behavioural therapy. One subsequent RCT found no significant difference in anxiety and depression at 24 months between applied relaxation with visualisation, cognitive therapy (with a behavioural component), and cognitive therapy (without a behavioural component).

Buspirone

RCTs found that buspirone improved symptoms over 4–9 weeks compared with placebo. RCTs found no significant difference in symptoms over 6–8 weeks ▶

between buspirone and antidepressants (venlafaxine), diazepam, or hydroxyzine, or kava, but the studies might have lacked power to detect clinically important differences among treatments. Adverse events associated with buspirone included increased nausea and somnolence.

Hydroxyzine

Three RCTs found that, compared with placebo, hydroxyzine improved symptoms of anxiety at 4, 5, or 12 weeks, although in one the RCTs the difference at 5 weeks was not significant. One of the RCTs found that hydroxyzine increased somnolence and headaches compared with placebo. One RCT found no significant difference between hydroxyzine and bromazepam in the proportion of people who responded after 6 weeks. Another RCT found no significant difference between hydroxyzine and buspirone in the proportion of people who responded after 4 weeks.

Pregabalin

Two RCTs found that pregabalin improved Hamilton Anxiety Scale scores at 4 weeks compared with placebo. One RCT found no significant difference in Hamilton Anxiety Scale scores between pregabalin and lorazepam at 4 weeks, whereas another RCT found that pregabalin improved anxiety compared with alprazolam at 4 weeks. Adverse effects associated with pregabalin included somnolence, dizziness, and headache.

TRADE OFF BETWEEN BENEFITS AND HARMS

Antipsychotic drugs (trifluoperazine)

One large RCT found that trifluoperazine reduced anxiety after 4 weeks compared with placebo, but caused more drowsiness, extrapyramidal reactions, and other movement disorders. We found no RCTs on antipsychotic drugs other than trifluoperazine.

Benzodiazepines

Two systematic reviews found that benzodiazepines reduced symptoms over 2–9 weeks compared with placebo. RCTs found no significant difference in symptoms over 3–8 weeks between alprazolam and bromazepam or mexazolam, or between benzodiazepines and buspirone, hydroxyzine, abecarnil, or antidepressants. One RCT found no significant difference in anxiety scores between lorazepam and pregabalin at 4 weeks, whereas another RCT found that alprazolam was less effective than pregabalin at improving anxiety scores at 4 weeks. RCTs and observational studies found that benzodiazepines increased the risk of dependence, sedation, industrial accidents, and road traffic accidents. If used in late pregnancy or while breast feeding, benzodiazepines may cause adverse effects in neonates. One systematic review of poor quality RCTs provided insufficient evidence to assess long term treatment with benzodiazepines.

Kava

One systematic review found that kava improved Hamilton Anxiety Scale scores from baseline compared with placebo at 4–24 weeks. However, one subsequent RCT found no significant difference in Anxiety Status Inventory scores at 4 weeks between kava and placebo. One RCT found no significant difference in Hamilton Anxiety Scale score or number of responses between kava and opopramol or buspirone at 8 weeks. Case report evidence has associated kava with liver damage.

Generalised anxiety disorder

UNKNOWN EFFECTIVENESS

Abecarnil

One RCT found limited evidence that low dose abecarnil improved symptoms compared with placebo. Another RCT found no significant difference in symptoms at 6 weeks between abecarnil and placebo or diazepam. Both RCTs found that at higher doses abecarnil increased drowsiness compared with placebo.

DEFINITION Generalised anxiety disorder (GAD) is defined as excessive worry and tension about every day events and problems, on most days, for at least 6 months, to the point where the person experiences distress or has marked difficulty in performing day to day tasks.[1] It may be characterised by the following symptoms and signs: increased motor tension (fatigability, trembling, restlessness, and muscle tension); autonomic hyperactivity (shortness of breath, rapid heart rate, dry mouth, cold hands, and dizziness); and increased vigilance and scanning (feeling keyed up, increased startling, and impaired concentration), but not panic attacks.[1] One non-systematic review of epidemiological and clinical studies found marked reduction in quality of life and psychosocial functioning in people with anxiety disorders (including GAD).[2] It also found that people with GAD had low overall life satisfaction and some impairment in ability to fulfil roles, social tasks, or both.[2]

INCIDENCE/ PREVALENCE One overview of observational studies found that 0.2–1.0% of adults in Europe had had GAD in the past month, 0.1–2.1% had had GAD in the past year, and 0.1–21.7% had had it during their lives.[3] It found that 4–7.9% of consecutive primary care attendees fulfilled DSM-IV criteria for GAD, and that 22% of people presenting with anxiety were diagnosed with GAD. GAD usually co-occurs with other diagnoses. The review found that up to 75% of people diagnosed with GAD had co-morbid conditions. One community survey in Germany found that 91% of people had co-morbid conditions,[3] and a community survey in Europe found that 51.6% of men and 75.7% of women had co-morbid conditions.[4] The reliability of the measures used to diagnose GAD in epidemiological studies is unsatisfactory.[5,6] One US study, with explicit diagnostic criteria (DSM-III-R), estimated that 5% of people will develop GAD at some time during their lives.[6] A recent cohort study of people with depressive and anxiety disorders found that 49% of people initially diagnosed with GAD retained this diagnosis over 2 years.[7] The incidence of GAD in men is half the incidence in women[8] and is lower in older people.[9] A non-systematic review (20 observational studies in younger and older adults) suggested that autonomic arousal to stressful tasks was decreased in older people, and that older people became accustomed to stressful tasks more quickly than did younger people.[10]

AETIOLOGY/ RISK FACTORS GAD is believed to be associated with an increase in the number of minor life events, independent of demographic factors,[11,12] but this finding is also common in people with other diagnoses.[7] One non-systematic review (5 case control studies) of psychological sequelae to civilian trauma found that rates of GAD reported in four of the five studies were significantly increased compared with a control population (RR 3.3, 95% CI 2.0 to 5.5).[13] One systematic review (search date 1997) of cross-sectional studies found that bullying (or peer victimisation) was associated with a significant increase in the incidence of GAD (effect size 0.21, CI not reported).[14] One systematic review (search date not reported, 2 family studies, 45 index cases, 225 first degree relatives) found a significant association between GAD in the index cases and in their first degree relatives (OR 6.1, 95% CI 2.5 to 14.9).[15] One systematic review of twin and family studies (search date 2003, 23 twin studies, 12 family studies) found an association between GAD, other anxiety disorders, and depression, and postulated that a common genetic factor was implicated.[16]

PROGNOSIS One systematic review found that 25% of adults with GAD will be in full remission after 2 years, and 38% will have a remission after 5 years.[17] The Harvard–Brown anxiety research program reported 5 year follow up of 167 people with GAD.[18] During this period, the weighted probability for full remission was 38% and for at least partial remission was 47%; the probability of relapse from full remission was 27% and relapse from partial remission was 39%.

Please refer to clinicalevidence.com for full text and references.

Obsessive compulsive disorder

Search date July 2005

G Mustafa Soomro

What are the effects of initial treatments in adults?

BENEFICIAL

Behavioural therapy

We found no RCTs comparing behavioural therapy versus no treatment. One systematic review and one subsequent RCT found that behavioural therapy improved symptoms compared with relaxation. The review and three subsequent RCTs found no consistent evidence of a difference in symptoms between behavioural therapy and cognitive or cognitive behavioural therapy. One small RCT found that behavioural therapy plus relaxation improved symptoms at 6 weeks compared with waiting list control. It found no significant difference between behavioural therapy plus relaxation and behavioural therapy plus cognitive therapy either at the end of 6 weeks' treatment or at 12 month follow up. One systematic review provided insufficient evidence from indirect comparisons to compare serotonin reuptake inhibitors versus behavioural therapy. RCTs provided insufficient evidence to assess the effects of adding serotonin reuptake inhibitors to behavioural or cognitive therapy.

Cognitive or cognitive behavioural therapy

We found no RCTs that compared cognitive therapy versus no treatment. Two RCTs found that cognitive behavioural therapy improved symptoms compared with no treatment or waiting list control after 6–12 weeks. One systematic review and three subsequent RCTs found no consistent evidence of a difference in symptoms between behavioural therapy and cognitive or cognitive behavioural therapy.

Serotonin reuptake inhibitors (citalopram, clomipramine, fluoxetine, fluvoxamine, paroxetine, sertraline)

RCTs found that selective and non-selective serotonin reuptake inhibitors (citalopram, clomipramine, fluoxetine, fluvoxamine, paroxetine) improved symptoms compared with placebo but increased adverse effects. Two systematic reviews found inconsistent results concerning the effects of sertraline compared with placebo. RCTs have found that selective and non-selective serotonin reuptake inhibitors (citalopram, clomipramine, fluoxetine, fluvoxamine, paroxetine, sertraline) improve symptoms compared with tricyclic antidepressants or monoamine oxidase inhibitors. RCTs found no consistent evidence of a difference in efficacy among serotonin reuptake inhibitors, but found that the non-selective serotonin reuptake inhibitor clomipramine was associated with more adverse effects than were selective serotonin reuptake inhibitors. One RCT found no significant difference in symptoms between clomipramine and venlafaxine, but it is likely to have been underpowered to detect a clinically important difference. One RCT found no significant difference in symptoms between venlafaxine and paroxetine. One systematic review provided insufficient evidence from indirect comparisons to compare serotonin reuptake inhibitors versus behavioural therapy. RCTs provided insufficient evidence to assess the effects of adding serotonin reuptake inhibitors to behavioural or cognitive therapy. Selective serotonin reuptake inhibitors have been linked to suicidal ideation. Abrupt withdrawal of selective serotonin reuptake inhibitors should be avoided.

UNKNOWN EFFECTIVENESS

Behavioural or cognitive therapy plus serotonin reuptake inhibitors (compared with behavioural or cognitive therapy alone)

RCTs provided insufficient evidence to assess the effects of adding serotonin reuptake inhibitors to behavioural or cognitive therapy.

Electroconvulsive therapy

We found no RCTs of electroconvulsive therapy in people with obsessive compulsive disorder.

What are the best forms of maintenance treatment in adults?

UNKNOWN EFFECTIVENESS

Optimum duration of maintenance treatment with serotonin reuptake inhibitors

RCTs provided insufficient evidence to define the optimum duration of maintenance treatment with serotonin reuptake inhibitors.

What are the effects of treatments in adults who have not responded to initial treatment with serotonin reuptake inhibitors?

LIKELY TO BE BENEFICIAL

Addition of antipsychotics to serotonin reuptake inhibitors

Five small RCTs in people unresponsive to serotonin reuptake inhibitors found that the addition of antipsychotics improved symptoms compared with serotonin reuptake inhibitors plus placebo. However, one small RCT found no significant difference between fluoxetine plus olanzapine compared with fluoxetine plus placebo after 6 weeks.

DEFINITION Obsessive compulsive disorder (OCD) involves obsessions, compulsions, or both, that are not caused by drugs or a physical disorder, and which cause significant personal distress or social dysfunction.[1,2] The disorder may have a chronic or an episodic course. **Obsessions** are recurrent and persistent ideas, images, or impulses that cause pronounced anxiety and that the person perceives to be self produced. **Compulsions** are repetitive behaviours or mental acts performed in response to obsessions or according to certain rules, which are aimed at reducing distress or preventing certain imagined dreaded events. People with OCD may have insight into their condition, in that obsessions and compulsions are usually recognised and resisted. There are minor differences in the criteria for OCD between the third, revised third, and fourth editions of the *Diagnostic and Statistical Manual* (DSM-III, DSM-III-R, and DSM-IV)[1] and *The ICD-10 Classification of Mental and Behavioural Disorders*.[2]

INCIDENCE/ PREVALENCE One national, community based survey of OCD in the UK (1993, 10 000 people) found that 1.0% of men and 1.5% of women reported symptoms in the previous month.[3] A survey of a random sample of people living in private households in the UK (2000, 8580 adults aged 16–74 years) found that 1.1% of those surveyed reported symptoms of OCD during the previous week.[4] An epidemiological catchment area survey carried out in the USA in 1984 (about 10 000 people) found an age and sex standardised annual prevalence of OCD in people aged 26–64 years of 1.3% and a lifetime

Obsessive compulsive disorder

prevalence of 2.3%.[5] Subsequent national surveys used similar methodology to the survey in the USA, and found broadly similar age and sex standardised annual and lifetime prevalence rates in Canada, Puerto Rico, Germany, Korea, and New Zealand, but slightly lower prevalence in Taiwan (see table 1) ❶.[5]

AETIOLOGY/ RISK FACTORS The cause of OCD is uncertain. Behavioural, cognitive, genetic, and neurobiological factors have been implicated.[6-12] Limited evidence from genetic studies in families and twins suggests that genetic factors may be involved, at least in some groups.[8,13-17] Risk factors include a family history of OCD, being single (which could be a consequence of the disorder), and belonging to a higher socioeconomic class.[18] The prevalence of OCD in the UK in 2000 was 1.3% in women and 9.0% in men.[4] The risk of OCD in women is higher than in men in most other countries.[5] Other risk factors include cocaine abuse, not being in paid employment, past history of alcohol dependence, affective disorder, and phobic disorder.[5]

PROGNOSIS One study (144 people followed for a mean of 47 years) found that an episodic course of OCD was more common during the initial years (about 1–9 years), but a chronic course was more common afterwards.[19] Over time, the study found that 39–48% of people had symptomatic improvement. A 1 year prospective cohort study found that 46% of people had an episodic course and 54% had a chronic course.[20]

Please refer to clinicalevidence.com for full text and references.

Panic disorder

Search date July 2004

Shailesh Kumar and Mark Oakley-Browne

What are the effects of treatments on panic disorder?

BENEFICIAL

Cognitive behavioural therapy

One RCT identified by a systematic review found that cognitive behavioural therapy improved symptoms after 3 and 6 months compared with placebo. Two subsequent RCTs found similar results after 6 months. Two RCTs found that cognitive behavioural therapy improved symptoms after 10—12 weeks compared with minimal contact control and to the same extent as applied relaxation. Three RCTs found different results for applied relaxation and cognitive behavioural therapy. One RCT found that applied relaxation improved symptoms to a greater extent than cognitive behavioural therapy over 12 weeks. Two RCTs found that applied relaxation improved symptoms less than cognitive behavioural therapy over 12 weeks. One small RCT found no significant difference in symptom improvement between cognitive behavioural therapy plus breathing retraining and cognitive behavioural therapy alone at the end of treatment or at 12 months. One RCT found no significant difference in improvement of symptoms between cognitive behavioural therapy and imipramine or between CBT plus imipramine and CBT alone at 6 months. One RCT found that cognitive behavioural therapy plus paroxetine increased the proportion of panic free people at 2 weeks compared with cognitive behavioural therapy alone. One RCT found no significant difference in symptom improvement over 3 months between fluvoxamine 150 mg, fluvoxamine plus cognitive behavioural therapy, and cognitive behavioural therapy alone compared with placebo but that the improvement was preserved in a larger proportion of people who received cognitive behavioural therapy compared with placebo or fluvoxamine alone at 6 months. We found insufficient evidence to compare the effects of buspirone versus cognitive behavioural therapy in people with panic disorder.

Selective serotonin reuptake inhibitors

Systematic reviews and one additional RCT found that selective serotonin reuptake inhibitors improved symptoms compared with placebo in panic disorder. One subsequent RCT found that discontinuation of sertraline in people with a good response increased exacerbation of symptoms. This RCT used treatment responders which is likely to bias the result in favour of the drug. A second methodologically weak subsequent RCT found that paroxetine plus cognitive behavioural therapy improved symptoms compared with placebo plus cognitive behavioural therapy. One RCT found no significant difference in symptom improvement over 3 months between fluvoxamine 150 mg, fluvoxamine plus cognitive behavioural therapy, and cognitive behavioural therapy alone and placebo but that the improvement was preserved in a smaller proportion of people who received fluvoxamine alone or placebo compared with cognitive behavioural therapy at 6 months.

Tricyclic antidepressants (imipramine)

One systematic review, two subsequent RCTs, and one additional RCT found that imipramine improved symptoms in people with panic disorder compared with placebo or a waiting list control. One subsequent RCT found that imipramine reduced relapse rates after 12 months in people with panic disorder compared with placebo.

Panic disorder

LIKELY TO BE BENEFICIAL

Applied relaxation

Two RCTs found that applied relaxation improved symptoms over 10—12 weeks compared with minimal contact controls and to the same extent as cognitive behavioural therapy. Three further RCTs found different results for applied relaxation compared with cognitive behavioural therapy. One RCT found that applied relaxation improved symptoms to a greater extent than cognitive behavioural therapy over 12 weeks. Two RCTs found that applied relaxation improved symptoms less than cognitive behavioural therapy over 12 weeks.

Client centred therapy

We found no RCTs comparing client centred therapy with placebo or no treatment. Two RCTs found that client centred therapy alone or in combination with exposure treatment improved symptoms over 14 weeks. One RCT found that client centred therapy plus exposure improved agoraphobic symptoms at 3 months compared with client centred therapy alone. However, one RCT found that a larger proportion of people felt less dependent on the expectations of others and less under stress with client centred therapy alone compared with client centred therapy plus exposure.

Cognitive restructuring

We found no RCTs comparing cognitive restructuring with placebo or no treatment. One RCT found no significant difference in improvement of symptoms between cognitive restructuring and interoceptive plus exteroceptive exposure therapy over 15 weeks.

Exposure in vivo and in vitro

One RCT found that exposure therapy improved symptoms compared with delayed treatment control at 10 weeks. The improvement was maintained at 6 months' follow up. One RCT found no significant difference in improvement in symptoms between exposure treatment and cognitive restructuring at 10 weeks. One RCT found that exposure plus alprazolam, alprazolam plus relaxation, placebo plus exposure, and placebo plus relaxation all improved symptoms at 8 weeks compared with baseline measures. However, symptoms remained improved at 6 months' follow up in a larger proportion of people treated with exposure plus placebo compared with other treatment groups.

TRADE OFF BETWEEN BENEFITS AND HARMS

Benzodiazepines

One systematic review and one additional RCT found that alprazolam reduced the number of panic attacks and improved symptoms compared with placebo. However, benzodiazepines are associated with a wide range of adverse effects, both during and after treatment.

UNKNOWN EFFECTIVENESS

Breathing retraining

One small RCT found that cognitive behavioural therapy plus breathing retraining and cognitive behavioural therapy alone improved symptoms compared with a delayed treatment control. It found no significant difference in symptom improvement between cognitive behavioural therapy plus breathing retraining and cognitive behavioural therapy alone at the end of treatment or at 12 months.

Buspirone

We found insufficient evidence to assess the effects of buspirone in people with panic disorder.

Couple therapy

We found no RCTs that compared couple therapy with placebo or no treatment. One RCT found that behavioural therapy with husband as co-therapist improved symptoms to the same extent as behavioural therapy with a female friend as co-therapist over 6 weeks. One RCT found that couples communication training improved symptoms more than couples relaxation training over 8 weeks. One RCT found that graded exposure with friends or spouses improved symptoms to the same extent as problem solving with friends or spouses over 4 weeks.

Insight oriented therapy

We found no RCTs comparing insight orientated therapy with placebo or no treatment. One RCT found that client centred therapy plus insight orientated therapy improved symptoms over 14 weeks more than client centred therapy alone during an inpatient anxiety treatment programme.

Monoamine oxidase inhibitors

We found no RCTs on the effects of monoamine oxidase inhibitors in panic disorder.

Psychoeducation

We found no systematic review or RCTs of psychoeducation in the treatment of panic disorder.

DEFINITION A panic attack is a period in which there is sudden onset of intense apprehension, fearfulness, or terror often associated with feelings of impending doom. Panic disorder occurs when there are recurrent, unpredictable attacks followed by at least 1 month of persistent concern about having another panic attack, worry about the possible implications or consequences of the panic attacks, or a significant behavioural change related to the attacks.[1] The term panic disorder excludes panic attacks attributable to the direct physiological effects of a general medical condition, a substance, or another mental disorder. Panic disorder is sometimes categorised as being with or without agoraphobia.[1] Alternative categorisations focus on phobic anxiety disorders and specify agoraphobia with or without panic disorder.[2] **Diagnosis:** Although panic attacks are a necessary feature of panic disorder, panic attacks on their own are not enough to make the diagnosis. Panic attacks may happen in the context of specific situations such as social or specific phobia which are different from panic disorder.[1] A diagnosis of panic disorder is made in the presence of recurrent unexpected panic attacks followed by at least 1 month of persistent concern about having another panic attack.[1]

INCIDENCE/ PREVALENCE Panic disorder often starts at about 20 years of age (between late adolescence and the mid-30s).[3] Lifetime prevalence is 1–3%, and panic disorder is more common in women than in men.[4] An Australian community study found 1 month prevalence rates for panic disorder (with or without agoraphobia) of 0.4% using International Classification of Diseases (ICD)-10 diagnostic criteria, and of 0.5% using Diagnostic and Statistical Manual (DSM)-IV diagnostic criteria.[5]

AETIOLOGY/ RISK FACTORS Stressful life events tend to precede the onset of panic disorder,[6,7] although a negative interpretation of these events in addition to their occurrence has been suggested as an important causal factor.[8] Panic disorder is associated with major depression,[9] social phobia, generalised anxiety disorder, obsessive

Panic disorder

compulsive disorder,[10] and a substantial risk of drug and alcohol abuse.[11] It is also associated with avoidant, histrionic, and dependent personality disorders.[10]

PROGNOSIS The severity of symptoms in people with panic disorder fluctuates considerably, and people commonly experience periods of no attacks, or only mild attacks with few symptoms. There is often a long delay between the initial onset of symptoms and presentation for treatment. Recurrent attacks may continue for several years, especially if associated with agoraphobia. Reduced social or occupational functioning varies among people with panic disorder and is worse in people with associated agoraphobia. Panic disorder is also associated with an increased rate of attempted, but unsuccessful, suicide.[12] One study analysing data from RCTs and systematic reviews found that co-existence of anxiety and depressive features adversely affected treatment response at 12 years compared with treatment of panic disorder alone.[13]

Please refer to clinicalevidence.com for full text and references.

Post-traumatic stress disorder

Search date December 2005

Jonathan Bisson

What are the effects of preventive interventions?

LIKELY TO BE BENEFICIAL

Multiple session cognitive behavioural therapy in people with acute stress disorder (reduced PTSD compared with supportive counselling)

Two small RCTs in people with acute stress disorder after a traumatic event (road traffic accident or non-sexual assault) found that five sessions of cognitive behavioural therapy reduced the proportion of people with post-traumatic stress disorder after 6 months compared with supportive counselling. One RCT in people with acute stress disorder found that cognitive behavioural therapy alone and cognitive behavioural therapy plus hypnosis reduced rates of post-traumatic stress disorder compared with supportive counselling. However, the differences between groups were not significant.

UNKNOWN EFFECTIVENESS

Hydrocortisone

One small RCT in people in intensive care with septic shock provided insufficient evidence to assess hydrocortisone in preventing post-traumatic stress disorder.

Multiple session cognitive behavioural therapy in all people exposed to a traumatic event

One RCT found that four sessions of cognitive behavioural therapy in people with psychological distress following physical injury reduced post-traumatic stress symptoms at 13 months compared with no psychological intervention. However, it found no significant difference in the proportion of people meeting the DSM-IV diagnostic criteria for post-traumatic stress disorder. Another RCT in bus drivers who had been attacked in the past 5 months found that cognitive behavioural therapy improved measures of anxiety and intrusive symptoms at 6 months compared with standard care. However, it found no significant difference in measures of depression or avoidance symptoms. One RCT provided insufficient evidence to assess cognitive behavioural therapy plus educational techniques in preventing post-traumatic stress disorder in road traffic accident survivors. Another small RCT provided insufficient evidence to compare memory structuring versus supportive listening in road traffic accident survivors.

Multiple session collaborative trauma support

Two RCTs provided insufficient evidence to assess multiple session collaborative trauma support interventions involving emotional, social, and practical support in people exposed to a traumatic event in the past 24 hours to 1 week.

Multiple session education

We found no systematic review or RCTs assessing the effects of multiple session education alone. One RCT provided insufficient evidence to assess educational techniques plus cognitive behavioural therapy in preventing post-traumatic stress disorder in road traffic accident survivors.

Propranolol

One small RCT provided insufficient evidence to assess propranolol in preventing post-traumatic stress disorder in people with early symptoms of post-traumatic stress disorder after a traumatic event.

BMJ Clin Evid Concise 2006;16:433–437.

Post-traumatic stress disorder

Single session group debriefing

One systematic review identified no RCTs comparing single session group debriefing versus no debriefing. One RCT found that early group debriefing (within 10 hours of the traumatic event) reduced post-traumatic stress disorder compared with delayed group debriefing (after 48 hours) at 2 weeks.

Temazepam

One small RCT provided insufficient evidence to assess temazepam in preventing post-traumatic stress disorder in people with acute stress disorder or early symptoms of post-traumatic stress disorder after a road traffic accident, industrial accident, or non-sexual assault.

UNLIKELY TO BE BENEFICIAL

Single session individual debriefing

One systematic review of RCTs in people who had been exposed to a traumatic event in the previous month found no significant difference between a single session of individual psychological debriefing and no debriefing in the rate of post-traumatic stress disorder at 3–6 months. The review found that individual psychological debriefing increased the rate of post-traumatic stress disorder compared with no debriefing at 13 months.

Supportive counselling

Three RCTs in people with acute stress disorder after a traumatic event (road traffic accident or non-sexual assault) found that supportive counselling was less effective than five sessions of cognitive behavioural therapy in reducing the proportion of people with post-traumatic stress disorder after 6 months.

What are the effects of treatments?

BENEFICIAL

Cognitive behavioural therapy

One systematic review and three subsequent RCTs found that cognitive behavioural therapy reduced rates of post-traumatic stress disorder compared with no treatment, stress management, supportive psychotherapy, psychodynamic psychotherapy, supportive counselling, or hypnotherapy. The review found no significant difference in rates of post-traumatic stress disorder between cognitive behavioural therapy and eye movement desensitisation and reprocessing. One RCT found that cognitive behavioural therapy produced similar reductions in PTSD scores compared with present centred therapy.

Eye movement desensitisation and reprocessing

One systematic review found that eye movement desensitisation and reprocessing improved symptoms compared with no treatment or usual treatment. The review found no significant difference in rates of post-traumatic stress disorder between eye movement desensitisation and reprocessing and stress management or cognitive behavioural therapies.

LIKELY TO BE BENEFICIAL

Fluoxetine

One systematic review of one large RCT found that fluoxetine reduced symptoms of post-traumatic stress disorder compared with placebo at 3 months. One subsequent RCT found that fluoxetine was more effective than placebo at reducing rates of relapse.

Paroxetine

One systematic review found that paroxetine improved symptoms compared with placebo at 3 months in people with post-traumatic stress disorder.

UNKNOWN EFFECTIVENESS

Affect management

One RCT provided insufficient evidence about the effects of affect management in improving symptoms in people with post-traumatic stress disorder.

Benzodiazepines

One systematic review identified no RCTs of sufficient quality of benzodiazepines in people with post-traumatic stress disorder.

Brofaromine

One RCT identified by a systematic review provided insufficient evidence about the effects of brofaromine in improving symptoms of post-traumatic stress disorder.

Carbamazepine

We found no systematic review or RCTs of carbamazepine in people with post-traumatic stress disorder.

Drama therapy

We found no systematic review or RCTs investigating the effects of drama therapy in improving symptoms of post-traumatic stress disorder.

Group therapy

RCTs identified by a systematic review provided insufficient evidence about the effects of group therapy in improving symptoms of post-traumatic stress disorder. One subsequent RCT found that a combination of group plus individual cognitive behavioural therapy was better than no treatment in improving symptoms of post-traumatic stress disorder.

Hypnotherapy

One RCT identified by a systematic review provided insufficient evidence about the effects of hypnotherapy in improving symptoms of post-traumatic stress disorder.

Inpatient treatment programmes

We found no systematic review or RCTs investigating the effects of inpatient treatment programmes in improving symptoms of post-traumatic stress disorder.

Internet based psychotherapy

One RCT provided insufficient evidence about the effects of internet based psychotherapy in improving symptoms of post-traumatic stress disorder.

Mirtazapine

One RCT identified by a systematic review provided insufficient evidence about the effects of mirtazapine in improving symptoms of post-traumatic stress disorder.

Nefazodone

We found insufficient evidence about the effects of nefazodone in improving symptoms of post-traumatic stress disorder.

Post-traumatic stress disorder

Olanzapine

One systematic review identified no good quality RCTs that assessed olanzapine in people with post-traumatic stress disorder.

Phenelzine

One RCT identified by a systematic review provided insufficient evidence about the effects of phenelzine in improving symptoms of post-traumatic stress disorder.

Propranolol

We found no systematic review or RCTs of propranolol in people with post-traumatic stress disorder.

Psychodynamic psychotherapy

One RCT identified by a systematic review provided insufficient evidence about the effects of psychodynamic psychotherapy in improving symptoms of post-traumatic stress disorder.

Risperidone

One RCT identified by a systematic review provided insufficient evidence about the effects of risperidone in improving symptoms of post-traumatic stress disorder versus placebo. However, two subsequent RCTs found that risperidone significantly reduced symptom scores for post-traumatic stress disorder compared with placebo.

Sertraline

One systematic review found that sertraline improved symptoms of post-traumatic stress disorder at 3–7 months compared with placebo but this did not quite reach significance.

SSRIs versus each other

Two RCTs comparing nefazodone with sertraline. The first found no significant difference in PTSD symptoms at 5 months, the second found similar reduction in PTSD scores between groups.

Supportive psychotherapy

One RCT provided insufficient evidence about the effects of supportive psychotherapy in improving symptoms in people with post-traumatic stress disorder.

Tricyclic antidepressants

RCTs identified by a systematic review provided insufficient evidence to assess imipramine or amitriptyline in people with post-traumatic stress disorder.

UNLIKELY TO BE BENEFICIAL

Venlafaxine

One large RCT identified by a systematic review found no significant difference in symptom severity at 12 weeks between venlafaxine and placebo in people with post-traumatic stress disorder.

DEFINITION **Post-traumatic stress disorder (PTSD)** can occur after any major traumatic event. Symptoms include upsetting thoughts and nightmares about the traumatic event, avoidance behaviour, numbing of general responsiveness, increased irritability, and hypervigilance.[1] To fulfil the *Diagnostic and statistical manual of mental disorders* (DSM-IV) criteria for PTSD, an individual must have been exposed to a traumatic event; have at least one re-experiencing, three avoidance, and two hyperarousal phenomena; have had the symptoms for at least 1 month; and the symptoms must cause clinically important distress or reduced day to day functioning.[1] People with sub-syndromal PTSD have all the criteria for PTSD except one of the re-experiencing, avoidance, or hyperarousal phenomena. **Acute stress disorder** occurs within the first month after a major traumatic event and requires the presence of symptoms for at least 2 days. It is similar to PTSD but dissociative symptoms are required to make the diagnosis. Treatments for PTSD may have similar effects, regardless of the traumatic event that precipitated PTSD. However, great caution should be applied when generalising from one type of trauma to another.

INCIDENCE/ PREVALENCE One large cross-sectional study in the USA found that 1/10 (10%) women and 1/20 (5%) men experience PTSD at some stage in their lives.[2]

AETIOLOGY/ RISK FACTORS Risk factors include major trauma, such as rape, a history of psychiatric disorders, acute distress and depression after the trauma, lack of social support, and personality factors.[3]

PROGNOSIS One large cross-sectional study in the USA found that over a third of people with previous PTSD continued to satisfy the criteria for PTSD 6 years after initial diagnosis.[2] However, cross-sectional studies provide weak evidence about prognosis.

Please refer to clinicalevidence.com for full text and references.

Schizophrenia

Search date September 2005

Zia Nadeem, Andrew McIntosh, and Stephen Lawrie

What are the effects of drug treatments for positive and negative symptoms?

TRADE OFF BETWEEN BENEFITS AND HARMS

Amisulpride

Two systematic reviews found that amisulpride improved symptoms more than did standard antipsychotic drugs. Like all antipsychotic drugs, the harms of amisulpride may include parkinsonism, dystonia, cholinergic effects, and weight gain. However, one review found that extrapyramidal adverse effects were less likely with amisulpride than with standard antipsychotic drugs. One RCT found no significant difference in symptoms between amisulpride and olanzapine. One systematic review found no significant difference in symptoms between amisulpride and risperidone.

Chlorpromazine

One systematic review found that, compared with placebo, chlorpromazine reduced the proportion of people with no improvement or with worse severity of illness at 6 months on a psychiatrist rated scale. The review found that, compared with placebo, chlorpromazine caused more adverse effects, such as sedation, acute dystonia, and parkinsonism.

Clozapine

One systematic review found that clozapine improved symptoms over 4–10 weeks compared with standard antipsychotic drugs (predominantly haloperidol and chlorpromazine) and was less likely to lead to antipsychotic induced movement disorders. RCTs provided insufficient evidence to compare clozapine versus other, newer antipsychotic drugs. RCTs found that clozapine may be associated with blood dyscrasias.

Depot bromperidol decanoate

One systematic review of three small RCTs found no significant difference between depot bromperidol decanoate and depot haloperidol or depot fluphenazine decanoate in the proportion of people who needed additional medication, left the trial early, or had movement disorders over 6–12 months. The review may have lacked power to detect a clinically important difference. Like all antipsychotic drugs, the harms of bromperidol may include parkinsonism, dystonia, cholinergic effects, and weight gain.

Depot haloperidol decanoate

One small RCT identified by a systematic review found no significant difference between depot haloperidol decanoate and oral haloperidol in global clinical state at 4 months, but it may have been too small to detect a clinically important difference. Haloperidol is associated with acute dystonia, akathisia, and parkinsonism.

Haloperidol

One systematic review found that haloperidol increased physician rated global improvement at 6 and 24 weeks compared with placebo, but was associated with acute dystonia, akathisia, and parkinsonism.

Loxapine

One systematic review found no significant difference between loxapine and standard antipsychotic drugs in symptom improvement and adverse events. Like all antipsychotic drugs, harms may include parkinsonism, dystonia, cholinergic effects, and weight gain.

Molindone

One systematic review found no significant difference in global clinical improvement or in the proportion of people who had adverse effects over 4–12 weeks between molindone and standard antipsychotic drugs. The harms of molindone may include parkinsonism, dystonia, cholinergic effects, and weight gain.

Olanzapine

One systematic review found no significant difference in persisting psychotic symptoms between olanzapine and standard antipsychotic drugs. Like all antipsychotic drugs, the harms of olanzapine may include parkinsonism, dystonia, cholinergic effects, and weight gain. However, the review found that olanzapine was associated with fewer extrapyramidal adverse effects than were standard antipsychotic drugs. RCTs found no clear difference in symptoms or adverse effects between olanzapine, amisulpride, risperidone, and clozapine.

Pimozide

One systematic review found no significant difference between pimozide and standard antipsychotic drugs in global clinical impression, and found that pimozide decreased sedation but increased tremor. It found no overall difference in cardiovascular adverse effects such as rise or fall in blood pressure or dizziness between pimozide and standard antipsychotic drugs. Pimozide has been associated with sudden cardiac death at doses above 20 mg daily.

Quetiapine

One systematic review found no significant difference in mental state between quetiapine and standard antipsychotic drugs (mainly haloperidol). Like all antipsychotic drugs, harms may include dystonia, cholinergic effects, and weight gain. However, the review found that quetiapine reduced akathisia, parkinsonism, and the proportion of people who left the trial early.

Risperidone

One systematic review found that risperidone increased the proportion of people with clinically important improvement in symptoms compared with standard antipsychotic drugs (mainly haloperidol), up to 12 and over 26 weeks. It found that risperidone decreased extrapyramidal adverse effects and the need for antiparkinsonian medication, but increased weight gain compared with standard antipsychotic drugs. One small additional RCT found no significant difference between risperidone and haloperidol in responders over 8 weeks. Systematic reviews found no significant difference in symptoms between risperidone and other new antipsychotic drugs (olanzapine, sulpiride, and clozapine).

Sulpiride

Systematic reviews found no significant difference between the newer antipsychotic drug, sulpiride, and standard antipsychotic drugs in symptom improvement, and that they have different profiles of adverse effects. However, like all antipsychotic drugs, harms may include parkinsonism, dystonia, cholinergic effects, and weight gain.

Ziprasidone

One systematic review found no significant difference in symptoms between ziprasidone and standard antipsychotic drugs (mainly haloperidol). Like all antipsychotic drugs, the harms of ziprasidone may include parkinsonism, cholinergic effects, and weight gain. However, one earlier systematic review found that ziprasidone reduced akathisia and acute dystonia but increased nausea and vomiting compared with haloperidol.

Zotepine

One systematic review found weak evidence that zotepine increased the proportion of people with a clinically important improvement in symptoms compared with standard antipsychotic drugs. This finding was not robust because removal of a single RCT from the analysis meant that the difference between zotepine and standard antipsychotic drugs was no longer significant. Like all antipsychotic drugs, the harms of zotepine may include parkinsonism, cholinergic effects, and weight gain. However, one systematic review found that zotepine reduced akasthesia, dystonia, and rigidity compared with other antipsychotic drugs.

UNKNOWN EFFECTIVENESS

Perazine

One weak RCT found no significant difference in global clinical impression over 28 days between perazine and haloperidol. Two small RCTs provided insufficient evidence to compare perazine versus zotepine, and one small RCT found no significant difference in mental state at 28 days between perazine and amisulpride. Like all antipsychotic drugs, the harms of perazine may include parkinsonism, dystonia, cholinergic effects, and weight gain. Three RCTs found no significant difference in extrapyramidal effects over 28 days between perazine and zotepine or amisulpride.

Which interventions reduce relapse rates?

BENEFICIAL

Continuation of antipsychotic drugs for at least 6 months after an acute episode

Systematic reviews found that continuing antipsychotic drugs for at least 6 months after an acute episode reduced relapse rates compared with no treatment or placebo. Eight systematic reviews found no significant difference in relapse rates among antipsychotic drugs. One systematic review found that clozapine reduced relapse rates over 12 weeks compared with standard antipsychotic drugs. Another review found that fewer people taking depot zuclopenthixol decanoate relapsed over 12 weeks to 1 year compared with people taking other depot preparations. A third review found that bromperidol increased the proportion of people who relapsed compared with haloperidol or fluphenazine. One systematic review found that risperidone reduced relapse rates compared with haloperidol at 1 year.

Multiple session family interventions

One systematic review found that multiple session family interventions reduced relapse rates at 12 months compared with usual care, single session family interventions, or psychoeducational interventions.

◀ Psychoeducational interventions

One systematic review found that psychoeducation reduced relapse rates at 9–18 months compared with usual care. There was heterogeneity of both interventions and outcomes. One systematic review found insufficient evidence on psychoeducational interventions compared with social skills training.

UNKNOWN EFFECTIVENESS

Cognitive behavioural therapy

Limited evidence from a systematic review found no significant difference in relapse rates between cognitive behavioural therapy plus standard care and standard care alone.

Social skills training

One systematic review of small RCTs provided insufficient evidence to assess the effect of social skills training on relapse rates.

Which interventions are effective in people who are resistant to standard antipsychotic drugs?

BENEFICIAL

Clozapine (compared with standard antipsychotic drugs)

One systematic review in people resistant to standard antipsychotic drugs found that clozapine improved symptoms after 12 weeks and after 2 years compared with standard antipsychotic drugs. One systematic review found no significant difference in symptoms between clozapine and other new antipsychotic drugs in people resistant to standard antipsychotic drugs. One small RCT identified by a systematic review found no significant difference in psychotic symptoms over 8 weeks between clozapine and olanzapine.

UNKNOWN EFFECTIVENESS

Olanzapine

Small RCTs identified by a systematic review found no significant difference in psychotic symptoms over 8 weeks between olanzapine and chlorpromazine or between olanzapine and clozapine.

Which interventions improve adherence to antipsychotic medication?

LIKELY TO BE BENEFICIAL

Behavioural therapy

One small RCT found limited evidence that behavioural interventions improved adherence to antipsychotic medication compared with usual treatment. Two RCTs found limited evidence that behavioural interventions improved adherence more than did psychoeducational therapy.

Compliance therapy

Two RCTs found limited evidence that compliance therapy increased adherence to antipsychotic drugs at 6 and 18 months compared with supportive or non-specific counselling. One RCT found no significant difference in adherence between compliance therapy and non-specific therapy, over 1 year. ▶

Schizophrenia

Psychoeducational interventions

One systematic review found limited evidence that psychoeducational interventions improved adherence to antipsychotic medication compared with usual care. Two RCTs found limited evidence that psychoeducational interventions improved adherence less than did behavioural therapy.

UNKNOWN EFFECTIVENESS

Multiple session family interventions

One systematic review found that "compliance with medication" over 9–24 months was higher in people who received multiple session family interventions compared with usual care, single family interventions, or psychoeducational interventions, but the difference was not significant.

DEFINITION Schizophrenia is characterised by the positive symptoms of auditory hallucinations, delusions, and thought disorder, and by the negative symptoms of demotivation, self neglect, and reduced emotion.[1] People are defined as being resistant to standard antipsychotic drugs if, over the preceding 5 years, they have not had a clinically important improvement in symptoms after 2–3 regimens of treatment with standard antipsychotic drugs for at least 6 weeks (from at least 2 classes at doses of ≥ 1000 mg/day chlorpromazine) and they have had no period of good functioning.[2,3] About 30% (10–45%) of people with schizophrenia meet these criteria.[3]

INCIDENCE/ PREVALENCE Onset of symptoms typically occurs in early adult life (average age 25 years) and is earlier in men than in women.[4,5] Prevalence worldwide is 2–4/1000. One in 100 people will develop schizophrenia in their lifetime.

AETIOLOGY/ RISK FACTORS Risk factors include a family history (although no major genes have been identified), obstetric complications, developmental difficulties, central nervous system infections in childhood, cannabis use, and acute life events.[4] The precise contributions of these factors, and ways in which they may interact, are unclear.

PROGNOSIS About three quarters of people suffer recurrent relapse and continued disability, although the proportion of people who improved significantly increased after the mid-1950s (mean: 48.5% from 1956–1985 *v* 35.4% from 1895–1956).[6] Outcome may be worse in people with insidious onset and delayed initial treatment, social isolation, or a strong family history; in people living in industrialised countries; in men; and in people who misuse drugs.[5] Drug treatment is generally successful in treating positive symptoms, but up to a third of people derive little benefit, and negative symptoms are notoriously difficult to treat. About half of people with schizophrenia do not adhere to treatment in the short term. The figure is even higher in the longer term.[7]

Please refer to clinicalevidence.com for full text and references.

Ankle sprain

Search date March 2005

Peter Struijs and Gino Kerkhoffs

What are the effects of treatment strategies for acute ankle ligament ruptures?

BENEFICIAL

Functional treatment (early mobilisation with use of an external support)

One systematic review and one subsequent RCT found evidence that functional treatment reduced the risk of the ankle giving way compared with minimal treatment. One systematic review and one subsequent RCT found that, compared with immobilisation, functional treatment improved symptoms and functional outcomes at short (< 6 weeks), intermediate (6 weeks to 1 year), or long term (> 1 year) follow up. However, effects were found to be less marked at long term follow up. One systematic review and one subsequent RCT provided insufficient evidence to compare functional treatment versus surgery. One systematic review and two additional RCTs provided insufficient evidence to compare different functional treatments.

LIKELY TO BE BENEFICIAL

Immobilisation

There is consensus that immobilisation is more effective than no treatment; however one systematic review and one subsequent RCT found that, compared with functional treatment, immobilisation was associated with less improvement in symptoms and functional outcomes at either short (< 6 weeks), intermediate (6 weeks to 1 year), or long term (> 1 year) follow up. Effects were less marked at long term follow up. One systematic review found no significant difference between immobilisation and surgery in pain, swelling, recurrence, or subjective instability. However, the review found that compared with immobilisation, surgery improved stability and increased the proportion of people able to return to sports. One RCT identified by a systematic review provided insufficient evidence to compare ultrasound versus immobilisation.

TRADE OFF BETWEEN BENEFITS AND HARMS

Surgery

One systematic review found no significant difference between surgery and immobilisation in pain, swelling, recurrence, or subjective instability. However, the review found that surgery increased the proportion of people able to return to sports and increased ankle stability compared with immobilisation. One systematic review and one subsequent RCT provided insufficient evidence to compare surgery versus functional treatment. Neurological injuries, infections, bleeding, osteoarthritis, and death are known harms of surgery.

UNKNOWN EFFECTIVENESS

Diathermy

One systematic review found insufficient evidence on the effects of diathermy compared with placebo on walking ability and reduction in swelling.

▶

Ankle sprain

Homeopathic ointment

One small RCT identified by a systematic review found limited evidence that homeopathic ointment improved outcome based on a "composite criteria of treatment success" compared with placebo.

UNLIKELY TO BE BENEFICIAL

Cold treatment

One RCT found no significant difference in symptoms between cold pack placement and placebo (simulated treatment). One RCT found less oedema with cold pack placement compared with heat or a contrast bath at 3–5 days after injury.

Ultrasound

One systematic review found no significant difference between ultrasound and sham ultrasound in the general improvement of symptoms or the ability to walk or bear weight at 7 days. Two RCTs identified by the review provided insufficient evidence to compare ultrasound versus immobilisation or electrotherapy.

DEFINITION Ankle sprain is an injury of the lateral ligament complex of the ankle joint. The injury is graded on the basis of severity.[1-5] Grade I is a mild stretching of the ligament complex without joint instability; grade II is a partial rupture of the ligament complex with mild instability of the joint (such as isolated rupture of the anterior talofibular ligament); and grade III involves complete rupture of the ligament complex with instability of the joint. Practically, this gradation may be considered as purely theoretical, because it has no therapeutic or prognostic consequences.[6] Unless otherwise stated, studies included in this topic did not specify the grades of injury included, or included a wide range of grades.

INCIDENCE/ PREVALENCE Ankle sprain is a common problem in acute medical care, occurring at a rate of about one injury per 10 000 people a day.[7] Injuries of the lateral ligament complex of the ankle form a quarter of all sports injuries.[7]

AETIOLOGY/ RISK FACTORS The usual mechanism of injury is inversion and adduction (usually referred to as supination) of the plantar flexed foot. Predisposing factors are a history of ankle sprains and specific malalignment, like crus varum and pes cavo-varus.

PROGNOSIS Some sports (e.g. basketball, football/soccer, and volleyball) are associated with a particularly high incidence of ankle injuries. Pain is the most frequent residual problem, often localised on the medial side of the ankle.[4] Other residual complaints include mechanical instability, intermittent swelling, and stiffness. People with more extensive cartilage damage have a higher incidence of residual complaints.[4] Long term cartilage damage can lead to degenerative changes, especially if there is persistent or recurrent instability. Every further sprain has the potential to add new damage.

Please refer to clinicalevidence.com for full text and references.

Bunions

Search date June 2006

Jill Ferrari

What are the effects of conservative treatments?

UNKNOWN EFFECTIVENESS

Antipronatory orthoses in children

One RCT in children found that antipronatory orthoses increased deterioration in metatarsophalangeal joint angles after 3 years compared with no treatment, although the difference was not statistically significant.

Night splints

One systematic review found no reliable RCTs comparing night splints with any other or no treatment.

Orthoses to treat hallux valgus in adults

One RCT in adults found that orthoses reduced pain compared with no treatment at 6 months but not at 1 year and that orthoses were less effective at improving outcomes than chevron osteotomy.

What are the effects of surgery?

LIKELY TO BE BENEFICIAL

Distal chevron osteotomy (more effective than no treatment or orthoses but insufficient evidence to compare with other osteotomies or arthrodesis)

One RCT identified by a systematic review found conflicting evidence on the effects of distal chevron osteotomy compared with other distal metatarsal osteotomies. One RCT found that distal chevron osteotomy reduced pain and improved functional outcomes compared with orthoses or no treatment after 1 year. One RCT identified by a systematic review found no significant difference between proximal osteotomy and distal chevron osteotomy in functional outcomes after 2 years. The RCT also found that proximal osteotomy significantly improved hallux abductus angle and intermetatarsal angle compared with distal chevron osteotomy after 2 years. One RCT identified by a systematic review found no significant difference in functional or radiographic outcomes between distal chevron osteotomy plus phalangeal (Akin) osteotomy versus phalangeal osteotomy plus distal soft tissue reconstruction. One RCT found no difference in outcomes when the Lapidus procedure was compared to a distal osteotomy.

UNKNOWN EFFECTIVENESS

Arthrodesis (Lapidus procedure)

We found no RCTs which compared arthrodesis versus no treatment. One RCT found no difference in outcomes when the Lapidus procedure was compared to a distal osteotomy (Hohmann procedure). One systematic review found insufficient evidence on the effects of arthrodesis compared to Keller's arthroplasty.

Arthrodesis (versus no treatment)

We found no RCTs which compared arthrodesis with no treatment.

Bunions

Chevron osteotomy plus adductor tenotomy versus chevron osteotomy alone (relative benefits unclear)

One RCT identified by a systematic review found no evidence that distal chevron osteotomy plus adductor tenotomy improved outcomes compared with distal chevron osteotomy alone.

Different methods of bone fixation (standard fixation, absorbable pin fixation, screw fixation plus early weight bearing, suture fixation plus delayed weight bearing)

One small RCT identified by a systematic review found no significant difference between standard fixation and absorbable pin fixation in clinical or radiological outcomes; however, it may have lacked power to detect a clinically significant difference. A second small RCT identified by the review found that screw fixation plus early weight bearing reduced time to return to work and social activity compared with suture fixation and later weight bearing, but found no significant difference in radiological outcomes.

Keller's arthroplasty

We found no RCTs comparing Keller's arthroplasty versus no treatment. One systematic review found insufficient evidence from limited RCTs on the effects of Keller's arthroplasty compared with other types of operation.

Keller–Lelievre arthroplasty

One systematic review found insufficient evidence from one small RCT on the effects of Keller–Lelievre arthroplasty compared with a modified version of the same operation. We found no RCTs comparing Keller-Lelievre arthroplasty versus no treatment.

Phalangeal (Akin) osteotomy plus distal chevron osteotomy

One RCT identified by a systematic review found no significant difference in functional or radiographic outcomes between Akin osteotomy plus distal chevron osteotomy and Akin osteotomy plus distal soft tissue reconstruction after 1 year. However, this RCT was small and may have lacked power to detect a clinically significant difference.

Proximal chevron osteotomy versus other types of proximal osteotomy (relative benefits unclear)

One RCT identified by a systematic review found no significant difference in functional or radiographic outcomes between proximal chevron osteotomy and proximal crescentic osteotomy after 22 months.

Proximal osteotomy versus distal chevron osteotomy (relative benefits unclear)

One RCT identified by a systematic review found no significant difference between proximal osteotomy and distal chevron osteotomy in functional outcomes after 2 years. The RCT also found that proximal osteotomy significantly improved hallux abductus angle and intermetatarsal angle compared with distal chevron osteotomy after 2 years.

What are the effects of postoperative care?

UNKNOWN EFFECTIVENESS

Continuous passive motion

One systematic review provided insufficient evidence on the effects of continuous passive motion on functional and radiographic outcomes.

Early weight bearing

One RCT from a systematic review found insufficient evidence on the effects of early weight bearing.

Slipper casts

One systematic review provided insufficient evidence on the effects of plaster slipper casts after either a Wilson osteotomy or a first metatarsophalangeal joint fusion.

DEFINITION **Hallux valgus** is a deformity of the great toe, whereby the hallux (great toe) moves towards the second toe, overlying it in severe cases. This abduction (movement away from the midline of the body) is usually accompanied by some rotation of the toe so that the nail is facing the midline of the body (valgus rotation). With the deformity, the metatarsal head becomes more prominent and the metatarsal is said to be in an adducted position as it moves towards the midline of the body.[1] Radiological criteria for hallux valgus vary, but a commonly accepted criterion is to measure the angle formed between the metatarsal and the abducted hallux. This is called the metatarsophalangeal joint angle or hallux abductus angle and it is considered abnormal when it is greater than 14.5°.[2] **Bunion** is the lay term used to describe a prominent and often inflamed metatarsal head and overlying bursa. Symptoms include pain, limitation in walking, and problems with wearing normal shoes.

INCIDENCE/ PREVALENCE The prevalence of hallux valgus varies in different populations. In a recent study of 6000 UK school children aged 9–10 years, 2.5% had clinical evidence of hallux valgus, and 2% met both clinical and radiological criteria for hallux valgus. An earlier study found hallux valgus in 48% of adults.[3] Differences in prevalence may result from different methods of measurement, varying age groups, or different diagnostic criteria (e.g. metatarsal joint angle $> 10°$ or $> 15°$).

AETIOLOGY/ RISK FACTORS Nearly all population studies have found that hallux valgus is more common in women. Footwear may contribute to the deformity, but studies comparing people who wear shoes with those who do not have found contradictory results. Hypermobility of the first ray and excessive foot pronation are associated with hallux valgus.[4]

PROGNOSIS We found no studies that looked at the progression of hallux valgus. While progression of deformity and symptoms is rapid in some people, others remain asymptomatic. One study found that hallux valgus is often unilateral initially, but usually progresses to bilateral deformity.[2]

Please refer to clinicalevidence.com for full text and references.

Carpal tunnel syndrome

Search date December 2005

Nigel Ashworth

What are the effects of drug treatments for carpal tunnel syndrome?

LIKELY TO BE BENEFICIAL

Corticosteroids (local injection)

Two small RCTs found that local corticosteroid injection (methylprednisone, hydrocortisone) improved symptoms after 4–6 weeks compared with placebo or no treatment. One small RCT identified by a systematic review found that local betamethasone injection improved symptoms after 1 month compared with betamethasone injection into the deltoid. Another small RCT identified by the same review found no significant difference in symptoms at 2 weeks between local methylprednisone injection and oral prednisone, but found that oral prednisone was less effective than local methylprednisone injection at improving symptoms after 8 and 12 weeks. One RCT found that local corticosteroid injection was more effective at improving symptoms and function at 3 months than carpal tunnel release surgery, although there was no significant difference at 6 and 12 months. Known serious adverse effects of local corticosteroid injection into the carpal tunnel include tendon rupture and injection into the median nerve.

Corticosteroids (systemic)

Two small RCTs identified by a systematic review and one subsequent RCT found that oral prednisone improved symptoms after 2 weeks compared with placebo, and two of the three RCTs found the improvement was maintained at 4–8 weeks. We found no systematic review or RCT that measured the effects of oral corticosteroids on symptoms in the longer term. One small RCT identified by a systematic review found that betamethasone injection into the deltoid was less effective at improving symptoms after 1 month, compared with local betamethasone injection. Another small RCT identified by the same review found no significant difference in symptoms at 2 weeks between oral prednisone and local methylprednisone injection. However, local methylprednisone injection was more effective than oral prednisone at improving symptoms after 8 and 12 weeks. One RCT found that oral prednisone reduced symptoms compared with a non-steroidal anti-inflammatory drug (tenoxicam) and a diuretic (trichlormethiazide) after 4 weeks.

UNKNOWN EFFECTIVENESS

Non-steroidal anti-inflammatory drugs

One RCT identified by a systematic review found no significant difference between a non-steroidal anti-inflammatory drug (tenoxicam) and placebo. It found that tenoxicam was less effective than oral prednisone after 4 weeks. It also found no significant difference between tenoxicam and a diuretic (trichlormethiazide) at 2 or 4 weeks.

Pyridoxine

One small RCT found a similar improvement in symptoms with pyridoxine compared with placebo or no treatment after 10 weeks. The RCT may have been too small to detect a clinically important difference between treatments. ▶

Another small RCT found no significant difference between pyridoxine and placebo in nocturnal pain, numbness, or tingling after 12 weeks.

UNLIKELY TO BE BENEFICIAL

Diuretics

Two small RCTs found no significant difference between diuretics and placebo in symptoms after 2 or 4 weeks. One of the RCTs found no significant difference in symptoms between a diuretic (trichlormethiazide) and a non-steroidal anti-inflammatory drug (tenoxicam) at 4 weeks. It found that trichlormethiazide was less effective than oral prednisone at reducing symptoms after 4 weeks.

What are the effects of non-drug treatments for carpal tunnel syndrome?

UNKNOWN EFFECTIVENESS

Nerve and tendon gliding exercises

One small RCT found no significant difference between 4 weeks of treatment with nerve and tendon gliding exercises plus neutral angle wrist splint and neutral angle wrist splint alone in symptom severity or function after 8 weeks.

Therapeutic ultrasound

One RCT provided limited evidence that ultrasound increased the proportion of wrists with satisfactory improvement or complete remission of symptoms after 6 months compared with placebo. One RCT found no significant difference in symptom severity after 2 weeks between high or low intensity ultrasound compared with placebo, or between high and low intensity ultrasound.

Wrist splints

One RCT found that a nocturnal hand brace improved symptoms after 2 and 4 weeks compared with no treatment. Two RCTs found that splinting was less effective than surgery at resolving symptoms at up to 18 months. One small RCT found no significant difference in symptoms after 2 weeks between neutral angle compared with 20° extension wrist splinting. One small RCT found no significant difference in symptoms at 6 weeks between full time compared with night time only neutral angle wrist splinting.

What are the effects of surgical treatments for carpal tunnel syndrome?

TRADE OFF BETWEEN BENEFITS AND HARMS

Endoscopic carpal tunnel release versus open carpal tunnel release

One systematic review provided limited evidence that endoscopic surgery improved grip and pinch strength at 12 weeks compared with open surgery. One RCT found that open surgery reduced wound pain at 2 and 4 weeks, but not after 8 weeks compared with endoscopic surgery, and one systematic review provided limited evidence of no significant difference in pain at 12 weeks between groups. A second systematic review concluded that carpal tunnel release was no more effective at relieving symptoms in the short or longer term than open carpal tunnel release. Seven RCTs found that endoscopic carpal tunnel release surgery reduced time to return to work, activities of daily living, or both compared with open release surgery. However, one RCT found that endoscopic release delayed return to work compared with open release, while one systematic review

Carpal tunnel syndrome

and four RCTs found no significant difference between groups. Two systematic reviews found that that reversible nerve injury seemed more common with endoscopic than with open surgery, and that scar tenderness was more common with open surgery.

Surgery versus local steroid injection

One RCT found that carpal tunnel release surgery was less effective than local steroid injection at improving symptoms and function at 3 months, although it found no significant difference at 6 and 12 months.

Surgery versus placebo

We found no RCTs comparing surgery with no treatment or placebo.

Surgery versus wrist splint

Two RCTs found that surgery increased symptom resolution compared with splinting at up to 18 months.

UNLIKELY TO BE BENEFICIAL

Internal neurolysis in conjunction with open carpal tunnel release

RCTs identified by a systematic review found no significant difference in symptoms between open carpal tunnel release alone and open carpal tunnel release plus internal neurolysis in symptoms.

What are the effects of postoperative treatments for carpal tunnel syndrome?

LIKELY TO BE INEFFECTIVE OR HARMFUL

Wrist splints after carpal tunnel release surgery

Two RCTs in people after carpal tunnel release surgery found no significant difference between wrist splinting and no splinting in grip strength or in the proportion of people who considered themselves "cured" at 2–4 weeks. A third RCT found that splinting increased pain at 1 month and the time to return to work compared with no splinting.

DEFINITION Carpal tunnel syndrome is a neuropathy caused by compression of the median nerve within the carpal tunnel.[1] Classical symptoms of carpal tunnel syndrome include numbness, tingling, burning, or pain in at least two of the three digits supplied by the median nerve (i.e. the thumb, index, and middle fingers).[2] The American Academy of Neurology has described diagnostic criteria that rely on a combination of symptoms and physical examination findings.[3] Other diagnostic criteria include results from electrophysiological studies.[2]

INCIDENCE/ PREVALENCE A general population survey in Rochester, Minnesota, found the age adjusted incidence of carpal tunnel syndrome to be 105 (95% CI 99 to 112) cases per 100 000 person years.[4,5] Age adjusted incidence rates were 52 (95% CI 45 to 59) cases per 100 000 person years for men and 149 (95% CI 138 to 159) cases per 100 000 person years for women. The study found incidence rates increased from 88 (95% CI 75 to 101) cases per 100 000 person years in 1961–1965 to 125 (95% CI 112 to 138) cases per 100 000 person years in 1976–1980. Incidence rates of carpal tunnel syndrome increased with age for men, whereas for women they peaked at the ages of 45–54 years. A general population survey in the Netherlands found prevalence to be 1% for men and 7% for women.[6] A more comprehensive study in southern Sweden found the general population prevalence for carpal tunnel syndrome was 3%

(95% CI 2% to 3%).[7] As in other studies, the overall prevalence in women was higher than in men (male to female ratio 1.0 < 1.4); however, among older people, the prevalence in women was almost four times that in men (age group 65–74 years: men 1%, 95% CI 0% to 4%; women 5%, 95% CI 3% to 8%).

AETIOLOGY/ RISK FACTORS Most cases of carpal tunnel syndrome have no easily identifiable cause (idiopathic).[4] Secondary causes of carpal tunnel syndrome include the following: space occupying lesions (tumours, hypertrophic synovial tissue, fracture callus, and osteophytes); metabolic and physiological causes (pregnancy, hypothyroidism, and rheumatoid arthritis); infections; neuropathies (associated with diabetes mellitus or alcoholism); and familial disorders.[4] One case control study found that risk factors in the general population included repetitive activities requiring wrist extension or flexion, obesity, very rapid dieting, shorter height, hysterectomy without oophorectomy, and recent menopause.[8]

PROGNOSIS One observational study (carpal tunnel syndrome defined by symptoms and electrophysiological study results) found that 34% of people with idiopathic carpal tunnel syndrome without treatment had complete resolution of symptoms (remission) within 6 months of diagnosis.[9] Remission rates were higher for younger age groups, for women, and in pregnancy. A more recent observational study of untreated idiopathic carpal tunnel syndrome also showed that symptoms may spontaneously resolve in some people. The main positive prognostic indicators were short duration of symptoms and young age, whereas bilateral symptoms and a positive Phalen's test were indicators of a poorer prognosis.[10]

Please refer to clinicalevidence.com for full text and references.

Chronic fatigue syndrome

Search date September 2005

Steven Reid, Trudie Chalder, Anthony Cleare, Matthew Hotopf, and Simon Wessely

What are the effects of treatments?

BENEFICIAL

Cognitive behavioural therapy

One systematic review found that cognitive behavioural therapy improved quality of life and physical functioning compared with standard medical care or relaxation therapy. One RCT found that cognitive behavioural therapy administered by therapists with no experience of treating chronic fatigue syndrome may also be effective compared with guided support groups or no interventions. One subsequent RCT found that cognitive behavioural therapy in adolescents reduced fatigue severity and functional impairment, and improved school attendance compared with no treatment.

Graded aerobic exercise

One systematic review of three RCTs found that a graded aerobic exercise programme improved measures of fatigue and physical functioning compared with flexibility training and relaxation training or general advice. One subsequent RCT found that graded exercise increased the proportion of people with self-reported improvement compared with standard medical treatment. The review identified one RCT, which found that an educational package to encourage graded exercise improved measures of physical functioning, fatigue, mood, and sleep at 1 year compared with written information alone.

UNKNOWN EFFECTIVENESS

Antidepressants

RCTs provided insufficient evidence about the effects of antidepressants in people with chronic fatigue syndrome.

Corticosteroids

RCTs provided insufficient evidence about the effects of corticosteroids in people with chronic fatigue syndrome.

Dietary supplements

One small RCT found no significant difference between a nutritional supplement (containing multivitamins, minerals, and coenzymes) and placebo in fatigue severity or functional impairment at 10 weeks.

Evening primrose oil

One small RCT found no significant difference between evening primrose oil and placebo in symptom scores at 3 months.

Homeopathy *New*

One RCT found insufficient evidence about the effects of homeopathy compared with placebo in people with chronic fatigue syndrome.

Magnesium (intramuscular)

One small RCT found that intramuscular magnesium injections improved symptoms at 6 weeks compared with placebo. However, we were unable to draw reliable conclusions from this small study.

Oral nicotinamide adenine dinucleotide

One RCT identified by a systematic review provided insufficient evidence about the effects of oral nicotinamide adenine dinucleotide in people with chronic fatigue syndrome.

Prolonged rest

We found no RCTs on the effects of prolonged rest. Indirect observational evidence in healthy volunteers and in people recovering from a viral illness suggests that prolonged rest may perpetuate or worsen fatigue and symptoms.

UNLIKELY TO BE BENEFICIAL

Galantamine *New*

One large RCT found no significant difference in symptomatic improvement between galantamine and placebo at 16 weeks.

LIKELY TO BE INEFFECTIVE OR HARMFUL

Immunotherapy

Small RCTs provided limited evidence that immunoglobulin G modestly improved physical functioning and fatigue at 3–6 months compared with placebo, but it was associated with considerable adverse effects. Small RCTs provided insufficient evidence on the effects of interferon alfa or aciclovir compared with placebo. One RCT found that staphylococcus toxoid improved symptoms at 6 months compared with placebo, although it was associated with local reaction and could cause anaphylaxis.

DEFINITION Chronic fatigue syndrome (CFS) is characterised by severe, disabling fatigue and other symptoms, including musculoskeletal pain, sleep disturbance, impaired concentration, and headaches. Two widely used definitions of CFS, from the US Centers for Disease Control and Prevention ([CDC], current criteria issued in 1994, which superseded CDC criteria issued in 1988)[1] and from Oxford, UK,[2] were developed as operational criteria for research (see table 1Ⓣ). There are important differences between these definitions. The UK criteria insist upon the presence of mental fatigue, whereas the US criteria include a requirement for several physical symptoms, reflecting the belief that CFS has an underlying immunological or infective pathology.

INCIDENCE/ PREVALENCE Community and primary care based studies have reported the prevalence of CFS to be from 0.007% to 2.8% in the general adult population and from 0.006% to 3.0% in primary care depending on the criteria used.[3]

AETIOLOGY/ RISK FACTORS Despite considerable research effort and several hypotheses, the cause of CFS remains poorly understood. Endocrine and immunological abnormalities have been found in many people, although it is unclear whether these changes are causal or part of the course of the syndrome. Women are at higher risk than men (RR 1.3–1.7, depending on diagnostic criteria used; confidence intervals not reported).[4] Population surveys in the US have found that white individuals have a lower risk of CFS compared with Latinos, African Americans, and Native Americans.[5,6]

PROGNOSIS Studies have focused on people attending specialist clinics. A systematic review of studies of prognosis (search date 1996) found that children with CFS had better outcomes than adults: 54–94% of children showed definite improvement in symptoms (after up to 6 years' follow up), whereas 20–50% of adults showed some improvement in the medium term (12–39 months) and only 6% returned to premorbid levels of functioning.[7] Despite the considerable burden of morbidity associated with CFS, we found no evidence of increased mortality. The systematic review found that a longer duration of illness, fatigue severity, comorbid depression and anxiety, and a physical attribution for CFS are factors associated with a poorer prognosis.[7]

Please refer to clinicalevidence.com for full text and references.

Fracture prevention in postmenopausal women

Search date January 2005

Leif Mosekilde, Peter Vestergaard, and Bente Langdahl

What are the effects of treatments to prevent fractures in postmenopausal women?

BENEFICIAL

Alendronate

One systematic review in postmenopausal women found that alendronate reduced vertebral and non-vertebral fractures compared with placebo at 1 year. One systematic review found that alendronate reduced vertebral and hip fractures at 1–4 years. One systematic review found no significant difference between alendronate and placebo in the proportion of women discontinuing alendronate because of adverse effects.

Parathyroid hormone

One RCT in women with prior vertebral fractures found that parathyroid hormone reduced the proportion of women with vertebral and non-vertebral fractures compared with placebo. One small RCT in women with osteoporosis found that parathyroid hormone plus oestrogen reduced vertebral fractures compared with oestrogen alone after 3 years. Parathyroid hormone increased transitory nausea and headache.

Raloxifene

One large RCT in postmenopausal women with osteoporosis found that raloxifene reduced vertebral fractures compared with placebo, but found no significant difference in non-vertebral fractures. One very small RCT found no significant difference between raloxifene and placebo in fractures. We found no RCTs examining the effects of other selective oestrogen receptor modulators. One large RCT found that raloxifene increased the number of women with venous thromboembolic events compared with placebo.

Risedronate

One systematic review in postmenopausal women found that, compared with control (placebo, calcium, or calcium plus vitamin D), risedronate reduced vertebral and non-vertebral fractures at 4 years. One systematic review found that risedronate reduced vertebral and hip fractures compared with placebo. One systematic review found no significant difference between risedronate and placebo, calcium, or calcium plus vitamin D in the proportion of women who withdrew due to side effects.

Strontium ranelate

One large RCT in postmenopausal women with osteoporosis found that strontium ranelate reduced vertebral fractures compared with placebo. One large RCT failed to show a reduction in non-vertebral fractures. This RCT found that strontium ranelate significantly increased the proportion of women with diarrhoea during the first 3 months of treatment.

Fracture prevention in postmenopausal women

LIKELY TO BE BENEFICIAL

Calcitonin

One systematic review found that calcitonin reduced vertebral fractures compared with placebo in postmenopausal women at 1–5 years after treatment, but found no significant difference between calcitonin and placebo in non-vertebral fractures. One systematic review found that doses of calcitonin between 50–400 IU daily reduced vertebral fractures, but not non-vertebral fractures. The first systematic review found that calcitonin increased headaches and climacteric symptoms.

Calcium plus vitamin D or vitamin D analogue

One large systematic review found that calcium plus vitamin D reduced non-vertebral and hip fractures compared with placebo or no intervention, but the results were of borderline significance. One systematic review found that calcium plus vitamin D reduced non-vertebral and hip fractures compared with placebo or calcium only when the dose of calcium exceeded 700 IU (17.5 μg). One systematic review found that calcium plus vitamin D reduced vertebral fractures compared with placebo or calcium, and that both calcium plus hydroxylated vitamin D and calcium plus vitamin D failed to significantly reduce non-vertebral fractures. The systematic reviews found that vitamin D or its analogues increased the risk of hypercalcaemia.

Clodronate

One small RCT found that clodronate reduced vertebral but not non-vertebral fractures compared with placebo. The RCT gave no information on adverse effects.

Etidronate

One systematic review in postmenopausal women found that etidronate reduced vertebral fractures compared with placebo, calcium, or calcium plus vitamin D over 2 years. One small systematic review found no significant difference between etidronate and placebo in vertebral fractures. One systematic review found no significant difference in non-vertebral fractures compared with placebo, calcium, or calcium plus vitamin D over 2 years. One systematic review did not report specifically on harms, but found no significant difference in dropout rates between etidronate and placebo.

Hip protectors

One systematic review found that hip protectors reduced hip fractures compared with no hip protectors in nursing home residents, although the result was of borderline significance. There was no significant difference between hip protectors and no hip protectors in any other fracture.

Ibandronate

One large RCT found that Ibandronate reduced vertebral but not non-vertebral fractures compared with placebo. It found no significant difference in side effects.

Pamidronate

One small RCT found that pamidronate reduced fractures compared with placebo, although the results for non-vertebral fractures did not reach significance. Another small RCT found similar results for vertebral fractures. It found no significant difference in side effects.

◀ **Vitamin D analogues (alphacalcidol or calcitriol)**

One systematic review in a mixed population of both sexes and various pathologies found vitamin D analogues reduced fractures compared with placebo. One systematic review found that vitamin D analogues reduced vertebral fractures compared with vitamin D in postmenopausal women. One systematic review found that vitamin D analogues increased the risk of hypercalcaemia compared with native vitamin D.

UNKNOWN EFFECTIVENESS

Calcium alone

One systematic review in postmenopausal women found no significant difference between calcium supplementation and placebo in vertebral or non-vertebral fractures at 1.5–4 years.

Environmental manipulation

We found no systematic review and no RCTs assessing environmental manipulation alone.

Exercise

Five small RCTs, in different populations that included many elderly patients, found no significant difference in peripheral fractures or falls resulting in peripheral fracture at 8 months to 2 years between exercise (advice to walk briskly three times weekly, balance and strength exercises plus walking, or low-intensity exercise plus incontinence care) and control. One small RCT in postmenopausal women found no significant difference between a 2 year back strengthening exercise programme and usual care in vertebral fractures over 10 years.

Multifactorial non-pharmacological interventions

Three RCTs found contradictory results on the effect of multifactorial non-pharmacological interventions on fractures. One RCT found that multifactorial non-pharmacological interventions reduced femoral fractures compared with placebo, whereas two RCTs found no significant difference in fractures between multifactorial non-pharmacological interventions and control.

UNLIKELY TO BE BENEFICIAL

Vitamin D alone

One systematic review found no significant difference in fractures between vitamin D (in doses up to 800 IU/day) and placebo. One systematic review found that vitamin D increased vertebral fractures compared with vitamin D analogues (alfacalcidol and calcitriol). One systematic review found that vitamin D increased the risk of hypercalcaemia compared with placebo.

LIKELY TO BE INEFFECTIVE OR HARMFUL

Hormone replacement therapy

Two systematic reviews and two large subsequent RCTs found that hormone replacement therapy (HRT) reduced non-vertebral and vertebral fractures compared with placebo, no intervention, or calcium and/or vitamin D. One systematic review found no significant difference in fractures between HRT and placebo. The pooled data from four large RCTs, one subsequent RCT, and one large observational study found that HRT increases the incidence of breast cancer compared with placebo, and four RCTs found that HRT also increases the risk of stroke and pulmonary embolism compared with placebo. One small RCT ▶

Fracture prevention in postmenopausal women

in women with osteoporosis found that oestrogen alone was less effective at reducing fractures compared with parathyroid hormone plus oestrogen.

DEFINITION This topic covers interventions to prevent fractures in postmenopausal women. A fracture is a break or disruption of bone or cartilage, and may be symptomatic or asymptomatic. Symptoms and signs may include immobility, pain, tenderness, numbness, bruising, joint deformity, joint swelling, limb deformity, and limb shortening.[1] **Diagnosis:** Fracture is usually diagnosed on the basis of a typical clinical picture (see above) combined with results from an appropriate imaging technique. Usually, in trials dealing with osteoporosis, menopause is considered to be present 12 months after the last menstruation.[2]

INCIDENCE/ PREVALENCE The lifetime risk of fracture in white women is 20% for the spine, 15% for the wrist, and 18% for the hip.[3] The incidence of postmenopausal fracture increases with age.[4] Observational studies found that age specific incidence rates for postmenopausal fracture of the hip increased exponentially beyond the age of 50 years. The incidence of fractures varies by ethnic group. The incidence of hip fractures is highest in Caucasians and then decreases successively in Hispanics, Asians, and African Americans.[5]

AETIOLOGY/ RISK FACTORS A fracture arises when load to the bone exceeds bone biomechanical competence (strength). Fractures usually arise from trauma, but may arise without any apparent injury. Risk factors are those factors that increase the risk of trauma and decrease bone biomechanical competence. An increased risk of trauma exists when the risk of falls is increased, such as in those with impaired vision, decreased postural balance, or neurological disorders (e.g. ataxia, stroke, epilepsy). Factors that decrease bone biomechanical competence and so induce osteoporosis include increasing age, low body mass index or weight, genetic predisposition, diseases (e.g. hyperthyroidism, hyperparathyroidism, and rheumatoid arthritis), drugs (e.g. corticosteroids), and environmental factors (e.g. smoking).[5] Postmenopausal women are at increased risk of fracture compared with premenopausal women and men of all ages because of hormone related bone loss.

PROGNOSIS Fractures may result in pain, short or long term disability, haemorrhage, thromboembolic disease (see thromboembolism), shock, and death. Vertebral fractures are associated with pain, physical impairment, muscular atrophy, changes in body shape, loss of physical function, and lower quality of life.[6] About 20% of women die in the first year after a hip fracture, representing an increase in mortality of 12–20% compared with women of similar age and no hip fracture. Half of all elderly women who have previously been independent become partly dependent after hip fracture. A third become totally dependent.

Please refer to clinicalevidence.com for full text and references.

Gout

Search date June 2005

Martin Underwood

What are the effects of treatments for acute gout?

UNKNOWN EFFECTIVENESS

Colchicine

One small RCT provided limited evidence that colchicine improved pain in people with gout. However, we were unable to draw reliable conclusions from this small RCT. The high incidence of adverse effects in people taking colchicine precludes its use as a routine treatment.

Corticosteroids

We found no RCTs on the effects of intra-articular, parenteral, or oral corticosteroids in people with gout.

Non-steroidal anti-inflammatory drugs

One small RCT provided limited evidence that tenoxicam reduced short term pain and tenderness in people with gout compared with placebo. However, this study was too small to provide reliable conclusions. We found no RCTs comparing other non-steroidal anti-inflammatory drugs versus placebo in people with gout. Five RCTs found no significant difference in effectiveness between different non-steroidal anti-inflammatory drugs. However, these RCTs may have lacked power to detect clinically relevant differences. Two equivalence studies found no difference in pain between etoricoxib and indometacin, but found that indometacin was associated with more adverse effects. The adverse effects of non-steroidal anti-inflammatory drugs include gastrointestinal ulceration and haemorrhage, and, for at least some cyclo-oxygenase-2 inhibitors, increased cardiovascular risk.

What are the effects of treatments to prevent gout in people with prior acute episodes?

UNKNOWN EFFECTIVENESS

Advice to lose weight

We found no RCTs on the effects of advice to lose weight to prevent attacks of gout in people with prior episodes.

Advice to reduce alcohol intake

We found no RCTs on the effects of advice to reduce alcohol intake to prevent attacks of gout in people with prior episodes.

Advice to reduce dietary intake of purines

We found no RCTs on the effects of advice to reduce dietary intake of purines to prevent attacks of gout in people with prior episodes.

Allopurinol

We found no RCTs on the effects of allopurinol to prevent attacks of gout in people with prior episodes.

Gout

Colchicine

One RCT provided limited evidence that colchicine reduces the incidence of recurrent gout when starting treatment with allopurinol.

Sulfinpyrazone

We found no RCTs on the effects of sulfinpyrazone to prevent attacks of gout in people with prior episodes.

DEFINITION Gout is a syndrome caused by deposition of urate crystals.[1] It typically presents as an acute monoarthritis of rapid onset. The first metatarsophalangeal joint is the most commonly affected joint (podagra). Gout also affects other joints: joints in the foot, ankle, knee, wrist, finger, and elbow are the most frequently affected. Crystal deposits (tophi) may develop around hands, feet, elbows, and ears. **Diagnosis:** This is usually made clinically. The American College of Rheumatology (ACR) criteria for diagnosing gout are as follows: (1) characteristic urate crystals in joint fluid; (2) a tophus proved to contain urate crystals; or (3) the presence of six or more defined clinical laboratory and x ray phenomena (see table 1Ⓣ).[2] We have included studies of people meeting the ACR criteria, studies in which the diagnosis was made clinically, and studies that used other criteria.

INCIDENCE/ PREVALENCE Gout is more common in older people and men.[3] In people aged 65–74 years in the UK, the prevalence is about 50/1000 in men and about 9/1000 in women.[4] The annual incidence of gout in people aged over 50 years in the USA is 1.6/1000 for men and 0.3/1000 for women.[5] One 12 year longitudinal study of 47 150 male health professionals with no previous history of gout estimated that annual incidence of gout ranged from 1/1000 for those aged 40–44 years to 1.8/1000 for those aged 55–64 years.[6] Gout may become more common because of increasing longevity, obesity, meat and fish consumption, and use of diuretics.[7] Gout may be more common in some non-white ethnic groups.[3] A pooled analysis of two cohort studies of former medical students found the annual incidence of gout to be 3.1/1000 in black men and 1.8/1000 in white men.[8] After correcting for the higher prevalence of hypertension among black men, which is a risk factor for gout, the relative risk of gout in black men compared with white men was 1.30 (95% CI 0.77 to 2.19).

AETIOLOGY/ RISK FACTORS Urate crystals form when serum urate concentration exceeds 0.42 mmol/L.[9] Serum urate concentration is the principal risk factor for a first attack of gout,[10] although 40% of people have normal serum urate concentration during an attack of gout.[9,11-13] A cohort study of 2046 men followed for about 15 years found that the annual incidence is about 0.4% in men with a urate concentration of 0.42–0.47 mmol/L, rising to 4.3% when serum urate concentration is 0.45–0.59 mmol/L.[14] A 5 year longitudinal study of 223 asymptomatic men with hyperuricaemia estimated the 5 year cumulative incidence of gout to be 10.8% for those with baseline serum urate of 0.42–0.47 mmol/L, 27.7% for baseline urate 0.48–0.53 mmol/L, and 61.1% for baseline urate levels of 0.54 mmol/L or more.[10] The study found that a 0.6 mmol/L difference in baseline serum urate increased the odds of an attack of gout by a factor of 1.8 (OR adjusted for other risk factors for gout: 1.84, 95% CI 1.24 to 2.72). One 12 year longitudinal study (47 150 male health professionals with no history of gout) estimated that the relative risks of gout associated with one additional daily serving of various foods (weekly for seafood) were as follows: meat 1.21 (95% CI 1.04 to1.41), seafood (fish, lobster, and shellfish) 1.07 (95% CI 1.01 to 1.12), purine rich vegetables 0.97 (95% CI 0.79 to 1.19), low fat dairy products 0.79 (95% CI 0.71 to 0.87), and high fat dairy products 0.99 (95% CI 0.89 to 1.10).[6,15] Alcohol consumption of greater than 14.9 g daily significantly increased the risk of gout compared with no alcohol consumption (compared with no alcohol consumption: RR for 15.0 g/day to 29.9 g/day:

1.49, 95% CI 1.14 to 1.94; RR for 30.0 g/day to 49.9 g/day: 1.96, 95% CI 1.48 to 2.60; RR for ≥ 50 g/day: 2.53, 95% CI 1.73 to 3.70).[15] The longitudinal study also estimated the relative risk of gout associated with an additional serving of beer (355 mL, 12.8 g alcohol), wine (118 mL, 11.0 g alcohol), and spirits (44 mL, 14.0 g alcohol). It found that an extra daily serving of beer or spirits was significantly associated with gout, but an extra daily serving of wine was not (RR for 355 mL/day beer: 1.49, 95% CI 1.32 to 1.70; RR for 44 mL/day spirits: 1.15, 95% CI 1.04 to 1.28; RR for 118 mL/day wine: 1.04, 95% CI 0.88 to 1.22).Other suggested risk factors for gout include obesity, insulin resistance, dyslipidaemia, hypertension, and cardiovascular disorders.[16,17]

PROGNOSIS We found few reliable data about prognosis or complications of gout.One study found that 3/11 (27%) people with untreated gout of the first metatarsophalangeal joint experienced spontaneous resolution after 7 days.[18] A case series of 614 people with gout who had not received treatment to reduce urate levels, and could recall the interval between first and second attacks, reported recurrence rates of 62% after 1 year, 78% after 2 years, and 84% after 3 years.[19] An analysis of two prospective cohort studies of 371 black and 1181 white male former medical students followed up for about 30 years found no significant difference in risk of coronary heart disease in men who had developed gout compared with men who had not (RR 0.85, 95% CI 0.40 to 1.81).[20]

Please refer to clinicalevidence.com for full text and references.

Herniated lumbar disc

Search date May 2005

Jo Jordan, Kika Konstantinou, Tamara Shawver Morgan, and James Weinstein

What are the effects of drug treatments?

UNKNOWN EFFECTIVENESS

Analgesics

We found no systematic review or RCTs on the use of analgesics for treatment of people with symptomatic herniated lumbar discs.

Antidepressants

We found no systematic review or RCTs on the use of antidepressants for treatment of people with symptomatic herniated lumbar discs.

Corticosteroids (epidural injections)

One systematic review provided limited evidence that epidural corticosteroid injections increased global improvement compared with placebo. However, one subsequent RCT found no significant difference between epidural corticosteroid injections plus conservative treatment and conservative treatment alone in pain, mobility, or ability to return to work at 6 months. Another subsequent RCT found no significant difference between epidural corticosteroid injection and control injection in pain, disability, or self rated improvement after 35 days. One RCT provided limited evidence that epidural corticosteroid injections were less effective at reducing leg pain and improving function than standard discectomy at 1–3 months, but found no significant differences between treatments at 2–3 years.

Muscle relaxants

We found no systematic review or RCTs on the use of muscle relaxants for treatment of people with symptomatic herniated lumbar discs.

UNLIKELY TO BE BENEFICIAL

Non-steroidal anti-inflammatory drugs

One systematic review found no significant difference in overall improvement between non-steroidal anti-inflammatory drugs and placebo in people with sciatica caused by disc herniation.

What are the effects of non-drug treatments?

LIKELY TO BE BENEFICIAL

Spinal manipulation

One RCT identified by a systematic review in people with sciatica caused by disc herniation found that spinal manipulation increased self perceived improvement after 2 weeks compared with a placebo of infrequent infrared heat. Another RCT identified by the review, comparing spinal manipulation, manual traction, exercise, and corsets, found no significant difference among groups in self perceived improvement after 1 month. One subsequent RCT found that spinal manipulation increased the proportion of people with improved symptoms compared with traction. Concerns exist regarding possible further herniation from spinal manipulation in people who are surgical candidates.

UNKNOWN EFFECTIVENESS

Acupuncture

One systematic review found insufficient evidence on the effects of acupuncture in people with herniated lumbar discs.

Advice to stay active

One systematic review of conservative treatments for sciatica caused by lumbar disc herniation found no RCTs on advice to stay active.

Exercise therapy

We found no systematic review or RCTs comparing exercise therapy versus placebo or no treatment. One small RCT identified by a systematic review found no significant difference in global improvement between isometric exercise and manual traction in people with sciatica caused by disc herniation. Another RCT identified by the review, comparing spinal manipulation, manual traction, exercise, and corsets, found no significant difference among groups in self perceived improvement after 1 month.

Heat or ice

One systematic review identified no RCTs of heat or ice for sciatica caused by lumbar disc herniation.

Massage

One systematic review identified no RCTs of massage in people with symptomatic lumbar disc herniation.

UNLIKELY TO BE BENEFICIAL

Bed rest

One systematic review of conservative treatment found no RCTs on bed rest in people with symptomatic herniated discs. One subsequent RCT in people with sciatica found no significant difference between bed rest and watchful waiting for 2 weeks in people's perceived improvement, mean pain scores, mean disability scores, or mean satisfaction scores after 12 weeks.

Traction

One systematic review found no significant difference in overall global improvement between traction and placebo in people with sciatica and herniated lumbar disc. One small RCT identified by the review found no significant difference in global measure of improvement between manual traction and isometric exercises in people with herniated lumbar disc. Another RCT identified by the review, comparing spinal manipulation, manual traction, exercise, and corsets, found no significant difference among groups in self perceived improvement after 1 month. One small RCT identified by the review found no significant difference in overall global improvement between autotraction and manual traction. Another small RCT identified by the review provided limited evidence that autotraction increased the proportion of people reporting a response immediately after treatment compared with passive traction.

Herniated lumbar disc

What are the effects of surgery?

LIKELY TO BE BENEFICIAL

Microdiscectomy (as effective as standard discectomy)

We found no RCTs comparing microdiscectomy versus conservative treatment. Three RCTs found no significant difference in clinical outcomes between microdiscectomy and standard discectomy. One RCT found no significant difference in satisfaction or pain between video assisted arthroscopic microdiscectomy and standard discectomy at about 30 months, although postoperative recovery was slower with standard discectomy. Two RCTs identified by a systematic review provided insufficient evidence on the effects of automated percutaneous discectomy compared with microdiscectomy.

Standard discectomy (short term benefit)

One RCT found that standard discectomy increased self reported improvement at 1 year, but not at 4 and 10 years, compared with conservative treatment (physiotherapy). One RCT provided limited evidence that standard discectomy improved leg pain and function at 1–3 months compared with epidural corticosteroid injections. It found no significant difference between treatments after 2–3 years. Three RCTs found no significant difference in clinical outcomes between standard discectomy and microdiscectomy. Adverse effects were similar with both procedures. One RCT found no significant difference in satisfaction or pain between standard discectomy and video assisted arthroscopic microdiscectomy at about 30 months, although postoperative recovery was slower with standard discectomy.

UNKNOWN EFFECTIVENESS

Automated percutaneous discectomy

We found no RCTs comparing automated percutaneous discectomy versus either conservative treatment or standard discectomy. Two RCTs identified by a systematic review provided insufficient evidence on the clinical effects of automated percutaneous discectomy compared with microdiscectomy.

Laser discectomy

We found no systematic review or RCTs on the use of laser discectomy for treatment of people with symptomatic herniated lumbar discs.

DEFINITION Herniated lumbar disc is a displacement of disc material (nucleus pulposus or annulus fibrosis) beyond the intervertebral disc space.[1] The diagnosis can be confirmed by radiological examination; however, magnetic resonance imaging findings of herniated disc are not always accompanied by clinical symptoms.[2,3] This review covers treatment of people who have clinical symptoms relating to confirmed or suspected disc herniation. It does not include treatment of people with spinal cord compression or people with cauda equine syndrome, which require emergency intervention. The management of non-specific acute low back pain and chronic low back pain are covered elsewhere in *Clinical Evidence*.

INCIDENCE/ PREVALENCE The prevalence of symptomatic herniated lumbar disc is about 1–3% in Finland and Italy, depending on age and sex.[4] The highest prevalence is among people aged 30–50 years,[5] with a male to female ratio of 2 : 1.[6] In people aged between 25 years and 55 years, about 95% of herniated discs occur at the lower lumbar spine (L4–L5 level); disc herniation above this level is more common in people over 55 years of age.[7,8]

AETIOLOGY/ RISK FACTORS Radiographical evidence of disc herniation does not reliably predict low back pain in the future or correlate with symptoms; 19–27% of people without symptoms have disc herniation on imaging.[2,9] Risk factors for disc herniation include smoking (OR 1.7, 95% CI 1.0 to 2.5), weight bearing sports (e.g. weight lifting, hammer throw etc), and certain work activities such as repeated lifting. Driving a motor vehicle has been suggested to be a risk factor for disc herniation, although evidence is not conclusive (OR 1.7, 95% CI 0.2 to 2.7).[6,10,11] This potential effect may be because the resonant frequency of the spine is similar to that of certain vehicles.

PROGNOSIS The natural history of disc herniation is difficult to determine because most people take some form of treatment for their back pain, and a formal diagnosis is not always made.[6] Clinical improvement is usual in most people, and only about 10% of people still have sufficient pain after 6 weeks to consider surgery. Sequential magnetic resonance images have shown that the herniated portion of the disc tends to regress over time, with partial to complete resolution after 6 months in two thirds of people.[12]

Please refer to clinicalevidence.com for full text and references.

Hip fracture

Search date December 2005

Helen Handoll and Martyn Parker

What are the effects of surgical interventions for hip fracture?

TRADE OFF BETWEEN BENEFITS AND HARMS

Internal fixation versus arthroplasty for intracapsular hip fracture

Two systematic reviews and four subsequent RCTs in older people with displaced intracapsular fractures found that internal fixation increased the need for subsequent revision surgery compared with arthroplasty. Internal fixation was, however, associated with less operative trauma, including reduced operative blood loss and transfusion requirements, and reduced deep wound sepsis. There were no clear differences in mortality. The larger review found no significant difference in functional outcomes between treatments. However, three of the subsequent RCTs provided limited evidence that arthroplasty improved short term functional outcomes in fitter older people compared with internal fixation. Most orthopaedic surgeons tend to favour arthroplasty in older people over internal fixation owing to the reduced reoperation rate. For people aged less than 60–70 years, preservation of the femoral head is generally preferred because the expected longer term survival may lead to a high revision rate if arthroplasty had been used. None of the RCTs identified were in younger people.

UNKNOWN EFFECTIVENESS

Arthroplasty versus internal fixation for extracapsular fracture

One RCT with weak methods identified by a systematic review and one subsequent RCT provided insufficient evidence to compare arthroplasty versus internal fixation in people with unstable extracapsular fractures.

Choice of implant for internal fixation of intracapsular hip fracture

One systematic review provided insufficient evidence to determine the best implant for internal fixation of intracapsular fractures.

Different types of arthroplasty for intracapsular hip fracture

One systematic review and two subsequent RCTs provided insufficient evidence to determine the best type of arthroplasty (cemented *v* uncemented prostheses; unipolar and bipolar hemiarthroplasty; or hemiarthroplasty and total hip replacement) for people with intracapsular fractures.

External fixation for extracapsular fracture

One systematic review provided insufficient evidence on the relative effects of external fixation compared with the sliding hip screw in people with extracapsular hip fracture.

Extramedullary implants other than older fixed nail plates versus sliding hip screw for extracapsular fracture

One systematic review provided insufficient evidence on the relative effects of extramedullary implants of both sliding and fixed designs (other than older fixed nail plates) in people with extracapsular hip fracture.

UNLIKELY TO BE BENEFICIAL

Conservative versus operative treatment for most types of hip fracture

One small RCT identified by a systematic review found limited evidence that conservative treatment of undisplaced intracapsular fractures increased the risk of non-union compared with internal fixation of the fracture. The review identified no RCTs in people with displaced intracapsular fracture. The review found limited evidence that conservative treatment of extracapsular fractures increased the proportion of people remaining in hospital after 12 weeks, the occurrence of leg shortening, and varus deformity compared with surgical treatment. The review provided insufficient evidence to assess whether significant differences exist between conservative and surgical treatment in medical complications, mortality, long term pain, or loss of independence.

Short cephalocondylic nail (e.g. Gamma nail) versus sliding hip screw for extracapsular hip fracture

One systematic review found no significant difference between intramedullary fixation with a short cephalocondylic nail (e.g. Gamma nail) and extramedullary fixation with a sliding hip screw in mortality, pain at follow up, ability to return to a previous residence, and ability to walk after 3–12 months. The review also found no significant difference between treatments in wound infection or cut-out of the implant, but found that cephalocondylic intramedullary fixation increased intraoperative and later femoral fractures and reoperation rates.

LIKELY TO BE INEFFECTIVE OR HARMFUL

Intramedullary fixation with condylocephalic nails (e.g. Ender nails) versus extramedullary fixation for extracapsular fracture

One systematic review found that intramedullary fixation with condylocephalic nails increased reoperation rates and the incidence of leg shortening and external rotation deformity compared with extramedullary fixation, although it found that condylocephalic nails (e.g. Ender nails) reduced length of surgery, the incidence of deep wound sepsis, and operative blood loss.

Older fixed nail plates for extramedullary fixation of extracapsular fracture (increased risk of fixation failure compared with sliding hip screws)

One systematic review found no significant difference between older fixed nail plates and sliding hip screws in mortality, pain at follow up, or impairment of mobility. It found that sliding hip screws reduced the risk of fixation failure in people with extracapsular hip fracture.

What are the effects of perisurgical medical interventions on surgical outcome and prevention of complications?

BENEFICIAL

Perioperative prophylaxis with antibiotics

One systematic review found that multiple dose perioperative and single dose preoperative antibiotic prophylaxis regimens reduced deep and superficial wound infection after hip surgery compared with placebo or no antibiotics.

Hip fracture

LIKELY TO BE BENEFICIAL

Cyclical compression of the foot or calf to reduce venous thromboembolism

One systematic review found that cyclical compression devices (foot or calf pumps) reduced deep venous thrombosis and pulmonary embolism compared with no compression, but were associated with non-compliance and skin abrasion.

Oral multinutrient feeds for nutritional supplementation after hip fracture

One systematic review found limited evidence that nutritional supplementation consisting of oral protein and energy multinutrient feeds reduced unfavourable outcome (postoperative complications or death) after surgery for hip fracture compared with control.

Perioperative prophylaxis with antiplatelet agents

One systematic review and one subsequent large RCT found that perioperative and postoperative antiplatelet prophylaxis reduced the incidence of deep venous thrombosis and pulmonary embolism compared with placebo or no prophylaxis. The RCT found no significant effect on mortality. Both the review and subsequent RCT found that more people having antiplatelet treatment had bleeding complications.

TRADE OFF BETWEEN BENEFITS AND HARMS

Perioperative prophylaxis with heparin to reduce venous thromboembolism

One systematic review found that perioperative prophylaxis with either unfractionated heparin or low molecular weight heparin reduced the incidence of deep venous thrombosis compared with placebo or no treatment. The review found insufficient evidence to determine whether heparin reduced pulmonary embolism, or mortality. It also found insufficient evidence to determine whether heparin increased bleeding and other complications, although another systematic review of unfractionated heparin in people having general, orthopaedic, and urological surgery found that, overall, heparin increased excessive bleeding or the need for transfusion compared with control.

UNKNOWN EFFECTIVENESS

Graduated elastic compression to prevent venous thromboembolism

We found no RCTs of thromboembolism stockings for prevention of thrombotic complications in people with hip fracture. Two systematic reviews in people having orthopaedic surgery (including elective total hip replacement) found that graduated elastic compression, either with or without other antithrombotic measures, reduced the risk of deep venous thrombosis compared with control.

Low molecular weight versus unfractionated heparin to reduce venous thromboembolism after hip fracture surgery

Five weak RCTs identified by a systematic review provided insufficient evidence to establish whether low molecular weight heparin reduced deep venous thrombosis compared with unfractionated heparin. A second systematic review in people having orthopaedic surgery found no evidence of a difference in bleeding complications between low molecular weight heparin and unfractionated heparin.

Nasogastric feeds for nutritional supplementation after hip fracture

One systematic review and one subsequent small RCT found no evidence that nasogastric multinutrient feeding reduced mortality compared with control. However, the RCTs were small, had flawed methods, and included people with differing nutritional status. There was insufficient evidence to assess other outcomes.

Nerve blocks for pain control before and after hip fracture

One systematic review of small RCTs found that nerve blocks reduced total analgesic intake (a surrogate measure of pain) compared with no nerve block. The RCTs, which tested different nerve blocks inserted at varying times, provided insufficient evidence on which to base conclusions.

Operative day (< 24 hours) versus longer duration multiple dose antibiotic regimens

Two systematic reviews provided limited evidence, from two or three RCTs respectively, that there was no significant difference in wound infection between extended and operative day multiple dose antibiotic prophylaxis in people having hip surgery.

Regional versus general anaesthesia for hip fracture surgery

One systematic review of people after hip fracture surgery found limited evidence that regional anaesthesia reduced the risk of acute postoperative confusion compared with general anaesthesia. It found insufficient evidence to draw conclusions regarding mortality or other outcomes.

Single dose (long acting) versus multiple dose antibiotic regimens

Two systematic reviews provided limited evidence of no significant difference in wound infection between some single and some multiple dose antibiotic regimens in people having hip surgery.

UNLIKELY TO BE BENEFICIAL

Preoperative traction to the injured limb

One systematic review found no significant difference in the relief of preoperative pain, or subsequent ease and quality of fracture reduction at time of surgery, between routine preoperative traction and control.

What are the effects of rehabilitation interventions and programmes after hip fracture?

LIKELY TO BE BENEFICIAL

Co-ordinated multidisciplinary approaches for inpatient rehabilitation of older people

One systematic review comparing co-ordinated multidisciplinary care for inpatient rehabilitation versus usual (often orthopaedic) care in older people found no significant difference in mortality or the combined outcomes of death or institutional care, death or deterioration in functional status, or death or readmission to hospital. However, there was a non-significant trend in favour of multidisciplinary care in these outcomes. The review provided limited evidence that multidisciplinary care resulted in fewer complications (pressure sores, chest infections, or cardiac problems). It was not possible to define the best method of multidisciplinary care from the various models assessed in the review.

Hip fracture

UNKNOWN EFFECTIVENESS

Early supported discharge followed by home based rehabilitation

Two of three RCTs found no significant difference in overall quality of life, mortality, falls, or readmissions between early supported discharge to home based rehabilitation and hospital based rehabilitation in less disabled people with a favourable home situation. One of these RCTs found that early supported discharge reduced carer burden at 12 months compared with hospital based rehabilitation. Both of these RCTs found that early supported discharge reduced length of hospital stay, but increased the overall length of rehabilitative care. A third RCT found limited evidence that home rehabilitation with a physiotherapist improved mobility at 12 months compared with institutional rehabilitation.

Mobilisation strategies applied soon after hip fracture surgery

One systematic review provided insufficient evidence to determine the effects of various mobilisation strategies started soon after hip fracture surgery.

Systematic multicomponent home based rehabilitation

One RCT comparing a systematic home based multicomponent rehabilitation programme versus usual care found no significant difference in recovery to pre-fracture levels of self care, home management, social activity, balance, or lower extremity strength after 12 months.

DEFINITION A hip or proximal femoral fracture refers to any fracture of the femur between the hip joint articular cartilage to a point 5 cm below the distal part of the lesser trochanter. Femoral head fractures are not included within this definition.[1] Hip fractures are divided into two groups according to their relationship to the capsular attachments of the hip joint. **Intracapsular fractures** occur proximal to the point at which the hip joint capsule attaches to the femur, and can be subdivided into displaced and undisplaced fractures.[2] Undisplaced fractures include impacted or adduction fractures. Displaced intracapsular fractures may be associated with disruption of the blood supply to the head of the femur leading to avascular necrosis. **Extracapsular fractures** occur distal to the hip joint capsule.[1] In the most distal part of the proximal femoral segment (below the lesser trochanter), the term "subtrochanteric" fracture is used. Numerous further subclassifications of intracapsular and extracapsular fractures exist.[1,2]

INCIDENCE/ PREVALENCE Hip fractures may occur at any age but are most common in older people (here defined as people aged > 65 years). In industrialised societies, the mean age of people with hip fracture is about 80 years and about 80% are female. In the USA, the lifetime risk after age 50 years of hip fracture is about 17% in white women and 6% in white men.[3] A study in the USA reported that prevalence increases from about 3/100 women aged 65–74 years to 12.6/100 women aged 85 years and above.[4] The age stratified incidence has also increased in some societies; not only are people living longer, but the incidence of fracture in each age group may have increased.[3] An estimated 1.26 million hip fractures occurred in adults in 1990 with predictions of numbers rising to 7.3–21.3 million by 2050.[5]

AETIOLOGY/ RISK FACTORS Hip fractures are usually sustained through a fall from standing height or less. The pattern of incidence is consistent with an increased risk of falling, loss of protective reflex mechanisms, and loss of skeletal strength from osteoporosis. All these increased risks are associated with aging.

PROGNOSIS Reported figures for mortality after a hip fracture in adults vary considerably. One year mortality figures vary from 12% to 37%[6] with about 9% of these deaths being directly attributed to the hip fracture.[7] After a hip fracture a 15–25% decline in the ability to perform daily activities is to be expected, and about 10–20% of the survivors will require a change to a more dependent residential status.[8]

Please refer to clinicalevidence.com for full text and references.

Leg cramps

Search date January 2006

Gavin Young

What are the effects of treatments for idiopathic leg cramps?

BENEFICIAL

Quinine

One systematic review found that quinine reduced the frequency of idiopathic nocturnal leg cramps compared with placebo over 4 weeks; this was supported by weaker evidence from a small crossover RCT where people acted as their own controls. We found no evidence about the optimal dose of quinine or length of treatment. One RCT found that people taking quinine had fewer nights of leg cramps than people taking vitamin E, but that severity of cramps was similar between groups. Another RCT found limited evidence that quinine alone was less effective in reducing idiopathic nocturnal leg cramps less than quinine plus theophylline over 2 weeks.

LIKELY TO BE BENEFICIAL

Quinine plus theophylline

One RCT found limited evidence that quinine plus theophylline reduced idiopathic nocturnal leg cramps compared with quinine alone or placebo over 2 weeks.

UNKNOWN EFFECTIVENESS

Analgesics

We found no systematic review or RCTs on the effects of analgesics on idiopathic leg cramps.

Antiepileptic drugs

We found no systematic review or RCTs on the effects of antiepileptic drugs on idiopathic leg cramps.

Compression hosiery

We found no systematic review or RCTs on the effects of compression hosiery in people with idiopathic leg cramps.

Magnesium salts

Two crossover RCTs provided insufficient evidence on the effects of magnesium salts on frequency, severity, or duration of idiopathic leg cramps.

Stretching exercises *New*

One RCT found that teaching people stretching "standing" exercises did not seem to be of benefit in reducing idiopathic leg cramps compared with teaching them passive non-stretching "lying" exercises.

Vitamin E

One small RCT found no significant difference between vitamin E and placebo in the frequency of nights disturbed by idiopathic leg cramps. Another small RCT found that people taking quinine had fewer nights of cramps than people taking vitamin E, but that severity of cramps was similar in both groups.

What are the effects of treatments for leg cramps in pregnancy?

LIKELY TO BE BENEFICIAL

Magnesium salts

One RCT identified by a systematic review found that magnesium tablets reduced leg cramps compared with placebo in pregnant women after 3 weeks.

UNKNOWN EFFECTIVENESS

Calcium salts

Two RCTs identified by a systematic review provided insufficient evidence on the effects of calcium salts on leg cramps in pregnant women.

Multivitamins and mineral supplements

One small RCT identified by a systematic review found no significant difference between a multivitamin plus mineral supplement and placebo given from 3 months' gestation in leg cramps in the ninth month of pregnancy. The RCT may have lacked power to detect a clinically important difference between groups.

Sodium chloride

One systematic review identified no RCTs on the effects of sodium chloride in pregnant women with leg cramps.

DEFINITION Leg cramps are involuntary, localised, and usually painful skeletal muscle contractions, which commonly affect calf muscles. Leg cramps typically occur at night and usually last only seconds to minutes. Leg cramps may be idiopathic (of unknown cause) or may be associated with a definable process or condition such as pregnancy, renal dialysis, or venous insufficiency. This chapter does not currently cover leg cramps associated with renal dialysis or venous insufficiency.

INCIDENCE/ PREVALENCE Leg cramps are common and their incidence increases with age. About half of people attending a general medicine clinic have had leg cramps within 1 month of their visit, and over two thirds of people over 50 years of age have experienced leg cramps.[1]

AETIOLOGY/ RISK FACTORS Very little is known about the causes of leg cramps. Risk factors include pregnancy, exercise, electrolyte imbalances, salt depletion, renal dialysis, peripheral vascular disease (both venous and arterial), peripheral nerve injury, polyneuropathies, motor neurone disease, muscle diseases, and certain drugs. Other causes of acute calf pain include, for example, trauma, deep venous thrombosis (see thromboembolism topic), and ruptured Baker's cyst.

PROGNOSIS Leg cramps may cause severe pain and sleep disturbance.

Please refer to clinicalevidence.com for full text and references.

Low back pain (acute)

Search date November 2004

Bart Koes and Maurits van Tulder

What are the effects of oral drug treatments?

BENEFICIAL

Non-steroidal anti-inflammatory drugs

One systematic review and one subsequent RCT found that non-steroidal anti-inflammatory drugs (NSAIDs) increased overall improvement after 1 week compared with placebo. One systematic review and additional RCTs found no significant difference among NSAIDs or between NSAIDs and other drug treatments (paracetamol [acetaminophen], opioids, muscle relaxants, NSAIDs plus muscle relaxants) in pain relief. One systematic review found insufficient evidence about effects of NSAIDs compared with non-drug treatments.

TRADE OFF BETWEEN BENEFITS AND HARMS

Muscle relaxants

One systematic review found that muscle relaxants reduced pain and improved overall clinical assessment compared with placebo, but the review found no significant difference among different muscle relaxants. The review found that both benzodiazepine and non-benzodiazepine muscle relaxants increased adverse effects compared with placebo, particularly drowsiness, dizziness, and nausea.

UNKNOWN EFFECTIVENESS

Analgesics (paracetamol, opioids)

We found no placebo controlled RCTs. Three small RCTs identified by a systematic review found no significant difference in symptoms or return to work between an opioid analgesic, paracetamol (acetaminophen), and a non-steroidal anti-inflammatory drug. Two small RCTs of low quality identified by another systematic review found limited evidence that paracetamol and unspecified analgesics were less effective in achieving pain relief than electroacupuncture and ultrasound treatment, respectively.

What are the effects of local injections?

UNKNOWN EFFECTIVENESS

Epidural steroid injections

One systematic review found no RCTs on the effects of epidural steroid injections in people with acute low back pain.

What are the effects of non-drug treatments?

BENEFICIAL

Advice to stay active

One systematic review and two subsequent RCTs found that advice to stay active reduced sick leave and chronic disability compared with no advice or traditional medical treatment (including analgesics as required, advice to rest, and "let ▶

pain be your guide"). One systematic review found that advice to stay active reduced pain and improved functional outcome compared with advice to rest in bed after 3–4 weeks and 12 weeks.

LIKELY TO BE BENEFICIAL

Multidisciplinary treatment programmes (for subacute low back pain)

One systematic review in people with subacute low back pain found limited evidence that multidisciplinary treatment, including a workplace visit, reduced sick leave compared with usual care.

Spinal manipulation (in the short term)

One systematic review and one subsequent RCT found that spinal manipulation slightly reduced pain within 6 weeks compared with sham treatment, but found no significant difference in functional outcomes. The review found no significant difference in pain or functional outcomes between spinal manipulative therapy and general practitioner care, physical therapy, exercises, or back school.

UNKNOWN EFFECTIVENESS

Acupuncture

One systematic review found insufficient evidence on the effects of acupuncture in people with acute low back pain.

Back schools

One systematic review found insufficient evidence on the effects of back schools in people with acute low back pain.

Behavioural therapy

One RCT identified by a systematic review found limited evidence that cognitive behavioural therapy reduced acute low back pain and disability after 9–12 months compared with traditional care.

Electromyographic biofeedback

We found no RCTs on the effects of electromyographic biofeedback.

Lumbar supports

We found no RCTs on the effects of lumbar supports.

Massage

One RCT identified by a systematic review found insufficient evidence about the effects of massage compared with spinal manipulation or electrical stimulation.

Multidisciplinary treatment programmes (for acute low back pain)

We found no RCTs on the effects of multidisciplinary treatment programmes in people with acute low back pain.

Temperature treatments (short wave diathermy, ultrasound, ice, heat)

Two systematic reviews identified no RCTs on the effects of temperature treatments.

Traction

Three systematic reviews found no RCTs on the effects of traction in people with acute low back pain.

Transcutaneous electrical nerve stimulation

We found no RCTs on the effects of transcutaneous electrical nerve stimulation.

Low back pain (acute)

UNLIKELY TO BE BENEFICIAL

Back exercises

One systematic review in acute low back pain (less than 6 weeks' duration) found no significant difference in pain or function between exercise and no treatment, and found no significant difference in pain or function between exercise and other conservative treatments. It found limited evidence in subacute low back pain (6–12 weeks' duration) that a graded activity exercise programme may reduce time off work in occupational settings compared with usual care, but found insufficient evidence in subacute low back pain otherwise.

LIKELY TO BE INEFFECTIVE OR HARMFUL

Bed rest

One systematic review found increased pain and poorer functional outcomes with advice to rest in bed compared with advice to stay active after 3–4 weeks and 12 weeks. RCTs in the review found limited evidence of no significant difference in outcomes between advice to rest in bed and exercise, or in outcomes between 3 days and 7 days of bed rest. One included RCT found limited evidence of no significant difference in pain between advice to rest in bed, exercise plus education, and no advice; whereas another included RCT found limited evidence of no significant difference in improvement between bed rest and manipulation, drug therapy, physiotherapy, back school, or placebo. One systematic review found that adverse effects of bed rest included joint stiffness, muscle wasting, loss of bone mineral density, pressure sores, and venous thromboembolism.

DEFINITION Low back pain is pain, muscle tension, or stiffness localised below the costal margin and above the inferior gluteal folds, with or without leg pain (sciatica),[1] and is defined as acute when it persists for less than 12 weeks.[2] Non-specific low back pain is low back pain not attributed to a recognisable pathology (such as infection, tumour, osteoporosis, rheumatoid arthritis, fracture, or inflammation).[1] This review excludes acute low back pain with symptoms or signs at presentation that suggest a specific underlying condition. People with sciatica (lumbosacral radicular syndrome) and herniated discs are also excluded. Unless otherwise stated, people included in this review have acute back pain (i.e. of less than 12 weeks' duration). Some included RCTs further subdivided acute low back pain of less than 12 weeks' duration into acute (< 6 weeks' duration) or subacute (6–12 weeks' duration).

INCIDENCE/ PREVALENCE Over 70% of people in developed countries will experience low back pain at some time in their lives.[3] Each year, 15–45% of adults suffer low back pain, and 1/20 (5%) people present to a health care professional with a new episode. Low back pain is most common between the ages of 35–55 years.[3] About 30% of European workers reported that their work caused low back pain. Prevalence rates from different countries range from 13% to 44%. About 70% of people with sick leave due to low back pain return to work within 1 week, and 90% return within 2 months. However, the longer the period of sick leave, the less likely return to work becomes. Less than half of people with low back pain who have been off work for 6 months will return to work.[3,4]

AETIOLOGY/ RISK FACTORS Symptoms, pathology, and radiological appearances are poorly correlated. Pain is non-specific in about 85% of people. About 4% of people with low back pain in primary care have compression fractures and about 1% have a tumour.[5] The prevalence of prolapsed intervertebral disc is about 1–3%.[3] Ankylosing spondylitis and spinal infections are less common.[5] Risk factors for the development of back pain include heavy physical work, frequent bending, twisting, lifting, and prolonged static postures. Psychosocial risk factors include anxiety, depression, and mental stress at work.[3,6]

PROGNOSIS Acute low back pain is usually self limiting (90% of people recover within 6 weeks), although 2–7% develop chronic pain. Acute low back pain has a high recurrence rate with symptoms recurring, to a lesser degree, in 50–80% of people within a year.[7]

Please refer to clinicalevidence.com for full text and references.

Low back pain (chronic)

Search date November 2004

Maurits van Tulder and Bart Koes

What are the effects of oral drug treatments?

LIKELY TO BE BENEFICIAL

Analgesics

One RCT found that tramadol (an opioid) decreased pain and increased function at 7 weeks compared with placebo. One RCT found that a combination of tramadol plus paracetamol (acetaminophen) decreased pain and increased function at 3 months compared with placebo. One small RCT identified by a systematic review found that diflunisal increased the proportion of people who rated the treatment as good or excellent compared with paracetamol.

Antidepressants

Two systematic reviews including almost the same RCTs found that antidepressants decreased pain compared with placebo, but found no consistent difference in function. One RCT found that maprotiline increased pain relief compared with paroxetine.

Non-steroidal anti-inflammatory drugs

One small RCT found that naproxen reduced pain compared with placebo. One systematic review and one subsequent RCT found no significant difference in symptoms between different non-steroidal anti-inflammatory drugs. One small RCT identified by the review found that diflunisal increased the proportion of people who rated the treatment as good or excellent compared with paracetamol. Two RCTs found that cyclo-oxygenase 2 inhibitors decreased pain and improved function at 4 and 12 weeks compared with placebo, but effects were small.

TRADE OFF BETWEEN BENEFITS AND HARMS

Muscle relaxants

Two RCTs identified by a systematic review found that tetrazepam reduced pain and increased overall improvement after 10–14 days compared with placebo. Two RCTs identified by a systematic review found that non-benzodiazepines (flupirtine and tolperisone) increased overall improvement at 7–21 days, but found no significant difference for pain. Adverse effects of muscle relaxants include dizziness and drowsiness.

What are the effects of injection therapy?

UNKNOWN EFFECTIVENESS

Epidural steroid injections

We found no systematic review or RCTs in people with chronic back pain who did not have sciatica.

Local injections

One systematic review found no significant difference between local injections (local anaesthetic and corticosteroids) and placebo in short term pain relief. ▶

LIKELY TO BE INEFFECTIVE OR HARMFUL

Facet joint injections

One RCT identified by a systematic review found no significant difference in pain relief and disability between corticosteroid and saline injections after 1 and 3 months.

What are the effects of non-drug treatments?

BENEFICIAL

Exercise

One systematic review found that exercise improved pain or function compared with placebo or no treatment or other conservative treatments.

Intensive multidisciplinary treatment programmes (evidence of benefit for intensive programmes but none for less intensive programmes)

One systematic review found that intensive (more than 100 hours of therapy) multidisciplinary biopsychosocial rehabilitation with functional restoration reduced pain and improved function compared with inpatient or outpatient non-multidisciplinary treatments or usual care. The review found no significant difference between less intensive multidisciplinary treatments and non-multidisciplinary treatment or usual care in pain or function.

LIKELY TO BE BENEFICIAL

Acupuncture

One systematic review found limited evidence of short term pain relief and functional improvement for acupuncture compared with no treatment or sham therapy. The review found insufficient evidence on the effects of acupuncture compared with other conventional therapies. It found limited evidence that acupuncture, added to other conventional therapies, relieved pain and improved function better than the conventional therapies alone.

Back schools

One systematic review found limited evidence that back schools reduced pain and disability compared with inactive treatments (waiting list control, placebo gel, or written advice) or no treatment within 6 months, although results suggested that benefits may not persist in the longer term. Three RCTs identified by the review compared back schools with other treatments and found mixed results.

Behavioural therapy

One systematic review found that behavioural therapy reduced pain and improved behavioural outcomes compared with no treatment, placebo, or waiting list control. The review and one subsequent RCT provided no evidence of a difference in functional status, pain, or behavioural outcomes between different types of behavioural therapy. The review found insufficient evidence to compare behavioural therapy with other treatments.

Spinal manipulative therapy

One systematic review found that spinal manipulative therapy reduced pain in the short and long term and improved short term function compared with sham manipulation, but found no significant difference in long term function after more than 6 weeks. The systematic review found no significant difference in pain or function between spinal manipulative therapy and general practitioner care,

Low back pain (chronic)

physical therapy, exercises, or back school. Two subsequent RCTs compared spinal manipulation with exercise or no treatment and found that spinal manipulation reduced pain at 6–12 months, but found different results for function. One of the RCTs found that spinal manipulation increased return to work at 12 months compared with exercise therapy. Another subsequent RCT found no significant difference in pain or function between spinal manipulation and exercises.

UNKNOWN EFFECTIVENESS

Electromyographic biofeedback

One systematic review of three small RCTs found no significant difference in pain relief or functional status between electromyographic biofeedback and placebo or waiting list control. The review found insufficient evidence on the effects of electromyographic biofeedback compared with other treatments.

Lumbar supports

We found insufficient evidence on the effects of lumbar supports.

Massage

One systematic review found insufficient evidence about effects of massage compared with inactive treatments or other treatments.

Traction

We found no RCTs on the effects of traction on chronic low back pain.

Transcutaneous electrical nerve stimulation

We found insufficient evidence on the effects of transcutaneous electrical nerve stimulation compared with placebo in chronic low back pain.

DEFINITION Low back pain is pain, muscle tension, or stiffness localised below the costal margin and above the inferior gluteal folds, with or without leg pain (sciatica),[1] and is defined as chronic when it persists for 12 weeks or more (see definition of low back pain and sciatica [acute]).[2] Non-specific low back pain is low back pain not attributed to a recognisable pathology (such as infection, tumour, osteoporosis, rheumatoid arthritis, fracture, or inflammation).[1] This review excludes low back pain with symptoms or signs at presentation that suggest a specific underlying condition. People with sciatica (lumbosacral radicular syndrome) or pain due to herniated discs are also excluded.

INCIDENCE/ PREVALENCE Over 70% of people in developed countries will experience low back pain at some time in their lives.[3] Each year, 15–45% of adults suffer low back pain, and 1/20 people present to hospital with a new episode. About 2–7% of people with acute low back pain will go on to become chronic. Low back pain is most common between the ages of 35 and 55 years.[3]

AETIOLOGY/ RISK FACTORS Symptoms, pathology, and radiological appearances are poorly correlated. Pain is non-specific in about 85% of people. About 4% of people with low back pain in primary care have compression fractures and about 1% have a tumour. The prevalence of prolapsed intervertebral disc among people with low back pain in primary care is about 1–3%.[3] Ankylosing spondylitis and spinal infections are less common.[4] This chapter only covers non-specific chronic low back pain. Risk factors for the development of non-specific low back pain include heavy physical work, frequent bending, twisting, lifting, and prolonged static postures. Psychosocial risk factors include anxiety, depression, and mental stress at work.[3,5] Having a previous history of low back pain and a longer duration of the present episode are significant risk factors for chronicity. A recently published systematic review of prospective cohort studies found that some psychological factors (distress, depressive mood, and somatisation) are associated with an increased risk of chronic low back pain.[6] Individual and workplace factors have also been reported to be associated with the transition to chronic low back pain.[7]

PROGNOSIS Generally, the clinical course of an episode of low back pain seems to be favourable, and most pain will resolve within 2 weeks. Back pain among people in a primary care setting typically has a recurrent course characterised by variation and change, rather than an acute, self limiting course.[8] Most people with back pain have experienced a previous episode, and acute attacks often occur as exacerbations of chronic low back pain. In general, recurrences will occur more frequently and be more severe if people have had frequent or long lasting low back pain complaints in the past. The course of sick leave due to low back pain is similarly favourable. One study reported that 67% of people with sick leave due to low back pain returned to work within 1 week, and 90% within 2 months. However, the longer the period of sick leave, the less likely the return to work becomes. Less than 50% of people with low back pain who have been off work for 6 months will return to work. After 2 years of work absenteeism, the chance of returning to work is almost zero.[9]

Please refer to clinicalevidence.com for full text and references.

Neck pain

Search date May 2006

Allan Binder

What are the effects of treatments for people with uncomplicated neck pain without severe neurological deficit?

LIKELY TO BE BENEFICIAL

Exercise

RCTs identified by systematic reviews and subsequent RCTs, primarily in people with chronic uncomplicated neck pain, found that strengthening exercise or active physical treatment including exercise reduced pain compared with usual care including drug treatment, stress management, or no specific exercise programme. RCTs identified by several systematic reviews provided insufficient evidence about the effects of exercise compared with traction. The reviews identified one RCT in people with chronic neck pain which compared low technology strengthening exercises plus manipulation, high technology strengthening exercises, and manipulation alone. It found that low technology strengthening exercises plus manipulation improved participant satisfaction, objective strength, and range of movement at 11 weeks compared with manipulation alone. At 1 and 2 years it found that both low technology strengthening exercises plus manipulation and high technology strengthening exercises improved pain and participant satisfaction compared with manipulation alone. The 2 year follow up was in a subset of participants only. Another RCT identified by a systematic review found no significant difference in pain after treatment or at 12 months among exercise, manipulation, or mobilisation. A third RCT found that exercise was less effective in improving pain than mobilisation in people with neck pain for over 2 weeks. One RCT found that exercise plus infrared reduced pain at 6 weeks and 6 months compared with infrared alone. One small RCT that compared exercise, McKenzie mobilisation, and control found no significant difference between groups in pain at 6 and 12 months. One RCT found no significant difference in pain between adding manual therapy (63% having mobilisation physiotherapy) to advice plus exercise or between adding pulsed short wave diathermy to advice plus exercise versus advice plus exercise alone at 6 weeks or 6 months.

Manipulation

One systematic review found no significant difference in symptoms between manipulation and other treatments (including usual care, diazepam, or anti-inflammatory drugs) in people with subacute or chronic neck or back pain. The meta-analysis performed by the review may have been underpowered to detect a clinically important difference. One RCT identified by systematic reviews found limited evidence that manual treatment (manipulation or mobilisation) may be more effective in reducing pain at 1 year than less active physical treatment (massage, pulsed electrical field treatment, and slight traction). Systematic reviews identified one RCT in people with chronic neck pain which compared manipulation plus low technology strengthening exercises, high technology strengthening exercises, and manipulation alone. It found that manipulation plus low technology strengthening exercises improved participant satisfaction, objective strength, and range of movement at 11 weeks compared with manipulation alone. At 1 and 2 years, it found that both manipulation plus low technology strengthening exercises and high technology strengthening exercises improved pain and patient satisfaction compared with manipulation alone. ▶

The 2 year follow up was in a subset of participants only. Two RCTs provided insufficient evidence to compare manipulation versus mobilisation in people with uncomplicated neck pain. Another RCT identified by the reviews found no significant difference in pain after treatment or at 12 months among manipulation, exercise, or mobilisation.

Manipulation plus exercise

Systematic reviews identified one RCT in people with chronic neck pain which compared low technology strengthening exercises plus manipulation, high technology strengthening exercises, and manipulation alone. It found that low technology strengthening exercises plus manipulation improved participant satisfaction, objective strength, and range of movement at 11 weeks compared with manipulation alone. At 1 and 2 years, it found that both low technology strengthening exercises plus manipulation and high technology strengthening exercises improved pain and patient satisfaction compared with manipulation alone. The 2 year follow up was in a subset of participants only. One RCT found no significant difference in pain between adding manual therapy (63% having mobilisation physiotherapy) to advice plus exercise and advice plus exercise alone at 6 weeks or 6 months.

Mobilisation

One RCT found that mobilisation improved symptoms compared with usual care (drug treatment) or exercise in people with neck pain for over 2 weeks. Another RCT identified by systematic reviews found no significant difference in pain after treatment or at 12 months among mobilisation, manipulation, or exercise. A third RCT identified by systematic reviews found limited evidence that manual treatment (mobilisation or manipulation) may be more effective in reducing pain at 1 year than less active physical treatment. Two RCTs provided insufficient evidence to compare mobilisation versus manipulation in people with uncomplicated neck pain. Weak RCTs, some identified by systematic reviews, provided insufficient evidence to compare mobilisation versus acupuncture or transcutaneous electrical nerve stimulation in people with uncomplicated neck pain. One small RCT that compared McKenzie mobilisation, exercise, and control found no significant difference between groups in pain at 6 and 12 months. One RCT found no significant difference in pain between adding manual therapy (63% having mobilisation physiotherapy) to advice plus exercise and advice plus exercise alone at 6 weeks or 6 months.

UNKNOWN EFFECTIVENESS

Acupuncture

Systematic reviews of weak RCTs provided insufficient evidence about the effects of acupuncture compared with a range of other treatments, including sham acupuncture, sham transcutaneous electrical nerve simulation, diazepam, traction, short wave diathermy, and mobilisation in people with acute or chronic uncomplicated neck pain.

Biofeedback

Three systematic reviews identified no RCTs of biofeedback in people with uncomplicated neck pain.

Neck pain

Drug treatments (analgesics, non-steroidal anti-inflammatory drugs, antidepressants, muscle relaxants)

We found insufficient evidence on the effects of analgesics, non-steroidal anti-inflammatory drugs, antidepressants, or muscle relaxants for neck pain, although they are widely used. Several drugs used to treat neck pain are associated with well documented adverse effects.

Heat or cold

Two systematic reviews identified no RCTs of sufficient quality of heat or cold in people with uncomplicated neck pain. One large RCT of people with chronic neck and back pain found that heat combined with other physical treatment was less effective in improving outcomes than manipulation or mobilisation. One RCT found that infrared alone was less effective at relieving pain than transcutaneous electrical nerve stimulation plus infrared or exercise plus infrared. One RCT found no significant difference in pain between adding pulsed short wave diathermy to advice plus exercise and advice plus exercise alone at 6 weeks or 6 months.

Multimodal treatment

One RCT identified by a systematic review and one subsequent RCT provided insufficient evidence to assess multimodal treatment in people with uncomplicated neck pain.

Patient education

Two RCTs in people with chronic neck, back, or shoulder pain found no significant difference among patient education (individual advice, pamphlets, or group instruction) with or without analgesics and no treatment, stress management, and cognitive behavioural therapy.

Pulsed electromagnetic field treatment

One RCT identified by three systematic reviews provided insufficient evidence to compare pulsed electromagnetic field treatment versus sham treatment in people with uncomplicated neck pain. RCTs in people with chronic neck and back pain identified by another systematic review found that pulsed electromagnetic field treatment combined with other physical treatments was less effective in improving outcomes than manipulation or mobilisation.

Soft collars and special pillows

We found no RCTs of sufficient quality on the effects of soft collars or special pillows in people with uncomplicated neck pain.

Spray and stretch

One RCT identified by several systematic reviews provided insufficient evidence about the effects of spray and stretch in people with uncomplicated neck pain.

Traction

Systematic reviews in people with acute or chronic neck pain provided insufficient evidence about the effects of traction compared with a range of other physical treatments, including sham traction, placebo tablets, exercise, acupuncture, heat, collar, and analgesics. Systematic reviews identified no RCTs of sufficient quality comparing traction versus manipulation or mobilisation.

Transcutaneous electrical nerve stimulation

Six systematic reviews identified no RCTs of transcutaneous electrical nerve stimulation of sufficient quality in people with uncomplicated neck pain. One subsequent RCT found that transcutaneous electrical nerve stimulation plus infrared reduced pain at 6 weeks compared with infrared alone, but found no significant difference between groups at 6 months.

What are the effects of treatments for acute whiplash injury?

LIKELY TO BE BENEFICIAL

Early mobilisation

Four RCTs identified by systematic reviews provided limited evidence that early mobilisation reduced pain compared with immobilisation or rest plus a collar.

Early return to normal activity

One RCT in people with acute whiplash identified by one systematic review provided limited evidence that advice to "act as usual" plus non-steroidal anti-inflammatory drugs improved some symptoms (including pain during daily activities, neck stiffness, memory, concentration, and headache) at 6 months compared with immobilisation plus 14 days' sick leave plus non-steroidal anti-inflammatory drugs. It found no significant difference in neck range or sick leave, and found that a similar proportion of people had severe neck pain.

UNKNOWN EFFECTIVENESS

Drug treatments (analgesics, non-steroidal anti-inflammatory drugs, antidepressant drugs, or muscle relaxants)

Three systematic reviews identified no RCTs of drug treatments in people with acute whiplash injury. One subsequent RCT found insufficient evidence comparing ketorolac versus manipulation in people with whiplash injuries.

Exercise

One RCT found no significant difference between two home exercise programmes in pain or disability. One RCT found limited evidence that early exercise reduced pain and self assessed disability compared with a soft collar at 6 weeks. Another RCT found no significant difference in pain, headache, or work activities between physiotherapy care (mainly exercise) and general practitioner care over 52 weeks in people with whiplash symptoms that had lasted for 4 weeks.

Multimodal treatment

One RCT identified by two systematic reviews found that multimodal treatment reduced pain at 1 and 6 months compared with physical treatments.

Pulsed electromagnetic field treatment

One small RCT identified by systematic reviews found limited evidence that electromagnetic field treatment reduced pain after 4 weeks but not after 3 months compared with sham treatment.

What are the effects of treatments for chronic whiplash injury?

UNKNOWN EFFECTIVENESS

Multimodal treatment

One small RCT identified by a systematic review found no difference between multimodal treatment and physical treatments in disability, pain, or range of movement at the end of treatment or at 3 months, but it may have been too small to detect a clinically important difference.

Percutaneous radiofrequency neurotomy

One RCT identified by systematic reviews found limited evidence that percutaneous radiofrequency neurotomy reduced pain after 27 weeks compared with sham treatment in people with chronic whiplash injury.

Physical treatments

One small RCT found no significant difference between physical treatments alone and multimodal treatment in disability, pain, or range of movement at the end of treatment or at 3 months, but it may have been too small to detect a clinically important difference.

What are the effects of treatments for neck pain with radiculopathy?

UNKNOWN EFFECTIVENESS

Drug treatments (epidural steroid injections, analgesics, non-steroidal anti-inflammatory drugs, or muscle relaxants)

We found no systematic review or RCTs examining the effects of analgesics, non-steroidal anti-inflammatory drugs, or muscle relaxants in people with neck pain with radiculopathy. Two RCTs found insufficient evidence on the effects of cervical epidural steroid injections.

Surgery versus conservative treatment

One RCT found no significant difference in pain at 1 year between surgery and conservative treatment in people with neck pain with radiculopathy.

DEFINITION In this chapter, we have differentiated uncomplicated neck pain from whiplash, although many studies, particularly in people with chronic pain (duration > 3 months), do not specify which types of people are included. Most studies of acute pain (duration < 3 months) are confined to whiplash. Uncomplicated neck pain is defined as pain with a postural or mechanical basis, often called cervical spondylosis. It does not include pain associated with fibromyalgia. Uncomplicated neck pain may include some people with a traumatic basis for their symptoms, but not people for whom pain is specifically stated to have followed sudden acceleration–deceleration injuries to the neck, that is, whiplash. Whiplash is commonly seen in road traffic accidents or sports injuries. It is not accompanied by radiographic abnormalities or clinical signs of nerve root damage. Neck pain often occurs in combination with limited movement and poorly defined neurological symptoms affecting the upper limbs. The pain can be severe and intractable, and can occur with radiculopathy or myelopathy. We have included under radiculopathy those studies involving people with predominantly radicular symptoms arising in the cervical spine.

INCIDENCE/ PREVALENCE About two thirds of people will experience neck pain at some time in their lives.[1,2] Prevalence is highest in middle age. In the UK, about 15% of hospital based physiotherapy and in Canada 30% of chiropractic referrals are for neck pain.[3,4] In the Netherlands, neck pain contributes up to 2% of general practitioner consultations.[5]

AETIOLOGY/ RISK FACTORS The aetiology of uncomplicated neck pain is unclear. Most uncomplicated neck pain is associated with poor posture, anxiety and depression, neck strain, occupational injuries, or sporting injuries. With chronic pain, mechanical and degenerative factors (often referred to as cervical spondylosis) are more likely. Some neck pain results from soft tissue trauma, most typically seen in whiplash injuries. Rarely, disc prolapse and inflammatory, infective, or malignant conditions affect the cervical spine and present with neck pain with or without neurological features.

PROGNOSIS Neck pain usually resolves within days or weeks but can recur or become chronic. In some industries, neck related disorders account for as much time off work as low back pain (see low back pain and sciatica [acute]).[6] The proportion of people in whom neck pain becomes chronic depends on the cause but is thought to be about 10%,[1] similar to low back pain. Neck pain causes severe disability in 5% of affected people.[2] Whiplash injuries are more likely to cause disability than neck pain because of other causes; up to 40% of sufferers reported symptoms even after 15 years' follow up.[7] Factors associated with a poorer outcome after whiplash are not well defined.[8] The incidence of chronic disability after whiplash varies among countries, although reasons for this variation are unclear.[9]

Please refer to clinicalevidence.com for full text and references.

Musculoskeletal disorders

Non-steroidal anti-inflammatory drugs

Search date December 2005

Peter C Gøtzsche

Are there any important differences between available non-steroidal anti-inflammatory drugs (NSAIDs)?

TRADE OFF BETWEEN BENEFITS AND HARMS

Choice between different non-steroidal anti-inflammatory drugs (NSAIDs)

Systematic reviews found no important differences in efficacy between different NSAIDs for the symptoms of musculoskeletal disorders. Systematic reviews found that cyclo-oxygenase (COX)-2 inhibitors reduced symptomatic ulcers compared with older NSAIDs. However, the COX-2 inhibitor rofecoxib was withdrawn from the market in 2004 after it was found to increase the risk of myocardial infarction, and there is good evidence that other COX-2 inhibitors may also increase cardiovascular risk.

UNLIKELY TO BE BENEFICIAL

Non-steroidal anti-inflammatory drugs (NSAIDs) in increased doses

Systematic reviews found that the benefits of NSAIDs increased toward a maximum value at high doses. Recommended doses are close to creating the maximum benefit. In contrast, three systematic reviews found no ceiling for adverse effects, which increased in an approximately linear fashion with dose.

What are the effects of co-treatments to reduce the risk of gastrointestinal adverse effects of non-steroidal anti-inflammatory drugs (NSAIDs)?

TRADE OFF BETWEEN BENEFITS AND HARMS

Misoprostol in people who cannot avoid non-steroidal anti-inflammatory drugs (NSAIDs)

One systematic review found that misoprostol reduced serious gastrointestinal complications and symptomatic ulcers compared with placebo. It did not assess adverse effects of misoprostol. However, another systematic review found that misoprostol increased withdrawals due to adverse events, mainly diarrhoea and abdominal pain, compared with placebo. RCTs provided insufficient evidence to compare the effects of misoprostol versus proton pump inhibitors or H_2 blockers.

UNKNOWN EFFECTIVENESS

H_2 blockers in people who cannot avoid non-steroidal anti-inflammatory drugs (NSAIDs)

One systematic review provided insufficient evidence about the effects of H_2 blockers on serious gastrointestinal complications and symptomatic ulcers. It found that H_2 blockers reduced endoscopically diagnosed ulcers compared with placebo, but the clinical relevance of these findings is uncertain. RCTs provided insufficient evidence to compare the effects of H_2 blockers versus misoprostol or proton pump inhibitors.

Proton pump inhibitors in people who cannot avoid non-steroidal anti-inflammatory drugs (NSAIDs)

One systematic review provided insufficient evidence about the effects of proton pump inhibitors compared with placebo on serious gastrointestinal complications and symptomatic ulcers. Another systematic review found that proton pump inhibitors reduced endoscopically diagnosed ulcers compared with placebo, but the clinical relevance of this finding is uncertain. RCTs provided insufficient evidence to compare the effects of proton pump inhibitors versus misoprostol or H_2 blockers.

What are the effects of topical non-steroidal anti-inflammatory drugs (NSAIDs)?

LIKELY TO BE BENEFICIAL

Topical non-steroidal anti-inflammatory drugs (NSAIDs) (for up to 2 weeks)

One systematic review in people with acute musculoskeletal pain conditions found limited evidence that topical NSAIDs reduced pain compared with placebo at 1 week. One systematic review in people with osteoarthritis found limited evidence that topical NSAIDs reduced pain compared with placebo at 2 weeks, but found no significant difference between treatments at 4 weeks.

UNKNOWN EFFECTIVENESS

Topical non-steroidal anti-inflammatory drugs (NSAIDs) (for longer than 2 weeks)

One systematic review in people with osteoarthritis found no significant difference between topical NSAIDs and placebo at 4 weeks. The review found no evidence about the effects of topical NSAIDs compared with placebo for longer than 4 weeks.

Topical versus systemic non-steroidal anti-inflammatory drugs (NSAIDs) or alternative analgesics

Two systematic reviews found insufficient evidence to compare topical versus oral NSAIDs for pain in acute musculoskeletal pain conditions or osteoarthritis. We found no systematic review or RCTs comparing topical NSAIDs versus paracetamol for musculoskeletal conditions.

DEFINITION Non-steroidal anti-inflammatory drugs (NSAIDs) have anti-inflammatory, analgesic and antipyretic effects, and they inhibit platelet aggregation. This chapter deals specifically with the use of NSAIDs for the treatment of the symptoms of musculoskeletal conditions. NSAIDs have no documented effect on the course of musculoskeletal diseases, such as osteoarthritis. NSAIDs inhibit the enzyme cyclo-oxygenase (COX), which has two known isoforms: COX-1 and COX-2. NSAIDs are often categorised according to their ability to inhibit the individual isoforms, with newer NSAIDs often predominantly inhibiting the COX-2 isoform and older NSAIDs often being less specific inhibitors.

INCIDENCE/ PREVALENCE Non-steroidal anti-inflammatory drugs (NSAIDs) are widely used. Almost 10% of people in The Netherlands used a non-aspirin NSAID in 1987, and the overall use was 11 defined daily doses per 1000 population per day.[1] In Australia in 1994, overall use was 35 defined daily doses per 1000 population per day, with 36% of the people receiving NSAIDs for osteoarthritis, 42% for sprain and strain or low back pain, and 4% for rheumatoid arthritis; 35% of the people receiving NSAIDs were aged over 60 years.[2]

Non-steroidal anti-inflammatory drugs

Please refer to clinicalevidence.com for full text and references.

Osteoarthritis of the hip

Search date November 2005

Jiri Chard, Claire Smith, Stefan Lohmander and David Scott

What are the effects of non-drug treatments for osteoarthritis of the hip?

UNKNOWN EFFECTIVENESS

Acupuncture New

One RCT found no significant difference between traditional Chinese acupuncture and sham acupuncture for pain, function, and quality of life in people with osteoarthritis of the hip.

Education to aid self management New

We found no systematic review of education to aid self management and no RCTs in which the data for osteoarthritis of the hip was provided separately.

Exercise New

One systematic review and subsequent RCTs found inconclusive evidence of the effects of exercise in people with osteoarthritis of the hip.

Physical aids New

We found no systematic review or RCTs of physical aids, including walking aids (stick/cane) and insoles.

What are the effects of drug treatments for osteoarthritis of the hip?

TRADE OFF BETWEEN BENEFITS AND HARMS

Oral non-steroidal anti-inflammatory drugs (including cyclo-oxygenase-2 inhibitors) New

Systematic reviews and RCTs found that non-steroidal anti-inflammatory drugs (including cyclo-oxygenase-2 inhibitors) were effective at reducing short term pain compared with placebo in people with osteoarthritis of the hip. One systematic review of people with mainly osteoarthritis of the knee found limited evidence that oral non-steroidal anti-inflammatory drugs were more effective than paracetamol (acetaminophen) in reducing pain. Studies have found that non-steroidal anti-inflammatory drugs increased the risk of gastrointestinal damage, including haemorrhage.

UNKNOWN EFFECTIVENESS

Capsaicin New

We found no systematic review or RCTs of capsaicin in people with osteoarthritis of the hip.

Chondroitin New

One systematic review of people with osteoarthritis of the hip or knee found that chondroitin reduced pain and improved function compared with placebo.

Osteoarthritis of the hip

Glucosamine *New*

One systematic review of people with osteoarthritis of multiple body sites found no significant difference between glucosamine and placebo in improving pain and function in those RCTs with adequate allocation concealment.

Opioid analgesics *New*

We found no systematic review and no RCTs of opioid analgesics in which the data for osteoarthritis of the hip was provided separately.

Oral NSAIDs plus simple oral or opioid analgesics *New*

One RCT found limited evidence that naproxen plus paracetamol (acetaminophen) was more effective than naproxen alone in reducing pain in people with osteoarthritis of the hip.

Simple oral analgesics (versus placebo — less effective versus non-steroidal anti-inflammatory drugs) *New*

We found no systematic review or RCTs for simple oral analgesics versus placebo or each other for which the data for osteoarthritis of the hip was provided separately. One systematic review of people with mainly osteoarthritis of the knee found limited evidence that paracetamol (acetaminophen) was less effective than oral non-steroidal anti-inflammatory drugs in reducing pain.

What are the effects of surgical treatments for osteoarthritis of the hip?

BENEFICIAL

Hip replacement *New*

We found many observational studies that reported the time to revision surgery, but less evidence on pain, function and quality-of-life outcomes. Studies have shown that total hip replacement is effective and beneficial in the treatment of osteoarthritis of the hip. We found insufficient evidence from RCTs or observational studies to predict responders and non-responders to treatment with total hip replacement.

UNKNOWN EFFECTIVENESS

Osteotomy *New*

We found no RCTs or comparative observational studies of osteotomy in people with osteoarthritis of the hip.

DEFINITION Osteoarthritis is a heterogeneous condition for which the prevalence, risk factors, clinical manifestations, and prognosis vary according to the joints affected. It most commonly affects knees, hips, hands, and spinal apophyseal joints. It is characterised by focal areas of damage to the cartilage surfaces of synovial joints, and is associated with remodelling of the underlying bone and mild synovitis. It is variously defined by a number of clinical and/or radiological features. Clinical features include pain, bony tenderness, and crepitus. When severe, there is often characteristic joint space narrowing and osteophyte formation, with visible subchondral bone changes on radiography. The hip is the second most common large joint to be affected by osteoarthritis. It is associated with significant pain, disability, and impaired quality of life.

INCIDENCE/PREVALENCE Osteoarthritis is a common and important cause of pain and disability in older adults.[1,2] Radiographical features are practically universal in at least some joints in people aged over 60 years, but significant clinical disease probably affects 10–20% of people. Hip disease is not as prevalent as knee disease in people aged over 60 years (about 5% *v* 10%).[3,4] The actual impact that osteoarthritis has on an individual person is the result of a combination of physical (including comorbidities), psychological, cultural, and social factors, and this may influence outcomes found in research — for example, if comorbidities are not accounted for in analysis.

AETIOLOGY/ RISK FACTORS There is moderate evidence for a positive association between osteoarthritis of the hip and obesity; participation in sporting activities, including running; and vocational activity, particularly involving a heavy physical workload, as characterised by farming (especially for more than 10 years) or lifting heavy loads (25 kg or more). Only limited evidence exists for a positive association between the occurrence of osteoarthritis of the hip and participation in athletics or presence of hip dysplasia in older persons.[5-8]

PROGNOSIS The natural history of osteoarthritis of the hip is poorly understood. Only a minority of people with clinical disease of the hip will progress to requiring surgery.

Please refer to clinicalevidence.com for full text and references.

Osteoarthritis of the knee

Search date October 2005

Jiri Chard, Claire Smith, Stefan Lohmander, and David Scott

What are the effects of non-surgical treatments for osteoarthritis of the knee?

BENEFICIAL

Exercise and physical therapy (pain relief and improved function)

Systematic reviews and subsequent RCTs found that exercise and physical therapy reduced pain and disability in people with knee osteoarthritis.

Oral non-steroidal anti-inflammatory drugs (short term pain relief only)

One systematic review and two subsequent RCTs found that oral non-steroidal anti-inflammatory drugs (NSAIDs) reduced short term pain compared with placebo, but found no evidence to support the long term use of NSAIDs. Systematic reviews and subsequent RCTs found evidence that oral NSAIDs are more effective than paracetamol (acetaminophen) in reducing pain symptoms. Three RCTs provided insufficient evidence to compare the effects of topical versus oral NSAIDs. A systematic review found limited evidence that NSAIDs were less effective at improving pain symptoms compared with glucosamine. A large population based observational study found an increased risk of myocardial infarction associated with current use of rofecoxib, diclofenac, and ibuprofen. Rofecoxib was withdrawn from the market in 2004 because of the increased risk of myocardial infarction. Studies have found that NSAIDs increased the risk of renal or gastrointestinal damage, including haemorrhage, particularly in the elderly and in people with intercurrent disease. Concerns exist relating to trial quality and commercial bias.

LIKELY TO BE BENEFICIAL

Acupuncture

Two systematic reviews and three subsequent RCTs found limited evidence that acupuncture improved pain and function compared with control.

Chondroitin

One systematic review and one subsequent RCT found that oral or intramuscular chondroitin reduced pain and improved function compared with placebo. Another systematic review reported five RCTs that found that chondroitin reduced pain and improved function compared with placebo. The review identified one RCT that found no significant difference between chondroitin and placebo.

Corticosteroids (intra-articular — short term pain relief)

One systematic review found that the pain relieving effects of intra-articular corticosteroid injections are rapid in onset but may be relatively short lived (about 1–3 weeks). One systematic review found no significant difference between intra-articular corticosteroids and hyaluronan and hyaluronan derivatives at up to 4 weeks after injection, suggesting a similar onset of effect. However, hyaluronan and hyaluronan derivatives had a longer lasting beneficial effect, and were more effective that corticosteroids for measures of pain and function at 5–13 weeks after injection.

◀ **Hyaluronan (intra-articular)**

One large systematic review and one subsequent RCT found that intra-articular hyaluronan and hyaluronan derivatives improved pain and function compared with placebo. The evidence for an effect was most convincing at 5–13 weeks after injection. Two subsequent RCTs found no significant difference between hyaluronan and placebo at up to 1 year. One systematic review found no significant difference between intra-articular corticosteroids and hyaluronan and hyaluronan derivatives at up to 4 weeks after injection, suggesting a similar onset of effect. However, hyaluronan and hyaluronan derivatives had a longer lasting beneficial effect, and were more effective than corticosteroids for measures of pain and function at 5–13 weeks after injection.

Joint bracing

One systematic review found limited evidence that a brace or neoprene sleeve improved pain and function compared with medical treatment alone. It also found that a brace improved pain and function compared with neoprene sleeve at 6 months.

Simple oral analgesics (short term pain relief only)

Systematic reviews and subsequent RCTs provided limited evidence that paracetamol (acetaminophen) reduced pain compared with placebo in the short term, but found that paracetamol was less effective than oral non-steroidal anti-inflammatory drugs for reducing pain.

Taping

One RCT found limited evidence that taping may improve symptoms compared with control treatment.

Topical non-steroidal anti-inflammatory drugs (short term pain relief)

One systematic review and one subsequent RCT found that topical non-steroidal anti-inflammatory drugs (NSAIDs) reduced pain compared with placebo at up to 2 weeks. The review found no significant difference in pain in weeks 3 and 4. However, two subsequent RCTs found that topical NSAIDs reduced pain and improved function at 4 and 12 weeks compared with placebo. We found no RCTs assessing the effects of topical NSAIDs for periods of longer than 12 weeks. Three RCTs provided insufficient evidence to compare the effects of topical versus oral NSAIDs.

UNKNOWN EFFECTIVENESS

Capsaicin

We found no systematic review or RCTs of capsaicin in which the data for osteoarthritis of the knee were provided separately.

Education (to aid self management)

One cluster randomised RCT found no significant difference between a primary care based education programme for people with osteoarthritis of the knee and waiting list control (routine care) in quality of life, pain, or disability. Another cluster randomised RCT found that a nurse directed self management programme could reduce reliance on non-steroidal anti-inflammatory drugs without any deterioration in pain control or function.

Glucosamine

Two systematic reviews in people with osteoarthritis of the knee found limited evidence that glucosamine may be more effective than placebo in improving pain and function. One more recent systematic review, mainly in people with ▶

Osteoarthritis of the knee

osteoarthritis of the knee, found no significant difference in pain or function between glucosamine and placebo in RCTs with adequate allocation concealment but found limited evidence that glucosamine improved pain symptoms compared with non-steroidal anti-inflammatory drugs. Glucosamine was found to be as safe as placebo and less likely than non-steroidal anti-inflammatory drugs to produce adverse events.

Insoles

One systematic review and subsequent RCTs provided insufficient evidence to assess the effects of insoles in osteoarthritis of the knee.

Opioid analgesics

Two RCTs provided limited evidence that tramadol improved some measures of pain and function but increased adverse events compared with placebo. We found no RCTs comparing opioid analgesics versus each other, or versus oral non-steroidal anti-inflammatory drugs. Opioid analgesics are associated with constipation, nausea, vomiting, and drowsiness, and can be associated with hypotension and respiratory depression at higher doses. Regular use can lead to tolerance and dependence. The potential for adverse effects means that opioid analgesics are not recommended as first line treatment for osteoarthritis.

What are the effects of surgical treatments for osteoarthritis of the knee?

LIKELY TO BE BENEFICIAL

Knee replacement (unicompartmental versus tricompartmental)

One RCT identified by a systematic review found limited evidence that unicompartmental knee replacement was more effective than tricompartmental knee replacement at 5 years' follow up.

Osteotomy

We found no RCTs comparing osteotomy versus conservative treatment. One systematic review of two RCTs provided limited evidence that high tibial osteotomy was as effective for treating medial compartment osteoarthritis of the knee as unicompartmental knee replacement.

DEFINITION Osteoarthritis is a heterogeneous condition for which the prevalence, risk factors, clinical manifestations, and prognosis vary according to the joints affected. It most commonly affects knees, hips, hands, and spinal apophyseal joints. It is characterised by focal areas of damage to the cartilage surfaces of synovial joints, and is associated with remodelling of the underlying bone and mild synovitis. It is variously defined by a number of clinical and or radiological features. Clinical features include pain, bony tenderness, and crepitus. When severe, there is often characteristic joint space narrowing and osteophyte formation, with visible subchondral bone changes on radiography. Osteoarthritis of the knee is common, causes considerable pain and frequent instability, and consequently often results in physical disability.[1] X ray changes are not strongly associated with disability.[2]

INCIDENCE/ PREVALENCE Osteoarthritis is a common and important cause of pain and disability in older adults.[3,4] Radiographical features are practically universal in at least some joints in people aged over 60 years, but significant clinical disease probably affects 10–20% of people. Knee disease is about twice as prevalent as hip disease in people aged over 60 years (about 10% knee *v* 5% hip).[5,6] In a general practice setting 1% of people aged over 45 years have a currently recorded clinical diagnosis of knee osteoarthritis; 5% will have had the clinical diagnosis made at some point.[7] A community based cohort study showed radiological features of knee osteoarthritis were very common: 13% of women aged 45–65 years developed new knee osteophytes, an incidence of 3% per year.[8]

AETIOLOGY/ RISK FACTORS Risk factors for osteoarthritis include abnormalities in joint shape, injury, and previous joint inflammation. Obesity is a major risk factor for osteoarthritis of the knee. Genetic factors modulate obesity and other risks.[9]

PROGNOSIS The natural history of osteoarthritis of the knee is poorly understood. Radiological progression is commonplace with 25% of osteoarthritic knees with initially normal joint space showing major damage after 10 years,[10] though x ray progression is not related to clinical features.[11] People with peripheral joint osteoarthritis of sufficient severity to lead to hospital referral have generally bad outcomes with high levels of physical disability, anxiety, and depression; they also have high levels of healthcare resources utilisation, including joint replacement, drugs, and walking aids.[12]

Please refer to clinicalevidence.com for full text and references.

Plantar heel pain and fasciitis

Search date October 2005

Fay Crawford

What are the effects of treatments for plantar heel pain?

UNKNOWN EFFECTIVENESS

Casted orthoses (custom made insoles)

One systematic review found no RCTs comparing the effects of casted orthoses versus placebo or no treatment. One RCT found no significant difference in pain between heel pad plus orthoses and corticosteroid injection plus local anaesthesia plus non-steroidal anti-inflammatory drugs. One RCT found that orthoses plus heel pads reduced pain compared with heel pads plus paracetamol at 8 weeks. One RCT found that heel pads plus stretching reduced pain compared with custom made orthoses plus stretching at 8 weeks. One RCT found that stretching plus heel pads (silicone, rubber, or felt insert) improved symptoms compared with stretching alone at 8 weeks. One RCT found no significant difference in pain between orthoses plus stretching (Achilles tendon stretching and plantar fascia stretching) and stretching alone after 8 weeks. One RCT provided insufficient evidence to compare orthoses versus night splints. One RCT found no significant difference in pain between functional and accommodative orthoses at 4 or 8 weeks.

Corticosteroid injection (in the short term)

One systematic review identified no RCTs comparing short term effects of corticosteroid injections versus placebo, orthoses, heel pads, analgesic medication, or corticosteroid injection plus local anaesthesia. Observational studies found a high rate of plantar fascia rupture and other complications associated with corticosteroid injections, which may lead to chronic disability in some people.

Corticosteroid injection plus local anaesthetic injection in the short term (with or without non-steroidal anti-inflammatory drugs or heel pads)

One systematic review identified no RCTs comparing short term effects of corticosteroid injections plus local anaesthesia versus placebo or no treatment. RCTs provided insufficient evidence about clinically important short term effects of corticosteroids plus local anaesthesia (alone or combined with non-steroidal anti-inflammatory drugs or heel pads) compared with other treatments. Observational studies found a high rate of plantar fascia rupture and other complications associated with corticosteroid injections, which may lead to chronic disability in some people.

Extracorporeal shock wave therapy

One systematic review compared extracorporeal shock wave therapy versus placebo, sham, or low dose extracorporeal shock wave therapy, in people with heel pain, and found a small but statistically significant difference in pain.

Heel pads and heel cups

One systematic review found no RCTs on the effects of heel pads and heel cups compared with placebo, no treatment, or corticosteroid injection. One RCT found insufficient evidence to compare pain relief between heel pads and heel pads plus corticosteroid injection. One RCT provided insufficient evidence about clinically important effects of heel pads compared with corticosteroids plus local anaesthesia (alone or combined with non-steroidal anti-inflammatory drugs or heel pads). One RCT found that stretching plus heel pad (silicone, rubber, or felt insert) improved symptoms compared with stretching alone at 8 weeks. One RCT found that heel pads plus stretching reduced pain compared with custom made orthoses plus stretching at 8 weeks. One RCT found that heel pads plus orthoses reduced pain compared with heel pads plus paracetamol at 8 weeks.

Lasers

One small RCT identified by a systematic review found no significant difference between laser treatment and placebo.

Local anaesthetic injection

One systematic review identified no RCTs comparing local anaesthesia versus placebo or no treatment. One RCT found that combining local anaesthetic with a corticosteroid injection compared with local anaesthetic injection alone slightly improved pain score at 1 month. However, it found no significant difference in pain thereafter. The clinical importance of this result is unclear.

Night splints plus non-steroidal anti-inflammatory drugs

One RCT found no significant difference in pain between a night splint plus non-steroidal anti-inflammatory drugs and non-steroidal anti-inflammatory drugs alone after 3 months. There was insufficient evidence from one RCT comparing night splints versus orthoses.

Stretching exercises

One systematic review identified no RCTs comparing stretching exercises versus no treatment in people with heel pain. One RCT found no significant difference in pain between stretching alone (Achilles tendon stretching and plantar fascia stretching) and stretching plus orthoses after 8 weeks. The same RCT also found that stretching plus heel pad (silicone, rubber, or felt insert) improved symptoms compared with stretching alone at 8 weeks. One RCT found no significant difference in pain between sustained and intermittent Achilles tendon stretching exercises. One RCT found that plantar fascia stretching plus heel pad was more effective at reducing morning heel pain than Achilles tendon stretching plus heel pad.

Surgery

One systematic review found no RCTs of surgery for heel pain.

Ultrasound

One small RCT identified by a systematic review found no significant difference in pain between ultrasound and sham ultrasound.

LIKELY TO BE INEFFECTIVE OR HARMFUL

Corticosteroid injection in the medium to long term (with or without heel pad)

One systematic review identified no RCTs comparing medium to long term effects of corticosteroid injections versus placebo, orthoses, heel pads, analgesic medication, or corticosteroid injection plus local anaesthesia. One small RCT provided insufficient evidence about the long term effects of corticosteroid injection plus heel pad compared with placebo plus heel pad. Observational studies found a high rate of plantar fascia rupture and other complications associated with corticosteroid injections, which may lead to chronic disability in some people.

Plantar heel pain and fasciitis

Corticosteroid injection plus local anaesthetic injection in the medium to long term (with or without non-steroidal anti-inflammatory drugs or heel pads)

One systematic review identified no RCTs comparing medium to long term effects of corticosteroid injections plus local anaesthesia versus placebo or no treatment. RCTs identified by the review provided insufficient evidence about clinically important long term effects of corticosteroids plus local anaesthesia (alone or combined with non-steroidal anti-inflammatory drugs or heel pads) compared with other treatments. Observational studies have found a high rate of plantar fascia rupture and other complications associated with corticosteroid injections, which may lead to chronic disability in some people.

DEFINITION Plantar heel pain is soreness or tenderness of the heel that is restricted to the sole of the foot. It often radiates from the central part of the heel pad or the medial tubercle of the calcaneum, but may extend along the plantar fascia into the medial longitudinal arch of the foot. Severity may range from an irritation at the origin of the plantar fascia, which is noticeable on rising after rest, to an incapacitating pain. This review excludes clinically evident underlying disorders, for example, infection, calcaneal fracture, and calcaneal nerve entrapment, which may be distinguished clinically — a calcaneal fracture may present after trauma, and calcaneal nerve entrapment gives rise to shooting pains and feelings of "pins and needles" on the medial aspect of the heel.

INCIDENCE/ PREVALENCE The incidence and prevalence of plantar heel pain is uncertain. Plantar heel pain primarily affects those in mid to late life.[1]

AETIOLOGY/ RISK FACTORS Unknown.

PROGNOSIS One systematic review found that almost all of the included trials reported an improvement in discomfort regardless of the intervention received (including placebo), suggesting that the condition is at least partially self limiting.[1] A telephone survey of 100 people treated conservatively (average follow up 47 months) found that 82 people had resolution of symptoms, 15 had continued symptoms but no limitations of activity or work, and three had persistent bilateral symptoms that limited activity or changed work status.[2] Thirty one people said that they would have seriously considered surgical treatment at the time that medical attention was sought.

Please refer to clinicalevidence.com for full text and references.

Raynaud's phenomenon (primary)

Search date October 2005

Janet Pope

What are the effects of treatments for primary Raynaud's phenomenon?

TRADE OFF BETWEEN BENEFITS AND HARMS

Nifedipine

One systematic review found that nifedipine reduced the frequency and severity of Raynaud's attacks compared with placebo. Some RCTs found that nifedipine was associated with higher rates of adverse effects compared with placebo, including flushing, headache, oedema, and tachycardia.

UNKNOWN EFFECTIVENESS

Amlodipine

We found no satisfactory RCTs of the effects of amlodipine.

Diltiazem

We found no satisfactory RCTs of the effects of diltiazem.

Exercise

We found no satisfactory RCTs of the effects of exercise.

Inositol nicotinate

Two RCTs provided insufficient evidence to assess inositol nicotinate.

Keeping warm

We found no satisfactory RCTs of the effects of keeping warm.

Moxisylyte (thymoxamine)

We found no satisfactory RCTs of the effects of moxisylyte (thymoxamine).

Naftidrofuryl oxalate

One RCT found that, compared with placebo, naftidrofuryl oxalate reduced the duration and intensity of Raynaud's attacks over 2 months and reduced the impact of attacks on daily activities. However, we were unable to draw a reliable conclusions from this single study.

Nicardipine

One RCT found that nicardipine decreased the frequency of Raynaud's attacks over 8 weeks after crossover compared with placebo, but found no significant difference in the severity of attacks. Another RCT found no significant difference in the frequency, severity, or duration of attacks with nicardipine compared with placebo, but it is likely to have been too small to detect a clinically important difference in outcomes.

Prazosin

One small crossover RCT found limited evidence that prazosin reduced the number and duration of attacks over 6 weeks after crossover compared with placebo, but found no significant difference in the severity of attacks. However, we were unable to draw a reliable conclusion from this single study.

Raynaud's phenomenon (primary)

DEFINITION Raynaud's phenomenon is episodic vasospasm of the peripheral arteries, causing pallor followed by cyanosis and redness with pain and sometimes paraesthesia, and, rarely, ulceration of the fingers and toes (and in some cases of the ears or nose). Primary or idiopathic Raynaud's phenomenon (Raynaud's disease) occurs without an underlying disease. Secondary Raynaud's phenomenon (Raynaud's syndrome) occurs in association with an underlying disease — usually connective tissue disorders such as scleroderma, systemic lupus erythematosus, rheumatoid arthritis, or polymyositis. This review excludes secondary Raynaud's phenomenon.

INCIDENCE/ PREVALENCE The prevalence of primary Raynaud's phenomenon varies by gender, country, and exposure to workplace vibration. One large US cohort study (4182 people) found symptoms in 9.6% of women and 8.1% of men, of whom 81% had primary Raynaud's phenomenon.[1] Smaller cohort studies in Spain have estimated the prevalence of Raynaud's phenomenon to be 3.7–4.0%, of which 90% is primary Raynaud's phenomenon.[2,3] One cohort study in Japan (332 men, 731 women) found symptoms of primary Raynaud's phenomenon in 3.4% of women and 3.0% of men.[4]

AETIOLOGY/ RISK FACTORS The cause of primary Raynaud's phenomenon is unknown.[5] There is evidence for genetic predisposition,[6,7] most likely in those people with early onset Raynaud's phenomenon (aged < 40 years).[8] One prospective observational study (424 people with Raynaud's phenomenon) found that 73% of sufferers first developed symptoms before age 40 years.[8] Women are more at risk than men (OR 3.0, 95% CI 1.2 to 7.8, in 1 US case control study [235 people]).[9] The other known risk factor is occupational exposure to vibration from tools (symptoms developed in about 8% with exposure *v* 2.7% with no exposure in 2 cohorts from Japan).[10,11] People who are obese may be less at risk.[9] Symptoms are often worsened by cold or emotion.

PROGNOSIS Attacks may last from several minutes to a few hours. One systematic review (search date 1996, 10 prospective observational studies, 639 people with primary Raynaud's phenomenon) found that 13% of long term sufferers later manifested an underlying disorder such as scleroderma.[12]

Please refer to clinicalevidence.com for full text and references.

Shoulder pain

Search date February 2006

Cathy Speed

What are the effects of oral drug treatment?

LIKELY TO BE BENEFICIAL

Oral non-steroidal anti-inflammatory drugs (reduce pain in people with acute tendonitis and/or subacromial bursistis)

We found inconclusive evidence on the effects of oral non-steroidal anti-inflammatory drugs (NSAIDs) in people with shoulder pain. One systematic review of two weak RCTs found no significant difference in pain at 4 weeks between oral NSAIDs and placebo in people with non-specific shoulder pain. However, three RCTs found that oral flurbiprofen, celecoxib, and naproxen all reduced pain in people with acute tendonitis and/or subacromial bursitis compared with placebo. The RCTs found no evidence that the incidence or nature of adverse effects varied among NSAIDs. Adverse effects were mostly gastrointestinal symptoms, skin rash, headache, or dizziness.

UNKNOWN EFFECTIVENESS

Corticosteroids (oral)

Three RCTs provided insufficient evidence to assess the effects of oral corticosteroids in people with shoulder pain. The adverse effects of corticosteroids are well documented.

Opioid analgesics

We found no systematic review or RCTs of opioid analgesics in people with shoulder pain.

Paracetamol

We found no systematic review or RCTs of paracetamol in people with shoulder pain.

What are the effects of topical drug treatment?

UNKNOWN EFFECTIVENESS

Non-steroidal anti-inflammatory drugs (topical)

We found no systematic review or RCTs about the effects of topical non-steroidal anti-inflammatory drugs in people with shoulder pain.

Phonophoresis

We found no systematic review or RCTs of phonophoresis solely in people with shoulder pain.

Transdermal glyceryl trinitrate

We found no systematic review or RCTs of sufficient quality assessing transdermal glyceryl trinitrate in people with shoulder pain.

Shoulder pain

What are the effects of local injections?

LIKELY TO BE BENEFICIAL

Nerve block *New*

One RCT found that suprascapular nerve block improved pain at 1 month compared with placebo and in people with adhesive capsulitis. Another RCT found similar results in people with degenerative disease and/or arthritis but it is unclear whether these results are generalisable to people with non-arthritic shoulder pain. One RCT found that suprascapular nerve block prolonged analgesia after non-arthroscopic shoulder surgery but did not improve outcome. We found no systematic review or RCTs in people with rotator cuff disease.

UNKNOWN EFFECTIVENESS

Intra-articular corticosteroid injections

RCTs provided insufficient evidence to assess intra-articular corticosteroids, with or without local anaesthetic or physiotherapy, compared with placebo or local anaesthetic alone in people with shoulder pain. RCTs also provided insufficient evidence to assess combined intra-articular and subacromial corticosteroid injections. RCTs found that intra-articular corticosteroids improved pain and function at 6–7 weeks compared with physiotherapy, but the difference between groups was no longer significant at 12 months.

Intra-articular guanethidine

We found no systematic review or RCTs of sufficient quality of intra-articular guanethidine in people with non-arthritic shoulder pain.

Intra-articular non-steroidal anti-inflammatory injections

We found no systematic review or RCTs about the effects of intra-articular non-steroidal anti-inflammatory injections in people with shoulder pain.

Subacromial corticosteroid injections

We found no RCTs comparing subacromial injection of corticosteroids versus placebo. Three small RCTs in people with rotator cuff tendinitis and two small RCTs in people with subacromial impingement provided insufficient evidence to compare the clinical effects of corticosteroid plus lidocaine or bupivacaine versus lidocaine or bupivacaine alone. RCTs also provided insufficient evidence to assess combined subacromial and intra-articular corticosteroid injections. One RCT found no significant difference between subacromial corticosteroid plus lidocaine and physiotherapy in terms of disability or successful outcome at 6 months in people attending their physician because of a new episode of unilateral shoulder pain, but found that corticosteroid injection increased the need for repeat consultation or other interventions.

What are the effects of non-drug treatment?

LIKELY TO BE BENEFICIAL

Extracorporeal shock wave therapy (in people with calcific tendinitis)

In people with calcific tendinitis, three RCTs found that both high energy and lower energy extracorporeal shock wave therapy reduced pain, improved shoulder function and reduced calcification compared with placebo. Results from one of these RCTs should be treated with caution because of the high withdrawal rate and lack of an intention to treat analysis. High energy extracorporeal shock wave therapy may be superior to lower energy extracorporeal shock wave therapy in these people. RCTs found no evidence of benefit in people with non-calcific rotator cuff tendinopathy. Extracorporeal shock wave therapy can be painful during treatment.

Laser treatment

One systematic review identified three small RCTs. Two of the RCTs found that laser improved pain after 2–3 weeks compared with placebo, and one RCT found no significant difference at 8 weeks between treatments, although it may have lacked power to detect a difference. One additional RCT found that laser increased recovery rates at 1 month compared with placebo.

Physiotherapy (manual treatment, exercises)

RCTs in people with mixed shoulder disorders found that physiotherapy improved pain and function compared with no treatment or sham laser. RCTs provided insufficient evidence to assess Maitland mobilisation or whether adding oral corticosteroids to home exercises was more effective than home exercises alone. One RCT found no significant difference in pain and function between physiotherapy and surgical arthroscopic decompression at 6 months or 2.5 years. Another RCT found no significant difference between physiotherapy and subacromial corticosteroid plus lidocaine in terms of disability or successful outcome at 6 months in people attending their physician because of a new episode of unilateral shoulder pain, but found that physiotherapy reduced the need for repeat consultations or other interventions. RCTs found that physiotherapy was less effective than intra-articular corticosteroids in improving pain and function at 6–7 weeks, but the difference between groups was no longer significant at 12 months.

UNKNOWN EFFECTIVENESS

Electrical stimulation

Three poor quality, small RCTs identified by a systematic review provided insufficient evidence about the effects of electrical stimulation in people with shoulder pain.

Ice

One small RCT provided insufficient evidence about the effects of ice in people with shoulder pain.

Multidisciplinary biopsychosocial rehabilitation

One systematic review found no good quality RCTs of multidisciplinary biopsychosocial rehabilitation in people with shoulder pain.

Ultrasound

One RCT identified by a systematic review found that ultrasound improved pain and quality of life at the end of treatment (6 weeks) in people with calcific tendinitis, but found no significant difference at 9 months. Four other RCTs identified by the review found no significant difference between ultrasound and sham ultrasound, but most may have been too small to detect a clinically important difference between groups.

Shoulder pain

What are the effects of surgical treatment?

LIKELY TO BE BENEFICIAL

Manipulation under anaesthesia plus intra-articular injection in people with frozen shoulder

One RCT found that, in people with adhesive capsulitis, manipulation under anaesthesia plus intra-articular hydrocortisone injection increased recovery rates compared with intra-articular hydrocortisone injection alone at 3 months. Another, weaker RCT found limited evidence that more people having manipulation under anaesthesia plus intra-articular saline injection than having manipulation alone or manipulation plus intra-articular injection of methylprednisolone had improvements in range of movement, pain relief, and return to normal activities. Potential adverse effects of manipulation under anaesthesia include intra-articular lesions within the glenohumeral joint.

Surgical arthroscopic decompression

One RCT found that arthroscopic decompression by experienced surgeons followed by physiotherapy improved pain and function compared with sham laser but not compared with supervised exercises at 6 months and 2.5 years in people with rotator cuff disease. One small RCT found that adding arthroscopic subacromial decompression did not improve functional outcome after arthroscopic repair of the rotator cuff.

UNKNOWN EFFECTIVENESS

Arthroscopic laser subacromial decompression

One systematic review found no RCTs on arthroscopic subacromial decompression.

DEFINITION Shoulder pain arises in or around the shoulder from its joints and surrounding soft tissues. Joints include the glenohumeral, acromioclavicular, sternoclavicular, "subacromial", and scapulothoracic. Regardless of the disorder, pain is the most common reason for consulting a practitioner. In adhesive capsulitis (frozen shoulder), pain is associated with pronounced restriction of movement. Rotator cuff disorders may affect one or more portions of the rotator cuff and can be further defined as rotator cuff tear (partial/full thickness), non-calcific tendinosis (previously termed tendinitis), or calcific tendinitis. A subacromial/subdeltoid bursitis may be associated with any of these disorders, or may occur in isolation. For most shoulder disorders, diagnosis is based on clinical features, with imaging studies playing a role in some people. Post-stroke shoulder pain and pain referred from the cervical spine are not addressed in this chapter.

INCIDENCE/ PREVALENCE Each year in primary care in the UK, about 1% of adults aged over 45 years present with a new episode of shoulder pain.[1] Prevalence is uncertain, with estimates from 4–20%.[2-6] One community survey (392 people) in the UK found a 1 month prevalence of shoulder pain of 34%.[7] A second survey (644 people aged ≥ 70 years) in a community based rheumatology clinic in the UK reported a point prevalence of 21%, with a higher frequency in women than men (25% *v* 17%).[8] Seventy per cent of cases involved the rotator cuff. Further analysis of 134 people included in the survey found that 65% of cases were rotator cuff lesions; 11% were caused by localised tenderness in the pericapsular musculature; 10% involved acromioclavicular joint pain; 3% involved glenohumeral joint arthritis; and 5% were referred pain from the neck.[9] Another survey in Sweden found that, in adults, the annual incidence of frozen shoulder was about 2%, with those aged 40–70 years most commonly affected.[10] The age distribution of specific shoulder disorders in the community is unknown.

AETIOLOGY/ RISK FACTORS Rotator cuff disorders are associated with excessive overloading, instability of the glenohumeral and acromioclavicular joints, muscle imbalance, adverse anatomical features (narrow coracoacromial arch and a hooked acromion), cuff degeneration with ageing, ischaemia, and musculoskeletal diseases that result in wasting of the cuff muscles.[11-14] Risk factors for adhesive capsulitis (frozen shoulder) include female sex, older age, shoulder trauma, surgery, diabetes, cardiorespiratory disorders, cerebrovascular events, thyroid disease, and hemiplegia.[10,15,16] Arthritis of the glenohumeral joint can occur in numerous forms, including primary and secondary osteoarthritis, rheumatoid arthritis, and crystal arthritides.[11] Shoulder pain can also be referred from other sites, in particular the cervical spine. It can also arise after stroke. Post-stroke shoulder pain and referred pain are not addressed in this chapter.

PROGNOSIS One survey in an elderly community found that most people with shoulder pain were still affected 3 years after the initial survey.[17] One prospective cohort study of 122 adults in primary care found that 25% of people with shoulder pain reported previous episodes and 49% reported full recovery at 18 months' follow up.[18]

Please refer to clinicalevidence.com for full text and references.

Tennis elbow

Search date August 2006

Rachelle Buchbinder, Sally Green, and Peter Struijs

What are the effects of treatments for tennis elbow?

LIKELY TO BE BENEFICIAL

Corticosteroid injections (for short term pain relief)

RCTs found limited evidence of a short term improvement in symptoms with corticosteroid injections compared with placebo or no treatment, local anaesthetic, orthoses (elbow strapping), physiotherapy, or oral non-steroidal anti-inflammatory drugs. Overall, we found no good evidence on long term effects of corticosteroids compared with placebo or no treatment, local anaesthetic, physiotherapy, or orthoses, although we did find limited evidence that corticosteroid injections were less effective than physiotherapy or oral non-steroidal anti-inflammatory drugs at improving symptoms in the long term. One RCT found limited evidence that corticosteroid injections were more effective than extracorporeal shock wave therapy at reducing pain at 3 months. We found limited data comparing one type of corticosteroid injection to another, or single versus repeated injections.

UNKNOWN EFFECTIVENESS

Acupuncture (for short term pain relief)

Small, methodologically weak RCTs provided conflicting evidence about the effects of needle acupuncture, laser acupuncture, or electroacupuncture in people with tennis elbow. Three out of five RCTs comparing acupuncture versus placebo or no treatment found a small short term benefit from acupuncture compared with placebo or no treatment, whereas two RCTs found no significant difference between groups.

Exercise and mobilisation

One RCT found that exercise improved pain and function after treatment and at 11 months compared with placebo. One RCT found that exercise improved pain at 6–8 weeks compared with ultrasound plus friction massage. We found limited evidence that physiotherapy was less effective than corticosteroid injections at improving symptoms in the short term, but more effective in the long term. One RCT found no significant difference between exercise and watchful waiting in the short or long term (6–52 weeks).

Oral non-steroidal anti-inflammatory drugs (for longer term pain relief)

One systematic review found limited evidence that oral non-steroidal anti-inflammatory drugs (NSAIDs) improved symptoms in the short term compared with placebo, although we also found limited evidence that they were less effective than corticosteroid injection in the short term. We found insufficient evidence to assess the longer term effects of NSAIDs compared with placebo. One RCT found that oral NSAIDs were more effective than corticosteroid injections in the long term. We found no RCTs comparing oral versus topical NSAIDs.

Orthoses (bracing)

One systematic review found insufficient evidence about the effects of orthoses (braces) compared with placebo, no treatment, physiotherapy, or non-steroidal ▶

anti-inflammatory cream. It found limited evidence of less short term improvement in symptoms with orthoses compared with corticosteroid injections. One additional RCT found that at 6 weeks, orthoses were less effective than physical therapy at improving pain outcomes or subjective satisfaction, but more effective at improving functional ability.

Surgery

One systematic review found no RCTs comparing surgery versus no treatment or other treatments. One small unblinded RCT in people who had failed 12 months of conservative treatment found that percutaneous tenotomy of the common extensor origin led to quicker recovery and return to work than open excision of the abnormal tissue.

Topical non-steroidal anti-inflammatory drugs (for longer term pain relief)

One systematic review found that topical non-steroidal anti-inflammatory drugs (NSAIDs) improve symptoms in the short term compared with placebo. Minor adverse effects were reported with NSAIDs. We found insufficient evidence to assess the longer term effects of NSAIDs compared with placebo. We found no RCTs comparing topical versus oral NSAIDs.

UNLIKELY TO BE BENEFICIAL

Extracorporeal shock wave therapy

One systematic review, which included a total of nine placebo controlled RCTs involving 1006 people, and an additional RCT of 62 people, found conflicting evidence about the benefits of shock wave therapy versus placebo. However, pooled analyses found no significant difference in pain outcomes between shock wave therapy and placebo. Side effects were mostly transient, and included local pain and reddening of the skin, and nausea. One RCT found limited evidence that extracorporeal shock wave therapy was less effective than corticosteroid injection at reducing pain at 3 months. We found no RCTs comparing early versus delayed shock wave treatment, or comparing different modes of delivery with each other.

DEFINITION Tennis elbow has many analogous terms, including lateral elbow pain, lateral epicondylitis, rowing elbow, tendonitis of the common extensor origin, and peritendinitis of the elbow. Tennis elbow is characterised by pain and tenderness over the lateral epicondyle of the humerus and pain on resisted dorsiflexion of the wrist, middle finger, or both. For the purposes of this review, tennis elbow is restricted to lateral elbow pain or lateral epicondylitis.

INCIDENCE/ PREVALENCE Lateral elbow pain is common (population prevalence 1–3%),[1] with peak incidence occurring at 40–50 years of age. In women aged 42–46 years, incidence increases to 10%.[2,3] In UK, the Netherlands, and Scandinavia the incidence of lateral elbow pain in general practice is 4–7/1000 people a year.[3-5]

AETIOLOGY/ RISK FACTORS Tennis elbow is considered to be an overload injury, typically after minor and often unrecognised trauma of the extensor muscles of the forearm. Despite the title tennis elbow, tennis is a direct cause in only 5% of those with lateral epicondylitis.[6]

Tennis elbow

PROGNOSIS Although lateral elbow pain is generally self limiting, in a minority of people symptoms persist for 18 months to 2 years, and in some cases for much longer.[7] The cost is therefore high, both in terms of lost productivity and healthcare use. In a general practice trial of an expectant waiting policy, 80% of the people with elbow pain already greater than 4 weeks' duration had recovered after 1 year.[8]

Please refer to clinicalevidence.com for full text and references.

Altitude sickness

Search date January 2006

David Murdoch

What are the effects of interventions to prevent acute mountain sickness?

BENEFICIAL

Acetazolamide

One systematic review and three RCTs found that acetazolamide reduced the incidence of acute mountain sickness compared with placebo. The reduction in mountain sickness in the smallest RCT did not reach statistical significance, but it may have lacked power to detect a clinically important difference. The review and subsequent RCTs found that acetazolamide caused polyuria, paraesthesia, or both in a large proportion of people. We found no RCTs of sufficient quality comparing acetazolamide versus dexamethasone. Two RCTs found that acetazolamide reduced the incidence of acute mountain sickness compared with ginkgo biloba, although the significance of this reduction was not assessed.

Dexamethasone

One systematic review and two RCTs found that dexamethasone was more effective than placebo for preventing acute mountain sickness. One RCT found no significant difference in the incidence of acute mountain sickness between dexamethasone and placebo, but it may have lacked power to detect a clinically significant difference. However, the review found that adverse effects (including depression) occurred in a quarter of people on withdrawal of dexamethasone. We found no RCTs of sufficient quality comparing dexamethasone versus acetazolamide.

Slow ascent (or acclimatisation)*

We found no systematic review or RCTs evaluating the effect on different rates of ascent or acclimatisation in preventing acute mountain sickness. Consensus opinion suggests that slower ascent reduces the risk of acute mountain sickness compared with faster ascent.

UNKNOWN EFFECTIVENESS

Ginkgo biloba *New*

Two RCTs found no significant difference in the incidence of acute mountain sickness between ginkgo biloba and placebo. One RCT found that ginkgo biloba reduced the incidence of severe acute mountain sickness, but not the overall incidence of acute mountain sickness, compared with placebo. Another RCT found that ginkgo biloba reduced the incidence of acute mountain sickness compared with placebo. Two RCTs found that acetazolamide reduced the incidence of acute mountain sickness compared with ginkgo biloba, although the significance of this difference was not assessed.

Altitude sickness

What are the effects of treatments for acute mountain sickness?

LIKELY TO BE BENEFICIAL

Descent compared with resting at the same altitude*

We found no systematic review or RCTs on the effects of descent compared with resting at the same altitude in people with acute mountain sickness. Consensus opinion suggests that people with acute mountain sickness should descend if possible. However, we found no RCTs examining the effects of different distances of descent, or about the balance of risks and benefits in people who might find it difficult to descend.

Dexamethasone

One small RCT in climbers with symptoms and signs of acute mountain sickness found that dexamethasone reduced mean acute mountain sickness symptom scores compared with placebo.

UNKNOWN EFFECTIVENESS

Acetazolamide

We found no systematic review or RCTs of sufficient quality on the effects of acetazolamide compared with placebo for treating people with acute mountain sickness.

*Although we found no RCTs on the effects of these interventions, there is a general consensus that they are effective.

DEFINITION Altitude sickness (or high altitude illness) includes acute mountain sickness, high altitude pulmonary oedema, and high altitude cerebral oedema. **Acute mountain sickness** typically occurs at altitudes greater than 2500 m (about 8000 feet) and is characterised by the development of some or all of the symptoms of headache, weakness, fatigue, listlessness, nausea, insomnia, and suppressed appetite. Symptoms may take days to develop or may occur within hours, depending on the rate of ascent and the altitude attained. More severe forms of altitude sickness have been identified. **High altitude pulmonary oedema** is characterised by symptoms and signs typical of pulmonary oedema, such as shortness of breath, coughing, and production of frothy or blood stained sputum. **High altitude cerebral oedema** is characterised by confusion, ataxia, and a decreasing level of consciousness. This review covers only acute mountain sickness.

INCIDENCE/ PREVALENCE The incidence of acute mountain sickness increases with absolute height attained and with the rate of ascent. One survey in Taiwan (93 people ascending above 3000 m) found that 27% of people experienced acute mountain sickness.[1] One survey in the Himalayas (278 unacclimatised hikers at 4243 m) found that 53% of people developed acute mountain sickness.[2] One survey in the Swiss Alps (466 climbers at 4 altitudes between 2850 m and 4559 m) found the prevalence of two or more symptoms of acute mountain sickness to be 9% of people at 2850 m; 13% of people at 3050 m; 34% of people at 3650 m; and 53% of people at 4559 m.[3]

AETIOLOGY/ RISK FACTORS One survey in the Himalayas identified the rate of ascent and absolute height attained as the only risk factors for acute mountain sickness.[2] It found no evidence of a difference in risk between men and women, or that previous episodes of altitude experience, load carried, or recent respiratory infections affected risk. However, the study was too small to exclude these as risk factors or to quantify risks reliably. One systematic review (search date 1999) comparing prophylactic agents versus placebo found that, among people receiving placebo, the incidence of acute mountain sickness was higher with a faster rate of ascent (54% of people at a mean ascent rate of 91 m/hour; 73% at a mean ascent rate of 1268 m/hour; 89% at a simulated ascent rate in a hypobaric chamber of 1647 m/hour).[4] One survey in Switzerland (827 mountaineers ascending to 4559 m) examined the effects of susceptibility, pre-exposure, and ascent rate on acute mountain sickness.[5] In this study, pre-exposure was defined as having spent more than 4 days above 3000 m in the preceding 2 months, and slow ascent was defined as ascending in more than 3 days. It found that, in susceptible people (who had previously had acute mountain sickness at high altitude), the prevalence of acute mountain sickness was 58% with rapid ascent and no pre-exposure, 29% with pre-exposure only, 33% with slow ascent only, and 7% with both pre-exposure and slow ascent.[5] In non-susceptible people, the corresponding values were 31%, 16%, 11%, and 4%. The overall odds ratio for developing acute mountain sickness in susceptible compared with non-susceptible people was 2.9 (95% CI 2.1 to 4.1).[5]

PROGNOSIS We found no reliable data on prognosis. It is widely held that if no further ascent is attempted, then the symptoms of acute mountain sickness tend to resolve over a few days. We found no reliable data about long term sequelae in people whose symptoms have completely resolved.

Please refer to clinicalevidence.com for full text and references.

Bell's palsy

Search date February 2006

Julian Holland

What are the effects of treatments in adults and children?

LIKELY TO BE BENEFICIAL

Corticosteroids plus antiviral treatment

One RCT identified by a systematic review found limited evidence that aciclovir plus prednisolone produced full recovery of facial function more often compared with prednisolone alone after 4 months.

UNKNOWN EFFECTIVENESS

Antiviral treatment

One systematic review identified no RCTs comparing aciclovir versus placebo. One RCT identified by the review found that prednisolone produced full recovery more often than aciclovir alone, but found no significant difference in motor synkinesis between treatment groups at 12 weeks. Another RCT identified by the review found limited evidence that aciclovir plus prednisolone produced full recovery of facial function more often compared with prednisolone alone after 4 months.

Corticosteroids

One systematic review found no significant difference between corticosteroids (cortisone acetate, prednisolone, methylprednisolone) and control in recovery of facial motor function or reduction of cosmetically disabling sequelae after 6 months. One RCT identified by the review found that prednisolone reduced the time to recover facial nerve function compared with placebo. However, the review found no significant difference between treatments in motor synkinesis and autonomic dysfunction at 12 months. One RCT identified by a systematic review found that prednisolone produced full recovery more often than aciclovir alone, but found no significant difference in motor synkinesis between treatment groups at 12 weeks. One RCT identified by a systematic review found limited evidence that aciclovir plus prednisolone produced full recovery of facial function more often compared with prednisolone alone after 4 months.

Facial nerve decompression surgery

One systematic review identified no RCTs of facial nerve decompression surgery for people with Bell's palsy.

DEFINITION Bell's palsy is an idiopathic, acute, unilateral paresis or paralysis of the face in a pattern consistent with peripheral facial nerve dysfunction, and may be partial or complete, occurring with equal frequency on the right and left sides of the face. While other possible causes need to be excluded, there is increasing evidence that Bell's palsy is caused by herpes viruses.[1] Additional symptoms of Bell's palsy may include mild pain in or behind the ear, oropharyngeal or facial numbness, impaired tolerance to ordinary levels of noise, and disturbed taste on the anterior part of the tongue.[2] Severe pain is more suggestive of herpes zoster virus infection (shingles) and possible progression to a Ramsay Hunt syndrome, but another cause should be carefully excluded. Up to 30% of people with an acute peripheral facial palsy will not have Bell's palsy; other causes may include stroke, tumour, trauma, middle ear disease and Lyme disease. Features such as sparing of movement in the upper face (central pattern) or weakness of a specific branch of the facial nerve (segmental pattern) suggest an alternative cause.[3] In children under 10 years of age, Bell's palsy is less common (under 40%) so an alternative cause should be carefully excluded.[4] The assessment should identify acute suppurative ear disease (including mastoiditis), a parotid mass or Lyme disease in endemic areas.[5]

INCIDENCE/ PREVALENCE The incidence is about 20/100 000 people a year, or about 1/60 people in a lifetime.[4] Bell's palsy has a peak incidence between the ages of 15 and 40 years. Men and women are equally affected, although the incidence may be increased in pregnant women.[4]

AETIOLOGY/ RISK FACTORS Bell's palsy is probably caused by reactivated herpes viruses from the cranial nerve ganglia. Herpes simplex virus-1 may be detected in up to 50% of cases and herpes zoster virus in approximately 30% of cases. Herpes zoster associated facial palsy more frequently presents as zoster sine herpete (without vesicles), although 6% of patients will subsequently develop vesicles (Ramsay Hunt syndrome).[6] Thus, treatment plans for the management of Bell's palsy should recognise the high incidence of herpes zoster virus, which is associated with worse outcomes.[7] Inflammation of the facial nerve initially results in reversible neuropraxia, but ultimately Wallerian degeneration ensues.

PROGNOSIS Overall, Bell's palsy has a fair prognosis without treatment. Significant improvement occurs within 3 weeks in 85% of people and within 3–5 months in the remaining 15%.[4] Patients failing to show signs of improvement by 3 weeks may have suffered significant degeneration of the facial nerve or have an alternative diagnosis that requires identification by specialist examination or investigations, such as computed tomography or magnetic resonance imaging. Overall, 71% of people will recover facial muscle function (61% of people with complete palsy, 94% of people with partial palsy).[4] The remaining 29% are left with mild to severe residual facial muscle weakness, 17% with contracture and 16% with hemifacial spasm or synkinesis.[4] Incomplete recovery of facial expression may have a long term impact on quality of life. The prognosis for children with Bell's palsy is generally good, with a high rate (> 90%) of spontaneous recovery, in part due to the high frequency of partial paralysis.[4] However, children with complete palsies may suffer poor outcomes as frequently as do adults.[8]

Please refer to clinicalevidence.com for full text and references.

Epilepsy

Search date November 2005

Anthony Marson and Sridharan Ramaratnam

What are the benefits and risks of starting antiepileptic drug treatment following a single seizure?

TRADE OFF BETWEEN BENEFITS AND HARMS

Antiepileptic drugs after a single seizure

Four RCTs found that treatment following a single seizure with antiepileptic drugs reduced seizure recurrence at 1–3 years compared with no treatment or placebo. One RCT in people with one or more seizures found that immediate treatment with antiepileptic drugs increased the time to first and second subsequent seizure, and reduced the time to achieve 2 year remission of seizures compared with no treatment. However, we found no evidence that treatment alters long term prognosis. Long term antiepileptic drug treatment is potentially harmful.

What are the effects of monotherapy in newly diagnosed partial epilepsy?

BENEFICIAL

Carbamazepine*

We found no placebo controlled RCTs of carbamazepine used as monotherapy in people with partial epilepsy, but widespread consensus holds that it is effective and placebo controlled trials would now be considered unethical. Systematic reviews found no reliable evidence on which to base a choice among antiepileptic drugs in terms of seizure control; carbamazepine is considered to be the drug of choice for partial epilepsy. Systematic reviews found that phenobarbital was more likely to be withdrawn than carbamazepine.

Phenobarbital*

We found no placebo controlled RCTs of phenobarbital used as monotherapy in people with partial epilepsy, but widespread consensus holds that it is effective and placebo controlled trials would now be considered unethical. Systematic reviews found no reliable evidence on which to base a choice among antiepileptic drugs in terms of seizure control. Systematic reviews found that phenobarbital was more likely to be withdrawn than phenytoin or carbamazepine.

Phenytoin*

We found no placebo controlled RCTs of phenytoin used as monotherapy in people with partial epilepsy, but widespread consensus holds that it is effective and placebo controlled trials would now be considered unethical. Systematic reviews found no reliable evidence on which to base a choice among antiepileptic drugs in terms of seizure control. Systematic reviews found that phenobarbital was more likely to be withdrawn than phenytoin.

Sodium valproate*

We found no placebo controlled RCTs of sodium valproate used as monotherapy in people with partial epilepsy, but widespread consensus holds that it is effective and placebo controlled trials would be considered unethical. Systematic reviews found no reliable evidence on which to base a choice among antiepileptic drugs in terms of seizure control.

What are the effects of monotherapy in newly diagnosed generalised epilepsy (tonic clonic type)?

BENEFICIAL

Carbamazepine*

We found no placebo controlled trials of carbamazepine used as monotherapy in people with generalised epilepsy, but widespread consensus holds that it is effective and a placebo controlled trial would be considered unethical. Systematic reviews found insufficient evidence on which to base a choice among antiepileptic drugs in terms of seizure control.

Phenobarbital*

We found no placebo controlled trials of phenobarbital used as monotherapy in people with generalised epilepsy, but widespread consensus holds that it is effective and a placebo controlled trial would now be considered unethical. Systematic reviews found insufficient evidence on which to base a choice among drugs in terms of seizure control.

Phenytoin*

We found no placebo controlled trials of phenytoin used as monotherapy in people with generalised epilepsy, but widespread consensus holds that it is effective and a placebo controlled trial would now be considered unethical. Systematic reviews found insufficient evidence on which to base a choice among antiepileptic drugs in terms of seizure control.

Sodium valproate*

We found no placebo controlled trials of sodium valproate used as monotherapy in people with generalised epilepsy, but widespread consensus holds that it is effective and a placebo controlled trial would now be considered unethical. Systematic reviews found insufficient evidence on which to base a choice among antiepileptic drugs in terms of seizure control.

What are the effects of additional treatments in people with drug resistant partial epilepsy?

BENEFICIAL

Addition of second line drugs (gabapentin, levetiracetam, lamotrigine, oxcarbazepine, tiagabine, topiramate, vigabatrin, or zonisamide)

Systematic reviews in people with drug resistant partial epilepsy found that adding gabapentin, levetiracetam, lamotrigine, oxcarbazepine, tiagabine, topiramate, vigabatrin, or zonisamide to usual treatment reduced seizure frequency compared with adding placebo. The reviews found that adding any of the drugs increased the frequency of adverse effects such as dizziness and somnolence compared with adding placebo. We found no RCTs of other antiepileptic drugs as second line treatment. We found no good evidence from RCTs on which to base a choice among drugs.

Epilepsy

Which people in remission from seizures are at risk of relapse on withdrawal of drug treatment?

TRADE OFF BETWEEN BENEFITS AND HARMS

Antiepileptic drug withdrawal for people in remission

One RCT in people who had been seizure free for at least 2 years found that further seizures were more likely if people stopped treatment than if they continued antiepileptic medication. Clinical predictors of relapse after drug withdrawal included age, seizure type, number of antiepileptic drugs being taken, whether seizures had occurred since antiepileptic drugs were started, and the period of remission before drug withdrawal.

What are the effects of behavioural and psychological treatments for people with epilepsy?

LIKELY TO BE BENEFICIAL

Educational programmes

One RCT found that a 2 day educational programme reduced seizure frequency at 6 months compared with waiting list control. However, it found no significant difference in health related quality of life. RCTs found that educational packages improved knowledge and understanding of epilepsy, adjustment to epilepsy, and psychosocial functioning compared with control.

UNKNOWN EFFECTIVENESS

Biofeedback

One systematic review provided insufficient evidence about the effects of electroencephalographic and galvanic skin response biofeedback.

Cognitive behavioural therapy

Two small RCTs provided insufficient evidence about the effects of cognitive behavioural therapy in people with epilepsy.

Family counselling

One small RCT with methodological weaknesses provided insufficient evidence about the effects of family counselling.

Relaxation plus behavioural modification therapy

One systematic review provided insufficient evidence about the effects of combined relaxation and behavioural modification treatment on seizures.

Relaxation therapy

One systematic review provided insufficient evidence about the effects of relaxation therapy compared with control in people with epilepsy.

Yoga

One systematic review provided insufficient evidence about the effects of yoga in people with epilepsy.

What are the effects of surgery in people with drug resistant temporal lobe epilepsy?

BENEFICIAL

Temporal lobectomy*

One RCT identified by a systematic review found that temporal lobectomy improved seizure control and quality of life after 1 year compared with continued medical treatment in people with poorly controlled temporal lobe epilepsy. There is consensus that temporal lobectomy is beneficial for people with drug resistant temporal lobe epilepsy.

LIKELY TO BE BENEFICIAL

Amygdalohippocampectomy*

We found no systematic review or RCTs that examined the effect of amygdalohippocampectomy in people with drug resistant temporal lobe epilepsy. However, there is consensus that amygdalohippocampectomy is likely to be beneficial for people with drug resistant temporal lobe epilepsy.

Vagus nerve stimulation as adjunctive therapy for partial seizures *New*

One systematic review of two RCTs found that high level vagus nerve stimulation reduced the frequency of seizures in people with medication resistant partial seizures compared with low level vagus nerve stimulation (control).

UNKNOWN EFFECTIVENESS

Lesionectomy

We found no systematic review or RCTs that examined the effects of lesionectomy in people with drug resistant temporal lobe epilepsy thought to be caused by a known cerebral lesion.

*Categorisation based on consensus.

DEFINITION Epilepsy is a group of disorders rather than a single disease. Seizures can be classified by type as partial or focal (categorised as simple partial, complex partial, and secondary generalised tonic clonic seizures) or generalised (categorised as generalised tonic clonic, absence, myoclonic, tonic, and atonic seizures).[1] A person is considered to have epilepsy if they have had two or more unprovoked seizures.

INCIDENCE/ PREVALENCE Epilepsy is common, with an estimated prevalence in the developed world of 5–10/1000, and an annual incidence of 50/100 000 people.[2] About 3% of people will be given a diagnosis of epilepsy at some time in their lives.[3]

AETIOLOGY/ RISK FACTORS Epilepsy is a symptom rather than a disease, and it may be caused by various disorders involving the brain. The causes/risk factors include birth/neonatal injuries, congenital or metabolic disorders, head injuries, tumours, infections of the brain or meninges, genetic defects, degenerative disease of the brain, cerebrovascular disease, or demyelinating disease. Epilepsy can be classified by cause.[1] **Idiopathic generalised** epilepsies (such as juvenile myoclonic epilepsy or childhood absence epilepsy) are largely genetic. **Symptomatic epilepsies** result from a known cerebral abnormality; for example, temporal lobe epilepsy may result from a congenital defect, mesial temporal sclerosis, or a tumour. **Cryptogenic epilepsies** are those that cannot be classified as idiopathic or symptomatic.

Epilepsy

PROGNOSIS About 60% of untreated people have no further seizures during the 2 years after their first seizure.[4] For most people with epilepsy the prognosis is good. About 70% go into remission, defined as being seizure free for 5 years on or off treatment. This leaves 20–30% who develop chronic epilepsy, which is often treated with multiple antiepileptic drugs.[5]

Please refer to clinicalevidence.com for full text and references.

Essential tremor

Search date March 2004

Joaquim Ferreira and Cristina Sampaio

What are the effects of drug treatments in people with essential tremor of the hand?

LIKELY TO BE BENEFICIAL

Propranolol

Small RCTs found that propranolol for up to 1 month improved clinical scores, tremor amplitude, and self evaluation of severity at up to 6 weeks compared with placebo. One RCT comparing propranolol versus clonidine found that the initial improvement in tremor from baseline was similar with both drugs and was maintained throughout follow up for 1 year. RCTs provided insufficient evidence to compare propranolol versus other beta-blockers.

Topiramate (improved tremor scores after 2 weeks' treatment but associated with appetite suppression, weight loss, and paraesthesia)

One RCT found limited evidence that topiramate improved observer rated tremor score after 2 weeks' treatment compared with placebo but was associated with adverse effects, including appetite suppression, weight loss, and paraesthesia. The clinical importance of the difference in tremor score is uncertain. We found no RCTs addressing long term outcomes.

TRADE OFF BETWEEN BENEFITS AND HARMS

Botulinum A toxin–haemagglutinin complex (improves clinical rating scales at 4–12 weeks but associated with hand weakness)

Two RCTs in people with essential hand tremor found that botulinum A toxin–haemagglutinin complex improved clinical rating scales at 4–12 weeks. They found no consistent improvement in motor tasks or functional disability. Hand weakness, which is dose dependent and transient, is a frequent adverse effect. We found no RCTs addressing long term outcomes.

Phenobarbital (improved tremor at 5 weeks but associated with depression and cognitive adverse effects)

One small RCT found that phenobarbital improved tremor at 5 weeks compared with placebo. However, another two RCTs found no significant difference in tremor scores at 4–5 weeks between phenobarbital and placebo. Phenobarbital is associated with depression and cognitive and behavioural adverse effects.

Primidone (improved tremor and function at 5 weeks compared with placebo and at 1 year compared with baseline but associated with depression and cognitive adverse effects)

Three small, short term RCTs found limited evidence that primidone improved tremor and functional ability over 4–10 weeks compared with placebo. One RCT comparing different doses of primidone found that it improved tremor from baseline at 1 year with no significant difference in outcome between groups. Primidone is associated with depression and cognitive and behavioural adverse effects.

Essential tremor

UNKNOWN EFFECTIVENESS

Benzodiazepines

Two small short term RCTs found weak evidence that alprazolam may improve tremor and function at 2–4 weeks compared with placebo. However, we were unable to draw reliable conclusions about effects. One very small RCT provided insufficient evidence to compare clonazepam versus placebo. Adverse effects with benzodiazepines, including dependency, sedation and cognitive and behavioural effects, have been well described for other conditions (see panic disorder).

Beta-blockers other than propranolol (atenolol, metoprolol, nadolol, pindolol, and sotalol)

Three small RCTs found weak evidence that atenolol or sotalol improved symptoms and self evaluated measures of tremor at 5 days to 4 weeks compared with placebo. One small RCT found no significant difference in symptoms between metoprolol and placebo and another small RCT found that pindolol worsened tremor amplitude compared with placebo. A third very small RCT provided insufficient evidence to compare nadolol versus placebo. RCTs provided insufficient evidence to compare other beta-blockers versus propranolol.

Calcium channel blockers (dihydropyridine)

Poor quality RCTs provided insufficient evidence to compare the dihydropyridine calcium channel blockers nicardipine and nimodipine versus placebo.

Carbonic anhydrase inhibitors

Small RCTs provided insufficient evidence to assess methazolamide or acetazolamide in people with essential tremor. We found no RCTs addressing long term outcomes.

Clonidine

One RCT found no significant difference between clonidine and placebo in essential hand tremor. However, the study lacked power to rule out a clinically important difference. Another RCT comparing clonidine versus propranolol found that the initial improvement in tremor from baseline was similar with both drugs and was maintained throughout follow up for 1 year.

Flunarizine

One small RCT found weak evidence that flunarizine reduced the symptoms of essential hand tremor after 1 months' treatment compared with placebo.

Gabapentin

Small RCTs provided insufficient evidence to compare gabapentin versus placebo. We found no RCTs addressing long term outcomes.

Isoniazid

One RCT found no significant difference between isoniazid and placebo in essential hand tremor, but it may have lacked power to detect a clinically important difference. We found no RCTs addressing long term outcomes.

LIKELY TO BE INEFFECTIVE OR HARMFUL

Mirtazapine

One RCT in people taking antitremor drugs such as propranolol, found no significant difference in tremor between adding mirtazapine and placebo and found that adverse effects were frequent.

DEFINITION Tremor is a rhythmic, mechanical oscillation of at least one body region. The term essential tremor is used when there is either a persistent bilateral tremor of hands and forearms, or an isolated tremor of the head without abnormal posturing, and when there is no evidence that the tremor arises from another identifiable cause. The diagnosis is not made if there are abnormal neurological signs, known causes of enhanced physiological tremor, a history or signs of psychogenic tremor, sudden change in severity, primary orthostatic tremor, isolated voice tremor, isolated position specific or task specific tremors, and isolated tongue, chin, or leg tremor.[1]

INCIDENCE/ PREVALENCE Essential tremor is one of the most common movement disorders throughout the world, with a prevalence of 0.4–3.9% in the general population.[2]

AETIOLOGY/ RISK FACTORS Essential tremor is sometimes inherited with an autosomal dominant pattern. About 40% of people with essential tremor have no family history. Alcohol ingestion provides symptomatic benefit in 50–70% of people.[3]

PROGNOSIS Essential tremor is a persistent and progressive condition. It usually begins during early adulthood and the severity of the tremor increases slowly. Only a small proportion of people with essential tremor seek medical advice, but the proportion in different surveys varies from 0.5–11%.[2] Most people with essential tremor are only mildly affected. However, most of the people who seek medical care are disabled to some extent, and most are socially handicapped by the tremor.[3] A quarter of people receiving medical care for the tremor change jobs or retire because of essential tremor induced disability.[4,5]

Please refer to clinicalevidence.com for full text and references.

Headache (chronic tension-type)

Search date July 2004

Nicholas Silver

What are the effects of treatments for chronic tension-type headache?

BENEFICIAL

Amitriptyline

One systematic review and three small, short duration RCTs found that amitriptyline reduced the duration and frequency of chronic tension-type headache compared with placebo. One RCT found that amitriptyline was more effective than citalopram in improving headache duration, frequency, and severity. Another RCT found comparable efficacy between amitriptyline and mirtazapine for the treatment of chronic tension-type headache, although amitriptyline was associated with a less favourable adverse effect profile. One RCT found no significant difference between amitriptyline and cognitive behavioural therapy in headache scores or frequency of clinically important improvement after six months.

Mirtazapine (only short term evidence)

One small RCT found that mirtazapine reduced the duration, frequency, and intensity of chronic tension-type headache compared with placebo. One RCT found comparable efficacy between mirtazapine and amitriptyline for the treatment of chronic tension-type headache, although mirtazapine was associated with a more favourable adverse effect profile.

LIKELY TO BE BENEFICIAL

Cognitive behavioural therapy

One systematic review and one subsequent RCT found limited evidence that cognitive behavioural therapy reduced the symptoms of chronic tension-type headache at 6 months compared with placebo. One RCT found no significant difference between cognitive behavioural therapy and amitriptyline or in headache scores or frequency of clinically important improvement after six months. One systematic review provided insufficient evidence to compare cognitive behavioural therapy versus relaxation or electromyographic biofeedback therapy.

UNKNOWN EFFECTIVENESS

Acupuncture

Two systematic reviews and one RCT provided insufficient evidence about the effects of acupuncture compared with sham acupuncture in people with episodic or chronic tension-type headache.

Relaxation and electromyographic biofeedback

Two systematic reviews and one subsequent RCT provided insufficient evidence about the effects of relaxation and electromyographic biofeedback on symptoms of chronic tension-type headache.

Serotonin reuptake inhibitor antidepressants

Two RCTs provided insufficient evidence about the effects of serotonin reuptake inhibitors on symptoms of chronic tension-type headache.

Tricyclic antidepressants other than amitriptyline

We found insufficient evidence about the effects of tricyclic antidepressants other than amitriptyline.

LIKELY TO BE INEFFECTIVE OR HARMFUL

Benzodiazepines

Two RCTs provided insufficient evidence about the effects of benzodiazepines compared with placebo or other treatments. Benzodiazepines are commonly associated with adverse effects if taken regularly.

Botulinum toxin

One systematic review provided no evidence that botulinum toxin improved the symptoms of chronic tension-type headache compared with placebo. However, botulinum toxin is associated with important adverse effects.

Regular acute pain relief medication

We found no systematic review or RCTs. One non-systematic review of observational studies provided insufficient evidence about the benefits of common analgesics in people with chronic tension-type headache. It found that sustained and frequent use of some analgesics was associated with chronic headache and reduced the effectiveness of prophylactic treatment.

DEFINITION Chronic tension-type headache (CTTH) is a disorder that evolves from episodic tension-type headache, with daily or very frequent episodes of headache lasting minutes to days.[1] The 2004 International Headache Society criteria for CTTH are: headaches on 15 or more days a month (180 days/year) for at least 3 months; pain that is bilateral, pressing, or tightening in quality and non-pulsating, of mild or moderate intensity, which does not worsen with routine physical activity such as walking or climbing stairs; presence of no more than one additional clinical feature (mild nausea, photophobia, or phonophobia) and without moderate/severe nausea or vomiting.[1] CTTH is to be distinguished from causes of chronic daily headache that require different treatment strategies (e.g. new daily persistent headache, medication overuse headache, chronic migraine, and hemicrania continua). In contrast to CTTH, episodic tension-type headache can last for 30 minutes to 7 days and occurs for fewer than 180 days a year. The greatest obstacle to studying tension-type headache is the lack of any single proven specific or reliable, clinical, or biological defining characteristic of the disorder. Terms based on assumed mechanisms (muscle contraction headache, tension headache) are not operationally defined. Old studies that used these terms may have included people with many different types of headache.

INCIDENCE/ PREVALENCE The prevalence of chronic daily headache from a survey of the general population in the USA was 4.1%. Half of sufferers met the International Headache Society criteria for CTTH.[2] In a survey of 2500 undergraduate students in the USA, the prevalence of CTTH was 2%.[3] The prevalence of CTTH was 2.5% in a Danish population based survey of 975 individuals.[4] One community based survey in Singapore (2096 people from the general population) found that the prevalence was 1.8% in females and 0.9% in males.[5]

AETIOLOGY/ RISK FACTORS Tension-type headache is more prevalent in women (65% of cases in one survey).[6] Symptoms begin before the age of 10 years in 15% of people with CTTH. Prevalence declines with age.[7] There is a family history of some form of headache in 40% of people with CTTH,[8] although a twin study found that the risk of CTTH was similar for identical and non-identical twins.[9]

Headache (chronic tension-type)

PROGNOSIS The prevalence of CTTH declines with age.[7]

Please refer to clinicalevidence.com for full text and references.

Multiple sclerosis

Search date January 2006

Richard Nicholas and Jeremy Chataway

What are the effects of interventions aimed at reducing relapse rates and disability?

LIKELY TO BE BENEFICIAL

Glatiramer acetate in people with relapsing and remitting multiple sclerosis

One RCT in people with relapsing and remitting multiple sclerosis found that glatiramer acetate reduced relapse rates over 2 years compared with placebo but found no effect on disability. One RCT in people with progressive multiple sclerosis found no significant difference in progression between glatiramer acetate and placebo at 2 years.

Interferon beta in people having a first demyelinating event or with relapsing and remitting multiple sclerosis

Two RCTs in people experiencing a first demyelinating event found that interferon beta-1a decreased the risk of conversion to clinically definite multiple sclerosis over 2–3 years compared with placebo. One systematic review in people with active relapsing and remitting multiple sclerosis found limited evidence that interferon beta-1a/b reduced exacerbations and disease progression over 2 years compared with placebo. One RCT in people with relapsing and remitting multiple sclerosis found that interferon beta-1b on alternate days reduced the proportion of people with relapse over 2 years compared with weekly interferon beta-1a. Another RCT found that both immunoglobulin and interferon beta-1a reduced relapse rates over 1 year in people with relapsing and remitting multiple sclerosis with no significant difference between groups.

Intravenous immunoglobulin in people having a first demyelinating event

One RCT in people experiencing a first demyelinating event found that intravenous immunoglobulin reduced the risk of a second clinical event and, therefore, of conversion to a definite diagnosis of multiple sclerosis after 1 year.

TRADE OFF BETWEEN BENEFITS AND HARMS

Azathioprine

One systematic review in people with relapsing and remitting or progressive multiple sclerosis comparing azathioprine versus placebo or no treatment found that it reduced relapse rates over 2 years but found no evidence of a difference in disability. However, we were unable to draw reliable conclusions because of clinical heterogeneity among the included RCTs. The review found that about 10% of people were unable to tolerate therapeutic doses of azathioprine. Well documented adverse effects include hepatotoxicity and bone marrow suppression and a large case control study raised concerns about long term cancer risk.

Mitoxantrone in people with relapsing and remitting multiple sclerosis

One systematic review in people with relapsing and remitting and progressive multiple sclerosis found that mitoxantrone reduced the progression of disability at 2 years compared with placebo, with a reduction in annualised relapse rate. However, it is associated with serious adverse effects including cardiotoxicity, amenorrhea, and treatment related leukaemias.

BMJ Clin Evid Concise 2006;16:527–530.

Multiple sclerosis

UNKNOWN EFFECTIVENESS

Interferon beta in people with secondary progressive multiple sclerosis

Four RCTs found variable effects of interferon beta compared with placebo on disease progression in people with secondary progressive multiple sclerosis; two found that it delayed disease progression and the other two found no significant difference between groups. In three of the RCTs, interferon beta reduced relapse rates.

Intravenous immunoglobulin in people with relapsing and remitting or secondary progressive multiple sclerosis

One RCT in people with relapsing and remitting multiple sclerosis found that intravenous immunoglobulin reduced disability over 2 years compared with placebo. However, the clinical importance of this reduction is unclear as the reduction in disability score was modest. Another RCT found that both immunoglobulin and interferon beta-1a reduced relapse rates over 1 year in people with relapsing and remitting multiple sclerosis with no significant difference between groups. One RCT in people with secondary progressive multiple sclerosis found no significant difference in time to progression and relapse rate between intravenous immunoglobulin and placebo.

Methotrexate

One small RCT identified by a systematic review provided insufficient evidence to assess the effects of methotrexate in reducing relapse rates and disability in people with primary or secondary multiple sclerosis.

What are the effects of interventions to improve symptoms during acute relapse?

LIKELY TO BE BENEFICIAL

Corticosteroids (methylprednisolone or corticotrophin)

One systematic review in people with multiple sclerosis requiring treatment for acute exacerbations found that corticosteroids (methylprednisolone or corticotrophin) improved symptoms compared with placebo within the first 5 weeks of treatment. The optimal dose, route, and duration of treatment are unclear.

UNKNOWN EFFECTIVENESS

Plasma exchange

Two RCTs provided insufficient evidence to assess plasma exchange in people with acute relapses of multiple sclerosis.

What are the effects of treatments for fatigue?

UNKNOWN EFFECTIVENESS

Amantadine

Four poor quality RCTs identified by two systematic reviews provided insufficient evidence to assess amantadine in people with multiple sclerosis related fatigue.

Behaviour modification

We found no systematic review or RCTs on the effects of behavioural modification treatment in people with multiple sclerosis related fatigue.

Exercise

One systematic review provided some evidence that exercise programmes can be beneficial for maintaining strength, physical fitness, and mobility related activities of daily living. There was no effect on fatigue. However, the results of the review should be treated with caution as its analysis was limited by the large variety of outcome measures assessed in the trials it identified.

Modafinil *New*

One small RCT found no improvement between modafinil and placebo in fatigue at 5 weeks in people with multiple sclerosis.

What are the effects of treatments for spasticity?

UNKNOWN EFFECTIVENESS

Botulinum toxin

One small RCT provided insufficient evidence about the effects of botulinum toxin on functional outcomes in people with spasticity owing to multiple sclerosis.

Gabapentin

We found no systematic review or RCTs on the effects of gabapentin on spasticity in people with multiple sclerosis.

Intrathecal baclofen

One small crossover RCT provided insufficient evidence to assess functional effects of intrathecal baclofen in people with spasticity owing to multiple sclerosis.

Oral drug treatments

One systematic review provided insufficient evidence about the effects of oral baclofen, dantrolene, tizanidine, or diazepam on functional outcomes in people with spasticity owing to multiple sclerosis. Two RCTs found no significant difference in spasticity between cannabinoids and placebo.

Physiotherapy

Two small RCTs provided insufficient evidence to assess physiotherapy in people with spasticity owing to multiple sclerosis. One of the RCTs found limited evidence that twice weekly hospital or home based physiotherapy for 8 weeks briefly improved mobility compared with no physiotherapy. The other, in people with progressive multiple sclerosis, found no significant difference between early and delayed physiotherapy in mobility or activities of daily living.

What are the effects of multidisciplinary care on disability?

LIKELY TO BE BENEFICIAL

Inpatient rehabilitation (reduces disability in the short term)

Two small RCTs found short term functional benefit but no reduction in neurological impairment. Longer term effects are uncertain.

Multiple sclerosis

UNKNOWN EFFECTIVENESS

Outpatient rehabilitation

Two small RCTs provided insufficient evidence to assess outpatient rehabilitation in people with multiple sclerosis.

DEFINITION Multiple sclerosis is a chronic inflammatory disease of the central nervous system. Diagnosis requires evidence of lesions that are separated in both time and space, and the exclusion of other inflammatory, structural, or hereditary conditions that might give a similar clinical picture. The disease takes three main forms: relapsing and remitting multiple sclerosis, characterised by episodes of neurological dysfunction interspersed with periods of stability; primary progressive multiple sclerosis, in which progressive neurological disability occurs from the outset; and secondary progressive multiple sclerosis, in which progressive neurological disability occurs later in the course of the disease. Axonal loss is the major determinant of the accumulation of irreversible (progressive) disability as a result of inflammation during both the relapsing and remitting and progressive phases of multiple sclerosis[1] but also owing to possible neurodegeneration through loss of trophic support.[2] The emergence of treatment for multiple sclerosis has led to the recognition of a first demyelinating event or "clinically isolated syndrome" (CIS), a single episode of neurological dysfunction lasting for greater than 24 hours that can be a prelude to multiple sclerosis. Characteristic episodes include optic neuritis, solitary brainstem lesions, and transverse myelitis that, when associated with magnetic resonance imaging changes, result in 30–70% risk of developing multiple sclerosis.[3] Increasingly recognised are other demyelinating syndromes thought to be distinct from multiple sclerosis. These include Devic's disease (neuromyelitis optica), relapsing optic neuritis, and relapsing myelitis. Apart from episodes of neurological dysfunction, chronic symptoms produce much of the disability in multiple sclerosis. Symptoms include fatigue (the main symptom in two thirds of people), spasticity, bladder/bowel problems, ataxia/tremor, visual problems, pain, depression/anxiety, dysphagia, and sexual dysfunction.

INCIDENCE/ PREVALENCE Prevalence varies with geography and racial group; it is highest in white populations in temperate regions.[4] In Europe and North America, prevalence is 1/800 people, with an annual incidence of 2–10/100 000, making multiple sclerosis the most common cause of neurological disability in young adults.[5,6] Age of onset is broad, peaking between 20 and 40 years.[7]

AETIOLOGY/ RISK FACTORS The cause remains unclear, although current evidence suggests that multiple sclerosis is an autoimmune disorder of the central nervous system resulting from an environmental stimulus in genetically susceptible individuals. Multiple sclerosis is currently regarded as a single disorder with clinical variants, but there is some evidence that it may consist of several related disorders with distinct immunological, pathological, and genetic features.[4,8]

PROGNOSIS In 90% of people, early disease is relapsing and remitting. Although some people follow a relatively benign course over many years, most develop secondary progressive disease, usually 6–10 years after onset. In 10% of people, initial disease is primary progressive. Apart from a minority of people with "aggressive" multiple sclerosis, life expectancy is not greatly affected and the disease course is often of more than 30 years' duration.

Please refer to clinicalevidence.com for full text and references.

Parkinson's disease

Search date August 2005

Carl E Clarke and A Peter Moore

What are the effects of drug treatments in people with early stage Parkinson's disease?

BENEFICIAL

Immediate release levodopa† (compared with placebo or no treatment)*

One RCT in people with early Parkinson's disease found that levodopa was effective in treating the motor impairments and disability compared with placebo. This is supported by many years of clinical experience, which has led to the consensus that levodopa is effective for early Parkinson's disease, but that long term use causes dyskinesias and motor fluctuations, which are irreversible. Two RCTs in people with early Parkinson's disease found no significant difference between immediate and modified release levodopa in dyskinesia, motor fluctuations, and motor impairment after 5 years. The first RCT found no significant difference between the Unified Parkinson's Disease Rating Score activities of daily living score. The second RCT found that modified release levodopa improved the activities of daily living score and was better tolerated than immediate release levodopa.

*Categorisation based on evidence and consensus opinion.

TRADE OFF BETWEEN BENEFITS AND HARMS

Dopamine agonists (reduced dyskinesia and motor fluctuations compared with levodopa,† but were associated with increased treatment withdrawal and poorer motor scores)

One systematic review and one subsequent RCT (published only as an abstract) found that dopamine agonist monotherapy (bromocriptine or pergolide) reduced the incidence of dyskinesias and motor complications compared with levodopa monotherapy. However, the review and the subsequent RCT found that dopamine agonist monotherapy was associated with greater motor impairment than was levodopa monotherapy, and an increased risk of treatment withdrawal.

Dopamine agonists plus levodopa† (reduced dyskinesia compared with levodopa alone, but increased disability)

One systematic review and additional RCTs provided evidence that dopamine agonists plus levodopa reduced dyskinesia or motor fluctuations compared with levodopa alone. One small additional RCT found no significant difference between lisuride (lysuride) plus levodopa and levodopa alone in motor complications at 5 years. However, some of the RCTs found that levodopa alone improved motor impairments and disability compared with dopamine agonists plus levodopa. One RCT found that pramipexole plus rescue levodopa increased somnolence and hallucinations compared with levodopa alone.

Monoamine oxidase B inhibitors

We found one systematic review in people with early Parkinson's disease, some of whom were taking levodopa or other anti-parkinsonian drugs, and one subsequent RCT in people not taking levodopa or other anti-parkinsonian drugs. The review and the subsequent RCT found that monoamine oxidase B inhibitors (MAOBIs) improved the symptoms of Parkinson's disease, reduced the need for levodopa, and reduced motor fluctuations compared with placebo or no MAOBI treatment. However, the review found an overall increase in adverse events with ▶

MAOBIs compared with placebo or no MAOBI treatment. Although one RCT identified by the systematic review found evidence of increased mortality in people treated with selegiline, pooled analysis of all available trials by the review did not find a significant increase in mortality. We found insufficient evidence to compare MAOBIs versus other drug classes in early Parkinson's disease.

UNLIKELY TO BE BENEFICIAL

Modified release levodopa† (no more effective than immediate release levodopa)

Two RCTs in people with early Parkinson's disease found no significant difference between modified and immediate release levodopa in dyskinesia, motor fluctuations, and motor impairment after 5 years. The first RCT found no significant difference between modified and immediate release levodopa in Unified Parkinson's Disease Rating Score activities of daily living score. The second RCT found that modified release levodopa improved the activities of daily living score and was better tolerated than immediate release levodopa.

What are the effects of adding other treatments in people with motor complications from levodopa?'

TRADE OFF BETWEEN BENEFITS AND HARMS

Adding a catechol-O-methyl transferase (COMT) inhibitor to levodopa

One systematic review found that in people taking levodopa, the catechol-O-methyl transferase inhibitors entacapone and tolcapone reduced "off" time, reduced levodopa dose, and modestly improved motor impairment and disability. Tolcapone was withdrawn from the European market and its use restricted in other countries because of three cases of fatal hepatic toxicity. It has recently been reintroduced for use in those who fail on entacapone, provided that stringent liver function test monitoring is performed.

Adding a dopamine agonist to levodopa†

Systematic reviews found that in people with response fluctuations to levodopa, certain dopamine agonists reduced "off" time, improved motor impairment and activities of daily living, and reduced levodopa dose, but increased dopaminergic adverse effects and dyskinesia.

What are the effects of surgery in people with later Parkinson's disease?

TRADE OFF BETWEEN BENEFITS AND HARMS

Pallidotomy

Two RCTs identified by two systematic reviews found that unilateral pallidotomy improved motor examination and activities of daily living compared with medical treatment. There is a high incidence of adverse effects with pallidotomy. One RCT found insufficient evidence to assess the effects of pallidotomy compared with those of pallidal deep brain stimulation. One RCT found that unilateral pallidotomy was less effective than bilateral subthalamic stimulation in improving parkinsonian symptoms.

UNKNOWN EFFECTIVENESS

Pallidal deep brain stimulation

We found no RCTs comparing pallidal deep brain stimulation versus medical treatment. One RCT found insufficient evidence to assess the effects of pallidal deep brain stimulation compared with those of pallidotomy. Adverse effects are probably less frequent with pallidal deep brain stimulation than with pallidotomy. Three RCTs provided insufficient evidence to assess the effects of pallidal deep brain stimulation compared with those of subthalamic nucleus deep brain stimulation.

Subthalamic nucleus deep brain stimulation

Three systematic reviews found no RCTs of sufficient quality comparing subthalamic nucleus deep brain stimulation versus medical treatment. Three RCTs provided insufficient evidence to assess the effects of subthalamic nucleus deep brain stimulation compared with those of pallidal deep brain stimulation. One RCT found that bilateral subthalamic stimulation was more effective than unilateral pallidotomy in improving parkinsonian symptoms.

Subthalamotomy

One systematic review found no RCTs of subthalamotomy in people with Parkinson's disease.

Thalamic deep brain stimulation

Two systematic reviews identified no RCTs comparing thalamic deep brain stimulation versus medical treatment. One RCT found that thalamic deep brain stimulation improved functional status and caused fewer adverse effects than thalamotomy.

Thalamotomy

Three systematic reviews found no RCTs comparing thalamotomy versus medical treatment. One RCT found that thalamic deep brain stimulation improved functional status and caused fewer adverse effects than thalamotomy. Case series found that, in 14–23% of people, thalamotomy was associated with permanent complications, including speech disturbance, apraxia, or death.

What are the effects of nursing and rehabilitation treatments in people with Parkinson's disease?

LIKELY TO BE BENEFICIAL

Parkinson's disease nurse specialist interventions

Two RCTs provided limited evidence of the benefits of Parkinson's disease nurse specialist interventions.

UNKNOWN EFFECTIVENESS

Occupational therapy

One systematic review provided insufficient evidence to assess the effects of occupational therapy in later Parkinson's disease.

Physiotherapy

Two systematic reviews and two subsequent RCTs found insufficient evidence of the effects of physiotherapy in Parkinson's disease.

Parkinson's disease

Speech and language therapy for speech disturbance

One systematic review provided insufficient evidence to assess the effects of speech and language therapy for speech disturbance in later Parkinson's disease.

Swallowing therapy for dysphagia

One systematic review identified no RCTs of swallowing therapy for dysphagia.

† We have used the term "levodopa" to refer to a combination of levodopa and a peripheral decarboxylase inhibitor.

DEFINITION Idiopathic Parkinson's disease is an age related neurodegenerative disorder, which is associated with a combination of asymmetrical bradykinesia, hypokinesia, and rigidity, sometimes combined with rest tremor and postural changes. Clinical diagnostic criteria have a sensitivity of 80% and a specificity of 30% (likelihood ratio +ve test 1.14, –ve test 0.67) compared with the gold standard of diagnosis at autopsy.[1] The primary pathology is progressive loss of cells that produce the neurotransmitter dopamine from the substantia nigra in the brainstem. Treatment aims to replace or compensate for the lost dopamine. A good response to treatment supports, but does not confirm, the diagnosis. Several other catecholaminergic neurotransmitter systems are also affected in Parkinson's disease. There is no consistent definition of early and late stage Parkinson's disease. In this chapter we consider people with early stage disease to be those who have not yet developed motor complications associated with long term levodopa treatment (such as dyskinesias and motor fluctuations, also known as "on/off" fluctuations). Late stage Parkinson's disease is taken to mean that motor complications of long term levodopa treatment are present.

INCIDENCE/ PREVALENCE Parkinson's disease occurs worldwide, with equal incidence in both sexes. In 5–10% of people who develop Parkinson's disease, the condition appears before the age of 40 years (young onset), and the mean age of onset is about 65 years. Overall age adjusted prevalence is 1% worldwide and 1.6% in Europe, rising from 0.6% at age 60–64 years to 3.5% at age 85–89 years.[2,3]

AETIOLOGY/ RISK FACTORS The cause is unknown. Parkinson's disease may represent different conditions with a final common pathway. People may be affected differently by a combination of genetic and environmental factors (viruses, toxins, 1-methyl-4-phenyl-1,2,3,6-tetrahydropyridine, well water, vitamin E, and smoking).[4-7] First degree relatives of affected people may have twice the risk of developing Parkinson's disease (17% chance of developing the condition in their lifetime) compared with people in the general population.[8-10] However, purely genetic varieties probably affect a small minority of people with Parkinson's disease.[11,12] The parkin gene on chromosome 6 may be associated with Parkinson's disease in families with at least one member with young onset Parkinson's disease, and multiple genetic factors, including the tau gene on chromosome 17q21, may be involved in idiopathic late onset disease.[13,14]

PROGNOSIS Parkinson's disease is currently incurable. Disability is progressive and associated with increased mortality (RR of death compared with matched control populations ranges from 1.6–3.0).[15] Treatment can reduce symptoms and slow progression but it rarely achieves complete control. The question of whether treatment reduces mortality remains controversial.[16] Levodopa seemed to reduce mortality in the UK for 5 years after its introduction, before a "catch up" effect was noted and overall mortality rose toward previous levels. This suggested a limited prolongation of life.[17] An Australian cohort study followed 130 people treated for 10 years.[18] The standardised mortality ratio was 1.58 ($P < 0.001$). At 10 years, 25% had been admitted to a nursing home and only four were still employed. The mean duration of disease until death was 9.1 years. In a similar Italian cohort study conducted over 8 years, the relative risk of death for affected people compared with healthy controls was 2.3 (95% CI 1.60 to 3.39).[19] Age at initial census date was the main predictor of outcome (for people aged < 75 years: RR of death 1.80, 95% CI 1.04 to 3.11; for people aged > 75 years: RR of death 5.61, 95% CI 2.13 to 14.80).

Please refer to clinicalevidence.com for full text and references.

Trigeminal neuralgia

Search date August 2005

Joanna M Zakrzewska and Benjamin C Lopez

What are the effects of treatments in people with trigeminal neuralgia?

LIKELY TO BE BENEFICIAL

Carbamazepine

One systematic review of three crossover RCTs found that carbamazepine increased pain relief compared with placebo, but also increased adverse effects (drowsiness, dizziness, constipation, and ataxia). One retrospective cohort study suggested that in the long term (5–16 years) only about one third of people who initially responded to carbamazepine continue to find it effective. One small RCT found insufficient evidence to compare carbamazepine versus tizanidine.[12]

UNKNOWN EFFECTIVENESS

Baclofen

We found no systematic review or RCTs of baclofen in people with trigeminal neuralgia.

Combined streptomycin and lidocaine nerve block

Small RCTs provided insufficient evidence about the effects of nerve block using streptomycin plus lidocaine compared with nerve block using lidocaine alone in people with trigeminal neuralgia.

Cryotherapy of peripheral nerves

We found no systematic review or RCTs of cryotherapy of the peripheral nerves in people with trigeminal neuralgia.

Lamotrigine

One weak crossover RCT identified by a systematic review provided insufficient evidence about the effects of lamotrigine in people with trigeminal neuralgia.

Nerve block

We found no systematic review or RCTs about the effects of nerve block in people with trigeminal neuralgia.

Other drugs (phenytoin, clonazepam, sodium valproate, gabapentin, mexiletine, oxcarbazepine, topiramate)

We found no systematic review or RCTs of sufficient quality of the antiepileptic drugs phenytoin, clonazepam, sodium valproate, gabapentin, oxcarbazepine, or topiramate and the antiarrhythmic drug mexiletine in people with trigeminal neuralgia.

Peripheral acupuncture

We found no systematic review or RCTs on the effects of peripheral acupuncture in people with trigeminal neuralgia.

Peripheral injection of alcohol

We found no systematic review or RCTs on the effects of injecting peripheral nerves with alcohol in people with trigeminal neuralgia.

◀ **Peripheral injection of phenol**

We found no systematic review or RCTs on the effects of peripheral nerve injection with phenol in people with trigeminal neuralgia.

Peripheral laser treatment

We found no systematic review or RCTs of sufficient quality of peripheral laser treatment in people with trigeminal neuralgia.

Peripheral neurectomy

We found no systematic review or RCTs on the effects of peripheral neurectomy in people with trigeminal neuralgia.

Peripheral radiofrequency thermocoagulation

We found no systematic review or RCTs on the effects of peripheral radiofrequency thermocoagulation in people with trigeminal neuralgia.

Stereotactic radiosurgery

Three systematic reviews identified no RCTs comparing stereotactic radiosurgery versus placebo or versus other treatments. One weak RCT provided insufficient evidence to compare different radiosurgery regimens.

Tizanidine

We found no systematic reviews or RCTs comparing tizanidine versus placebo. One systematic review of one small RCT provided insufficient evidence to compare tizanidine versus carbamazepine.

UNLIKELY TO BE BENEFICIAL

Proparacaine eye drops (single application)

One RCT found no significant difference in pain at 30 days between placebo and a single application of proparacaine hydrochloride eye drops to the eye on the same side as the pain.

DEFINITION Trigeminal neuralgia is a characteristic pain in the distribution of one or more branches of the fifth cranial nerve. The diagnosis is made on the history alone, based on characteristic features of the pain.[1-3] It occurs in paroxysms with each pain, lasting a few seconds to 2 minutes. The frequency of paroxysms is highly variable, ranging from hundreds of attacks a day to long periods of remission that can last years. Between paroxysms, the person is asymptomatic. The pain is severe and described as intense, sharp, superficial, stabbing, shooting, often like an electric shock. In any individual, the pain has the same character in different attacks. It is triggered by light touch in a specific area or by eating, talking, washing the face, or cleaning the teeth. Other causes of facial pain may need to be excluded.[1-3] In trigeminal neuralgia, the neurological examination is usually normal.[1-3]

INCIDENCE/ PREVALENCE Most evidence about the incidence and prevalence of trigeminal neuralgia is from the USA.[4] The annual incidence (age adjusted to the 1980 age distribution of the USA) is 5.9/100 000 women and 3.4/100 000 men. The incidence tends to be slightly higher in women at all ages, and increases with age. In men aged over 80 years, the incidence is 45.2/100 000.[5] Other published surveys are small. One questionnaire survey of neurological disease in a single French village found one person with trigeminal neuralgia among 993 people.[6]

AETIOLOGY/ RISK FACTORS The cause of trigeminal neuralgia remains unclear.[7,8] It is more common in people with multiple sclerosis (RR 20.0, 95% CI 4.1 to 59.0).[5] Hypertension is a risk factor in women (RR 2.1, 95% CI 1.2 to 3.4) but the evidence is less clear ▶

Trigeminal neuralgia

for men (RR 1.53, 95% CI 0.30 to 4.50).[5] One case control study in the USA found that people with trigeminal neuralgia smoked less, consumed less alcohol, had fewer tonsillectomies, and were less likely than matched controls to be Jewish or an immigrant.[9]

PROGNOSIS One retrospective cohort study found no reduction in 10 year survival in people with trigeminal neuralgia.[10] We found no evidence about the natural history of trigeminal neuralgia. The illness is characterised by recurrences and remissions. Many people have periods of remission with no pain for months or years.[8] Anecdotal reports suggest that in many people it becomes more severe and less responsive to treatment with time.[11] Most people with trigeminal neuralgia are initially managed medically, and a proportion eventually have a surgical procedure.[8] We found no good evidence about the proportion of people who require surgical treatment for pain control. Anecdotal evidence indicates that pain relief is better after surgery than with medical treatment.[8,11]

Please refer to clinicalevidence.com for full text and references.

Aphthous ulcers (recurrent)

Search date April 2004

Stephen Porter and Crispian Scully CBE

What are the effects of treatments for recurrent aphthous ulcers?

LIKELY TO BE BENEFICIAL

Chlorhexidine

RCTs found that chlorhexidine gluconate mouth rinses reduced the severity of each episode of ulceration, but did not affect the incidence of ulceration. Limited evidence from one RCT suggested that 0.2% chlorhexidine gel may reduce the incidence and duration of ulceration compared with a control preparation. RCTs found that chlorhexidine reduced the mean severity of pain compared with an inert preparation.

UNKNOWN EFFECTIVENESS

Topical corticosteroids

Small RCTs found that topical corticosteroids reduced the number of ulcer days compared with control preparations. RCTs found no consistent effect of topical corticosteroids on the incidence of new ulcers compared with control preparations. They found weak evidence that topical corticosteroids may reduce the duration and pain of ulcers and hasten pain relief without causing notable local or systemic adverse effects.

UNLIKELY TO BE BENEFICIAL

Hexitidine

Limited evidence from RCTs found no significant difference in any of the reported outcomes between hexitidine mouthwash or a proprietary antibacterial mouthwash and control mouthwashes.

DEFINITION Recurrent aphthous ulcers are superficial and rounded, painful mouth ulcers usually occurring in recurrent bouts at intervals of a few days to a few months.[1]

INCIDENCE/ PREVALENCE The point prevalence of recurrent aphthous ulcers in Swedish adults has been reported as 2%.[1] Prevalence may be 5–10% in some groups of children. Up to 66% of young adults give a history consistent with recurrent aphthous ulceration.

AETIOLOGY/ RISK FACTORS The causes of aphthous ulcers remain unknown. Associations with deficiency of iron, folic acid and vitamins, infections, gluten sensitive enteropathy, food sensitivities and psychological stress have rarely been confirmed. Similar ulcers are seen in Behçet's syndrome. Local physical trauma may initiate ulcers in susceptible people. Recurrent aphthous ulcers are uncommon on keratinised oral mucosal surfaces, and the frequency of recurrent aphthous ulcers may fall if people cease any tobacco smoking habit.[1]

PROGNOSIS About 80% of people with recurrent aphthous ulcers develop a few ulcers smaller than 1 cm in diameter that heal within 5–14 days without scarring (the pattern known as minor aphthous ulceration). The episodes recur typically after an interval of 1–4 months. One in 10 people with recurrent ulceration may have multiple minute ulcers (herpetiform ulceration). Likewise, one in 10 sufferers has a more severe form (major aphthous ulceration), with lesions larger than ▶

BMJ Clin Evid Concise 2006;16:539–540.

Aphthous ulcers (recurrent)

1 cm that may recur after a shorter interval and can cause scarring. Most of the trials in this review have focused upon the treatment of minor aphthous ulceration.[1]

Please refer to clinicalevidence.com for full text and references.

Burning mouth syndrome

Search date February 2006

John Buchanan and Joanna Zakrzewska

What are the effects of treatments?

LIKELY TO BE BENEFICIAL

Cognitive behavioural therapy

One small RCT identified by a systematic review found that cognitive behavioural therapy reduced symptom intensity in people with resistant burning mouth syndrome after 6 months compared with placebo treatment. However, the study had important flaws in its methods.

TRADE OFF BETWEEN BENEFITS AND HARMS

Anticonvulsants (topical clonazepam) *New*

One small RCT found that topical clonazepam reduced pain in people with burning mouth syndrome compared with placebo over 2 weeks. However, the RCT found evidence of low level systemic absorption of clonazepam (a benzodiazepine); systemic absorption could lead to benzodiazepine dependence if used in the long term.

UNKNOWN EFFECTIVENESS

Antidepressants

One RCT found no significant difference in pain or related symptoms between trazodone and placebo at 8 weeks. One small RCT found a similar reduction in pain score between sertraline, paroxetine, and amisulpride at 8 weeks. However, it was too small to detect a clinically important difference among treatments.

Benzydamine hydrochloride

One small RCT identified by a systematic review provided insufficient evidence on the effects of benzydamine hydrochloride in people with burning mouth syndrome.

Dietary supplements

Three small RCTs with weak methods provided insufficient evidence to draw reliable conclusions about the effects of alphalipoic acid in people with burning mouth syndrome. We found limited evidence from one small weak RCT that oryzanol plus vitamin E was less effective than tibolone in improving symptoms at 6 months.

Hormone replacement therapy in postmenopausal women

We found limited evidence from one small RCT with weak methods that tibolone improved symptoms compared with oryzanol plus vitamin E at 6 months.

DEFINITION Burning mouth syndrome is an idiopathic burning discomfort or pain affecting people with clinically normal oral mucosa in whom a medical or dental cause has been excluded.[1-3] Terms previously used to describe what is now called burning mouth syndrome include glossodynia, glossopyrosis, stomatodynia, stomatopyrosis, sore tongue, and oral dysaesthesia.[4] A survey of 669 men and 758 women randomly selected from 48 500 people aged 20–69 years found that people with burning mouth also have subjective dryness (66%), take some form of medication (64%), report other systemic illnesses (57%), and have altered taste (11%).[5] Many studies of people with symptoms of ▶

Burning mouth syndrome

burning mouth do not distinguish those with burning mouth syndrome (i.e. idiopathic disease) from those with other conditions (such as vitamin B deficiency), making results unreliable. Local and systemic factors (such as infections, allergies, ill fitting dentures,[6] hypersensitivity reactions,[7] and hormone and vitamin deficiencies[8-10]) may cause the symptom of burning mouth and should be excluded before diagnosing burning mouth syndrome. This chapter deals only with idiopathic burning mouth syndrome.

INCIDENCE/ PREVALENCE Burning mouth syndrome mainly affects women,[11-13] particularly after the menopause, when its prevalence may be 18–33%.[14] One study in Sweden found a prevalence of 4% for the symptom of burning mouth without clinical abnormality of the oral mucosa (11/669 [2%] men, mean age 59 years; 42/758 [6%] women, mean age 57 years), with the highest prevalence (12%) in women aged 60–69 years.[5] Reported prevalence in general populations varies from 1%[14] to 15%.[11] Incidence and prevalence vary according to diagnostic criteria,[4] and many studies included people with the symptom of burning mouth rather than with burning mouth syndrome as defined above.

AETIOLOGY/ RISK FACTORS The cause is unknown, and we found no good aetiological studies. Possible causal factors include hormonal disturbances associated with the menopause,[12-14] psychogenic factors (including anxiety, depression, stress, life events, personality disorders, and phobia of cancer),[6,15,16] and neuropathy in so-called supertasters.[17] Support for a neuropathic aetiology comes from studies that have shown altered sensory and pain thresholds in people with burning mouth syndrome.[18] Two studies using blink reflex and thermal quantitative sensory tests have demonstrated signs of neuropathy in most people with burning mouth syndrome.[19,20]

PROGNOSIS We found no prospective cohort studies describing the natural history of burning mouth syndrome.[21] We found anecdotal reports of at least partial spontaneous remission in about 50% of people with burning mouth syndrome within 6–7 years.[15] However, a recent retrospective study assessing 53 people with burning mouth syndrome (48 women and 5 men, mean duration of burning mouth syndrome 5.5 years, mean follow up 56 months) found a complete spontaneous resolution of oral symptoms in 11% of people (2/19) who received no treatment. Overall, 30% of people (15/53) experienced a moderate improvement, with or without treatment.[22]

Please refer to clinicalevidence.com for full text and references.

Candidiasis (oropharyngeal)

Search date June 2005

Caroline L Pankhurst

What are the effects of interventions to prevent and treat oropharyngeal candidiasis in adults having treatment causing immunosuppression?

BENEFICIAL

Antifungal prophylaxis with absorbed or partially absorbed antifungal drugs in adults having anticancer drugs (more effective than placebo or non-absorbed drugs)

One systematic review and one RCT found that absorbed antifungal drugs (ketoconazole, itraconazole, fluconazole) prevented oropharyngeal candidiasis compared with placebo or no drug treatment, or compared with non-absorbed antifungal drugs (nystatin alone, nystatin plus chlorhexidine, amphotericin B alone, or amphotericin B combined with nystatin, norfloxacin, natamycin, thymostimulin, or chlorhexidine). The review also found that partially absorbed antifungal drugs (miconazole, clotrimazole) prevented oropharyngeal candidiasis compared with placebo or no drug treatment. The review found no significant difference in the rates of oropharyngeal candidiasis between non-absorbed antifungal drugs and placebo. However, there was heterogeneity among studies for the non-absorbed drugs. The review found no significant difference in adverse effects between antifungal drugs of any type and placebo or between absorbed and non-absorbed antifungals.

UNKNOWN EFFECTIVENESS

Antifungal prophylaxis in adults having tissue transplants

Two small RCTs in people with liver transplant found no significant difference in the risk of oropharyngeal candidiasis between nystatin and fluconazole or clotrimazole. However, the trials may have lacked power to detect clinically important differences. We found insufficient evidence from two RCTs about the effects of prophylactic chlorhexidine mouth rinse with or without nystatin compared with placebo in people having bone marrow transplant. One RCT provided insufficient evidence to compare adding different topical suspensions to systemic fluconazole in people having bone marrow transplants.

Antifungal treatment in adults having chemotherapy, radiotherapy, or both treatments for cancer

One systematic review and one subsequent RCT provided insufficient evidence about the clinical effects of antifungals compared with placebo for treating oropharyngeal candidiasis in people having chemotherapy or radiotherapy, or about the effects of different antifungal agents or doses in people with oropharyngeal candidiasis having radiotherapy or chemotherapy. ▶

Candidiasis (oropharyngeal)

What are the effects of interventions to prevent and treat oropharyngeal candidiasis in infants and children?

BENEFICIAL

Antifungal treatment with miconazole or fluconazole in immunocompetent and immunocompromised infants and children (more effective than nystatin)

RCTs found that miconazole and fluconazole increased clinical cure of oropharyngeal candidiasis compared with nystatin in immunocompetent and immunocompromised infants and children.

LIKELY TO BE BENEFICIAL

Antifungal prophylaxis with fluconazole in immunocompromised infants and children (more effective than oral nystatin or amphotericin B)

One large RCT in immunocompromised infants and children found that fluconazole reduced the incidence of oropharyngeal candidiasis compared with oral nystatin, amphotericin B, or both.

What are the effects of interventions to prevent and treat oropharyngeal candidiasis in people with diabetes?

UNKNOWN EFFECTIVENESS

Antifungal prophylaxis or treatment in people with diabetes mellitus

We found no systematic review or RCTs assessing preventive interventions or treatments for oropharyngeal candidiasis in people with diabetes.

What are the effects of interventions to prevent and treat oropharyngeal candidiasis in people with dentures?

UNKNOWN EFFECTIVENESS

Antifungal treatment for denture stomatitis

We found no systematic review or RCTs of antifungal treatment for preventing oropharyngeal candidiasis in people with dentures. We found insufficient evidence from small RCTs to compare effects of antifungal agents versus placebo or versus each other for treating oropharyngeal candidiasis in people who wear dentures.

Denture hygiene

We found no RCTs evaluating the effect of denture hygiene or removing dentures at night on preventing denture stomatitis, although observational evidence suggests that poor oral hygiene and wearing dentures at night may increase the risk of developing denture stomatitis. We found insufficient evidence from three RCTs, two of which were underpowered, to assess clinical effects on oropharyngeal candidiasis of mouth rinses, disinfectants, denture soaks, denture scrubbing, and microwave irradiation of dentures. Microwave treatment is not suitable for all dentures.

What are the effects of interventions to prevent and treat oropharyngeal candidiasis in people with HIV infection?

BENEFICIAL

Antifungal prophylaxis with fluconazole, itraconazole, or nystatin in people with advanced HIV disease

RCTs in people with HIV infection found that daily or weekly antifungal prophylaxis with fluconazole, itraconazole, or nystatin reduced incidence and relapse of oropharyngeal candidiasis compared with placebo. One large RCT found that fluconazole reduced recurrence of oropharyngeal candidiasis compared with clotrimazole.

Topical antifungals (absorbed, partially absorbed, and non-absorbed antifungals in people with HIV infection)

RCTs found that topical preparations of miconazole nitrate, clotrimazole, and oral suspensions of itraconazole, used in a swish and swallow mode effectively treated oropharyngeal candidiasis in people with HIV infection. One RCT found that fluconazole suspension reduced symptoms and signs of oropharyngeal candidiasis compared with nystatin suspension.

Which treatments reduce the risk of acquiring resistance to antifungal drugs?

UNKNOWN EFFECTIVENESS

Continuous prophylaxis versus intermittent treatment in people with HIV infection and acute episodes of oropharyngeal candidiasis (in preventing antifungal resistance)

One RCT in people with HIV infection and acute episodes of oropharyngeal candidiasis found no significant difference between continuous antifungal prophylaxis with fluconazole and intermittent antifungal treatment with fluconazole in terms of the emergence of antifungal resistance.

DEFINITION Oropharyngeal candidiasis is an opportunistic mucosal infection caused, in most cases, by *Candida albicans*. The four main types of oropharyngeal candidiasis are: (1) pseudomembranous (thrush), consisting of white discrete plaques on an erythematous background, on the buccal mucosa, throat, tongue, or gingivae; (2) erythematous, consisting of smooth red patches on the hard or soft palate, dorsum of tongue, or buccal mucosa; (3) hyperplastic, consisting of white, firmly adherent patches or plaques, usually bilaterally distributed on the buccal mucosa; and (4) denture induced stomatitis, presenting as either a smooth or granular erythema confined to the denture bearing area of the hard palate and often associated with an angular cheilitis.[1] Symptoms vary, ranging from none to a sore and painful mouth with a burning tongue and altered taste. Oropharyngeal candidiasis can impair speech, nutritional intake, and quality of life.

INCIDENCE/ PREVALENCE *Candida* species are commensals in the gastrointestinal tract. Transmission occurs directly between infected people or on fomites (objects that can harbour pathogenic organisms). *Candida* is found in the mouth of 31–60% of healthy people in developed countries.[2] Denture stomatitis associated with *Candida* is prevalent in 65% of denture wearers.[2] Oropharyngeal candidiasis affects 15–60% of people with haematological or oncological malignancies during periods of immunosuppression.[3] Oropharyngeal candidiasis occurs in 7–48% of people with HIV infection and in over 90% of those with advanced

Candidiasis (oropharyngeal)

disease. In severely immunosuppressed people, relapse rates are high (30–50%) and relapse usually occurs within 14 days of stopping treatment.[4]

AETIOLOGY/ RISK FACTORS Risk factors associated with symptomatic oropharyngeal candidiasis include local or systemic immunosuppression; haematological disorders; broad spectrum antibiotic use; inhaled or systemic steroids; xerostomia; diabetes; and wearing dentures, obturators, or orthodontic appliances.[1,5] The same strain may persist for months or years in the absence of infection. In people with HIV infection, there is no direct correlation between the number of organisms and the presence of clinical disease. Symptomatic oropharyngeal candidiasis associated with *in vitro* resistance to fluconazole occurs in 5% of people with advanced HIV disease.[6] Resistance to azole antifungals is associated with severe immunosuppression (≤ 50 CD4 cells/mm^3), more episodes treated with antifungal drugs, and longer median duration of systemic azole treatment.[7]

PROGNOSIS In most people, untreated candidiasis persists for months or years unless associated risk factors are treated or eliminated. In neonates, spontaneous cure of oropharyngeal candidiasis usually occurs after 3–8 weeks.

Please refer to clinicalevidence.com for full text and references.

Halitosis

Search date December 2005

Crispian Scully CBE and Stephen Porter

What are the effects of treatments in people with physiological halitosis?

LIKELY TO BE BENEFICIAL

Regular use mouthwash

Three RCTs found that regular use of a mouthwash (one mouthwash containing chlorhexidine plus cetylpyridinium chloride plus zinc lactate, another mouthwash containing cetylpyridinium chloride, and a third containing zinc chloride plus sodium chloride) reduced breath odour at 2–4 weeks compared with placebo.

Single use mouthwash (short term benefit only)

Three small RCTs found limited evidence that single use mouthwash reduced odour unpleasantness and odour intensity between 1 and 8 hours after use compared with distilled water or placebo. One of these RCTs found no significant difference between single use mouthwash and distilled water in odour unpleasantness or odour intensity after 24 hours.

UNKNOWN EFFECTIVENESS

Artificial saliva

We found no systematic review or RCTs on the effects of artificial saliva in people with halitosis.

Diet modification (drinking plenty of liquids; chewing herbs; eating fresh, fibrous vegetables such as carrots; avoiding coffee)

We found no systematic review or RCTs of diet change (drinking plenty of liquids; chewing herbs; eating fresh, fibrous vegetables such as carrots; avoiding coffee) in people with halitosis.

Sugar free chewing gums

We found no systematic review or RCTs on the effects of sugar free chewing gum in people with halitosis.

Tongue cleaning, brushing, or scraping

We found no systematic review or RCTs on the effects of tongue cleaning, brushing, or scraping in people with halitosis.

Zinc toothpastes

We found no systematic review or RCTs on the effects of zinc toothpaste in people with halitosis.

DEFINITION Halitosis is an unpleasant odour emitted from the mouth. It may be caused by oral conditions, including poor oral hygiene, oral and periodontal disease,[1,2] or conditions such as chronic sinusitis, tonsillitis and bronchiectasis. In this topic, we deal only with physiological halitosis (i.e. confirmed persistent bad breath in the absence of systemic, oral or periodontal disease). We have excluded halitosis due to underlying systemic disease, which would require disease specific treatment, pseudo-halitosis (in people who believe they have bad breath but whose breath is not considered malodourous by others), and artificially induced halitosis (e.g. in studies requiring people to stop brushing ▶

their teeth). This topic is only applicable, therefore, to people in whom such underlying causes have been ruled out, and in whom pseudo-halitosis has been excluded. There is no consensus regarding duration of bad breath for diagnosis of halitosis, although the standard organoleptic test for bad breath involves smelling the breath on at least two or three different days.[1]

INCIDENCE/ PREVALENCE We found no reliable estimate of prevalence, although several studies report the population prevalence of halitosis (physiological or because of underlying disease) to be about 50%.[1,3-5] One cross-sectional study of 491 people found that about 5% of people with halitosis have pseudo-halitosis and about 40% of people with halitosis have physiological bad breath not due to underlying disease.[6] We found no reliable data about age or sex distribution of physiological halitosis.

AETIOLOGY/ RISK FACTORS We found no reliable data about risk factors for physiological bad breath. Mass spectrometric and gas chromatographic analysis of expelled air from the mouth of people with any type of halitosis have shown that the main malodourants are volatile sulphur compounds, including hydrogen sulphide, methyl mercaptan, and dimethyl suphide.[7,8]

PROGNOSIS We found no evidence on the prognosis of halitosis.

Please refer to clinicalevidence.com for full text and references.

Impacted wisdom teeth

Search date August 2005

Marco Esposito

Should asymptomatic and disease-free impacted wisdom teeth be removed prophylactically?

LIKELY TO BE INEFFECTIVE OR HARMFUL

Prophylactic extraction

Two RCTs identified by a systematic review found no evidence that prophylactic extraction of asymptomatic impacted wisdom teeth improved outcomes compared with no extraction. Based on non-RCT evidence, one treatment guideline suggested that extraction is not advisable in people with deeply impacted wisdom teeth who have no history of pertinent local or systemic pathology. Removal of lower wisdom teeth causes permanent numbness of the lower lip or tongue in about 1% of people.

DEFINITION Wisdom teeth are third molars that develop in the majority of adults and generally erupt between the ages of 18 and 24 years, although there is wide variation in the age of eruption. In some people, the teeth become partially or completely impacted below the gum line because of lack of space, obstruction, or abnormal position. Impacted wisdom teeth may be diagnosed because of pain and swelling or incidentally by routine dental radiography.

INCIDENCE/ PREVALENCE Third molar impaction is common. Over 72% of Swedish people aged 20–30 years have at least one impacted lower third molar.[1] The surgical removal of impacted third molars (symptomatic and asymptomatic) is the most common procedure performed by oral and maxillofacial surgeons. It is performed on about 4/1000 people each year in England and Wales, making it one of the top 10 inpatient and day case procedures.[2-4] Up to 90% of people on oral and maxillofacial surgery hospital waiting lists are awaiting removal of wisdom teeth.[3]

AETIOLOGY/ RISK FACTORS Retention and impaction of wisdom teeth may be more common than it was previously because the modern diet tends to be softer than in the past.[5]

PROGNOSIS Impacted wisdom teeth can cause pain, swelling, and infection, and may destroy adjacent teeth and bone. The removal of diseased and symptomatic wisdom teeth alleviates pain and suffering and improves oral health and function. We found no good evidence on untreated prognosis in people with asymptomatic impacted wisdom teeth.

Please refer to clinicalevidence.com for full text and references.

Postoperative pulmonary infections

Search date May 2006

Michelle Conde and Valerie Lawrence

What are the effects of interventions to prevent postoperative pulmonary infections?

BENEFICIAL

Prophylactic lung expansion techniques

One systematic review of strategies to reduce postoperative pulmonary complications after non-cardiothoracic surgery concluded that various prophylactic lung expansion techniques reduced pulmonary risk in people undergoing abdominal surgery compared with no prophylactic treatment. It found no evidence that any single technique was superior to any other in preventing clinically significant postoperative pulmonary complications following abdominal surgery. An additional RCT in people undergoing open abdominal surgery found no significant difference in pulmonary complications between a standardised physiotherapist directed program of early mobilisation and a standardised physiotherapist directed program of early mobilisation plus deep breathing exercises and secretion clearing techniques. Two RCTs identified by a systematic review in people undergoing cardiac surgery found insufficient evidence on the effects of prophylactic lung expansion techniques.

LIKELY TO BE BENEFICIAL

Regional (epidural or spinal) anaesthesia

One systematic review found that spinal or epidural anaesthesia (alone or in combination with general anaesthesia) reduced postoperative pneumonia compared with general anaesthesia alone. One smaller systematic review in people undergoing hip fracture surgery found no significant difference in postoperative pneumonia rates between people having neuraxial blockade and people having general anaesthesia alone.

UNKNOWN EFFECTIVENESS

Advice to stop smoking preoperatively

Two RCTs identified by a systematic review found insufficient evidence on the effects of smoking cessation advice in reducing postoperative pulmonary infections. Three observational studies found that people who smoked were more likely to develop postoperative pulmonary complications of all kinds than those who did not. One study suggested that people who had stopped smoking 6 months prior to surgery reverted to the risk of those who had never smoked.

DEFINITION A working diagnosis of postoperative pulmonary infection may be based on three or more new findings from: cough, phlegm, shortness of breath, chest pain, temperature above 38 °C, and pulse rate above 100 a minute.[1] In this chapter, we are dealing strictly with pneumonia that is regarded to be a complication of the operation. We examine a selection of pre-, intra-, and postoperative techniques to reduce the risk of this complication. In this chapter, the diagnosis of pneumonia implies consolidation observed in a chest radiograph.[2]

INCIDENCE/ PREVALENCE Reported morbidity for chest complications depends on how carefully they are investigated and the type of surgery performed. One observational study found blood gas and chest radiograph abnormalities in about 50% of people after open cholecystectomy.[3] However, fewer than 20% of these had abnormal clinical signs and only 10% had a clinically significant chest infection. One observational study found the incidence of pneumonia to be 17.5% after thoracic and abdominal surgeries.[4] Another observational study found the incidence of pneumonia to be 2.8% (using a more restrictive definition of pneumonia) after laparotomy.[5]

AETIOLOGY/ RISK FACTORS Risk factors include increasing age (> 50 years), with the odds of developing postoperative pneumonia systematically increasing with each decile above the age of 50 years; functional dependency; a history of chronic obstructive pulmonary disease; weight loss > 10% in last 6 months; impaired sensorium (acute confusion / delirium associated with current illness); cigarette smoking; recent alcohol use; and blood urea nitrogen level > 7.5 mmol/L.[6,7] Serum albumin level < 35 g/l is also a risk factor for the development of overall postoperative pulmonary complications.[7] The strongest risk factor, however, is the type of surgery (particularly aortic aneurysm repair, thoracic surgery, abdominal surgery, neurosurgery, head and neck surgery, and vascular surgery).[6,7] Interestingly, obesity was not found to be an independent risk factor in a recent systematic review of preoperative pulmonary risk stratification for non-cardiothoracic surgery.[7]

PROGNOSIS In one large systematic review (search date 1997, 141 RCTs, 9559 people), 10% of people with postoperative pneumonia died.[8] If systemic sepsis ensues, mortality is likely to be substantial.[9] Pneumonia delays recovery from surgery and poor tissue oxygenation may contribute to delayed wound healing. In a cohort of 160 805 United States veterans undergoing major non-cardiac surgery, 1.5% of people developed postoperative pneumonia, and the 30 day mortality rate was 10-fold higher in these people compared with those without postoperative pneumonia.[6]

Please refer to clinicalevidence.com for full text and references.

Poisoning

Carbon monoxide poisoning (acute)

Search date August 2004

Nicholas Phin

What are the effects of oxygen treatments for acute carbon monoxide poisoning?

BENEFICIAL

Oxygen 100% via non-re-breather mask (compared with air)*

We found no systematic review, RCTs, or analytical observational studies comparing oxygen 100% by non-re-breather mask versus air for clinically relevant outcomes of interest. Such an RCT in people with suspected acute carbon monoxide poisoning would be considered unethical. One retrospective chart review in people with various levels of severity of acute carbon monoxide poisoning receiving oxygen 100% either by non-re-breather mask or by ventilation if intubated in a tertiary teaching hospital setting found that oxygen 100% reduced carboxyhaemoglobin half life. We found no systematic review or RCTs for other clinical outcomes of interest in people with acute carbon monoxide poisoning. Based on physiological studies, the benefits of oxygen 100% by non-re-breather mask in the emergency situation are universally accepted but there is still considerable debate about the optimum duration of treatment in secondary or tertiary care settings.

LIKELY TO BE BENEFICIAL

Hyperbaric oxygen 100% at 2–3 ATA (compared with normobaric oxygen 100% in moderate to severe poisoning)

One RCT in people with moderate to severe acute carbon monoxide poisoning found limited evidence that, compared with normobaric oxygen 100%, hyperbaric oxygen 100% delivered within 24 hours of presentation at pressures of 2–3 atmospheres reduced cognitive sequelae at 6 weeks. However, it is unclear which the types of people will benefit, the optimum treatment regime, and how long after exposure the treatment has an effect. The size of the effect derived from hyperbaric oxygen treatment may be highly sensitive to the pressure at which the oxygen is delivered, the number of treatment sessions, and the oxygen content of control treatments.

Oxygen 28% (compared with air)*

We found no systematic review, RCTs, or analytical observational studies comparing 28% normobaric oxygen versus air in people with carbon monoxide poisoning for clinically relevant outcomes of interest. It may be considered unethical to conduct analytical studies. Oxygen 28% will affect carboxyhaemoglobin levels but may not be as effective as higher concentrations of oxygen for reducing carboxyhaemoglobin half life. UK paramedics routinely use oxygen 28% so that individuals who may be dependent on their hypoxic drive are not adversely affected.

UNKNOWN EFFECTIVENESS

Hyperbaric oxygen 100% (compared with oxygen 100% in mild poisoning)

We found no systematic review or RCTs only in people with mild carbon monoxide poisoning. Two RCTs in people with mild to moderate acute carbon monoxide poisoning found insufficient evidence to draw conclusions about the ▶

effects of hyperbaric oxygen versus oxygen 100% via non-re-breather mask for prevention of delayed neurological complications. We found no systematic review or RCTs for other clinical outcomes of interest.

*Categorisation is based on consensus and physiological studies.

DEFINITION Carbon monoxide is an odourless, colourless gas and poisoning causes hypoxia, cell damage, and death.[1,2] **Diagnosis of carbon monoxide poisoning:** Exposure to carbon monoxide is measured either directly from blood samples and expressed as a percentage of carboxyhaemoglobin or indirectly using the carbon monoxide in expired breath. Percentage carboxyhaemoglobin is the most frequently used biomarker of carbon monoxide exposure. Although the diagnosis of carbon monoxide poisoning can be confirmed by detecting elevated levels of blood carboxyhaemoglobin levels, the presence of clinical signs and symptoms after known exposure to carbon monoxide should not be ignored. The signs and symptoms of carbon monoxide poisoning are mainly associated with the brain and heart which are most sensitive to hypoxia. The symptoms of carbon monoxide poisoning are non-specific and varied and include headache, fatigue,[3] malaise, "trouble thinking", confusion, nausea, dizziness, visual disturbances, chest pain, shortness of breath, loss of consciousness, and seizures.[4-6] In people suffering from coexisting morbidities, symptoms such as shortness of breath or chest pain may be more evident. The classical signs of carbon monoxide poisoning, described as cherry-red lips, peripheral cyanosis, and retinal haemorrhages, are in reality rarely seen.[7] **Interpretation of carboxyhaemoglobin levels:** Non-smokers living away from urban areas have carboxyhaemoglobin levels of between 0.4% and 1.0% reflecting endogenous carbon monoxide production whereas levels of up to 5% may be considered normal in a busy urban or industrial setting.[8] Smokers are exposed to increased levels of carbon monoxide in cigarettes and otherwise healthy heavy smokers can tolerate levels of carboxyhaemoglobin of up 15%.[9] The use of percentage carboxyhaemoglobin as a measure of severity of carbon monoxide poisoning or to predict treatment options is limited because carboxyhaemoglobin levels are affected by the removal from the source of carbon monoxide and any oxygen treatment given before measurement of percentage carboxyhaemoglobin. In addition, people with co-morbidities that make them more sensitive to the hypoxia associated with carbon monoxide can present with symptoms of poisoning at carboxyhaemoglobin levels that are either low or within the normal range.[10] Attempts have been made in the literature to equate symptoms and signs to different carboxyhaemoglobin levels[11] but it is accepted that carboxyhaemoglobin levels in an acutely poisoned person only roughly correlate with the clinical signs and symptoms, especially those relating to neurological function.[12] Earlier studies attempted to differentiate between smokers and non- smokers. Attempts have also been made in the literature to divide carbon monoxide poisoning into mild, moderate, and severe based on percentage carboxyhaemoglobin levels and clinical symptoms,[13] but there is no clear clinical consensus or agreement on this issue. The degree of poisoning has been described in the literature as *mild carbon monoxide poisoning:* a carboxyhaemoglobin level of greater than 10% without clinical signs or symptoms of carbon monoxide poisoning; *moderate carbon monoxide poisoning:* a carboxyhaemoglobin level of greater than 10% and less than 20–25% with minor clinical signs and symptoms of poisoning such as headache, lethargy or fatigue; and *severe carbon monoxide poisoning:* a carboxyhaemoglobin level of greater than 20–25%, loss of consciousness and confusion or signs of cardiac ischaemia, or both. **Population:** For the purpose of this review, we have included adults presenting to health care professionals with suspected carbon monoxide poisoning. Although there is as yet no clear consensus on this issue, most studies examining carbon monoxide poisoning and its

Carbon monoxide poisoning (acute)

management use a carboxyhaemoglobin level of 10% or more or the presence of clinical signs and symptoms after known exposure to carbon monoxide to be indicative of acute carbon monoxide poisoning. Unless otherwise stated this is the definition of acute carbon monoxide poisoning that has been used throughout this chapter. Where appropriate, the terms mild, moderate, or severe have been used to reflect the descriptions of populations in individual studies.

INCIDENCE/ PREVALENCE Carbon monoxide poisoning is considered to be one of the leading causes of death and injury worldwide and a major public health problem.[14] In 2000, there were 521 deaths where carbon monoxide was the recorded cause of death (ICD 9 – E986) in England and Wales[15] compared with 1363 deaths recorded in 1985;[16] a trend that has also been observed in the US.[17] Of the 521 deaths attributed to carbon monoxide poisoning, 148 were accidental and the remaining 373 the result of suicide or self inflicted injury. Poisoning by carbon monoxide is almost certainly underdiagnosed because of the varied ways in which it can present and it has been estimated in the US that there are over 40 000 emergency department visits a year; many presenting with a flu-like illness.[18] In 2003, there were 534 recorded medical episodes in English hospitals involving people suffering from the toxic effects of carbon monoxide.[19] This may be a substantial underestimate if the US experience reflects the true morbidity associated with carbon monoxide poisoning. Studies in the US have shown that the incidence of accidental carbon monoxide poisoning peaks during the winter months,[20,21] and is associated with increased use of indoor heating and petrol powered generators and reduced external ventilation. This seasonal rise in numbers coincides with the annual increase in influenza notifications and given the similarity in symptoms many cases of mild carbon monoxide poisoning are probably misdiagnosed.

AETIOLOGY/ RISK FACTORS **People at high risk:** People who are most at risk from carbon monoxide poisoning include those with coronary heart disease, vascular disease, or anaemia; pregnant women and their fetus; infants; and the elderly. In people with coronary heart disease, experimentally induced blood carboxyhaemoglobin levels of 4.5% shorten the period of exercise before the onset of anginal pain and the duration of pain is prolonged.[22-24] In people with anaemia the oxygen carrying capacity of the blood is already compromised and therefore they will be more sensitive to carbon monoxide.[25] The elderly are at risk because of existing co-morbidities such as heart disease or respiratory disease and because of a reduced compensatory response to hypoxic situations. During pregnancy, a woman's oxygen carrying capacity is reduced because of an increased endogenous carbon monoxide production and additional endogenous carbon monoxide from the developing fetus leading to an increased carboxyhaemoglobin concentration.[26] A higher ventilation rate during pregnancy will lead to increased uptake of carbon monoxide at any given carbon monoxide concentration.[27] The fetus is also at risk and there have been occasional fetal deaths in non-fatal maternal exposures.[26,28,29] In the developing fetus, oxygen is released at a lower oxygen partial pressure and fetal haemoglobin binds with carbon monoxide more quickly compared with adults. Carbon monoxide may be a teratogen where there is a significant increase in maternal carboxyhaemoglobin or where there is moderate to severe maternal toxicity.[30] Infants may be more susceptible to the effect of carbon monoxide because of their greater oxygen consumption in relation to adults and their response and symptoms are more variable. There are recorded instances of children travelling in the same car and having varying symptoms with similar carboxyhaemoglobin levels or widely varying carboxyhaemoglobin levels with similar carbon monoxide exposure.[31] **Sources of carbon monoxide:** Carbon monoxide is produced by the incomplete combustion of carbon containing fuel, such as gas (domestic or bottled), charcoal, coke, oil, and wood. Gas stoves, fires, and boilers; gas powered water heaters; car exhaust fumes; charcoal barbeques; paraffin heaters; solid fuel powered stoves; boilers; and room heaters that are faulty or inadequately ventilated are all potential sources. A sometimes overlooked source of carbon monoxide is methylene chloride in some paint strippers and sprays. Methylene chloride is readily absorbed through the skin and lungs and once in the liver, is converted to carbon monoxide. Methylene chloride is stored in body tissues and released gradually; the carbon monoxide elimination half life in people exposed to methylene chloride is more than twice that of inhaled carbon monoxide. Natural background levels of carbon monoxide in the outdoor environment range from 0.01–0.23 mg/m^3 (0.009–.0.2 ppm)[32] but in urban traffic in the UK the 8 hour mean concentrations are higher at about 20 mg/m^3 (17.5 ppm);[33] exposure to this level for prolonged periods could result in a carboxyhaemoglobin level of about 3%.

PROGNOSIS The data regarding prognosis in carbon monoxide poisoning are inconclusive and contradictory. However, there is general agreement that outcome and prognosis are related to the level of carbon monoxide that a person is exposed to, the duration of exposure, and the presence of underlying risk factors.[33] A poor outcome is predicted by lengthy carbon monoxide exposure, loss of consciousness, and advancing age. In addition, hypotension and cardiac arrest independently predict permanent disability and death. After acute carbon monoxide poisoning the organs most sensitive to hypoxia will be most affected; i.e. the brain and the heart. Pre-existing co-morbidities that affect these organs will to an extent influence the clinical presentation and the prognosis; an individual with pre-existing heart disease may present with myocardial ischaemia that could lead to infarction and death. The prognosis for people resuscitated after experiencing cardiac arrest with carbon monoxide poisoning is poor. In a small retrospective study,[34] 18 people with carboxyhaemoglobin levels of 31.7 ± 11.0% given hyperbaric oxygen after resuscitation after cardiac arrest all died. The effects on the brain are more subtle given that different sections of the brain are more sensitive to hypoxic insults either as a consequence of reduced oxygen delivery or by direct effects on intracellular metabolism.[35] Therefore, in addition to the acute neurological sequelae leading to loss of consciousness, coma and death, neurological sequelae such as poor concentration and memory problems may be apparent in people recovering from carbon monoxide poisoning (persistent neurological sequelae) or develop after a period of apparent normality (delayed neurological sequelae). Delayed neurological sequelae develop between 2 days to 240 days after exposure and are reported to affect 10–32% of people recovering from carbon monoxide poisoning.[36,37] Symptoms include cognitive changes, personality changes, incontinence, psychosis, and Parkinsonism.[38] Fortunately 50–75% of people recover within 1 year.[39]

Please refer to clinicalevidence.com for full text and references.

Organophosphorus poisoning (acute)

Search date August 2005

Michael Eddleston, Surjit Singh, and Nick Buckley

What are the effects of treatments for acute organophosphorus poisoning?

LIKELY TO BE BENEFICIAL

Atropine*

Atropine is considered the mainstay of treatment, and many case series found that it reversed the early muscarinic effects of acute organophosphorus poisoning. We found no RCTs comparing atropine versus placebo but it would now be considered unethical to perform such an RCT. One small RCT found no significant difference in mortality or ventilation rate between atropine and glycopyrronium bromide, but it may have lacked power to detect clinically important differences.

Benzodiazepines to control organophosphorus induced seizures*

Diazepam is considered standard treatment for organophosphorus induced seizures. We found no RCTs comparing diazepam or other benzodiazepines versus placebo or another anticonvulsant. It would now be considered unethical to perform an RCT comparing benzodiazepines versus placebo in people with seizures.

Glycopyrronium bromide (glycopyrrolate)*

We found no RCTs comparing glycopyrronium bromide (glycopyrrolate) versus placebo, but it is unlikely that such a trial would be considered ethical unless glycopyrronium bromide and placebo were given in addition to atropine. One small RCT found no significant difference in mortality or ventilation rate between glycopyrronium bromide and atropine, but it may have lacked power to detect clinically important differences. Glycopyrronium bromide has been used instead of atropine because it is thought to have fewer adverse effects on the central nervous system.

Washing the poisoned person and removing contaminated clothes*

We found no RCTs or observational studies of sufficient quality that evaluated washing the poisoned person and removing contaminated clothes. However, this seems to be an obvious way to reduce further dermal and mucocutaneous exposure and is widely recommended. An RCT would therefore be considered unethical. Healthcare workers should ensure that washing does not distract them from other treatment priorities and they should also protect themselves through the use of gloves, aprons, and eye protection, with careful disposal of contaminated equipment and clothes.

*Based on consensus, RCTs would be considered unethical.

UNKNOWN EFFECTIVENESS

Activated charcoal (single or multiple dose)

We found no systematic review, RCTs, or observational studies of sufficient quality evaluating activated charcoal, in either single or multiple dose regimens, in people with acute organophosphorus poisoning.

Alpha$_2$ adrenergic receptor agonists (clonidine)

We found no RCTs or observational studies of sufficient quality evaluating clonidine in people with acute organophosphorus poisoning.

Fresh frozen plasma

We found one systematic review of fresh frozen plasma that found no RCTs in people with acute organophosphorus poisoning.

Gastric lavage

We found no RCTs or observational studies of sufficient quality evaluating gastric lavage in people with acute organophosphorus poisoning. Adverse effects are common when gastric lavage is performed in physically restrained, non-consenting people without careful control of the airway. If the person cannot be sedated and intubated, the risk of harm owing to aspiration is likely to outweigh its potential benefits.

Magnesium sulphate

We found no systematic review, RCTs, or observational studies of sufficient quality evaluating magnesium sulphate in people with acute organophosphorus poisoning.

Milk or other home remedy immediately after ingestion

We found no RCTs or observational studies of sufficient quality that assessed giving a "home remedy" soon after the ingestion.

N-methyl-D-aspartate receptor antagonists

We found no RCTs or observational studies of sufficient quality evaluating N-methyl-D-aspartate receptor antagonists in people with acute organophosphorus poisoning.

Organophosphorus hydrolases

We found no systematic review, RCTs, or observational studies of sufficient quality evaluating organophosphorus hydrolases in people with acute organophosphorus poisoning.

Oximes

One systematic review of two small RCTs with methodological weaknesses provided insufficient evidence to assess oximes in people with acute organophosphorus poisoning.

Sodium bicarbonate

One systematic review found insufficient evidence to assess sodium bicarbonate in people with acute organophosphorus poisoning.

LIKELY TO BE INEFFECTIVE OR HARMFUL

Cathartics

We found no systematic review, RCTs, or observational studies of sufficient quality evaluating cathartics in people with acute organophosphorus poisoning. Organophosphorus poisoning itself causes diarrhoea, which can lead to electrolyte imbalance. This may be exacerbated by cathartics, suggesting that the risk of harm may outweigh its potential benefits.

Ipecacuanha (ipecac)

We found no systematic review, RCTs, or observational studies of sufficient quality evaluating ipecacuanha (ipecac) in people with acute organophosphorus poisoning. Clinical consensus suggests that the risk of harm, although not quantified, probably outweighs any potential benefits.

Organophosphorus poisoning (acute)

DEFINITION Acute organophosphorus poisoning occurs after dermal, respiratory, or oral exposure to either low volatility pesticides (e.g. chlorpyrifos, dimethoate) or high volatility nerve gases (e.g. sarin, tabun). Inhibition of acetylcholinesterase at synapses results in accumulation of acetylcholine and over-activation of acetylcholine receptors at the neuromuscular junction and in the autonomic and central nervous systems.[1] Early clinical features reflect involvement of the parasympathetic system: bronchorrhoea, miosis, salivation, lachrymation, defecation, urination, and hypotension. Features indicating involvement of the neuromuscular junction (muscle weakness and fasciculations) and central nervous system (seizures [with nerve gases], coma, and respiratory failure) are also common at this stage. An intermediate syndrome has been described (cranial nerve palsies and proximal muscle weakness with preserved distal muscle power after resolution of early cholinergic symptoms), but its definition, pathophysiology, and incidence are still unclear. A late motor or motor/sensory peripheral neuropathy may also develop after recovery from acute poisoning with some organophosphorus compounds.[1] Acute poisoning may result in long term neurological and psychiatric effects but the evidence is also still unclear.[2,3] There are differences between pesticides in the clinical syndrome they produce and in the frequency and timing of respiratory failure and death.[4,5]

INCIDENCE/ PREVALENCE Most cases occur in the developing world as a result of occupational or deliberate exposure to organophosphorus pesticides.[6] Although data are sparse, organophosphorous pesticides appear to be the most important cause of death from deliberate self poisoning worldwide.[7] For example, in Sri Lanka, about 10 000–20 000 admissions to hospital for organophosphorus poisoning occur each year. Of these, at least 10% die. In most cases, the poisoning is intentional.[8] Case mortality rates across the developing world are commonly greater than 20%.[7] In Central America, occupational poisoning is reported to be more common than intentional poisoning, and deaths are fewer.[9] Extrapolating from limited data, the World Health Organization has estimated that each year more than 200 000 people worldwide die from pesticide poisoning,[10] but these figures are old and widely contested.[6] Most deaths occur in Asia, and organophosphorus pesticides probably cause at least 50% of cases.[7] Deaths from organophosphorus nerve gases occurred during the Iran-Iraq war.[11] Military or terrorist action with these chemical weapons remains possible. Twelve people died in a terrorist attack in Tokyo and probably thousands died in Iran after military use.

AETIOLOGY/ RISK FACTORS The widespread accessibility of pesticides in rural parts of the developing world makes them easy options for acts of self harm.[7] Occupational exposure is usually because of insufficient or inappropriate protective equipment.[6]

PROGNOSIS There are no validated scoring systems for categorising severity or predicting outcome, although many have been proposed. The highly variable natural history and difficulty in determining ingested dose make predicting outcome for an individual inaccurate and potentially hazardous, because people admitted in good condition can deteriorate rapidly and require intubation and mechanical ventilation. Prognosis in acute self poisoning is likely to depend on dose and toxicity of the ingested organophosphorus (e.g. neurotoxicity potential, half life, rate of aging, whether activation to the toxic compound is required [pro-poison], and whether dimethylated or diethylated [see comment under oximes]).[5,12] Prognosis in occupational exposure is better because the dose is normally smaller and the route is dermal.

Please refer to clinicalevidence.com for full text and references.

Paracetamol (acetaminophen) poisoning

Search date March 2006

Nick Buckley and Michael Eddleston

What are the effects of treatments for acute paracetamol poisoning?

BENEFICIAL

_N_-acetylcysteine

One small RCT identified by a systematic review found that *N*-acetylcysteine reduced mortality in people with established paracetamol induced liver failure, compared with placebo after 21 days. One cohort study found that people given early treatment with *N*-acetylcysteine were less likely to develop liver damage than untreated historical controls. We found no RCTs comparing different regimens of *N*-acetylcysteine with each other, or comparing *N*-acetylcysteine with methionine. There are clear animal data, observational evidence, and clinical experience that the introduction of *N*-acetylcysteine has dramatically changed the natural history of paracetamol poisoning favourably.

LIKELY TO BE BENEFICIAL

Methionine

One small RCT identified by a systematic review found no significant difference in mortality between methionine and supportive care, although it lacked power to detect a clinically important difference. It found limited evidence that methionine reduced hepatotoxicity compared with supportive care. We found no RCTs comparing methionine versus *N*-acetylcysteine.

UNKNOWN EFFECTIVENESS

Activated charcoal (single or multiple dose)

One systematic review found no RCTs that examined the clinical effects of activated charcoal, whether in single or multiple dose regimens, in people poisoned by paracetamol. One large case series found that clinically significant complications of multiple dose activated charcoal were rare.

Gastric lavage

One systematic review found no RCTs examining the clinical effects of gastric lavage in people with paracetamol poisoning.

Ipecacuanha

One systematic review found no RCTs examining the clinical effects of ipecacuanha in people with paracetamol poisoning.

Liver transplant *New*

One systematic review found no RCTs examining the role of liver transplant in people with fulminant hepatic failure after paracetamol poisoning.

DEFINITION Paracetamol poisoning occurs as a result of either accidental or intentional overdose with paracetamol (acetaminophen).

INCIDENCE/ PREVALENCE Paracetamol is the most common drug used for self poisoning in the UK.[1] It is also a common means of self poisoning in the rest of Europe, North America, and Australasia. In 1968, there were only 10 deaths and 150 hospital admissions in England and Wales for paracetamol poisoning.[2] An exponential rise resulted in an estimated 41 200 cases of poisoning with ▶

Paracetamol (acetaminophen) poisoning

products containing paracetamol in 1989–1990 in England and Wales, with a mortality of 0.40% (95% CI 0.38% to 0.46%). Overdoses from paracetamol alone result in an estimated 150–200 deaths and 15–20 liver transplants each year in England and Wales (data from routinely collected health and coronial statistics).[3,4] More recent studies suggest that paracetamol poisoning is slightly less common now in the UK, with 25 000 admissions from paracetamol poisoning recorded in 2001.[4] There is limited evidence that, in the UK, there have been modest reductions in large overdoses, liver transplants, and deaths since packaging restrictions were instituted in 1998.[3]

AETIOLOGY/ RISK FACTORS Most cases in the UK are impulsive acts of self harm in young people.[1,5] In one cohort study of 80 people who had overdosed with paracetamol, 42 had obtained the tablets for the specific purpose of taking an overdose and 33 had obtained them less than 1 hour before the act.[5]

PROGNOSIS People with blood paracetamol concentrations above the standard treatment line (defined in the UK as a line joining 200 mg/L at 4 hours and 30 mg/L at 15 hours on a semilogarithmic plot) have a poor prognosis without treatment (see figure 1 Ⓕ).[6-9] In one cohort study of 57 untreated people with blood concentrations above this line, 33/57 [58%] developed severe liver damage and 3/57 [5%] died.[7] People with a history of chronic alcohol misuse, use of enzyme inducing drugs, eating disorders, or multiple paracetamol overdoses may be at risk of liver damage with blood concentrations below this line.[9] In the USA, a lower line is used as an indication for treatment, but we found no data relating this line to prognostic outcomes.[10] More recently, a modified nomogram specifically designed to estimate prognosis (not need for treatment) has been developed by modelling data from a large cohort.[11] This takes into account time to initiation of *N*-acetylcysteine treatment and the effect of alcohol use. However, it has not yet been validated, and is not widely used. **Dose effect:** The dose ingested also indicates the risk of hepatotoxicity. A case series showed people ingesting less than 125 mg/kg had no significant hepatotoxicity, with a sharp dose dependent rise for higher doses.[12] The threshold for toxicity after acute ingestion may be higher in children, where a single dose of less than 200 mg/kg has not been reported to lead to death and rarely causes hepatotoxicity.[13] The higher threshold for toxicity in children may relate to different metabolic pathways or their larger relative liver size.[14] For people who present later than 24 hours or an unknown time after ingestion, several other prognostic indicators have been proposed, including prothrombin time and abnormal liver function tests.[15,16] These have not been validated prospectively.

Please refer to clinicalevidence.com for full text and references.

Ectopic pregnancy

Search date June 2006

Rajesh Varma and Janesh Gupta

What treatments improve outcomes in women with unruptured tubal ectopic pregnancy?

BENEFICIAL

Salpingectomy (in women not desiring future fertility) *New*

One cohort study found that initial treatment failure was lower with salpingectomy than with salpingotomy or methotrexate. One non-systematic review and cohort studies found limited evidence that subsequent intrauterine pregnancy rates were lower with salpingectomy than salpingotomy in women with contralateral tubal disease; however they did not find this for women without contralateral tubal disease.

LIKELY TO BE BENEFICIAL

Prophylactic methotrexate (systemic) following salpingotomy *New*

One RCT found that methotrexate after salpingotomy reduced persistent trophoblast compared with no methotrexate.

Systemic methotrexate (single or multiple dose) *New*

One systematic review found that treatment failure was higher with single dose methotrexate compared with multiple doses. One systematic review found no significant difference between methotrexate and salpingotomy in primary treatment success, but found that methotrexate was less effective in other outcomes.

UNKNOWN EFFECTIVENESS

Expectant management of unruptured ectopic pregnancies *New*

One cohort study found that subsequent intrauterine pregnancy rates were similar between expectant management and surgery. Cohort studies without a control group found that ectopic pregnancies can spontaneously resolve. Expectant management is confined to a selected subgroup of unruptured ectopic pregnancies.

Salpingotomy (compared with laparoscopic salpingectomy) *New*

One systematic review found that primary treatment success was lower with salpingotomy by laparoscopy than with laparotomy, but found no significant difference for future fertility or repeat ectopic pregnancy. One cohort study found that initial treatment failure with salpingotomy than with salpingectomy but lower than with methotrexate. One non-systematic review and cohort studies found limited evidence that subsequent intrauterine rates were higher with salpingotomy than with salpingectomy in women with contralateral tubal disease; however they did not find this for women without contralateral tubal disease. One systematic review found no significant difference between salpingotomy and methotrexate in primary treatment success, but found that salpingotomy was more effective in other outcomes. One cohort study found that subsequent intrauterine pregnancy rates were similar between expectant management and surgery.

BMJ Clin Evid Concise 2006;16:561–563.

Ectopic pregnancy

UNLIKELY TO BE BENEFICIAL

Systemic methotrexate plus mifepristone (versus systemic methotrexate alone) *New*

RCTs found no significant difference in treatment success between methotrexate plus mifepristone and methotrexate alone; however, one of the RCTs found that treatment success was increased by adding mifepristone to methotrexate in women with higher progesterone levels.

DEFINITION Ectopic pregnancy is defined as a conceptus implanting outside the uterine endometrium. The most common implantation site is within the fallopian tube (95.5%), followed by ovarian (3.2%) and abdominal (1.3%) sites. The sites of tubal implantation in descending order of frequency are ampulla (73.3%), isthmus (12.5%), fimbrial (11.6%), and interstitial (2.6%).[1] **Population:** In this systematic review, we will consider haemodynamically stable women with unruptured tubal ectopic pregnancy, diagnosed by non-invasive or invasive techniques.

INCIDENCE/ PREVALENCE Around 10 000 ectopic pregnancies are diagnosed annually in the UK. The incidence of ectopic pregnancy in the UK (11.0/1000 pregnancies) is similar to that in other countries, such as Norway (14.9/1000) and Australia (16.2/1000).[2-4] Since 1994, the overall rate of ectopic pregnancy and mortality rate (0.4/1000 ectopic pregnancies) have been static in the UK.[4] Until recently, most epidemiological studies have failed to distinguish between ectopic pregnancies occurring in women who did not use contraception (reproductive failure) and women who used contraception (contraceptive failure).[5,6] A French population study undertaken from 1992–2002 found that, over the duration of the study, the rate of reproductive failure ectopic pregnancies increased by 17%, whereas the rate of contraceptive failure ectopic pregnancies decreased by 29%.[6] Increasing rates of chlamydia infection, smoking, and assisted reproductive technology usage may have contributed to the disproportionate increase in reproductive failure ectopic pregnancy rate over contraceptive failure ectopic pregnancy rate. Widespread use of dedicated early pregnancy assessment units and non-invasive diagnostic algorithms are likely to have contributed to increasing rates of ectopic pregnancy diagnosis.[7,8]

AETIOLOGY/ RISK FACTORS The aetiology of ectopic pregnancy is unclear. Ectopic pregnancy arising from reproductive failure or contraceptive failure should be considered as separate entities with differing aetiology, risk factors, and reproductive outcomes.[5,6,9] The main risk factors for reproductive failure are a history of pelvic inflammatory disease, previous ectopic pregnancy, pelvic and tubal surgery, infertility, smoking, and assisted conception.[5,10] The main risk factor for contraceptive failure ectopic pregnancy is intrauterine contraceptive device (IUD) failure. IUDs do not increase the absolute risk of ectopic pregnancy, but a pregnancy occurring with IUD is more likely to be ectopic than intrauterine. Other risk factors for ectopic pregnancy include prior spontaneous abortion, prior induced abortion, endometriosis, uterotubal anomalies, and prior in utero exposure to diethylstilbestrol. However, fewer than half of the ectopic pregnancies diagnosed are associated with risk factors.[11]

PROGNOSIS **Ectopic pregnancies:** As the pregnancy advances, tubal pregnancies may either diminish in size and spontaneously resolve, or increase in size and eventually lead to tubal rupture with consequent maternal morbidity and mortality. There are no reliable clinical, sonographic, or biological markers (e.g. serum beta human chorionic gonadotrophin or serum progesterone) that can predict rupture of tubal ectopic pregnancy.[12,13] Maternal mortality following ectopic pregnancy is an uncommon short term outcome in developed countries. The recent UK Confidential Enquiry into Maternal Deaths cited ectopic pregnancy as a cause of 11 maternal deaths (0.4/1000 ectopic pregnancies).[4] Short term maternal morbidity relates to pain, transfusion requirement, and operative complications. Primary treatment success and long term fertility outcomes depend on the clinical characteristics of the ectopic pregnancy (e.g. whether the ectopic pregnancy occurred in a woman using contraception or not, tubal rupture or not, contralateral tubal disease) and the type of surgical or medical treatment chosen. A 10 year follow up of ectopic pregnancies showed that the rate of repeat ectopic pregnancy was much higher in women with an IUD in place at the time of the index ectopic pregnancy compared with women whose ectopic pregnancy was not associated with IUD use. By contrast, the rate of intrauterine pregnancy was 1.7-fold higher (fecundity rate ratio [FRR] 1.7, 95% CI 1.3 to 2.3) in women who had an IUD in place at the time of the index ectopic pregnancy compared with women whose index ectopic pregnancy was not associated with IUD use.[9] Short and long term consequences on health related quality of life and psychological issues (e.g. bereavement) are also important, but are rarely quantified. **Pregnancies of unknown location:** Pregnancy of unknown location is the absence of pregnancy localisation (either intrauterine or extrauterine) by transvaginal sonography when serum beta human chorionic gonadotrophin levels are below the discriminatory zone (1000–1500 IU/L). An observational study of pregnancies of unknown location has shown that 55% spontaneously resolve, 34% are subsequently diagnosed as viable, and 11% are subsequently diagnosed as ectopic pregnancies.[14]

Please refer to clinicalevidence.com for full text and references.

Nausea and vomiting in early pregnancy

Search date September 2005

Mario Festin

What are the effects of treatment for nausea and vomiting in early pregnancy?

BENEFICIAL

Ginger

Two RCTs identified by a systematic review found that ginger reduced nausea and vomiting in early pregnancy compared with placebo. One RCT identified by the review found that ginger reduced nausea and dry retching compared with placebo, but found that ginger had no effect on episodes of vomiting. Two RCTs identified by the review found that both ginger and pyridoxine were effective in reducing nausea and vomiting from baseline, with no significant difference between treatments.

LIKELY TO BE BENEFICIAL

Acupressure

One systematic review found limited evidence that P6 acupressure may reduce self reported morning sickness compared with sham acupressure or no treatment. Three additional RCTs found that P6 acupressure reduced the duration, but not necessarily the intensity, of nausea and vomiting. In one RCT, 63% of women having P6 acupressure and 90% of women having sham acupressure experienced problems with using the wristband.

Antihistamines (H_1 antagonists)

Two systematic reviews found limited evidence that antihistamines (buclizine, dimenhydrinate, doxylamine, hydroxyzine, meclozine) reduced nausea and vomiting compared with placebo, with no evidence of teratogenicity. One RCT found similar rates of emesis episodes and self reported response with a phenothiazine (prochlorperazine) and an antihistamine (promethazine), but did not provide a statistical comparison.

Pyridoxine (vitamin B_6)

Two systematic reviews of pyridoxine found limited evidence that pyridoxine reduced nausea compared with placebo but found no evidence of an effect on vomiting. One review found no evidence of teratogenicity. Two RCTs identified by a systematic review found that both pyridoxine and ginger were effective in reducing nausea and vomiting from baseline, with no significant difference between treatments.

UNKNOWN EFFECTIVENESS

Acupuncture

One systematic review identified two RCTs. The first RCT found that acupuncture reduced nausea and retching compared with no acupuncture, with no evidence of adverse effects. However, an improvement was also found with sham acupuncture compared with no treatment. The second smaller RCT found no significant difference in nausea between acupuncture and sham acupuncture.

Dietary interventions (other than ginger)

We found no RCTs of dietary interventions (other than ginger) in women with nausea and vomiting in early pregnancy.

Phenothiazines

One systematic review found no significant difference between phenothiazine and placebo in nausea. The review found no evidence of teratogenicity. One RCT found similar rates of emesis episodes and self reported response with a phenothiazine (prochlorperazine) and an antihistamine (promethazine), but did not provide a statistical comparison.

What are the effects of treatments for hyperemesis gravidarum?

UNKNOWN EFFECTIVENESS

Acupuncture

One small crossover RCT found a faster reduction in nausea after active PC6 acupuncture compared with sham acupuncture in women with hyperemesis gravidarum. Episodes of vomiting were also reduced.

Corticosteroids

One small RCT identified by two systematic reviews and one subsequent RCT found no significant improvement in persistent vomiting or readmission to hospital after 1 week of treatment with prednisolone compared with placebo in women with hyperemesis gravidarum. Another small RCT identified by the review found no significant difference in persistence of vomiting between prednisolone and the antihistamine promethazine. However, it found that prednisolone reduced admission to hospital. Another subsequent RCT found that prednisolone was not as fast as promethazine in reducing symptoms of hyperemesis gravidarum, but that, during prolonged treatment, prednisolone had at least the same effects on the symptoms and caused fewer adverse effects.

Corticotrophins

One small RCT found no significant difference in nausea and vomiting between intramuscular corticotrophin and placebo in women with hyperemesis gravidarum.

Diazepam

One small RCT provided insufficient evidence to assess diazepam compared with placebo in women with hyperemesis gravidarum.

Dietary interventions (other than ginger)

One small crossover RCT provided insufficient evidence to assess dietary supplementation with carob seed flour compared with placebo in women with hyperemesis gravidarum.

Ginger

One small crossover RCT identified by two systematic reviews provided insufficient evidence on the effects of ginger in women with hyperemesis gravidarum.

Ondansetron

We found no systematic review or RCTs that compared ondansetron versus placebo. One small RCT provided insufficient evidence to compare the effects of ondansetron versus antihistamines in women with hyperemesis gravidarum.

Nausea and vomiting in early pregnancy

DEFINITION **Nausea and vomiting** are common problems in early pregnancy. Although often called "morning sickness", nausea and vomiting can occur at any time of the day and may persist through the day.[1] Symptoms usually begin between 4 weeks and 7 weeks' gestation (1 study found this to be the case in 70% of affected women)[2] and disappear by 16 weeks in about 90% of women.[1-3] One study found that fewer than 10% of affected women suffer nausea, vomiting, or both before the first missed period.[3] Most women do not require treatment. However, if nausea and vomiting are severe and persistent, the condition can progress to hyperemesis, especially if the woman is unable to maintain adequate hydration, fluid and electrolyte balance, and nutrition. **Hyperemesis gravidarum** is a diagnosis of exclusion, characterised by prolonged and severe nausea and vomiting, dehydration, and weight loss.[1] Laboratory investigation may show ketosis, hyponatraemia, hypokalaemia, hypouricaemia, metabolic hypochloraemic alkalosis, and ketonuria.

INCIDENCE/ PREVALENCE Nausea affects about 70% and vomiting about 60% of pregnant women.[1] The true incidence of hyperemesis gravidarum is not known. It has been documented to range from 3 in 1000 to 20 in 1000 pregnancies. However, most authors report an incidence of 1 in 200.[2]

AETIOLOGY/ RISK FACTORS The causes of nausea and vomiting in pregnancy are unknown. One theory, that they are caused by the rise in human chorionic gonadotrophin concentration, is compatible with the natural history of the condition, its severity in pregnancies affected by hydatidiform mole, and its good prognosis (see prognosis below).[4] The aetiology of hyperemesis gravidarum is also uncertain. Again, endocrine and psychological factors are suspected, but evidence is inconclusive.[4] One prospective study found that *Helicobacter pylori* infection was more common in women with hyperemesis gravidarum (95/105 [90.5%] had positive serum *Helicobacter pylori* IgG concentrations) than in pregnant women without hyperemesis gravidarum (60/129 [46.5%] had positive serum *Helicobacter pylori* IgG concentrations).[5] However, it was not clear whether this link was causal.

PROGNOSIS One systematic review (search date 1988) found that nausea and vomiting were associated with a reduced risk of miscarriage (6 studies, 14 564 women; OR 0.36, 95% CI 0.32 to 0.42) but found no association with perinatal mortality.[6] Nausea and vomiting and hyperemesis usually improve over the course of pregnancy, but in one cross-sectional observational study 13% of women reported that nausea and vomiting persisted beyond 20 weeks' gestation.[7]

Please refer to clinicalevidence.com for full text and references.

Perineal care

Search date April 2006

Chris Kettle

What are the effects of intrapartum surgical interventions on rates of perineal trauma?

BENEFICIAL

Restrictive use of episiotomy (reduced risk of posterior trauma compared with routine use)

One systematic review found that restricting episiotomy to specific fetal and maternal indications reduced the rates of posterior perineal trauma, need for suturing, and healing complications compared with routine use, but increased the rates of anterior perineal trauma, which carry minimal morbidity. The review found no significant difference in overall rates of severe vaginal or perineal trauma, dyspareunia, or urinary incontinence. One subsequent RCT found that restricting episiotomy to specific fetal indications increased the proportion of women with intact perineum compared with a liberal (routine) episiotomy policy, but it found no significant difference in rates of anterior perineal trauma or third degree tears.

TRADE OFF BETWEEN BENEFITS AND HARMS

Vacuum extraction (less perineal trauma than with forceps but newborns have increased risk of cephalhaematoma)

One systematic review and subsequent RCTs found that vacuum extraction reduced the rate of severe perineal trauma compared with forceps delivery but increased the incidence of neonatal cephalhaematoma and retinal haemorrhage. One subsequent RCT found that symptoms of altered faecal continence were more common following forceps delivery at 3 months after birth.

UNLIKELY TO BE BENEFICIAL

Midline episiotomy incision (associated with higher risk of third or fourth degree tears compared with mediolateral incision)

We found no evidence that midline episiotomy incision improved perineal pain or wound dehiscence compared with mediolateral incision. Limited evidence from one quasi-randomised trial suggested that midline incision may increase the risk of third and fourth degree tears compared with mediolateral incision.

LIKELY TO BE INEFFECTIVE OR HARMFUL

Epidural analgesia (increased instrumental delivery, which is associated with increased rates of perineal trauma)

One systematic review found that epidural analgesia increased the risk of instrumental delivery compared with non-epidural analgesia or no analgesia in labour; instrumental delivery is in turn associated with an increased risk of perineal trauma.

Perineal care

What are the effects of intrapartum non-surgical interventions on rates of perineal trauma?

BENEFICIAL

Continuous support during labour (reduced instrumental delivery, which is associated with increased perineal trauma)

One systematic review found that providing continuous support for women during childbirth reduced the rate of assisted vaginal birth (vacuum extraction or forceps) compared with usual care. It found no significant difference in the overall rates of episiotomy or perineal trauma (defined as episiotomy or laceration requiring suturing).

TRADE OFF BETWEEN BENEFITS AND HARMS

Upright position during delivery (fewer episiotomies but more second degree tears than supine or lithotomy positions)

One systematic review found limited evidence that any upright position for delivery marginally reduced episiotomies compared with supine or lithotomy positions, but this was offset by an increase in second degree tears. Rates of assisted vaginal delivery were slightly reduced in the upright group.

"Hands poised" method of delivery (fewer episiotomies, but increased pain and need for manual delivery of placenta compared with "hands on" method)

One multicentre RCT and one quasi-randomised trial found that the "hands poised" method (not touching the baby's head or supporting the mother's perineum) reduced episiotomy rates compared with the conventional "hands on" method (applying pressure to the baby's head during delivery and supporting the mother's perineum). Both trials found no evidence of an effect on the risk of perineal trauma requiring suturing, and the RCT found that the "hands poised" group had an increased risk of requiring manual removal of the placenta and higher rates of short term perineal pain.

UNKNOWN EFFECTIVENESS

Passive descent in the second stage of labour (no difference in perineal trauma compared with active pushing)

One RCT comparing passive fetal descent versus immediate active pushing found no significant difference in perineal trauma.

Sustained breath holding (Valsalva) method of pushing (no difference in perineal trauma compared with spontaneous pushing)

One systematic review of two poor quality controlled clinical trials found no significant difference in the extent or rate of perineal trauma between sustained breath holding (Valsalva) and spontaneous exhalatory methods of pushing during the second stage of labour.

What are the effects of different methods and materials for primary repair of first and second degree tears and episiotomies?

BENEFICIAL

Absorbable synthetic sutures for perineal repair of first and second degree tears and episiotomies (reduced short term analgesic use compared with catgut sutures)

One large systematic review found that absorbable synthetic sutures reduced analgesic use at up to 10 days after birth compared with catgut sutures. Two subsequent RCTs found no significant difference in perineal pain at 3 days or analgesia use after 24–48 hours and 10–14 days; however, they may have lacked power to detect clinically important effects. The systematic review and one subsequent RCT found no significant difference between absorbable synthetic sutures and catgut sutures in pain or dyspareunia at 3 months. However, one RCT with 12 months' follow up, which was included in the review, found lower rates of dyspareunia with absorbable synthetic sutures. Two RCTs found no significant difference between rapidly absorbed and standard absorbable synthetic sutures in overall perineal pain, pain on sitting, or dyspareunia. These RCTs also found reduced perineal pain on walking and a reduction in suture material removal with rapidly absorbed synthetic sutures.

Continuous sutures for first and second degree tears and episiotomies (reduced short term pain compared with interrupted sutures)

One systematic review found that continuous subcuticular sutures for perineal skin reduced short term pain and need for suture removal compared with interrupted sutures, but found no significant difference in perineal pain or dyspareunia at 3 months postpartum. One RCT found that a loose continuous technique for repair of all layers reduced perineal pain at 10 days and reduced the need for suture removal up to 3 months postpartum compared with interrupted sutures.

LIKELY TO BE BENEFICIAL

Non-suturing of perineal skin alone in first and second degree tears and episiotomies (reduced dyspareunia compared with conventional suturing)

One large RCT found no significant difference between leaving the perineal skin alone unsutured (vagina and perineal muscle were sutured) compared with conventional suturing in pain at 10 days after birth. A second RCT found that non-suturing of the perineal skin reduced pain for up to 3 months after delivery. Both RCTs found that non-suturing of the perineal skin reduced dyspareunia at 3 months after birth.

LIKELY TO BE INEFFECTIVE OR HARMFUL

Non-suturing of muscle and skin in first and second degree perineal tears (poorer wound healing than with suturing)

Two small RCTs found no significant difference in short term perineal pain between non-suturing and suturing of muscle and skin in first and second degree tears. One of the RCTs, which had methodological weaknesses, found no significant difference in healing between groups but the second RCT found that a greater proportion of women in the non-sutured group had poorer wound healing at 6 weeks after birth.

Perineal care

What are the effects of different methods and materials for primary repair of obstetric anal sphincter injuries (third and fourth degree tears)?

UNKNOWN EFFECTIVENESS

Different methods and materials for primary repair of obstetric anal sphincter injuries (third and fourth degree tears)

One small RCT comparing the overlap method versus the end-to-end method for primary repair of the external anal sphincter following childbirth (third degree obstetric tears) found no significant difference in perineal discomfort, and a non-significant reduction in the rate of reported faecal urgency and anal incontinence with the overlap technique compared with the end-to-end method.

DEFINITION Perineal trauma is any damage to the genitalia during childbirth that occurs spontaneously or intentionally by surgical incision (episiotomy). Anterior perineal trauma is injury to the labia, anterior vagina, urethra, or clitoris, and is usually associated with little morbidity. Posterior perineal trauma is any injury to the posterior vaginal wall, perineal muscles, or anal sphincter. First degree spontaneous tears involve only skin; second degree tears involve perineal muscles; third degree tears partially or completely disrupt the anal sphincter; and fourth degree tears completely disrupt the external and internal anal sphincter and epithelium.[1]

INCIDENCE/ PREVALENCE Over 85% of women having a vaginal birth sustain some form of perineal trauma,[2] and 60–70% receive stitches — equivalent to 400 000 women a year in the UK in 1997.[2,3] There are wide variations in rates of episiotomy: 8% in The Netherlands, 14% in England, 50% in the USA, and 99% in East European countries.[4-6] Sutured spontaneous tears are reported in about a third of women in the USA[6] and the UK,[7] but this is probably an underestimate because of inconsistencies in reporting and classification of perineal trauma. The incidence of anal sphincter tears varies between 0.5% in the UK, 2.5% in Denmark, and 7% in Canada.[8]

AETIOLOGY/ RISK FACTORS Perineal trauma occurs during spontaneous or assisted vaginal delivery and is usually more extensive after the first vaginal delivery.[1] Associated risk factors also include increased fetal size, mode of delivery, and malpresentation and malposition of the fetus. Other maternal factors that may increase the extent and degree of trauma are ethnicity (white women are probably at greater risk than black women), older age, abnormal collagen synthesis, and poor nutritional state.[9] Clinicians' practices or preferences in terms of intrapartum interventions may influence the severity and rate of perineal trauma (e.g. use of ventouse *v* forceps).

PROGNOSIS Perineal trauma affects women's physical, psychological, and social wellbeing in the immediate postnatal period as well as in the long term. It can also disrupt breast feeding, family life, and sexual relations. In the UK, about 23–42% of women continue to have pain and discomfort for 10–12 days postpartum, and 7–10% of women continue to have long term pain (3–18 months after delivery);[2,3,10] 23% of women experience superficial dyspareunia at 3 months; 3–10% report faecal incontinence;[11,12] and up to 24% have urinary problems.[2,3] Complications depend on the severity of perineal trauma and on the effectiveness of treatment.

Please refer to clinicalevidence.com for full text and references.

Postnatal depression

Search date September 2005

Louise Howard

What are the effects of drug treatments for postnatal depression?

LIKELY TO BE BENEFICIAL

Selective serotonin reuptake inhibitor antidepressants (fluoxetine and paroxetine)*

One small RCT found limited evidence that fluoxetine plus one or six sessions of cognitive behavioural therapy may improve postnatal depression at 4 and 12 weeks compared with placebo plus one or six sessions of cognitive behavioural therapy. The RCT had methodological weaknesses, a high withdrawal rate, and it excluded breastfeeding women. A second small RCT found limited evidence of no significant difference in improvement of postnatal depression between paroxetine plus 12 sessions of cognitive behavioural therapy compared with paroxetine alone. The RCT was very small and excluded women who were suicidal or substance misusers. Despite a lack of evidence in postnatal depression, selective serotonin reuptake inhibitors are known to be effective in treating depression in the general population and are therefore considered likely to be beneficial for the treatment of postnatal depression.

UNKNOWN EFFECTIVENESS

Antidepressants other than fluoxetine and paroxetine

We found no RCTs on the effects of other antidepressants in women with postnatal depression, and no RCTs that compared other antidepressants with psychological treatments.

Hormones

One small RCT in women with severe postnatal depression found that oestrogen treatment improved postnatal depression at 3 and 6 months compared with placebo.

What are the effects of non-drug treatments for postnatal depression?

LIKELY TO BE BENEFICIAL

Cognitive behavioural therapy (individual)

One small RCT found limited evidence that individual cognitive behavioural therapy (CBT) and ideal standard care both improved depressive symptoms immediately and at 6 months, but that there was no significant difference between the two interventions. Limited evidence from one RCT suggested that individual CBT may improve postnatal depression in the short term (immediately after treatment) compared with routine primary care. The RCT found no clear longer term benefits (9 months to 5 years postpartum) from individual CBT compared with routine primary care, non-directive counselling, or psychodynamic therapy.

Interpersonal psychotherapy

One RCT found that interpersonal psychotherapy improved postnatal depression compared with waiting list controls at 12 weeks.

Postnatal depression

Non-directive counselling

Limited evidence from two RCTs suggested that in the short term (immediately after treatment), non-directive counselling improved postnatal depression compared with routine primary care. One RCT with follow up beyond 12 weeks, found no clear longer term benefits (from 9 months to 5 years postpartum) from non-directive counselling compared with routine primary care, individual cognitive behavioural therapy, or psychodynamic therapy.

Psychodynamic therapy

One RCT provided limited evidence that psychodynamic therapy may improve postnatal depression in the short term (immediately after treatment) compared with routine primary care. The RCT found no clear longer term benefits (9 months to 5 years postpartum) from psychodynamic therapy compared with routine primary care, non-directive counselling, or cognitive behavioural therapy.

UNKNOWN EFFECTIVENESS

Cognitive behavioural therapy (group)

One small RCT in women with a high level of depressive symptoms on screening found that group cognitive behavioural therapy improved symptoms at 6 months compared with routine primary care.

Light therapy

We found no RCTs on the effects of light therapy.

Mother–infant interaction coaching

One RCT found that mother–infant interaction coaching had no significant effect on maternal depression scores compared with usual treatment, but found that it improved maternal responsiveness to the infant within 10 weeks of starting treatment.

Psychoeducation with partner

One small RCT found that psychoeducation with partner reduced patients' depression scores and partners' psychiatric morbidity at 10 weeks compared with psychoeducation without partner.

Telephone based peer support (mother to mother)

One small RCT found that telephone based peer support reduced depression scores compared with usual treatment at 4 months.

*Fluoxetine and paroxetine are categorised on the evidence of their effectiveness in the treatment of depression in general.

DEFINITION Postnatal depression (PND) has been variously defined as non-psychotic depression occurring during the first 6 months, the first 4 weeks postpartum, or the first 3 months postpartum. Recently 3 months postpartum was suggested in the UK as a useful clinical definition.[1] Puerperal mental disorders have only recently been categorised separately in psychiatric classifications, but both the International Classification of Diseases (ICD-10)[2] and the *Diagnostic and statistical manual of mental disorders*, fourth edition (DSM-IV) (see table 1)❶ require certain qualifications to be met that limit their use: ICD-10 categorises mental disorders that occur postpartum as puerperal, but only if they cannot otherwise be classified, and DSM-IV allows "postpartum onset" to be specified for mood disorders starting within 4 weeks' postpartum.[3] In clinical practice and research, the broader definition above is often used, because whether or not PND is truly distinct from depression in general, depression in the postpartum period raises treatment issues for the nursing mother and has implications for the developing infant (see prognosis below). However, there is increased recognition that many PNDs start during pregnancy.[4,5] The symptoms are similar to symptoms of depression at other times of life, but in addition to low mood, sleep disturbance, change in appetite, diurnal variation in mood, poor concentration, and irritability, women with PND also experience guilt about their inability to look after their new baby. In many countries, health visitors screen for PND using the Edinburgh Postnatal Depression Scale,[6,7] which identifies depressive symptoms.

INCIDENCE/ PREVALENCE The prevalence of depression in women postpartum is similar to that found in women generally. However, the incidence of depression in the first month after childbirth is three times the average monthly incidence in non-childbearing women.[8] A meta-analysis of studies mainly based in the developed world found the incidence of PND to be 12–13%;[9] with higher incidence in developing countries.[10,11]

AETIOLOGY/ RISK FACTORS Four systematic reviews have identified the following risk factors for PND: past history of any psychopathology (including history of previous PND), low social support, poor marital relationship, and recent life events.[9,12-14] Recent studies from India also suggest that spousal disappointment with the gender of the newborn child, particularly if the child is a girl, is associated with the development of PND.[10,15]

PROGNOSIS Most episodes of PND resolve spontaneously within 3–6 months,[16] but about one in four affected mothers are still depressed on the child's first birthday.[17] In the developed world, suicide is now the main cause of maternal deaths in the first year postpartum,[18] but the suicide rate is lower at this time than in age matched non-postpartum women.[19] PND is also associated with reduced likelihood of secure attachment,[20] deficits in maternal–infant interactions,[21] and impaired cognitive and emotional development of the child, particularly in boys living in areas of socioeconomic deprivation.[22,23] These associations remain significant even after controlling for subsequent episodes of depression in the mother. However there is also evidence to suggest that later effects on the child are related to chronic or recurrent maternal depression, rather than postpartum depression per se.[24] Women whose depression persists beyond 6 months postpartum have been found to have fewer positive interactions with their infants than women who were depressed but whose depressive symptoms ended before 6 months,[25] suggesting that the timing of depression is an important factor in determining its effect on the mother–infant relationship.

Please refer to clinicalevidence.com for full text and references.

Postpartum haemorrhage: prevention

Search date May 2005

David Chelmow and Barbara O'Brien

What are the effects of interventions to prevent primary postpartum haemorrhage?

BENEFICIAL

Active management of the third stage of labour

One systematic review found that active management of the third stage of labour consisting of controlled cord traction, early cord clamping plus drainage, and a prophylactic oxytocic agent reduced postpartum haemorrhage of 500 or 1000 mL or greater, and reduced related morbidities including mean blood loss, postpartum haemoglobin less than 9 g/dL, blood transfusion, need for supplemental iron postpartum, and length of third stage. Although active management increased adverse effects such as nausea, vomiting, and headache, one RCT identified by the review found that women were less likely to be dissatisfied when their third stage was actively managed.

Oxytocin

One systematic review found that, compared with placebo, oxytocin reduced the need for further medication and most outcomes of blood loss, except low maternal haemoglobin postpartum. Another systematic review found a higher rate of postpartum haemorrhage and a slightly increased need for additional treatment of postpartum haemorrhage with oxytocin compared with an oxytocin plus ergometrine combination. However, rates of adverse effects such as diastolic hypertension, nausea, and vomiting were lower with oxytocin alone. The review found no significant difference between interventions in the rates of severe postpartum haemorrhage or transfusion. The first systematic review and one additional RCT found no significant difference in outcomes of blood loss between oxytocin and ergot alkaloids. They found that oxytocin causes less nausea, and may reduce the risk of retained placenta and hypertension. One systematic review found a lower rate of postpartum haemorrhage and fewer adverse effects, particularly fever, shivering, and diarrhoea with oxytocin compared with oral misoprostol. Limited evidence from one RCT found similar results in measured blood loss between oxytocin and an injectable prostaglandin (prostaglandin E2).

LIKELY TO BE BENEFICIAL

Controlled cord traction

One RCT found that controlled cord traction reduced risk of retained placenta and further medical treatment compared with minimal intervention; however, the timing of oxytocin administration was different in the two groups and may have affected the results. It found no significant difference between interventions in rates of shock and need for transfusion. One RCT found a smaller drop in haemoglobin with controlled cord traction plus immediate cord drainage compared with expectant management. It found no significant difference between interventions in postpartum haemoglobin levels, need for transfusion, or for manual removal of the placenta.

TRADE OFF BETWEEN BENEFITS AND HARMS

Ergot compounds

Limited evidence from one RCT found no significant difference in risk of severe postpartum haemorrhage and in need for further treatment or transfusion between oral ergotamine and placebo. One systematic review found no significant difference in outcomes of blood loss between ergot alkaloids and oxytocin. It found that ergot alkaloids caused more nausea, and may increase the risk of retained placenta and hypertension. One additional RCT found similar results. One systematic review and one additional RCT found no significant difference in outcomes assessing blood loss or need for manual placenta removal between ergot compounds alone and in combination with oxytocin. Three RCTs found no significant difference in measures of blood loss between ergot compounds and prostaglandin analogues. They found that ergot compounds reduced the risk of adverse effects such as shivering or fever.

Injectable prostaglandins

Limited evidence from one additional RCT found no significant difference in measured blood loss between an injectable prostaglandin and oxytocin. RCTs found no significant difference in measures of blood loss between prostaglandin analogues and ergot. They found that prostaglandins increased the risk of adverse effects such as shivering or fever. RCTs comparing injectable prostaglandins with an oxytocin plus ergometrine combination found no difference between interventions in measures of blood loss, but a higher risk of diarrhoea with injectable prostaglandins. Two RCTs were stopped early, one for unacceptably high rates of gastrointestinal adverse effects with prostaglandin.

Oxytocin plus ergometrine combinations

One systematic review found a lower rate of postpartum haemorrhage and a slightly reduced need for additional treatment of postpartum haemorrhage with an oxytocin plus ergometrine combination compared with oxytocin alone. However, rates of adverse effects such as diastolic hypertension, nausea, and vomiting were higher with the combination. The review found no significant difference between interventions in the rates of severe postpartum haemorrhage or transfusion. One systematic review found no significant difference between oxytocin plus ergometrine and ergot compounds alone in outcomes assessing blood loss or need for manual placenta removal. One systematic review found that an oxytocin plus ergometrine reduced the need for additional medical treatment and the risk of shivering compared with oral misoprostol. One RCT comparing a fixed combination of oxytocin plus ergometrine versus rectal misoprostol found no difference between interventions, whereas another RCT found that a fixed combination of oxytocin plus ergometrine reduced the risk of postpartum haemorrhage, severe postpartum haemorrhage, need for transfusion, and shivering compared with rectal misoprostol. RCTs comparing an oxytocin plus ergometrine combination with injectable prostaglandins found no difference between interventions in effect, and a lower risk of diarrhoea with the combination. Two RCTs were stopped early, one for unacceptably high rates of gastrointestinal adverse effects with prostaglandin.

UNKNOWN EFFECTIVENESS

Uterine massage

We found no RCTs on the effects of uterine massage for the prevention of postpartum haemorrhage.

Postpartum haemorrhage: prevention

UNLIKELY TO BE BENEFICIAL

Immediate breastfeeding

One quasi-randomised trial found no significant difference in the rate of postpartum haemorrhage or mean blood loss between immediate breastfeeding after expectant management of the third stage of labour and expectant management alone.

LIKELY TO BE INEFFECTIVE OR HARMFUL

Misoprostol

One systematic review found no significant difference between prostaglandins and placebo or no intervention in most measures of blood loss, and found that oral misoprostol increased the rate of severe postpartum haemorrhage. In addition, it found that oral misoprostol increased the rate of adverse effects, in particular fever and shivering. One systematic review found a higher rate of postpartum haemorrhage and more adverse effects, particularly fever, shivering, and diarrhoea with oral misoprostol compared with oxytocin. One systematic review found that oral misoprostol increased the need for additional medical treatment and the risk of shivering compared with an oxytocin plus ergometrine combination. One RCT comparing rectal misoprostol with a fixed combination of oxytocin plus ergometrine found no difference between interventions, whereas another RCT found that rectal misoprostol increased the risk of postpartum haemorrhage, severe postpartum haemorrhage, need for transfusion, and shivering.

DEFINITION Postpartum haemorrhage is characterised by an estimated blood loss greater than 500 mL. The leading cause of postpartum haemorrhage is uterine atony, the failure of the uterus to contract fully after delivery of the placenta. Postpartum haemorrhage is divided into immediate (primary) and delayed (secondary). Primary postpartum haemorrhage occurs within the first 24 hours after delivery, whereas secondary postpartum haemorrhage occurs after 24 hours and before 6 weeks after delivery. This topic will address the effects of strategies for prevention of postpartum haemorrhage after vaginal delivery in low and high risk women, specifically looking at strategies to prevent uterine atony. Future updates will examine strategies to prevent postpartum haemorrhage owing to other causes, as well as treatment strategies.

INCIDENCE/ PREVALENCE Postpartum haemorrhage complicates 10.5% of deliveries worldwide, and is responsible for 132 000 deaths with a case fatality of 1%.[1] It is the leading direct cause of maternal mortality with most maternal deaths occurring in the poorest countries, most numerous in Africa and Asia.[1] The imbalance between developed and undeveloped areas probably stems from a combination of: increased prevalence of risk factors like grand multiparity, safe blood banking not being available, no routine use of prophylaxis against haemorrhage, and measures for drug and surgical management of atony not being available.

AETIOLOGY/ RISK FACTORS In addition to uterine atony, immediate postpartum haemorrhage is frequently caused by retained placental tissue, trauma such as laceration of the perineum, vagina, or cervix, rupture of the uterus, or coagulopathy. Risk factors for uterine atony include use of general anaesthetics, an overdistended uterus, particularly from twins, a large foetus, or polyhydramnios, prolonged labour, precipitous labour, use of oxytocin for labour induction or augmentation, high parity, chorioamnionitis, history of atony in a previous pregnancy, or retained placental tissue.

◀ **PROGNOSIS** Most postpartum haemorrhage, particularly in Europe and the US, is well tolerated by women. However, in low resource settings, where women may already be significantly anaemic during pregnancy, blood loss of 500 mL may be significant. Although death from pregnancy is rare in the US, postpartum haemorrhage was responsible for 29% of deaths.[2] Maternal death is 50–100 times more frequent in developing nations, with postpartum haemorrhage responsible for a similar proportion as in the US. Other significant morbidities associated with postpartum haemorrhage include renal failure, respiratory failure, multiple organ failure, need for transfusion, need for surgery including dilatation and curettage or, rarely, hysterectomy. Some women with large blood loss will later develop Sheehan's syndrome.

Please refer to clinicalevidence.com for full text and references.

Pre-eclampsia and hypertension

Search date November 2004

Lelia Duley

What are the effects of preventive interventions in women at risk of pre-eclampsia?

BENEFICIAL

Antiplatelet drugs

One systematic review and one subsequent RCT found evidence that, in women considered at risk of pre-eclampsia, antiplatelet drugs (mainly aspirin) reduced the risk of pre-eclampsia, death of the baby, and delivery before 37 completed weeks compared with placebo or no treatment. The RCTs found no significant difference in other important outcomes. The systematic review found no evidence that aspirin increased the risk of bleeding in mother or baby compared with placebo.

Calcium supplementation

One systematic review found that calcium supplementation (mainly 2 g/day) reduced the risk of pre-eclampsia and reduced the risk of having a baby with birth weight under 2500 g compared with placebo. It found no significant difference between calcium supplements and placebo on the risk of caesarean section, preterm delivery, or stillbirth or death of the baby before discharge from hospital.

UNKNOWN EFFECTIVENESS

Antioxidants

Two RCTs found limited evidence that antioxidants (vitamins C plus E, or lycopene) reduced the risk of pre-eclampsia compared with placebo. The RCTs provided insufficient evidence on other clinically important outcomes.

Atenolol

One RCT comparing atenolol with placebo was too small to allow any reliable conclusions to be drawn.

Fish oil, evening primrose oil, or both

We found insufficient evidence from six small RCTs about effects on pre-eclampsia or preterm birth of fish oil, evening primrose oil, or both, compared with either placebo or each other. One small RCT provided insufficient evidence on the effects of supplementation with protein, fish oil, and calcium, plus rest in the left lateral position compared with iron supplementation.

Glyceryl trinitrate

Two RCTs comparing glyceryl trinitrate patches versus placebo or no treatment and one RCT comparing glyceryl trinitrate versus aspirin and dipyridamole provided insufficient evidence on the effects of glyceryl trinitrate.

Magnesium supplementation

One systematic review found insufficient evidence about the effects of magnesium supplements on the risk of pre-eclampsia or its complications.

Salt restriction

Limited evidence from one systematic review found no significant difference in the risk of pre-eclampsia with a low salt diet compared with a normal diet. ▶

What are the effects of interventions in women who develop mild–moderate hypertension during pregnancy?

UNKNOWN EFFECTIVENESS

Antihypertensive drugs for mild to moderate hypertension

Two systematic reviews found that antihypertensive agents may halve the risk of severe hypertension but the effects of antihypertensive agents on other important outcomes are unclear. Systematic reviews found that angiotensin converting enzyme inhibitors used in pregnancy were associated with fetal renal failure, and found that beta blockers increased the risk of the baby being small for its gestational age. It remains unclear whether treatment of mild to moderate hypertension during pregnancy is worthwhile with any antihypertensive agent compared with no treatment.

Bed rest/admission *v* day care

We found insufficient evidence about hospital admission or bed rest compared with outpatient or day care or normal activities in hospital.

What are the effects of interventions in women who develop severe pre-eclampsia or very high blood pressure during pregnancy?

BENEFICIAL

Prophylactic magnesium sulphate in severe pre-eclampsia

One systematic review found that prophylactic magnesium sulphate halved the risk of eclampsia compared with placebo in women with severe pre-eclampsia. It found that magnesium sulphate reduced maternal mortality compared with placebo, although differences between groups did not reach significance. The review found no significant difference between magnesium sulphate and placebo on the risk of stillbirth or neonatal death in babies born to women with severe pre-eclampsia. The review also found that magnesium sulphate reduced the risk of eclampsia compared with phenytoin or nimodipine. A quarter of women given magnesium sulphate reported adverse effects (mainly flushing) compared with 5% of those given placebo. The review found insufficient evidence about the effects of diazepam compared with magnesium sulphate in women with severe pre-eclampsia.

LIKELY TO BE BENEFICIAL

Antihypertensive drugs for very high blood pressure*

Consensus opinion is that women with severe hypertension during pregnancy should have antihypertensive treatment. Placebo trials would therefore be unethical. One systematic review and one subsequent RCT in women with blood pressures high enough to merit immediate treatment found that all of the included antihypertensives reduced blood pressure, but found no evidence of a difference in the control of blood pressure by various antihypertensive drugs. The studies were too small to draw any further conclusions about the relative effects of different agents. Ketanserin and diazoxide may be associated with more adverse effects than hydralazine and labetalol, respectively.

*Consensus opinion is that women with severe hypertension during pregnancy should have antihypertensive treatment. Placebo controlled trials would therefore be unethical.

Pre-eclampsia and hypertension

UNKNOWN EFFECTIVENESS

Antioxidants in severe pre-eclampsia

One RCT found insufficient evidence about the effects of a combination of vitamin E plus vitamin C plus allopurinol compared with placebo.

Choice of analgesia during labour with severe pre-eclampsia

Two RCTs in women with severe pre-eclampsia or pregnancy induced hypertension found that epidural analgesia during labour reduced pain compared with patient controlled intravenous analgesia, although epidural analgesia increased the length of the second stage of labour, the risk of intrapartum fever and the risk of a forceps delivery.

Early delivery for severe early onset pre-eclampsia

One systematic review based on two small RCTs found no evidence that interventionist obstetric management reduced stillbirth or perinatal death rates compared with expectant management in babies born to mothers with severe early onset pre-eclampsia. However, it found that interventionist management increased rates of admission to neonatal intensive care and increased the risk of necrotising enterocolitis and respiratory distress in the baby compared with expectant management. The review found insufficient evidence about the effects of interventionist compared with expectant management in the mother.

Plasma volume expansion in severe pre-eclampsia

One systematic review comparing plasma volume expansion versus no expansion found insufficient evidence to draw reliable conclusions.

What is the best choice of anticonvulsant for women with eclampsia?

BENEFICIAL

Magnesium sulphate for eclampsia (better and safer than other anticonvulsants)

Systematic reviews and one subsequent RCT found that magnesium sulphate reduced the risk of further fits in women with eclampsia compared with phenytoin, diazepam, or lytic cocktail. One systematic review found that magnesium sulphate reduced the risk of maternal death compared with diazepam. Two other systematic reviews found lower maternal death rates with magnesium sulphate compared with phenytoin or lytic cocktail, although differences between groups did not reach significance.

DEFINITION Hypertension during pregnancy may be associated with one of several conditions. **Pregnancy induced hypertension** is a rise in blood pressure, without proteinuria, during the second half of pregnancy. **Pre-eclampsia** is a multisystem disorder, unique to pregnancy, which is usually associated with raised blood pressure and proteinuria. It rarely presents before 20 weeks' gestation. **Eclampsia** is one or more convulsions in association with the syndrome of pre-eclampsia. **Pre-existing hypertension** (not covered in this chapter) is known hypertension before pregnancy or raised blood pressure before 20 weeks' gestation. It may be essential hypertension or, less commonly, secondary to underlying disease.[1]

Pre-eclampsia and hypertension

INCIDENCE/ PREVALENCE Pregnancy induced hypertension affects 10% of pregnancies, and pre-eclampsia complicates 2–8% of pregnancies.[2] Eclampsia occurs in about 1/2000 deliveries in developed countries.[3] In developing countries, estimates of the incidence of eclampsia vary from 1/100–1/1700.[4,5]

AETIOLOGY/ RISK FACTORS The cause of pre-eclampsia is unknown. It is likely to be multifactorial, and may result from deficient placental implantation during the first half of pregnancy.[6] Pre-eclampsia is more common among women likely to have a large placenta, such as those with multiple pregnancy, and among women with medical conditions associated with microvascular disease, such as diabetes, hypertension, and collagen vascular disease.[7,8] Other risk factors include genetic susceptibility, increased parity, and older maternal age.[9] Cigarette smoking seems to be associated with a lower risk of pre-eclampsia, but this potential benefit is outweighed by an increase in adverse outcomes such as low birth weight, placental abruption, and perinatal death.[10]

PROGNOSIS The outcome of pregnancy in women with pregnancy induced hypertension alone is at least as good as that for normotensive pregnancies.[7,11] However, once pre-eclampsia develops, morbidity and mortality rise for both mother and child. For example, perinatal mortality for women with severe pre-eclampsia is double that for normotensive women.[7] Perinatal outcome is worse with early gestational hypertension.[7,9,11] Perinatal mortality also increases in women with severe essential hypertension.[12]

Please refer to clinicalevidence.com for full text and references.

Preterm birth

Search date June 2005

David M. Haas

What are the effects of preventive interventions in women at high risk of preterm delivery?

LIKELY TO BE BENEFICIAL

Prophylactic cervical cerclage for women at risk of preterm labour in whom cervical changes have not been identified

Five RCTs found different results for women in whom cervical changes had not been identified. One large RCT found that cerclage at 9–29 weeks reduced delivery before 33 weeks' gestation in women with a previous preterm delivery or previous cervical surgery, but increased the risk of puerperal pyrexia compared with no cerclage. The other four smaller RCTs found no significant difference in delivery before 34 weeks between cerclage at 10–30 weeks and no cerclage in women with a variety of risk factors for preterm delivery.

UNLIKELY TO BE BENEFICIAL

Enhanced antenatal care programmes for socially deprived population groups/high risk groups

RCTs carried out in a range of countries found no significant difference between enhanced antenatal care and usual care in reducing the risk of preterm delivery.

Prophylactic cervical cerclage for women at risk of preterm labour in whom cervical changes have been identified

Five RCTs found different results when cervical changes had been identified. Three RCTs found no significant difference in delivery before 33,34 and 35 weeks between cerclage and no cerclage. One RCT found that, compared with bed rest alone, cerclage plus bed rest significantly reduced preterm delivery before 34 weeks but found no significant difference in neonatal survival between cerclage plus bed rest and no cerclage. One small RCT found that, compared with bedrest, emergency cerclage reduced preterm delivery and improved neonatal morbidity when cerclage was done in the presence of protruding membranes at or beyond the cervical os.

What are the effects of interventions to improve outcome after preterm rupture of the membranes?

LIKELY TO BE BENEFICIAL

Antibiotic treatment for premature rupture of the membranes (prolongs gestation and may reduce infection, but unknown effect on perinatal mortality)

One systematic review in women with premature rupture of membranes has found that antibiotics prolong pregnancy and reduce the risk of neonatal morbidity, such as neonatal infection, requirement for treatment with oxygen, and abnormal cerebral ultrasound, compared with placebo. It found that co-amoxiclav (amoxycillin plus clavulanic acid) increased the risk of neonatal necrotising enterocolitis compared with placebo.

UNKNOWN EFFECTIVENESS

Amnioinfusion for preterm rupture of the membranes

One systematic review found insufficient evidence from one small RCT about the effects of amnioinfusion compared with no amnioinfusion in improving neonatal outcomes after preterm rupture of the membranes.

What are the effects of treatments to stop contractions in preterm labour?

LIKELY TO BE BENEFICIAL

Calcium channel blockers

We found no systematic review or RCTs comparing calcium channel blockers versus placebo. One systematic review has found that calcium channel blockers significantly reduce deliveries within 48 hours, neonatal morbidity, and withdrawals caused by maternal adverse effects compared with other tocolytics (mainly beta agonists).

UNKNOWN EFFECTIVENESS

Oxytocin receptor antagonists (atosiban)

One systematic review identified two RCTs that compared atosiban with placebo and found different results. The larger RCT found that atosiban prolonged pregnancy compared with placebo, but found that atosiban increased fetal deaths below 28 weeks' gestation compared with placebo, but the statistical significance of this finding was not reported. The other RCT found that atosiban increased delivery within 48 hours compared with placebo, but the statistical significance of this finding was not reported.

Prostaglandin inhibitors (indometacin)

One systematic review of three small RCTs found limited evidence that indometacin reduced delivery within 48 hours and 7 days, and delivery before 37 weeks' gestation compared with placebo. However, it found no significant difference between indometacin and placebo or no treatment in perinatal mortality, respiratory distress syndrome, bronchopulmonary dysplasia, necrotising enterocolitis, neonatal sepsis, or low birth weight. The review may have lacked power to detect a clinically important adverse effect.

UNLIKELY TO BE BENEFICIAL

Magnesium sulphate

One systematic review found no significant difference between magnesium sulphate and placebo or no treatment in delivery before 36 weeks, perinatal mortality or respiratory distress syndrome. A second systematic review found no significant difference between magnesium sulphate and other tocolytics (betamimetics, calcium channel blockers, prostaglandin synthetase inhibitors, nitroglycerine, alcohol, and dextrose infusion) in delivery within 48 hours, although results were statistically heterogeneous. It also found that, compared with other tocolytics, magnesium sulphate increased fetal, neonatal and infant mortality.

LIKELY TO BE INEFFECTIVE OR HARMFUL

Beta mimetics

One systematic review found no significant difference between $beta_2$ agonists and placebo or no treatment in perinatal mortality, neonatal mortality or

Preterm birth

respiratory distress syndrome; however, $beta_2$ agonists reduced delivery within 48 hours compared with placebo or no treatment . The review found that $beta_2$ agonists increased fetal tachycardia and maternal adverse effects such as chest pain, palpitations, dyspnoea, tremor, nausea, vomiting, headache, hyperglycaemia, and hypokalaemia compared with placebo or no treatment.

What are the effects of elective compared with selective caesarean delivery for women in preterm labour?

UNLIKELY TO BE BENEFICIAL

Elective rather than selective caesarean delivery in preterm labour

One systematic review has found that elective caesarean delivery increases maternal morbidity compared with selective caesarean delivery, and found no significant difference in neonatal morbidity or mortality. The RCTs may have been underpowered to detect a clinically important neonatal benefit.

What are the effects of interventions to improve outcome in preterm delivery?

BENEFICIAL

Antenatal corticosteroids

One systematic review found that antenatal corticosteroids significantly reduced respiratory distress syndrome, intraventricular haemorrhage, and neonatal mortality compared with placebo or no treatment.

LIKELY TO BE INEFFECTIVE OR HARMFUL

Antibiotic treatment for preterm labour with intact membranes

One systematic review found no significant difference between antibiotics and no antibiotics in delivery within 48 hours and 7 days, or perinatal mortality. It found that antibiotics reduced maternal infection compared with no antibiotics. One subsequent RCT found no significant difference between antibiotics and no antibiotics in delivery at 7 days or before 37 weeks.

Thyrotropin releasing hormone plus corticosteroids before preterm delivery

One systematic review found no significant difference in improving neonatal outcomes between thyrotropin releasing hormone plus corticosteroids and corticosteroids alone. The review found that thyrotropin releasing hormone plus corticosteroids increased maternal and fetal adverse events compared with corticosteroids alone.

DEFINITION Preterm or premature birth is defined by the World Health Organization as delivery of an infant before 37 completed weeks of gestation.[1] There is no set lower limit to this definition, but 23–24 weeks' gestation is widely accepted,[1] which approximates to an average fetal weight of 500 g.

INCIDENCE/ PREVALENCE Preterm birth occurs in about 5–10% of all births in developed countries,[2-4] but in recent years the incidence seems to have increased in some countries, particularly the USA.[5] We found little reliable evidence for incidence (using the definition of premature birth given above) in less developed countries. The rate in northwestern Ethiopia has been reported to vary between 11–22% depending on the age group of mothers studied, and is highest in teenage mothers.[6]

Preterm birth

AETIOLOGY/ RISK FACTORS About 30% of preterm births are unexplained and spontaneous.[4,7,8] Preterm labour usually results in preterm birth. One systematic review (search date not reported), which compared tocolysis versus placebo, found that about 27% of preterm labours resolved spontaneously and about 70% progressed to preterm delivery.[9] The two strongest risk factors for idiopathic preterm labour are low socioeconomic status and previous preterm delivery. Multiple pregnancy accounts for about another 30% of cases.[4,7] Other known risk factors include genital tract infection, preterm rupture of the membranes, antepartum haemorrhage, cervical incompetence, and congenital uterine abnormalities, which collectively account for about 20–25% of cases. The remaining cases (15–20%) are attributed to elective preterm delivery secondary to hypertensive disorders of pregnancy, intrauterine fetal growth restriction, congenital abnormalities, trauma and medical disorders of pregnancy.[4,5,7,8]

PROGNOSIS Preterm birth is the leading cause of neonatal death and infant mortality, often as a result of respiratory distress syndrome as a consequence of immature lung development.[10] Children who survive are also at high risk of neurologic disability.[11] Observational studies have found that one preterm birth significantly raises the risk of another in a subsequent pregnancy.[12]

Please refer to clinicalevidence.com for full text and references.

Acute respiratory distress syndrome

Search date November 2004

Satyendra Sharma

What are the effects of interventions in adults with ARDS?

BENEFICIAL

Low tidal volume mechanical ventilation *New*

Two RCTs found that low tidal volume ventilation decreased mortality at 28 and 180 days compared with high tidal volume ventilation. One RCT also found that low tidal volume ventilation increased ventilator free days. The target low tidal volume was 6 mL/kg of predicted body weight. One RCT found no significant difference between low tidal volume and high tidal volume ventilation in the duration of hospital stay. Low tidal volume ventilation may lead to respiratory acidosis, which may require treatment with either high respiratory rates and/or sodium bicarbonate infusion.

LIKELY TO BE BENEFICIAL

Protective ventilation *New*

Three RCTs found no significant difference between higher and lower positive end expiratory pressure (PEEP) strategies in overall mortality, although two of the RCTs found that protective ventilation improved other outcomes, including weaning rates. One RCT found no significant difference between high PEEP and lower PEEP ventilation strategies in people managed with low tidal volume ventilation. There is consensus that PEEP is effective in people with acute respiratory distress syndrome (ARDS). Protective ventilation uses PEEP to keep the alveoli open throughout the entire respiratory cycle but current evidence does not support the routine application of a high PEEP strategy in people with acute lung injury/ARDS.

TRADE OFF BETWEEN BENEFITS AND HARMS

Prone position *New*

Prone position can improve oxygenation, but this benefit must be carefully weighed against the lack of any good evidence of benefit or mortality, and uncommon but potentially serious harms. One systematic review found that prone positioning improved oxygenation in 69% of people with acute respiratory distress syndrome. However, the review and one subsequent RCT found no difference in mortality at 10 days and at 6 months between supine and prone positioning. One small controlled clinical trial found that both prone positioning and positive end expiratory pressure improved oxygenation compared with supine positioning alone. Subgroup analysis found that only prone positioning improved oxygenation in those with localised infiltrates, compared with supine positioning or positive end expiratory pressure. Adverse effects of prone positioning include increased sedation, facial oedema, and accidental extubation. Spinal instability is an absolute contraindication to prone positioning. Relative contraindications include haemodynamic and cardiac instability and recent thoracic or abdominal surgery.

UNKNOWN EFFECTIVENESS

Corticosteroids *New*

There is insufficient evidence to assess corticosteroids in people with acute respiratory distress syndrome (ARDS). One RCT found no significant difference ▶

between methylprednisolone and placebo in mortality or reversal of ARDS at day 45. However, another weak RCT found that methylprednisolone significantly reduced mortality in the intensive care unit and increased the proportion of people discharged at day 10. Although RCT evidence is lacking, corticosteroids are sometimes used in people with persistent ARDS.

UNLIKELY TO BE BENEFICIAL

Nitric oxide *New*

One systematic review and one subsequent RCT found no significant difference between nitric oxide and placebo in mortality, ventilator free days, or duration of hospital admission. One RCT identified by the review found that nitric oxide improved oxygenation compared with placebo, but the improvement was modest and not sustained.

DEFINITION Acute respiratory distress syndrome (ARDS), originally described by Ashbaugh et al in 1967, is a clinical syndrome that represents the severe end of the spectrum of acute lung injury (ALI).[1] In 1994, the following definitions were recommended by the American-European Consensus Conference on ARDS; widespread acceptance of these definitions by the clinicians and researchers has improved standardisation of clinical research. **Acute lung injury (ALI):** a syndrome of acute and persistent inflammatory disease of the lungs and characterised by three clinical features: 1) bilateral pulmonary infiltrates on the chest radiograph; 2) a ratio of the partial pressure of arterial oxygen to the fraction of inspired oxygen (PaO_2/FiO_2) of less than 300; 3) absence of clinical evidence of left atrial hypertension (if measured, the pulmonary capillary wedge pressure is 18 mm Hg or less).[2] **Acute respiratory distress syndrome (ARDS):** The definition of ARDS is the same as that of acute lung injury, except that the hypoxia is severe: a PaO_2/FiO_2 ratio of 200 mm Hg or less.[2] The distinction between ALI and ARDS is arbitrary, because the severity of hypoxia does not correlate reliably with the extent of the underlying pathology and does not influence predictably the clinical course or survival. ARDS is an acute disorder, which typically develops over 4–48 hours and persists for days to weeks. Subacute or chronic lung diseases, such as sarcoidosis and idiopathic pulmonary fibrosis, are excluded from the definition of ARDS. The early pathological features of ARDS are generally described as diffuse alveolar damage. Recognition of diffuse alveolar damage requires histological examination of the lung tissue, which is not necessary to make a clinical diagnosis. **Population:** For the purpose of this chapter, we have defined ARDS as including people with ALI and ARDS. It therefore includes adults with ALI and ARDS from any cause and with any level of severity. Neonates and children less than 12 years of age have been excluded.

INCIDENCE/ PREVALENCE Ten to fifteen per cent of all people admitted to an intensive care unit and up to 20% of mechanically ventilated people meet the criteria for ARDS.[3] The incidence of ALI in the USA (17–64/100 000 person-years) appears to be higher than in Europe, Australia, and other developed countries (17–34/ 100 000 person-years).[4] One prospective, population based cohort study (1113 people in Washington, aged over 15 years) found the crude incidence of ALI to be 78.9/100 000 person-years and the age adjusted incidence to be 86.2/100 000 person-years.[5]

AETIOLOGY/ RISK FACTORS ARDS encompasses many distinct disorders that share common clinical and pathophysiological features. More than 60 causes of ARDS have been identified. Although the list of possible aetiologies is long, most episodes of ARDS are associated with a few common causes or predisposing conditions, either individually or in combination. These include sepsis, aspiration of gastric contents, infectious pneumonia, severe trauma, surface burns, lung contusion, fat embolism syndrome, massive blood transfusion, lung and bone marrow

Acute respiratory distress syndrome

transplantation, drugs, acute pancreatitis, near drowning, cardiopulmonary bypass, and neurogenic pulmonary oedema.[6,7] One or more of these predisposing conditions are often evident at the onset of ALI. When ARDS occurs in the absence of common risk factors such as trauma, sepsis, or aspiration, an effort should be made to identify a specific cause for lung injury. In such cases, a systematic review of the events that immediately preceded the onset of ARDS is normally undertaken to identify the predisposing factors.

PROGNOSIS **Mortality:** Survival for people with ARDS has improved remarkably in recent years, and cohort studies have found mortality to range from 34–58%.[4,8,9] The mortality rate varies with the cause; however, by far the most common cause of death is multiorgan system failure rather than acute respiratory failure. In a prospective cohort study (207 at risk of developing ARDS, of which 47 developed ARDS during the trial), only 16% of all deaths were considered to be due to irreversible respiratory failure. Most deaths in the first 3 days of being diagnosed with ARDS could be attributed to the underlying illness or injury. The majority of late deaths (after 3 days, 16/22 [72.7%]) were related to sepsis syndrome.[10] One prospective cohort study (902 mechanically ventilated people with ALI) found that an age of 70 years or younger significantly increased the proportion of people who survived at 28 days (74.6% aged 70 years or younger *v* 50.3% aged 71 years or older, $p < 0.001$).[11] **Lung function and morbidity:** One cohort study of 16 long term survivors of severe ARDS (lung injury score ≥ 2.5) found that only mild abnormalities in pulmonary function (and often none) were observed. Restrictive and obstructive ventilatory defects (each noted in 4/16 [25.0%] of people) were observed in ARDS survivors treated with low or conventional tidal volumes.[12] One cohort study of 109 people found no significant difference between various ventilatory strategies and long term abnormalities in pulmonary function or health related quality of life. However, it did find an association between abnormal pulmonary function and decreased quality of life at 1 year follow up.[13] One retrospective cohort study (41 people with ARDS) found that duration of mechanical ventilation and severity of ARDS were important determinants of persistent symptoms 1 year after recovery.[14] Better lung function was observed when no illness was acquired during the intensive care unit stay and with rapid resolution of multiple organ failure (e.g. pneumonia during ARDS: 7/41 [17.1%] people with long term impairment *v* 2/41 [4.9%] with no long term impairment; significance assessment not performed).[14] Persistent disability 1 year after discharge from the intensive care unit in survivors of ARDS is secondary to extrapulmonary conditions, most importantly the muscle wasting and weakness.[13] **Cognitive morbidity:** One cohort study (55 people 1 year after ARDS) found that 17/55 [30.1%] exhibited generalised cognitive decline and 43/55 [78.2%] had all, or at least one, of the following: impaired memory, attention, concentration, and/or decreased mental processing speed. These deficits may be related to hypoxaemia, drug toxicity, or complications of critical illness.[15] To date, no association between different ventilatory strategies and long term neurological outcomes has been demonstrated.

Please refer to clinicalevidence.com for full text and references.

Bronchitis (acute)

Search date July 2005

Peter Wark

What are the effects of treatments for acute bronchitis in people without chronic respiratory disease?

TRADE OFF BETWEEN BENEFITS AND HARMS

Antibiotics versus placebo and other treatments

One systematic review found that antibiotics (doxycycline, erythromycin, cefuroxime, amoxicillin plus clavulanic acid, and trimethoprim plus sulphamethoxazole) modestly reduced cough at follow up compared with placebo. However, the magnitude of improvement was of questionable clinical importance. There were small reductions in the proportion of people with cough at 1–2 weeks, a reduction in the mean days of coughing (by about half a day), a reduction in the proportion of people with night time cough at follow up, and an increase in the proportion of people judged improved by their treating physicians. People receiving antibiotics had fewer mean days with impaired activities and days feeling ill than people receiving placebo, but the difference between groups did not quite reach significance. There was no significant difference between antibiotics and placebo in productive cough at follow up or quality of life scores. More people taking antibiotics than placebo had adverse events such as nausea, vomiting, rash, headache, and vaginitis, although the difference between groups was not significant. Widespread antibiotic use may lead to bacterial resistance to antibiotics.

UNKNOWN EFFECTIVENESS

Amoxicillin, cephalosporins, and macrolides versus each other (no significant difference in clinical cure among different antibiotics; insufficient evidence on adverse effects)

RCTs found no significant difference in clinical improvement or cure between amoxicillin and cefuroxime or roxithromycin. RCTs found no significant difference in clinical improvement or cure between the macrolides azithromycin and clarithromycin, among different cephalosporins, or between cefuroxime and amoxicillin plus clavulanic acid. However, two RCTs found that adverse effects were less common with cefuroxime than with amoxicillin plus clavulanic acid. One small RCT identified by a systematic review found limited evidence that erythromycin was less effective than beta$_2$ agonists in reducing cough but may cause less shaking and tremor. Widespread antibiotic use may lead to bacterial resistance to antibiotics.

Antihistamines

One RCT identified by a systematic review provided insufficient evidence about the effects of antihistamines compared with placebo in people with acute bronchitis.

Antitussives

Three RCTs, one in children and two in adults with acute bronchitis, identified by a systematic review found no significant difference in cough severity between codeine or dextromethorphan and placebo in children or adults with acute bronchitis. It found that moguisteine modestly reduced cough severity compared with placebo in adults, but was associated with more gastrointestinal adverse effects.

Bronchitis (acute)

Beta$_2$ agonists (inhaled)

One systematic review combined data for inhaled and oral beta$_2$ agonists and found no significant difference in cough or ability to return to work between beta$_2$ agonists and placebo in adults with acute bronchitis. It found no RCTs assessing inhaled beta$_2$ agonists in children. It found limited evidence from one small RCT that inhaled beta$_2$ agonists reduced cough compared with erythromycin. The review found that beta$_2$ agonists (oral or inhaled) were more frequently associated with shaking and tremor than placebo or oral antibiotics (erythromycin).

Beta$_2$ agonists (oral)

One RCT identified by a systematic review found no significant difference in cough between oral salbutamol and placebo in children with acute bronchitis. The review combined data for oral and inhaled beta$_2$ agonists when assessing adults and found no significant difference in cough or ability to return to work between beta$_2$ agonists and placebo. The review found that oral or inhaled beta$_2$ agonists were more frequently associated with shaking and tremor than placebo.

Expectorants

One systematic review identified no RCTs about the effects of expectorants in people with acute bronchitis.

UNLIKELY TO BE BENEFICIAL

Amoxicillin plus clavulanic acid (no significant difference in clinical cure compared with cephalosporins but increased adverse effects)

Two RCTs found no significant difference in clinical improvement or cure between amoxicillin plus clavulanic acid and cefuroxime. However, they found that adverse effects were more common with amoxicillin plus clavulanic acid than with cefuroxime. There is no evidence to support the use of amoxicillin plus clavulanic acid in people with acute bronchitis.

DEFINITION Acute bronchitis is a transient inflammation of the trachea and major bronchi. Clinically, it is diagnosed on the basis of cough and occasionally sputum, dyspnoea, and wheeze. This review is limited to episodes of acute bronchitis in people (smokers and non-smokers) with no pre-existing respiratory disease such as a pre-existing diagnosis of asthma or chronic bronchitis, evidence of fixed airflow obstruction, or both, and excluding those with clinical or radiographic evidence of pneumonia. However, the reliance on a clinical definition for acute bronchitis implies that people with conditions such as transient/mild asthma or mild chronic obstructive pulmonary disease may have been recruited in some of the reported studies.

INCIDENCE/ PREVALENCE Acute bronchitis affects 44/1000 adults (> 16 years old) each year in the UK, with 82% of episodes occurring in autumn or winter.[1] One survey found that acute bronchitis was the fifth most common reason for people of any age to present to a general practitioner in Australia.[2]

AETIOLOGY/ RISK FACTORS Infection is believed to be the trigger for acute bronchitis. However, pathogens have been identified in fewer than 55% of people.[1] Community studies that attempted to isolate pathogens from the sputum of people with acute bronchitis found viruses in 8–23%, typical bacteria (*Streptococcus pneumoniae*, *Haemophilus influenzae*, *Moraxella catarrhalis*) in 45%, and atypical bacteria (*Mycobacterium pneumoniae*, *Chlamydia pneumoniae*, *Bordetella pertussis*) in 0–25%.[1,3,4] It is unclear whether smoking affects the risk for developing acute bronchitis.

PROGNOSIS Acute bronchitis is regarded as a mild, self limiting illness but there are limited data on prognosis and rates of complications such as chronic cough or progression to chronic bronchitis or pneumonia. One prospective longitudinal study reviewed 653 previously well adults who presented to suburban general practices over a 12 month period with symptoms of acute lower respiratory tract infection.[1] It found that within the first month of the illness 20% of people re-presented to their general practitioner with persistent or recurrent symptoms, mostly persistent cough. One prospective study of 138 previously well adults found that 34% had symptoms consistent with either chronic bronchitis or asthma 3 years after initial presentation with acute bronchitis.[5] It is also unclear whether acute bronchitis plays a causal role in the progression to chronic bronchitis or is simply a marker of predisposition to chronic lung disease. Although smoking has been identified as the most important risk factor for chronic bronchitis,[6,7] it is unclear whether the inflammatory effects of cigarette smoke and infection causing acute bronchitis have additive effects in leading to chronic inflammatory airway changes. In children, exposure to parental environmental tobacco smoke (ETS) is associated with an increase in risk for community lower respiratory infection in children aged 0–2 years and an increase in symptoms of cough and phlegm in those aged 5–16 years.[8]

Please refer to clinicalevidence.com for full text and references.

Common cold

Search date May 2005

Bruce Arroll

What are the effects of treatments?

LIKELY TO BE BENEFICIAL

Antihistamines (may improve runny nose and sneezing, no significant difference in overall symptoms)

One systematic review found that chlorpheniramine or doxylamine reduced runny nose and sneezing after 2 days compared with placebo in people with common cold, but the clinical benefit was small. Another review, that assessed a wide variety of antihistamines, found no significant difference in overall cold symptoms at 1–10 days between antihistamines and placebo and found that first generation antihistamines increased adverse effects, including sedation.

Decongestants (norephedrine, oxymetazoline, or pseudoephedrine) provided short term (3–10 hour) relief of congestive symptoms

One systematic review found that, compared with placebo, decongestants (norephedrine, oxymetazoline, or pseudoephedrine) reduced nasal congestion over 3–10 hours after a single dose in adults with common cold. The review identified no RCTs of other decongestants. One case control study found weak evidence that phenylpropanolamine may increase the risk of haemorrhagic stroke.

UNKNOWN EFFECTIVENESS

Analgesics or anti-inflammatory drugs

We found no RCTs of analgesics or anti-inflammatory drugs in people with common cold.

Decongestants (insufficient evidence to assess longer term [> 10 hours] effects on congestive symptoms)

One systematic review provided insufficient evidence to assess the effects of longer use of decongestants in people with colds.

Echinacea

Systematic reviews of weak RCTs found inconsistent evidence on the effects of echinacea in treating colds. One subsequent RCT found no significant difference between echinacea and placebo in the severity or duration of cold symptoms.

Steam inhalation

One systematic review provided insufficient evidence to assess steam inhalation in people with common cold.

Vitamin C

One systematic review found no significant difference between vitamin C and placebo initiated after the onset of cold symptoms in the duration or severity of cold.

Zinc (intranasal gel or lozenges)

One systematic review found limited evidence that zinc gluconate or acetate lozenges may reduce duration of cold symptoms at 7 days compared with placebo. Another review found no significant difference in duration of symptoms. Both reviews found that symptoms were unchanged at 3 or 5 days. One ▶

subsequent small RCT identified by a third review found that zinc lozenges reduced the duration of cold compared with placebo, while another subsequent larger RCT identified by the review found no significant difference between groups in cold duration or severity. Two RCTs found that zinc intranasal gel reduced the mean duration of cold symptoms compared with placebo. A third RCT found no significant difference in overall symptom duration between intranasal zinc and placebo.

LIKELY TO BE INEFFECTIVE OR HARMFUL

Antibiotics

Systematic reviews and one additional RCT found no significant difference between antibiotics and placebo in cure or general improvement at 6–14 days in people with colds. The additional RCT found that, in a subgroup of people (20%) with nasopharyngeal culture positive *Haemophilus influenzae*, *Moraxella catarrhalis*, or *Streptococcus pneumoniae*, antibiotics increased recovery at 5 days compared with placebo. However, we have no methods currently of easily identifying such people at first consultation.

DEFINITION Common colds are defined as upper respiratory tract infections that affect the predominantly nasal part of the respiratory mucosa. Since upper respiratory tract infections can affect any part of the mucosa, it is often arbitrary whether an upper respiratory tract infection is called a "cold" or "sore throat" ("pharyngitis" or "tonsillitis"), "sinusitis", "acute otitis media", or "bronchitis" (see figure 1 in sore throat). Sometimes all areas (simultaneously or at different times) are affected in one illness. Symptoms include sneezing, rhinorrhoea (runny nose), headache, and general malaise. In addition to nasal symptoms, half of sufferers experience sore throat and 40% experience cough.[1] This review does not include treatments for people with acute sinusitis (see acute sinusitis), acute bronchitis, (see acute bronchitis), or sore throat (see sore throat).

INCIDENCE/ PREVALENCE Upper respiratory tract infections, nasal congestion, throat complaints, and cough are responsible for 11% of general practice consultations in Australia.[2] Each year, children suffer about five such infections and adults two to three infections.[2-4] One cross-sectional study in Norwegian children aged 4–5 years found that 48% experienced more than two common colds annually.[5]

AETIOLOGY/ RISK FACTORS Transmission of common cold infection is mostly through hand to hand contact with subsequent passage to the nostrils or eyes rather than, as commonly perceived, through droplets in the air.[1] The organisms for common colds are mainly viruses (typically rhinovirus, but also coronavirus and respiratory syncytial virus, or metapneumovirus and others). For many colds, no infecting organism can be identified.

PROGNOSIS Common colds are usually short lived, lasting a few days, with a few lingering symptoms lasting longer, especially cough. Symptoms peak within 1–3 days and generally clear by 1 week, although cough often persists.[1] Although they cause no mortality or serious morbidity, common colds are responsible for considerable discomfort, lost work, and medical costs.

Please refer to clinicalevidence.com for full text and references.

Community acquired pneumonia

Search date April 2005

Mark Loeb

What are the effects of preventive interventions?

LIKELY TO BE BENEFICIAL

Influenza vaccine (in elderly people)

We found no RCTs that assessed the effects of influenza vaccine in preventing community acquired pneumonia. Observational studies suggest that influenza vaccine may reduce the incidence of pneumonia and may reduce mortality in the elderly.

UNLIKELY TO BE BENEFICIAL

Pneumococcal vaccine (for all cause pneumonia and mortality in immunocompetent adults)

One systematic review found no significant difference in all cause pneumonia or all cause mortality between pneumococcal vaccination and no pneumococcal vaccination in immunocompetent adults. The review provided limited evidence that pneumococcal vaccine may reduce definitive pneumococcal pneumonia compared with no vaccination in immunocompetent adults.

What are the effects of interventions in outpatient settings?

BENEFICIAL

Antibiotics in outpatient settings

One systematic review that evaluated different oral antibiotics in outpatient settings found no significant difference between different antibiotics (clarithromycin, erythromycin, or sparfloxacin) in clinical cure or improvement, which was observed in 80% or more of people regardless of antibiotic taken. One subsequent RCT found no significant difference in clinical cure rates between telithromycin and clarithromycin. Most trials were designed to show equivalence between treatments rather than superiority of one antibiotic over another.

What are the effects of treatments in people admitted to hospital?

BENEFICIAL

Antibiotics in hospital

One systematic review found no significant difference in mortality or clinical cure between antibiotic regimens containing antibiotics active against atypical pathogens (predominantly quinolones and macrolides) and regimens without atypical coverage (predominantly beta lactams and cephalosporins). RCTs that compared different oral or intravenous antibiotics in people admitted to hospital found clinical cure or improvement in 73–96% of people. Two RCTs found no significant difference in clinical cure or improvement among different antibiotics. Two RCTs found that quinolones may increase clinical cure compared with co-amoxiclav (amoxicillin plus clavulanic acid) or cephalosporins. However, most trials were small and were designed to show equivalence between treatments rather than superiority of one antibiotic over another.

LIKELY TO BE BENEFICIAL

Early mobilisation (reduced hospital stay compared with usual care)

One RCT found that early mobilisation reduced hospital stay compared with usual care. One RCT in people receiving antibiotics and usual medical care found that early mobilisation plus bottle blowing physiotherapy plus encouragement to sit up regularly and take deep breaths reduced mean hospital stay compared with early mobilisation alone. It found no significant difference in duration of fever.

UNLIKELY TO BE BENEFICIAL

Intravenous antibiotics in immunocompetent people in hospital without life threatening illness (compared with oral antibiotics)

One systematic review found no significant difference for clinical cure rates or mortality between oral and intravenous antibiotics in people hospitalised with non-severe community acquired pneumonia. One small RCT found that inpatient regimens consisting of staged intravenous and oral antibiotic treatment reduced hospital stay compared with regimens consisting of intravenous antibiotics alone.

What are the effects of treatments in people with community acquired pneumonia receiving intensive care?

LIKELY TO BE BENEFICIAL

Prompt administration of antibiotics in people admitted to intensive care with community acquired pneumonia (improved outcomes compared with delayed antibiotic treatment)

We found no systematic review and no RCTs comparing prompt versus delayed antibiotic treatment. Two retrospective observational studies found that prompt administration of antibiotics improved survival. It would be considered unethical to perform an RCT of delayed antibiotic treatment.

UNKNOWN EFFECTIVENESS

Different combinations of antibiotics in intensive care settings

We found no RCTs that compared one combination of antibiotics versus another in intensive care units.

DEFINITION Community acquired pneumonia is pneumonia contracted in the community rather than in hospital. It is defined by clinical symptoms (such as cough, sputum production, and pleuritic chest pain) and signs (such as fever, tachypnoea, and rales), with radiological confirmation.

INCIDENCE/ PREVALENCE In the northern hemisphere, community acquired pneumonia affects about 12/1000 people a year, particularly during winter and at the extremes of age (annual incidence in people < 1 year old: 30–50/1000; 15–45 years old: 1–5/1000; 60–70 years old: 10–20/1000; 71–85 years old: 50/1000).[1-6]

AETIOLOGY/ RISK FACTORS More than 100 microorganisms have been implicated in community acquired pneumonia, but most cases are caused by *Streptococcus pneumoniae* (see table 1) T.[4-7] Smoking is probably an important risk factor.[8] One large cohort study conducted in Finland (4175 people aged ≥ 60 years) suggested that risk factors for pneumonia in older people included alcoholism (RR 9.0, 95% CI 5.1 to 16.2), bronchial asthma (RR 4.2, 95% CI 3.3 to 5.4), immunosuppression (RR 3.1, 95% CI 1.9 to 5.1), lung disease (RR 3.0, 95% CI 2.3 to 3.9), heart

Community acquired pneumonia

disease (RR 1.9, 95% CI 1.7 to 2.3), institutionalisation (RR 1.8, 95% CI 1.4 to 2.4), and increasing age (≥ 70 years *v* 60–69 years; RR 1.5, 95% CI 1.3 to 1.7).[9]

PROGNOSIS Severity varies from mild to life threatening illness within days of the onset of symptoms. One systematic review of prognosis studies for community acquired pneumonia (search date 1995, 33 148 people) found overall mortality to be 13.7%, ranging from 5.1% for ambulant people to 36.5% for people who required intensive care.[10] The following prognostic factors were significantly associated with mortality: male sex (OR 1.3, 95% CI 1.2 to 1.4), absence of pleuritic chest pain (OR 2.00, 95% CI 1.25 to 3.30); hypothermia (OR 5.0, 95% CI 2.4 to 10.4); systolic hypotension (OR 4.8, 95% CI 2.8 to 8.3); tachypnoea (OR 2.9, 95% CI 1.7 to 4.9); diabetes mellitus (OR 1.3, 95% CI 1.1 to 1.5); neoplastic disease (OR 2.8, 95% CI 2.4 to 3.1); neurological disease (OR 4.6, 95% CI 2.3 to 8.9); bacteraemia (OR 2.8, 95% CI 2.3 to 3.6); leucopenia (OR 2.5, 95% CI 1.6 to 3.7); and multilobar radiographic pulmonary infiltrates (OR 3.1, 95% CI 1.9 to 5.1).

Please refer to clinicalevidence.com for full text and references.

Sore throat

Search date May 2005

Tim Kenealy

What are the effects of interventions to reduce symptoms of acute infective sore throat?

LIKELY TO BE BENEFICIAL

Non-steroidal anti-inflammatory drugs

RCTs identified by a systematic review found that non-steroidal anti-inflammatory drugs reduced sore throat symptoms both at 24 hours or less and at 2–5 days compared with placebo. The range of benefit was 25–75% over 24 hours or less, and 33–93% at 2–5 days. Non-steroidal anti-inflammatory drugs are associated with gastrointestinal and renal adverse effects.

Paracetamol

Two RCTs identified by a systematic review found that a single dose of paracetamol reduced acute sore throat pain at 2–3 hours compared with placebo. Another RCT identified by the review found that paracetamol three times daily reduced sore throat pain at 2 days compared with placebo. We found no RCTs of other analgesics in people with sore throat.

TRADE OFF BETWEEN BENEFITS AND HARMS

Antibiotics

One systematic review found that antibiotics reduced the proportion of people with sore throat, fever, and headache at 3 days compared with placebo. The review found limited evidence from indirect comparisons that the absolute and relative reduction in sore throat symptoms at 3 days was greater in people with positive throat swabs for *Streptococcus* than in people with negative swabs. The review gave no information on adverse effects. One subsequent RCT in children found no significant difference in the duration of sore throat between penicillin (3 or 7 day course) and placebo. We found no RCTs that assessed the effects of antibiotics in reducing the severity of sore throat symptoms. Antibiotics may increase the risk of nausea, vomiting, rash, headache, and vaginitis. Widespread antibiotic use may lead to bacterial resistance to antibiotics.

Corticosteroids

One RCT in children and adolescents with moderate to severe sore throat, but without group A beta haemolytic streptococcal infection, found that oral dexamethasone reduced time to initial pain relief and duration of throat pain compared with placebo. One RCT identified by a systematic review and one subsequent RCT found that adding corticosteroids to antibiotics improved short term pain relief compared with adding placebo. The RCT included by the review provided limited evidence that adding corticosteroids to antibiotics reduced the duration of pain in adults. However, the subsequent RCT found that adding corticosteroids to antibiotics did not significantly reduce pain duration in children and adolescents with group A beta haemolytic streptococcal infection. The RCTs provided insufficient evidence to assess adverse effects of corticosteroids in people with sore throat. However, data from systematic reviews in people with other disorders suggest that corticosteroids may be associated with serious adverse effects, although this may be only after long term use.

Sore throat

UNKNOWN EFFECTIVENESS

Probiotics

RCTs suggested that super-colonisation with *Streptococcus* isolated from healthy individuals apparently resistant to infections from *Streptococcus* may reduce recurrent sore throat over 2–3 months compared with placebo. However, at present, super-colonisation with *Streptococcus* is available only experimentally. We found no RCTs of other probiotics. We found no RCTs examining the effects of probiotics on the symptoms of acute sore throat.

What are the effects of interventions to prevent complications of acute infective sore throat?

TRADE OFF BETWEEN BENEFITS AND HARMS

Antibiotics

One systematic review found that antibiotics reduced suppurative and non-suppurative complications of beta haemolytic streptococcal pharyngitis compared with placebo. However, in industrialised countries, non-suppurative complications are extremely rare. Widespread antibiotic use may lead to bacterial resistance to antibiotics.

DEFINITION Sore throat is an acute upper respiratory tract infection that affects the respiratory mucosa of the throat. Since infections can affect any part of the mucosa, it is often arbitrary whether an acute upper respiratory tract infection is called "sore throat" ("pharyngitis" or "tonsillitis"), "common cold", "sinusitis", "otitis media", or "bronchitis" (see figure 1)Ⓕ. Sometimes, all areas are affected (simultaneously or at different times) in one illness. In this chapter, we aim to cover people whose principal presenting symptom is sore throat. This may be associated with headache, fever, and general malaise. Suppurative complications include acute otitis media (most commonly), acute sinusitis, and peritonsillar abscess (quinsy). Non-suppurative complications include acute rheumatic fever and acute glomerulonephritis.

INCIDENCE/ PREVALENCE There is little seasonal fluctuation in sore throat. About 10% of the Australian population present to primary healthcare services annually with an upper respiratory tract infection consisting predominantly of sore throat.[1] This reflects about one fifth of the overall annual incidence.[1] However, it is difficult to distinguish between the different types of upper respiratory tract infection.[2] A Scottish mail survey found 31% of adult respondents reported a severe sore throat in the previous year, for which 38% of these people visited a doctor.[3]

AETIOLOGY/ RISK FACTORS The causative organisms of sore throat may be bacteria (*Streptococcus*, most commonly group A beta haemolytic, although sometimes others: *Haemophilus influenzae*, *Moraxella catarrhalis*, and others) or viruses (typically rhinovirus, but also coronavirus, respiratory syncytial virus, metapneumovirus, Ebstein-Barr, and others). It is difficult to distinguish bacterial from viral infections clinically. Some features are thought to predict the probability of the infection being caused by *Streptococcus* (fever > 38.5 °C; exudate on the tonsils; anterior neck lymphadenopathy; absence of cough).[4] Sore throat can be caused by processes other than primary infections, including gastro-oesophageal reflux, physical or chemical irritation (e.g. from nasogastric tubes or smoke), and occasionally hay fever. However, we do not consider causes other than primary infection here.

PROGNOSIS Sore throat infections usually last a few days, with a few symptoms lasting longer, especially cough.[5] The untreated symptoms of sore throat disappear by 3 days in about 40% of people and untreated fevers in about 85%. By 1 week, 85% of people are symptom free. This natural history is similar in *Streptococcus* positive, negative, and untested people.

Please refer to clinicalevidence.com for full text and references.

Spontaneous pneumothorax

Search date April 2006

Abel Wakai

What are the effects of treatments in people presenting with spontaneous pneumothorax?

LIKELY TO BE BENEFICIAL

Chest tube drainage

We found no RCTs comparing chest tube drainage versus observation. One systematic review found that chest tube drainage was associated with longer hospital stay than needle aspiration but found no significant difference between treatments in treatment success or recurrence at one year. One RCT and one controlled clinical trial found no significant difference in rate of resolution of pneumothorax whether chest tube drainage bottles were connected to suction or not. However, both trials were too small to rule out a clinically important difference.

Needle aspiration

One small RCT provided insufficient evidence to compare needle aspiration versus observation. One systematic review found that needle aspiration was associated with shorter hospital stay than chest tube drainage but found no significant difference between groups in treatment success or recurrence at 1 year.

UNKNOWN EFFECTIVENESS

Chest tube drainage plus suction

One RCT and one controlled clinical trial found no significant difference in rate of resolution of pneumothorax whether chest tube drainage bottles were connected to suction or not. However, both trials were too small to detect a clinically important difference between groups.

One way valves on chest tubes

One RCT found no significant difference in rate of resolution between one way valves and drainage bottles with underwater seals, but it is likely to have been too small to detect a clinically important difference. It found that people treated with one way valves used less analgesia and were less likely to be admitted to hospital than people treated with drainage bottles.

Small versus standard sized chest tubes

We found no RCTs assessing small or standard sized tubes for chest drainage. Limited evidence of one small non-randomised trial found no difference between small gauge catheters and standard chest tubes in duration of drainage but found that, in people with large pneumothoraces, successful resolution was less likely with small chest tubes. However, small chest tubes were also less likely to result in subcutaneous emphysema.

What are the effects of interventions to prevent recurrence in people with previous spontaneous pneumothorax?

TRADE OFF BETWEEN BENEFITS AND HARMS

Pleurodesis

Two RCTs found that adding chemical pleurodesis to chest tube drainage reduced the rate of recurrence of spontaneous pneumothorax compared with chest tube drainage alone. One of the RCTs found that chemical pleurodesis injection was intensely painful. The RCTs found no significant difference in length of hospital stay. One RCT found that thoracoscopic surgery with talcum powder instillation reduced the rate of recurrence at 5 years compared with chest tube drainage. Two RCTs provided insufficient evidence to compare video assisted thoracoscopic surgery versus thoracotomy. We found no RCTs comparing chemical versus surgical pleurodesis.

UNKNOWN EFFECTIVENESS

Optimal timing of pleurodesis (after first, second, or subsequent episodes)

We found no RCTs or high quality cohort studies assessing whether pleurodesis should take place after the first, second, or subsequent episodes of spontaneous pneumothorax.

DEFINITION A pneumothorax is air in the pleural space. A **spontaneous pneumothorax** occurs when there is no provoking factor, such as trauma, surgery, or diagnostic intervention. It implies a leak of air from the lung parenchyma through the visceral pleura into the pleural space, which causes the lung to collapse and results in pain and shortness of breath. This review does not include people with **tension pneumothorax**.

INCIDENCE/ PREVALENCE In a survey in Minnesota, USA, the incidence of spontaneous pneumothorax was 7/100 000 for men and 1/100 000 for women.[1] In England and Wales, the overall rate of people consulting with pneumothorax (in both primary and secondary care combined) is 24/100 000 a year for men and 9.8/100 000 a year for women.[2] The overall annual incidence of emergency hospital admissions for pneumothorax in England and Wales is 16.7/100 000 for men and 5.8/100 000 for women.[2] Smoking increases the likelihood of spontaneous pneumothorax by 22 times for men and 8 times for women. The incidence is directly related to the amount smoked.[3]

AETIOLOGY/ RISK FACTORS Primary spontaneous pneumothorax is thought to result from congenital abnormality of the visceral pleura and is typically seen in young, otherwise fit people. Secondary spontaneous pneumothorax is caused by underlying lung disease, typically affecting older people with emphysema or pulmonary fibrosis.[4]

PROGNOSIS Death from spontaneous pneumothorax is rare with UK mortality of 1.26 per million a year for men and 0.62 per million a year for women.[5] Published recurrence rates vary. One cohort study in Denmark found that, after a first episode of primary spontaneous pneumothorax, 23% of people suffered a recurrence within 5 years, most of them within 1 year.[6] Recurrence rates had been thought to increase substantially after the first recurrence, but one retrospective case control study (147 US military personnel) found that 28% of men with a first primary spontaneous pneumothorax had a recurrence; 23% of the 28% had a second recurrence; and 14% of that 23% had a third recurrence, resulting in a total recurrence rate of 35%.[7]

Please refer to clinicalevidence.com for full text and references.

Asthma

Search date May 2005

Rodolfo J Dennis, Ivan Solarte, and J Mark FitzGerald

What are the effects of treatments for chronic asthma?

BENEFICIAL

Adding long acting inhaled beta$_2$ agonists in people with mild to moderate, persistent asthma that is poorly controlled by inhaled corticosteroids

RCTs found that, in people with asthma that is poorly controlled with inhaled corticosteroids, adding regular long acting inhaled beta$_2$ agonists improved symptoms and lung function compared with placebo and reduced the need for rescue medication. There was no significant difference in exacerbation rates between the two groups in any of the RCTs. One systematic review and additional RCTs found that adding regular doses of long acting inhaled beta$_2$ agonists improved lung function and symptoms, decreased exacerbation episodes, and reduced the need for rescue medication compared with increasing the dose of inhaled corticosteroids. However, one further RCT found that adding a long acting inhaled beta$_2$ agonist was less effective than increasing inhaled corticosteroid dose in reducing exacerbations. One small RCT found that adding salmeterol improved quality of life compared with doubling the dose of fluticasone. We found insufficient evidence about effects of adding long acting inhaled beta$_2$ agonists on mortality. One RCT found that salmeterol was associated with an increase in asthma related mortality, possibly by making asthma episodes more severe. This has been supported by regulatory warnings. Thus, long acting inhaled beta$_2$ agonists are not a substitute for controller medications (corticosteroids) at appropriate doses. RCTs found that adding long acting inhaled beta$_2$ agonists improved lung function compared with adding leukotriene antagonists.

Low dose, inhaled corticosteroids in mild, persistent asthma

Systematic reviews and subsequent RCTs found that, in people with mild, persistent asthma, low doses of inhaled corticosteroids improved symptoms and lung function compared with placebo or regular inhaled beta$_2$ agonists.

Short acting inhaled beta$_2$ agonists as needed for symptom relief (as effective as regular use) in mild to moderate, persistent asthma

One systematic review and one subsequent RCT found no significant difference between regular and as needed short acting inhaled beta$_2$ agonists in lung function, use of relief medication, or exacerbation rates.

LIKELY TO BE BENEFICIAL

Adding leukotriene antagonists in people with mild to moderate, persistent asthma not taking inhaled corticosteroids (likely to be better than adding no treatment, but less effective than adding inhaled corticosteroids)

RCTs in people taking beta$_2$ agonists alone found that leukotriene antagonists (zafirlukast or montelukast) reduced asthma symptoms and beta$_2$ agonist use compared with placebo. One systematic review found that adding leukotriene antagonists was generally less effective for symptom control than adding inhaled corticosteroids and led to increased exacerbations or reduced lung function. These results were not supported by three underpowered subsequent RCTs, which found no significant difference between leukotriene antagonists and inhaled corticosteroids. Two out of four RCTs found that an inhaled corticosteroid plus a long acting $beta_2$ agonist improved symptoms, lung function, and decreased exacerbations compared with a leukotriene antagonist alone at 12 weeks.

Adding theophylline in people with mild to moderate, persistent asthma poorly controlled by inhaled corticosteroids

One RCT found that adding theophylline improved peak expiratory flow rate compared with continuing low dose corticosteroids plus placebo after 6 months in people with mild to moderate, persistent asthma that was poorly controlled with inhaled corticosteroids alone. One small RCT found no significant difference in lung function or symptoms between theophylline and formoterol (a long acting $beta_2$ agonist) or between theophylline and zafirlukast (a leukotriene antagonist) after 3 months.

UNKNOWN EFFECTIVENESS

Adding leukotriene antagonists to inhaled corticosteroids in people with mild to moderate, persistent asthma

One systematic review in people taking inhaled corticosteroids found no significant difference between leukotriene antagonists and placebo for exacerbation rates at 4–16 weeks. However, one subsequent RCT in people taking a stable dose of budesonide found that adding montelukast increased asthma free days and decreased nocturnal waking compared with placebo at 16 weeks. One RCT in people taking inhaled corticosteroids found no significant difference between adding montelukast and doubling the dose of budesonide in peak expiratory flow rate, daytime symptoms, nocturnal wakening, days with asthma exacerbations, or quality of life.

What are the effects of treatments for acute asthma?

BENEFICIAL

Controlled oxygen supplementation (28% oxygen better than 100% oxygen)

One RCT found that 28% oxygen increased lung function in people with acute asthma compared with 100% oxygen.

Education about acute asthma

One systematic review and four subsequent RCTs provided evidence that education to facilitate self management of asthma in adults reduced hospital admission, unscheduled visits to the doctor, and days off work compared with usual care. The RCTs provided insufficient evidence about effects of asthma education on quality of life or social functioning at 6 months.

Inhaled corticosteroids

One systematic review found that inhaled corticosteroids given in the emergency department reduced hospital admission rates in adults compared with placebo. One systematic review and one subsequent RCT found no significant difference in relapse rates after emergency department discharge between oral and inhaled steroids at 7–10 days. One systematic review found no significant difference in relapse rates between inhaled plus oral corticosteroids and oral corticosteroids alone up to 24 days. One RCT showed that the addition of inhaled corticosteroids to salbutamol and ipratropium bromide improved lung function but had no significant effect on hospital admissions.

Asthma

Inhaled plus oral corticosteroid for acute asthma (as effective as oral corticosteroid alone)

One systematic review found no significant difference in relapse rates for inhaled plus oral corticosteroid compared with oral corticosteroids alone at up to 24 days.

Ipratropium bromide added to beta$_2$ agonists

Two systematic reviews and one subsequent RCT found that ipratropium bromide plus salbutamol improved lung function compared with salbutamol alone and was likely to reduce hospital admission in people with severe acute asthma. One RCT found that adding ipratropium bromide to beta$_2$ agonists plus flunisolide improved lung function at 3 hours.

Short courses of systemic corticosteroids

Two systematic reviews and one subsequent RCT found that early treatment with systemic corticosteroids reduced admission and relapse rates compared with placebo in people with acute asthma. One subsequent RCT found no significant difference in relapse rates between oral and intramuscular corticosteroids after discharge. One systematic review and one small subsequent RCT found no significant difference between oral and inhaled steroids after emergency department discharge in relapse rates at 7–10 days in adults with acute asthma.

Spacer devices for delivering beta$_2$ agonists from pressurised metered dose inhalers (as good as nebulisers)

One systematic review in people with acute, but not life threatening exacerbations of asthma found no significant difference between beta$_2$ agonists delivered by spacer device compared with nebulisers in rates of hospital admission, time spent in the emergency department, peak expiratory flow rate, or forced expiratory volume in 1 second.

LIKELY TO BE BENEFICIAL

Adding isotonic nebulised magnesium to inhaled salbutamol

One systematic review found that isotonic nebulised magnesium sulphate plus salbutamol improved lung function compared with beta$_2$ agonists.

Continuous nebulised short acting beta$_2$ agonists (more effective than intermittent nebulised short acting beta$_2$ agonists)

One systematic review found that continuous nebulised short acting beta$_2$ agonists reduced admission rates and improved pulmonary function in adults with severe acute asthma compared with intermittent nebulised short acting beta$_2$ agonists.

Magnesium sulphate (intravenous) for people with severe acute asthma (better than placebo)

We found limited evidence from one systematic review and one subsequent RCT that intravenous magnesium improved lung function compared with placebo in people with severe acute asthma. One subsequent RCT found that intravenous magnesium did not improve lung function compared with placebo. The review and three subsequent RCTs found no significant difference between intravenous magnesium sulphate and placebo for hospital admission rates.

Mechanical ventilation for people with severe acute asthma*

We found no RCTs comparing mechanical ventilation with or without inhaled beta$_2$ agonists versus no mechanical ventilation in people with severe acute asthma. Evidence from cohort studies support its use, although observational studies suggest that ventilation is associated with a high level of morbidity.

Specialist care (more effective than generalist care)

One systematic review and one subsequent RCT found limited evidence that specialist care improved outcomes in people with acute asthma compared with generalist care.

*Categorisation based on consensus. RCTs are unlikely to be conducted.

UNKNOWN EFFECTIVENESS

Magnesium sulphate alone versus $beta_2$ agonists

One RCT provided insufficient data to compare magnesium sulfate alone versus $beta_2$ agonists.

UNLIKELY TO BE BENEFICIAL

Helium–oxygen mixture

One systematic review found no significant difference between helium–oxygen mixture and air or oxygen in pulmonary function tests at 60 minutes for adults and children.

Intravenous short acting $beta_2$ agonists (no more effective than nebulised short acting $beta_2$ agonists)

One systematic review found that intravenous delivery of short acting $beta_2$ agonists was no more effective than nebulised delivery in improving peak expiratory flow rate at 60 minutes. Intravenous delivery is more invasive than nebulised delivery.

DEFINITION Asthma is characterised by variable airflow obstruction and airway hyperresponsiveness. Symptoms include dyspnoea, cough, chest tightness, and wheezing. The normal diurnal variation of peak expiratory flow rate is increased in people with asthma. **Chronic asthma** is defined here as asthma requiring maintenance treatment. Asthma is classified differently in the USA and UK (see table 1)Ⓣ. Where necessary, the text specifies the system of classification used.[1,2] **Acute asthma** is defined here as an exacerbation of underlying asthma requiring urgent treatment.

INCIDENCE/ PREVALENCE Reported prevalence of asthma is increasing worldwide. About 10% of people have suffered an attack of asthma.[3-5] Epidemiological studies have also found marked variations in prevalence in different countries.[6,7]

AETIOLOGY/ RISK FACTORS Most people with asthma are atopic. Exposure to certain stimuli initiates inflammation and structural changes in airways causing airway hyperresponsiveness and variable airflow obstruction, which in turn cause most asthma symptoms. There are a large number of such stimuli; the more important include environmental allergens, occupational sensitising agents, and respiratory viral infections.[8,9]

PROGNOSIS **Chronic asthma:** In people with mild asthma, prognosis is good and progression to severe disease is rare. However, as a group, people with asthma lose lung function faster than those without asthma, although less quickly than people without asthma who smoke.[10] People with chronic asthma can improve with treatment. However, some people (possibly up to 5%) have severe disease that responds poorly to treatment. These people are most at risk of morbidity and death from asthma. **Acute asthma:** About 10–20% of people presenting to the emergency department with asthma are admitted to hospital. Of these, fewer than 10% receive mechanical ventilation.[11,12] Those who are ventilated are at 19-fold increased risk of ventilation for a subsequent episode.[13] It is unusual for people to die unless they have suffered respiratory arrest before they reach hospital.[14] One prospective study of 939 people discharged from emergency care found that 106/641 (17%, 95% CI 14% to 20%) relapsed by 2 weeks.[15]

Please refer to clinicalevidence.com for full text and references.

Bronchiectasis

Search date June 2005

Nick ten Hacken, Huib Kerstjens, and Dirkje Postma

What are the effects of treatments in people with bronchiectasis but without cystic fibrosis?

LIKELY TO BE BENEFICIAL

Exercise or physical training

One systematic review of two small RCTs found that inspiratory muscle training improved quality of life and exercise endurance compared with no intervention in people with non-cystic fibrosis bronchiectasis. We found no other types of exercise or physical training and no RCTs comparing exercise versus other treatments in people with non-cystic fibrosis bronchiectasis.

UNKNOWN EFFECTIVENESS

Anticholinergic therapy

One systematic review identified no RCTs comparing anticholinergic therapy versus placebo or other treatments in people with non-cystic fibrosis bronchiectasis.

Bronchopulmonary hygiene physical therapy

One systematic review found no high quality RCTs of bronchopulmonary hygiene physical therapy in people with non-cystic fibrosis bronchiectasis.

Hyperosmolar agents (inhaled)

One systematic review found no high quality RCTs of inhaled hyperosmolar agents in people with non-cystic fibrosis bronchiectasis.

Leukotriene receptor antagonists

One systematic review identified no RCTs comparing leukotriene receptor antagonists versus placebo or other treatments in people with non-cystic fibrosis bronchiectasis.

Long acting $beta_2$ agonists

One systematic review identified no RCTs comparing long acting $beta_2$ agonists versus placebo or other treatments in people with non-cystic fibrosis bronchiectasis.

Methyl-xanthines (oral)

One systematic review identified no RCTs comparing oral methyl-xanthines versus placebo or other active treatments in people with non-cystic fibrosis bronchiectasis.

Mucolytics (bromhexine or deoxyribonuclease)

One systematic review found insufficient evidence from three RCTs to compare the effects of bromhexine or recombinant human deoxyribonuclease versus placebo in people with non-cystic fibrosis bronchiectasis. We found no RCTs comparing mucolytics versus other treatments in people with non-cystic fibrosis bronchiectasis.

BMJ Clin Evid Concise 2006;16:607–608.

Bronchiectasis

Short acting beta$_2$ agonists

One systematic review identified no RCTs comparing short acting beta$_2$ agonists versus placebo or other treatments in people with non-cystic fibrosis bronchiectasis.

Steroids (inhaled)

One systematic review found insufficient evidence from two small RCTs to compare inhaled steroids versus placebo in people with bronchiectasis not due to a specific congenital disease. One subsequent RCT found that fluticasone improved 24 hour sputum volume at 12 months compared with placebo but found no significant difference between groups in exacerbations or lung function.

Steroids (oral)

One systematic review found no RCTs comparing oral steroids versus placebo, no treatment, or other treatments in people with non-cystic fibrosis bronchiectasis.

Surgery

One systematic review found no RCTs comparing surgery versus non-surgical treatment for non-cystic fibrosis bronchiectasis.

DEFINITION Bronchiectasis is defined as irreversible widening of medium sized airways (bronchi) in the lung. It is characterised by inflammation, destruction of bronchial walls, and chronic bacterial infection. The condition may be limited to a single lobe or lung segment, or it may affect one or both lungs more diffusely. Clinically, the condition manifests as chronic cough and chronic overproduction of sputum (up to about 500 mL/day), which is often purulent.[1] People with severe bronchiectasis may have life threatening haemoptysis and may develop features of chronic obstructive airways disease, such as wheezing, chronic respiratory failure, pulmonary hypertension, and right sided heart failure.

INCIDENCE/ PREVALENCE We found few reliable data. Incidence has declined over the past 50 years and prevalence is low in higher income countries. Prevalence is much higher in poorer countries and is a major cause of morbidity and mortality.

AETIOLOGY/ RISK FACTORS Bronchiectasis is most commonly a long term complication of previous lower respiratory infections such as measles pneumonitis, pertussis, and tuberculosis. Foreign body inhalation and allergic, autoimmune, and chemical lung damage also predispose to the condition.[2] Underlying congenital disorders such as cystic fibrosis, cilial dysmotility syndromes, alpha$_1$ antitrypsin deficiency, and congenital immunodeficiencies may also predispose to bronchiectasis and may be of greater aetiological importance than respiratory infection in higher income countries. Cystic fibrosis is the most common congenital cause. This chapter does not deal with bronchiectasis in people with cystic fibrosis.

PROGNOSIS Bronchiectasis is a chronic condition with frequent relapses of varying severity. Long term prognosis is variable. Data on morbidity and mortality are sparse.[3] Bronchiectasis frequently coexists with other respiratory disease, making it difficult to distinguish prognosis for bronchiectasis alone.

Please refer to clinicalevidence.com for full text and references.

Chronic obstructive pulmonary disease

Search date March 2005

Huib Kerstjens, Dirkje Postma, and Nick ten Hacken

What are the effects of maintenance drug treatment in stable chronic obstructive pulmonary disorder?

BENEFICIAL

Inhaled anticholinergics (improved exacerbation rate, symptoms, and FEV_1 compared with placebo)

RCTs found that inhaled anticholinergics improved forced expiratory volume in 1 second, exercise capacity, and symptoms compared with placebo. One large RCT found that adding ipratropium to a smoking cessation programme had no significant impact on decline in forced expiratory volume in 1 second over 5 years compared with the smoking cessation programme alone. RCTs identified by a systematic review found that inhaled tiotropium (a long acting anticholinergic drug) improved exacerbation rates, health related quality of life, and forced expiratory volume in 1 second compared with placebo or ipratropium.

Inhaled anticholinergics plus $beta_2$ agonists (improved FEV_1 compared with either drug alone)

A systematic review found that combining a short acting $beta_2$ agonist with an anticholinergic drug (ipratropium) for 12 weeks improved exacerbations compared with the $beta_2$ agonist alone but not ipratropium alone. One RCT found that combining a long acting $beta_2$ agonist with an anticholinergic drug did not improve symptoms but modestly improved some measures of lung function compared with the long acting $beta_2$ agonist alone. One RCT found that, when combined with an anticholinergic drug, a long acting $beta_2$ agonist improved forced expiratory volume in 1 second and peak expiratory flow more than a short acting $beta_2$ agonist. We found no RCTs of long term treatment comparing anticholinergics plus $beta_2$ agonists with placebo.

Inhaled $beta_2$ agonists (improved FEV_1, quality of life and exacerbation rates compared with placebo)

RCTs found that treatment with inhaled $beta_2$ agonists for 1 week to 12 months improved forced expiratory volume in 1 second compared with placebo. A systematic review and RCTs found that long acting $beta_2$ agonists for 12–52 weeks improved quality of life and exacerbation rates compared with placebo.

Inhaled corticosteroids plus long acting $beta_2$ agonists (improved exacerbation rate, symptoms, quality of life, FEV_1 compared with placebo)

RCTs found that the combination of an inhaled corticosteroid plus a long acting $beta_2$ agonist reduced exacerbation rates and improved lung function, symptoms, and health related quality of life compared with placebo in people with moderate to severe disease. In general, the combination was more effective than inhaled corticosteroid alone or long acting $beta_2$ agonist alone, although this difference was not significant for all outcomes.

LIKELY TO BE BENEFICIAL

Inhaled anticholinergics compared with $beta_2$ agonists (improved FEV_1 compared with $beta_2$ agonists in long term)

RCTs found inconsistent evidence about the effects of short acting inhaled anticholinergics compared with long acting $beta_2$ agonists for up to 3 months. ▶

BMJ Clin Evid Concise 2006;16:609–612.

Chronic obstructive pulmonary disease

Two RCTs identified by a systematic review found that 6 months of a long acting inhaled anticholinergic improved forced expiratory volume in 1 second compared with a long acting inhaled $beta_2$ agonist. The RCTs found mixed results for health related quality of life and one of the RCTs found no significant difference between a long acting inhaled anticholinergic and a long acting inhaled $beta_2$ agonist in quality of life or exacerbation rates at 6 months.

Long term domiciliary oxygen (beneficial in people with severe hypoxaemia)

One RCT in people with severe daytime hypoxaemia found that domiciliary oxygen improved survival compared with no domiciliary oxygen. A second RCT in people with severe hypoxaemia found that continuous oxygen reduced mortality compared with nocturnal oxygen. Three RCTs in people with milder hypoxaemia or with nocturnal hypoxaemia only, found no significant difference in mortality between long term domiciliary oxygen and no oxygen.

TRADE OFF BETWEEN BENEFITS AND HARMS

Inhaled corticosteroids (improved exacerbation rates, but may have long term harms)

RCTs found no significant difference between inhaled corticosteroids and placebo in lung function (forced expiratory volume in 1 second) over 10 days to 10 weeks. One systematic review and one subsequent RCT found no significant difference in decline in forced expiratory volume in 1 second between inhaled corticosteroids and placebo after 24 months. However, a second systematic review that examined effects of high dose inhaled corticosteroids and four subsequent RCTs found that inhaled corticosteroids slightly reduced the decline in forced expiratory volume in 1 second compared with placebo after 12–24 months. Two systematic reviews and one subsequent RCT found that long term inhaled steroids reduced the frequency of exacerbations compared with placebo. Two subsequent RCTs found no significant difference in exacerbation rates. Long term inhaled steroids may predispose to adverse effects, including skin bruising and oral candidiasis.

Theophyllines

One systematic review found that theophyllines slightly improved forced expiratory volume in 1 second compared with placebo after 3 months. One large RCT found that theophyllines improved forced expiratory volume in 1 second compared with placebo after 12 months' treatment. The usefulness of these drugs is limited by adverse effects and the need for frequent monitoring of blood concentrations.

UNKNOWN EFFECTIVENESS

$Alpha_1$ antitrypsin

One RCT in people with $alpha_1$ antitrypsin deficiency and moderate emphysema found no significant difference between $alpha_1$ antitrypsin infusion and placebo in the decline in forced expiratory volume in 1 second after 1 year.

Mucolytics

Two systematic reviews in chronic bronchitis found limited evidence that mucolytics for 3–24 months reduced the frequency and duration of exacerbations compared with placebo. Two RCTs in chronic obstructive pulmonary disease found no significant difference in decline in forced expiratory volume in 1 second and exacerbations.

Prophylactic antibiotics

One systematic review found limited evidence of a small reduction in exacerbation rates and days with disability with prophylactic antibiotics. These benefits probably do not outweigh the harms of antibiotics, especially the development of antibiotic resistance. All of the identified RCTs were conducted more than 30 years ago, and the results are unlikely to apply to current practice.

UNLIKELY TO BE BENEFICIAL

Oral corticosteroids (evidence of harm but no evidence of long term benefits)

We found no RCTs on long term benefits. One systematic review found that treatment with oral corticosteroids for 2–4 weeks improved forced expiratory volume in 1 second compared with placebo. Long term systemic corticosteroids are associated with serious adverse effects, including osteoporosis and diabetes.

What are the effects of non-drug interventions in stable chronic obstructive pulmonary disease?

BENEFICIAL

Psychosocial plus pharmacological interventions for smoking cessation

One large RCT in people with mild chronic obstructive pulmonary disease found that nicotine gum plus a psychosocial smoking cessation and abstinence maintenance programme (with or without ipratropium) slowed the decline of forced expiratory volume in 1 second, and reduced respiratory symptoms and lower respiratory illnesses, but increased weight gain compared with usual care (without psychosocial intervention). The RCT found no significant difference between treatments in all cause mortality at 5 years, but it found that smoking cessation reduced all cause mortality compared with usual care at 14.5 years.

Pulmonary rehabilitation

Two systematic reviews found that multi-modality pulmonary rehabilitation improved quality of life, maximal exercise capacity, and functional exercise capacity.

LIKELY TO BE BENEFICIAL

General physical activity

One systematic review found that general physical activity enhancement (walking, cycling, or swimming) improved exercise tolerance compared with control. It found no consistent evidence of a difference in quality of life and dyspnoea.

Inspiratory muscle training

One systematic review found that inspiratory muscle training improved inspiratory muscle strength and endurance, and dyspnoea at rest and during exercise compared with control, but it found no significant difference in exercise capacity between groups. The review found that adding inspiratory muscle training to general exercise reconditioning improved inspiratory muscle strength and endurance, but did not have any additional beneficial effects on exercise capacity.

Peripheral muscle training

One systematic review found that peripheral muscle training improved upper body and leg strength compared with no treatment or other exercise training. It found that pulmonary function, maximal exercise capacity, walking endurance, cycling endurance, and psychological wellbeing were similar in both groups.

UNKNOWN EFFECTIVENESS

Pharmacological interventions alone for smoking cessation

One systematic review found no RCTs of pharmacological interventions alone for smoking cessation in people with chronic obstructive pulmonary disease.

Psychosocial interventions alone for smoking cessation

We found no systematic review or RCTs of psychosocial interventions alone for smoking cessation in people with chronic obstructive pulmonary disease.

UNLIKELY TO BE BENEFICIAL

Nutritional supplementation

Two systematic reviews found no consistent evidence that nutritional supplementation improves lung function or exercise capacity in people with stable chronic obstructive pulmonary disease.

DEFINITION Chronic obstructive pulmonary disease (COPD) is a disease state characterised by airflow limitation that is not fully reversible. The airflow limitation is usually both progressive and associated with an abnormal inflammatory response of the lungs to noxious particles or gases.[1] Classically, it has been thought to be a combination of emphysema and chronic bronchitis, although only one of these may be present in some people with COPD. Emphysema is abnormal permanent enlargement of the air spaces distal to the terminal bronchioles, accompanied by destruction of their walls and without obvious fibrosis. Chronic bronchitis is chronic cough or mucus production for at least 3 months in at least 2 successive years when other causes of chronic cough have been excluded.[2]

INCIDENCE/ PREVALENCE COPD mainly affects middle aged and elderly people. In 1998, the World Health Organization estimated that COPD was the fifth most common cause of death worldwide, responsible for 4.8% of all mortality (estimated 2 745 816 deaths in 2002),[3] and morbidity is increasing. Estimated prevalence in the USA rose by 41% between 1982 and 1994 and age adjusted death rates rose by 71% between 1966 and 1985. All cause age adjusted mortality declined over the same period by 22% and mortality from cardiovascular diseases by 45%.[2] In the UK, physician diagnosed prevalence was 2% in men and 1% in women between 1990 and 1997.[4]

AETIOLOGY/ RISK FACTORS COPD is largely preventable. The main cause in developed countries is exposure to tobacco smoke. In developed countries, 85–90% of people with COPD have smoked at some point.[1] The disease is rare in lifelong non-smokers (estimated prevalence 5% in 3 large representative US surveys of non-smokers from 1971–1984), in whom "passive" exposure to environmental tobacco smoke has been proposed as a cause.[5,6] Other proposed causes include bronchial hyperresponsiveness, indoor and outdoor air pollution, and allergy.[7-9]

PROGNOSIS Airway obstruction is usually progressive in those who continue to smoke, resulting in early disability and shortened survival. Smoking cessation reverts the rate of decline in lung function to that of non-smokers.[10] Many people will need medication for the rest of their lives, with increased doses and additional drugs during exacerbations.

Please refer to clinicalevidence.com for full text and references.

Lung cancer

Search date September 2005

Alan Neville

What are the effects of treatment for resectable non-small cell lung cancer?

LIKELY TO BE BENEFICIAL

Postoperative chemotherapy (cisplatin based or uracil plus tegafur based regimens) in resected stage 1–3 non-small cell lung cancer

One systematic review and two subsequent RCTs found that postoperative cisplatin based regimens and uracil plus tegafur regimens improved survival compared with surgery alone. A third subsequent RCT found no significant difference in survival with uracil plus tegafur compared with no further treatment. RCTs found that chemotherapy was associated with more toxic effects than no chemotherapy, including a small risk of treatment related death.

UNKNOWN EFFECTIVENESS

Preoperative chemotherapy in resectable non-small cell lung cancer

One systematic review of small, weak RCTs and one subsequent RCT provided inconclusive evidence about the effects of preoperative chemotherapy in people with resectable non-small cell lung cancer.

What are the effects of treatments for unresectable non-small cell lung cancer?

BENEFICIAL

Palliative chemotherapy in unresectable and metastatic non-small cell lung cancer (improves survival compared with supportive care)

Systematic reviews and one subsequent RCT in people with unresectable and metastatic non-small cell lung cancer found that adding chemotherapy regimens containing cisplatin to supportive care increased survival at 1 year compared with supportive care alone. RCTs provided limited evidence that chemotherapy plus best supportive care may improve quality of life compared with best supportive care alone. Many studies found that chemotherapy was associated with adverse effects.

Thoracic irradiation plus chemotherapy (compared with thoracic irradiation alone)

Systematic reviews and subsequent RCTs in people with unresectable stage 3 non-small cell lung cancer found that adding chemotherapy to irradiation improved survival at 2–5 years compared with irradiation alone. One subsequent RCT found no significant difference in median survival between radical radiotherapy plus chemotherapy and radiotherapy alone. One subsequent RCT suggested that concurrent chemoradiotherapy increased survival compared with sequential chemoradiotherapy. Observational evidence suggests that, in people aged over 70 years with unresectable stage 3 non-small cell lung cancer, chemotherapy plus radiotherapy may reduce quality adjusted survival compared with radiotherapy alone. We found insufficient evidence about effects on quality of life.

Lung cancer

UNKNOWN EFFECTIVENESS

Different palliative chemotherapy regimens in unresectable and metastatic non-small cell lung cancer (relative benefits of different regimens unclear)

One systematic review found that two drug chemotherapy improved survival compared with single drug chemotherapy. One subsequent RCT found that paclitaxel plus carboplatin improved response but not overall survival compared with paclitaxel alone. One systematic review provided inconclusive evidence on the effects of single agent non-platinum based chemotherapy compared with combination platinum based first line treatment. In people previously treated with platinum chemotherapy, one RCT identified by a systematic review and one subsequent RCT found that adding docetaxel to supportive care improved survival at 1 year and reduced pain. One RCT found that second line docetaxel improved survival compared with vinorelbine or ifosfamide. RCTs found no significant difference in survival between second line docetaxel and pemetrexed or docetaxel plus irinotecan. Many studies found that chemotherapy was associated with adverse effects.

Hyperfractionated radiotherapy in unresectable stage 3 non-small cell lung cancer

One systematic review found no clear evidence that altered fractionation regimens, accelerated, hyperfractionated, or hyperfractionated split course regimens were more effective than conventional radiotherapy, whether or not people also received chemotherapy. One RCT identified by the review found that continuous, hyperfractionated, accelerated radiotherapy reduced mortality at 2 years compared with conventional radiotherapy in people with stage 1, 2, 3A, or 3B non-small cell lung cancer.

What are the effects of treatments for small cell lung cancer?

BENEFICIAL

Thoracic irradiation plus chemotherapy in limited stage small cell lung cancer (improves survival compared with chemotherapy alone)

Two systematic reviews in people with limited stage small cell lung cancer found that adding thoracic irradiation to chemotherapy improved survival at 3 years and local control compared with chemotherapy alone. However, one of these reviews found that chemotherapy plus thoracic irradiation increased treatment related death compared with chemotherapy alone. One systematic review found no significant difference in survival at 2 years between early and late chest radiotherapy.

LIKELY TO BE BENEFICIAL

Prophylactic cranial irradiation for people in complete remission from limited or extensive stage small cell lung cancer

One systematic review in people with small cell lung cancer in complete remission found that prophylactic cranial irradiation improved survival at 3 years and reduced the risk of developing brain metastases compared with no irradiation. Although long term cognitive dysfunction after cranial irradiation has been described in non-randomised studies, RCTs did not find a cumulative increase in neuropsychological dysfunction.

UNKNOWN EFFECTIVENESS

Dose intensification of chemotherapy

Two systematic reviews and additional RCTs provided no clear evidence that intensifying chemotherapy increased survival. Two RCTs found that dose intensive chemotherapy increased deaths related to toxicity compared with standard chemotherapy.

DEFINITION Lung cancer (bronchogenic carcinoma) is an epithelial cancer arising from the bronchial surface epithelium or bronchial mucous glands. It is broadly divided into small cell (about 25% of all lung cancers) and non-small cell lung cancer (about 75% of all lung cancers). For a description of the stages of lung cancer see table 1 Ⓣ.[1,2]

INCIDENCE/ PREVALENCE Lung cancer is the leading cause of cancer death in both men and women annually, affecting about 100 000 men and 80 000 women in the USA and about 40 000 men and women in the UK. Small cell lung cancer constitutes about 20–25% of all lung cancers, the remainder being non-small cell lung cancers of which adenocarcinoma is now the most prevalent form.[3]

AETIOLOGY/ RISK FACTORS Smoking remains the major preventable risk factor, accounting for about 80–90% of all cases.[4] Other respiratory tract carcinogens have been identified that may enhance the carcinogenic effects of tobacco smoke, either in the workplace (e.g. asbestos and polycyclic aromatic hydrocarbons) or in the home (e.g. indoor radon).[5]

PROGNOSIS At the time of diagnosis, 10–15% of people with lung cancer have localised disease. Of these, half will have died at 5 years despite potentially curative surgery. Over half of people have metastatic disease at the time of diagnosis. Surgery is the treatment of choice in people with stage 1 and stage 2 non-small cell lung cancer, unless they are not well enough to have surgery. People with stage 1A disease have an excellent overall survival with surgery alone. Complete resection of the cancer with or without chemotherapy and radiotherapy may be performed in some people with locally advanced stage 3 disease, but the disease is inoperable in others and they have a poorer prognosis. People with inoperable stage 3 or metastatic disease can be offered palliative chemotherapy. See table 1 Ⓣ for 5 year survival in non-small cell lung cancer (estimates include both treated and untreated people).[2] Chemotherapy is the mainstay of treatment in the 25% of people with small cell lung cancer, which has a high risk of metastases. See table 1 Ⓣ for median survival in small cell lung cancer.[6] About 5–10% of people with small cell lung cancer present with central nervous system involvement, and half develop symptomatic brain metastases by 2 years. Of these, only half respond to palliative radiotherapy, and their median survival is less than 3 months.[1]

Please refer to clinicalevidence.com for full text and references.

Bacterial vaginosis

Search date March 2004

M Riduan Joesoef and George Schmid

What are the effects of different antibacterial regimens in non-pregnant women with symptomatic bacterial vaginosis on cure rates and symptom relief?

BENEFICIAL

Antibacterial treatment with metronidazole or clindamycin (short term benefit)

One systematic review found that more women having antibacterial treatment (intravaginal clindamycin cream or intravaginal metronidazole gel) achieved cure than women using placebo. One systematic review found no significant difference in cure rates or adverse effects at 5–10 days or 4 weeks between intravaginal clindamycin and oral metronidazole. However, comparison of results across RCTs found that yeast vulvovaginitis may be less common with intravaginal clindamycin than with oral metronidazole. Intravaginal clindamycin has been associated, rarely, with mild to severe colitis and vaginal candidiasis in non-pregnant women. Another systematic review found that a 7 day course of twice daily oral metronidazole increased cure rates compared with a single 2 g dose; it gave no information on adverse effects. Limited evidence from RCTs found no significant difference in cure rates between oral clindamycin and oral metronidazole, and found that both treatments were associated with nausea and metallic taste. One RCT found no significant difference in cure rates at 35 days between 3 day treatment with intravaginal clindamycin ovules and 7 day treatment with intravaginal clindamycin cream. It found that the proportion of people who had adverse effects was similar in both groups, but ovules were associated with a higher incidence of vaginal pain and headache, and cream with a higher incidence of flu syndrome. Another RCT found no significant difference in cure rates or adverse effects between once and twice daily dosing with intravaginal metronidazole gel. We found no evidence on long term outcomes. One small RCT suggested that more than 50% of women had recurrent bacterial vaginosis 2 months after antibacterial treatment.

What are the effects of antibacterial treatments in pregnant women to reduce adverse outcomes of pregnancy and prevent neonatal complications?

LIKELY TO BE BENEFICIAL

Antibacterial treatment (except intravaginal clindamycin) in pregnant women who have had a previous preterm birth

One systematic review found that antibiotics reduced the risk of low birth weight in women with bacterial vaginosis who had a previous preterm delivery, although results for preterm delivery varied widely between trials. One subsequent RCT found that oral clindamycin given early in the second trimester reduced miscarriages or preterm deliveries compared with placebo in women with previous late miscarriage or preterm delivery.

UNKNOWN EFFECTIVENESS

Antibacterial treatment in low risk pregnancy

One systematic review in general populations of pregnant women found no significant difference between antibiotics (oral or vaginal) and placebo or no treatment in the risk of preterm delivery, low birth weight, neonatal sepsis, or perinatal death. However, subsequent RCTs in women with bacterial vaginosis or abnormal genital tract flora (may or may not have included bacterial vaginosis) found that oral or intravaginal clindamycin given early in the second trimester reduced miscarriages or preterm deliveries compared with placebo.

LIKELY TO BE INEFFECTIVE OR HARMFUL

Intravaginal clindamycin cream

In studies that assessed women regardless of previous preterm delivery, three RCTs found a non-significant increase in preterm birth and low birth weight in women with bacterial vaginosis treated with clindamycin cream compared with placebo. However, one subsequent RCT found limited evidence in women with abnormal genital tract flora (may or may not have included bacterial vaginosis) that intravaginal clindamycin cream given early in the second trimester reduced preterm birth compared with placebo.

Does treating male partners prevent recurrence?

LIKELY TO BE INEFFECTIVE OR HARMFUL

Treating a woman's male sexual partner with metronidazole or clindamycin (did not reduce the woman's risk of recurrence)

One systematic review found that in women receiving antibacterial agents, and who have one steady male sexual partner, treating the partner with an oral antibacterial agent did not reduce the woman's risk of recurrence.

What are the effects of treatment before gynaecological procedures?

LIKELY TO BE BENEFICIAL

Oral or intravaginal antibacterial treatment before surgical abortion

Three RCTs found a lower rate of post operative pelvic inflammatory disease with oral or intravaginal antibacterial treatment compared with placebo given to women with bacterial vaginosis who were about to have surgical abortion, but the difference was significant only in the largest RCT. The RCTs gave no information on adverse effects. In RCTs in non-pregnant women with bacterial vaginosis, intravaginal clindamycin was associated, rarely, with mild to severe colitis and vaginal candidiasis. Oral metronidazole was associated with nausea and metallic taste.

UNKNOWN EFFECTIVENESS

Antibacterial treatment before gynaecological procedures other than abortion

We found no RCTs on the effects of antibacterial treatment in women with bacterial vaginosis about to have gynaecological procedures other than abortion.

Bacterial vaginosis

DEFINITION Bacterial vaginosis is a microbial disease characterised by a change in the bacterial flora of the vagina from mainly *Lactobacillus* species to high concentrations of anaerobic bacteria. The condition is asymptomatic in 50% of infected women. Women with symptoms have an excessive white to grey, or malodorous vaginal discharge, or both; the odour may be particularly noticeable during sexual intercourse. Commonly practised clinical diagnosis requires three out of four features: the presence of clue cells on microscopy; a homogenous discharge adherent to the vaginal walls; pH of vaginal fluid greater than 4.5; and a "fishy" amine odour of the vaginal discharge before or after addition of 10% potassium hydroxide. Some experts prefer other methods of diagnosis, (e.g. Gram stain of vaginal secretions), particularly in a research setting. Gram stain using Nugent's criteria[1] categorise the flora of vagina into three categories – normal, intermediate, and flora consistent with bacterial vaginosis. Abnormal vaginal flora includes intermediate flora and bacterial vaginosis.

INCIDENCE/ PREVALENCE Bacterial vaginosis is the most common infectious cause of vaginitis, being about twice as common as candidiasis.[2] Prevalences of 10–61% have been reported among unselected women from a range of settings.[3] Data on incidence are limited but one study found that, over a 2 year period, 50% of women using an intrauterine contraceptive device had at least one episode, as did 20% of women using oral contraceptives.[4] Bacterial vaginosis is particularly prevalent among lesbians.[5]

AETIOLOGY/ RISK FACTORS The cause of bacterial vaginosis is not fully understood. Risk factors include new or multiple sexual partners[2,4,6] and early age of sexual intercourse,[7] but no causative microorganism has been shown to be transmitted between partners. Use of an intrauterine contraceptive device[4] and douching[6] have also been reported as risk factors. Infection seems to be most common around the time of menstruation.[8]

PROGNOSIS The course of bacterial vaginosis varies and is poorly understood. Without treatment, symptoms may persist or resolve in both pregnant and non-pregnant women. Recurrence after treatment occurs in about a third of women. A history of bacterial vaginosis is associated with increased rates of complications in pregnancy: low birth weight;[7] preterm birth (pooled OR from 10 cohort studies: 1.8, 95% CI 1.5 to 2.6);[9] preterm labour; premature rupture of membranes;[7] late miscarriage; chorioamnionitis;[10] endometritis after normal delivery (8.2% *v* 1.5%; OR 5.6, 95% CI 1.8 to 17.2);[11] endometritis after caesarean section (55% *v* 17%; OR 5.8, 95% CI 3.0 to 10.9);[12] and surgery to the genital tract.[13,14] Women who have had a previous preterm delivery are especially at risk of complications in pregnancy, with a sevenfold increased risk of preterm birth (24/428 [5.6%] in all women *v* 10/24 [41.7%] in women with a previous preterm birth).[15] Bacterial vaginosis can also increase the risk of HIV acquisition and transmission.[16]

Please refer to clinicalevidence.com for full text and references.

Chlamydia (uncomplicated, genital)

Search date January 2006

Nicola Low

What are the effects of antibiotic treatment in men and non-pregnant women with uncomplicated genital chlamydial infection?

BENEFICIAL

Azithromycin (single dose)

One systematic review of 12 blinded and open label RCTs found high microbiological cure rates with both a single dose of azithromycin and a 7 day course of doxycycline. The SR found no significant difference in microbiological cure of *C trachomatis* between a single dose of azithromycin and a 7 day course of doxycycline. Rates of adverse effects were similar.

Doxycycline, tetracycline (multiple dose regimens)

Multiple dose regimens of tetracyclines (doxycycline, tetracycline) achieve microbiological cure in at least 95% of people with genital chlamydia. These RCTs are mostly small, with short term follow up and high withdrawal rates. A systematic review of 12 blinded and open label RCTs found no significant difference in microbiological cure of *C trachomatis* between a 7 day course of doxycycline and a single dose of azithromycin. Rates of adverse effects were similar. Data pooling of two RCTs found that doxycycline reduced microbiological failure compared with ciprofloxacin.

LIKELY TO BE BENEFICIAL

Erythromycin (multiple dose regimens)

Three small RCTs found that erythromycin achieved microbiological cure in 77–100% of people, with the highest cure rate with a 2 g rather than a 1 g daily dose.

UNKNOWN EFFECTIVENESS

Amoxicillin, ampicillin, clarithromycin, lymecycline, minocycline, ofloxacin, pivampicillin, rifampicin, roxithromycin, sparfloxacin, trovafloxacin (multiple dose regimens)

We found limited evidence on the effects of these regimens.

UNLIKELY TO BE BENEFICIAL

Ciprofloxacin (multiple dose regimens)

Two RCTs found that ciprofloxacin cured 63–92% of people. Meta-analysis of these two RCTs found that ciprofloxacin increased microbiological failure compared with doxycycline.

Chlamydia (uncomplicated, genital)

What are the effects of treatment for pregnant women with uncomplicated genital chlamydial infection?

LIKELY TO BE BENEFICIAL

Azithromycin (single dose)

One systematic review found that a single dose of azithromycin increased microbiological cure and decreased the risk of an adverse effect sufficient to stop treatment compared with a 7 day course of erythromycin. Two subsequent open label RCTs found no significant difference in cure rates between single dose azithromycin and multiple dose amoxicillin. Azithromycin should only be used in pregnancy if no adequate alternative is available.

Erythromycin, amoxicillin (multiple dose regimens)

One small RCT identified in a systematic review found that erythromycin increased microbiological cure compared with placebo. The review found that a 7 day course of erythromycin reduced microbiological cure and increased the risk of an adverse event sufficient to stop treatment, compared with a single dose of azithromycin. Two subsequent open label RCTs found no significant difference in cure rates between multiple dose amoxicillin and single dose azithromycin. Other RCTs in the review found high cure rates with erythromycin and amoxicillin and no significant difference in microbiological cure between the two drugs.

UNKNOWN EFFECTIVENESS

Clindamycin (multiple dose regimens)

One small RCT found no significant difference in cure rates between clindamycin and erythromycin.

DEFINITION Genital chlamydia is a sexually transmitted infection of the urethra in men, and of the endocervix or urethra (or both) in women. It is defined as **uncomplicated** if it has not ascended to the upper genital tract. Infection in women is asymptomatic in up to 80% of cases, but may cause non-specific symptoms, including vaginal discharge and intermenstrual bleeding. Infection in men causes urethral discharge and urethral irritation or dysuria, but may also be asymptomatic in up to half of cases.[1] **Complicated** chlamydial infection includes spread to the upper genital tract (causing pelvic inflammatory disease in women (see pelvic inflammatory disease, p 636) and epididymo-orchitis in men) and extragenital sites, such as the eye. Interventions for complicated chlamydial infection are not included in this chapter.

INCIDENCE/ PREVALENCE Genital chlamydia is the most commonly reported bacterial sexually transmitted infection in developed countries[1] and reported rates increased by around 20% in the UK and USA between 2000 and 2002.[2,3] In women, infection occurs most commonly between the ages of 16 and 19 years. In this age group, about 1300/100 000 new infections are reported each year in the UK,[2] compared with 1900/100 000 in Sweden,[4] and 2536/100 000 in the USA.[3] The peak age group for men is 20–24 years, with about 1000/100 000 new infections a year in the UK and USA and 1200/100 000 in Sweden.[2-4] Rates decline markedly with increasing age. Reported rates are highly dependent on the level of testing. The population prevalence of uncomplicated genital chlamydia in 16–24 year olds in the UK has been estimated to be between 2% and 6% in both men and women.[5,6]

Chlamydia (uncomplicated, genital)

AETIOLOGY/ RISK FACTORS Infection is caused by the bacterium *C trachomatis* serotypes D–K. It is transmitted primarily through sexual intercourse, but also perinatally and through direct or indirect oculogenital contact.[1]

PROGNOSIS In women, untreated chlamydial infection that ascends to the upper genital tract causes pelvic inflammatory disease (see pelvic inflammatory disease, p 636).[7] Tubal infertility has been found to occur in about 11% of women after a single episode of pelvic inflammatory disease, and the risk of ectopic pregnancy is increased six to sevenfold.[8] Ascending infection in men causes epididymitis, but evidence that this causes male infertility is limited.[9] Maternal to infant transmission can lead to neonatal conjunctivitis and pneumonitis.[1] Chlamydia may coexist with other genital infections and may facilitate transmission and acquisition of HIV infection.[1] Untreated chlamydial infection persists in most women for at least 60 days and for a shorter period in men.[10] Spontaneous remission also occurs at an estimated rate of 5% a month.[11]

Please refer to clinicalevidence.com for full text and references.

Genital herpes

Search date December 2004

Eva Jungmann

What are the effects of interventions to prevent sexual transmission of herpes simplex virus?

LIKELY TO BE BENEFICIAL

Antiviral treatment of infected sexual partner (reduced transmission to uninfected partner)

One RCT found that daily use of valaciclovir reduced the risk of transmission of herpes simplex virus-2 to a previously uninfected sexual partner compared with placebo.

Male condom use to prevent sexual transmission from infected men to uninfected sexual partners*

One prospective cohort study found limited evidence that condom use by men infected with genital herpes reduced transmission of herpes simplex virus-2 to their uninfected sexual partners.

UNKNOWN EFFECTIVENESS

Female condoms

We found no systematic review or RCTs on the effects of female condoms to prevent sexual transmission.

Male condom use to prevent sexual transmission from infected women to uninfected men

Subgroup analysis of one prospective cohort study found no significant difference between male condom use and no male condom use in transmission of herpes simplex virus-2 to uninfected men from their infected female partners.

Vaccines other than recombinant glycoprotein vaccines

We found no systematic review or RCTs.

UNLIKELY TO BE BENEFICIAL

Recombinant glycoprotein vaccines (gB2 and gD2) in people at high risk of infection (no effect except in women known to be HSV-1 and HSV-2 negative before vaccination)

One RCT found no significant difference between recombinant glycoprotein vaccine (gB2 plus gD2) and placebo in preventing genital herpes simplex virus-2 infection in people at high risk of infection. Subgroup analysis in a second RCT found that recombinant herpes simplex virus-2 glycoprotein-D-adjuvant vaccine reduced the risk of genital herpes infection compared with placebo in women who had been seronegative for herpes simplex virus-1 and herpes simplex virus-2 at baseline and who had regular sexual partners with clinically confirmed genital herpes. Subgroup analyses also found no significant difference between the vaccine and placebo in infection rate for men or in women who had been seropositive for herpes simplex virus-1 and who had regular sexual partners with genital herpes.

What are the effects of interventions to prevent transmission of herpes simplex virus from mother to neonate?

UNKNOWN EFFECTIVENESS

Caesarean delivery in women with genital lesions at term

We found no systematic review or RCTs on the effects of caesarean delivery on mother to baby transmission of genital herpes in mothers with genital lesions at term. The procedure carries the risk of increased maternal morbidity and mortality.

Oral antiviral maintenance treatment in late pregnancy (36 or more weeks of gestation) in women with a history of genital herpes

One systematic review provided insufficient evidence to assess the effects of oral antiviral agents during pregnancy on transmission of infection to neonates. The review found that aciclovir reduced the recurrence of infection at term in women with first or recurrent episodes of genital herpes simplex virus during pregnancy, and reduced the need for caesarean delivery because of genital herpes.

Serological screening and counselling to prevent acquisition of herpes simplex virus in late pregnancy

We found no systematic review or RCTs on the effects of either serological screening or counselling to prevent maternal infection in late pregnancy.

What are the effects of antiviral treatment in people with a first episode of genital herpes?

BENEFICIAL

Oral antiviral treatment in first episodes of genital herpes

Three RCTs found that oral aciclovir treatment decreased the duration of lesions, symptoms, and viral shedding compared with placebo.

UNKNOWN EFFECTIVENESS

Different types of oral antiviral treatment for first episodes of genital herpes

One RCT found no difference in clinical outcomes between oral aciclovir and valaciclovir.

What are the effects of interventions to reduce the impact of recurrence?

BENEFICIAL

Oral antiviral maintenance treatment in people with high rates of recurrence

RCTs found that daily maintenance treatment with oral antiviral agents (valaciclovir, aciclovir, or famciclovir) reduced the frequency of recurrences, and that oral aciclovir and oral valaciclovir improved quality of life compared with placebo.

Genital herpes

◀ Oral antiviral treatment taken at the start of recurrence

One systematic review, one non-systematic review, and one RCT found that oral antiviral treatment (aciclovir, famciclovir, or valaciclovir) taken at the start of recurrence reduced the duration of lesions and viral shedding, and increased the rate of aborted recurrences compared with placebo in people with recurrent genital herpes. RCTs found that aciclovir, famciclovir, and valaciclovir were similarly effective in reducing symptom duration, lesion healing time, and viral shedding compared with placebo. Two RCTs found no difference between valaciclovir taken for 3 days or 5 days.

UNKNOWN EFFECTIVENESS

Psychotherapy to reduce recurrence

One systematic review of poor quality studies provided insufficient evidence about the effects of psychosocial interventions to prevent recurrence of genital herpes.

What are the effects of treatments in people with genital herpes and HIV?

LIKELY TO BE BENEFICIAL

Oral antiviral maintenance treatment for preventing recurrence of genital herpes

One RCT found that valaciclovir was more effective than placebo in preventing herpes simplex virus infection. One RCT found no significant difference between valaciclovir and aciclovir in preventing recurrent herpes simplex virus infections over 48 weeks.

Oral antiviral treatment for an acute recurrent episode of genital herpes (compared with no treatment)*

We found no placebo controlled RCTs in people with HIV. However, consensus regards antiviral treatment as effective for treating recurrences in people with HIV, based on evidence in people without immunocompromise and in immunocompromised people without HIV.

Oral antiviral treatment for first episode genital herpes*

We found no RCTs on the treatment of first episode genital herpes in people with HIV. Current consensus is that oral antiviral treatment is effective for the treatment of first episode genital herpes in people with HIV.

UNKNOWN EFFECTIVENESS

Different types of oral antiviral treatment (relative benefits of different treatments unclear)

Two RCTs found no significant differences in duration of lesions and symptoms between famciclovir, valaciclovir, and aciclovir in the treatment of acute recurrent episodes of genital herpes. One RCT found no significant difference between valaciclovir and acyclovir maintenance treatment in preventing recurrent herpes simplex virus infections over 48 weeks.

*Categorisation based on observational or non-randomised evidence or consensus in the context of practical and ethical problems of performing RCTs. ▶

Genital herpes

DEFINITION Genital herpes is an infection with herpes simplex virus type 1 (HSV-1) or type 2 (HSV-2). The typical clinical features include painful shallow anogenital ulceration. Herpes simplex virus infections can be confirmed on the basis of virological and serological findings. Types of infection include **first episode primary infection**, which is defined as herpes simplex virus confirmed in a person without prior findings of HSV-1 or HSV-2 antibodies; **first episode non-primary infection**, which is HSV-2 confirmed in a person with prior findings of HSV-1 antibodies or vice versa; **first recognised recurrence**, which is HSV-1 (or HSV-2) confirmed in a person with prior findings of HSV-1 (or HSV-2) antibodies; and **recurrent genital herpes**, which is caused by reactivation of latent herpes simplex virus. HSV-1 can also cause gingivostomatitis and orolabial ulcers; HSV-2 can also cause other types of herpes infections, such as ocular herpes; and both virus types can cause infection of the central nervous system (e.g. encephalitis).

INCIDENCE/ PREVALENCE Genital herpes infections are among the most common sexually transmitted diseases. Seroprevalence studies showed that 22% of adults in the USA had HSV-2 antibodies.[1] A UK study found that 23% of adults attending sexual medicine clinics and 7.6% of blood donors in London had antibodies to HSV-2.[2] Seroprevalence of HSV-2 increased by 30.0% (95% CI 15.8% to 45.8%) between the periods 1976–1980 and 1988–1994.[1] However, it should be noted that although antibody levels prove the existence of present or past infections, they do not differentiate between possible manifestations of HSV-2 infections (e.g. genital/ocular). Thus, the figures must be treated with caution when applied to genital herpes only.

AETIOLOGY/ RISK FACTORS Both HSV-1 and HSV-2 can cause a first episode of genital infection, but HSV-2 is more likely to cause recurrent disease.[3] Most people with HSV-2 infection have only mild symptoms and remain unaware that they have genital herpes. However, these people can still pass on the infection to sexual partners and newborns.[4,5]

PROGNOSIS Sequelae of herpes simplex virus infection include neonatal herpes simplex virus infection, opportunistic infection in immunocompromised people, recurrent genital ulceration, and psychosocial morbidity. HSV-2 infection is associated with an increased risk of HIV transmission and acquisition.[6] The most common neurological complications are aseptic meningitis (reported in about 25% of women during primary infection) and urinary retention (reported in up to 15% of women during primary infection).[5] The absolute risk of neonatal infection is high (41%, 95% CI 26% to 56%) in babies born to women who acquire infection near the time of labour and low (< 3%) in women with established infection, even in those who have a recurrence at term.[7,8] About 15% of neonatal infections result from postnatal transmission from oral lesions of relatives or hospital personnel.[5]

Please refer to clinicalevidence.com for full text and references.

Genital warts

Search date February 2006

Henry W Buck, Jr

What are the effects of treatments for external genital warts?

BENEFICIAL

Imiquimod in people without HIV

One systematic review and two subsequent RCTs found that 5% or 1% imiquimod cream increased wart clearance and reduced recurrence compared with placebo in people without HIV. One RCT in women without HIV found that twice daily doses of imiquimod 5% did not increase wart clearance over 20 weeks compared with once daily or three times weekly doses, but found that it increased skin erythema. One RCT in people without HIV found that imiquimod 5% increased moderate to severe erythema, erosion, excoriation, oedema, and scabbing compared with placebo. Two RCTs in people without HIV found that imiquimod 5% cream increased wart clearance, but also increased local adverse reactions, compared with 1% imiquimod cream.

Interferon, topical

Three RCTs found that topical interferon increased wart clearance at 4 weeks after treatment compared with placebo. One of the RCTs also found that topical interferon increased wart clearance at 4 weeks after treatment compared with podophyllotoxin.

Podophyllotoxin

RCTs found that podophyllotoxin increased wart clearance within 16 weeks compared with placebo. Six RCTs provided no consistent evidence of a difference between podophyllotoxin and podophyllin in wart clearance or recurrence. One RCT found that podophyllotoxin was less effective than topical interferon in clearing warts at 4 weeks.

LIKELY TO BE BENEFICIAL

Bi- and trichloroacetic acid*

We found no RCTs comparing bi- and trichloroacetic acid versus placebo, but there is clinical consensus that bi- and trichloroacetic acid are effective for clearing genital warts. Two RCTs found no significant difference between trichloroacetic acid and cryotherapy in clearance of warts after 6–10 weeks' treatment, and one of the RCTs found no significant difference in the recurrence of warts 2 months after the end of treatment.

Cryotherapy*

We found no RCTs comparing cryotherapy versus placebo or no treatment, but there is clinical consensus that cryotherapy is effective for clearing genital warts. Two RCTs found no significant difference between cryotherapy and trichloroacetic acid in clearance of warts after 6–10 weeks' treatment. One of the RCTs found no significant difference in recurrence of warts 2 months after the end of treatment. One RCT found no significant difference in wart clearance at 3 months between cryotherapy and electrosurgery.

Electrosurgery

One RCT found that electrosurgery increased clearance of warts at 6 months compared with no treatment. One RCT found that electrosurgery increased clearance of warts at 6 months compared with systemic interferon but the ▶

increase was not significant. One RCT found no significant difference in wart clearance at 3 months between electrosurgery and cryotherapy.

Podophyllin (probably as effective as podophyllotoxin or surgical excision)*

We found no RCTs comparing podophyllin versus placebo, but there is consensus that podophyllin is effective for clearing genital warts. Six RCTs provided no consistent evidence of a difference between podophyllotoxin and podophyllin in wart clearance or recurrence. RCTs found no significant difference between surgical (scissor) excision and podophyllin in wart clearance. However, they found that surgical excision was more effective than podophyllin in preventing recurrence at 6–12 months. One RCT found that podophyllin was more effective than systemic interferon in clearing warts at 3 months.

Surgical excision (as effective as podophyllin in clearing warts; more effective than podophyllin in preventing recurrence)

We found no RCTs comparing surgical excision versus no treatment. Two RCTs found no significant difference between surgical (scissor) excision and podophyllin in wart clearance. However, they found that surgical excision was more effective than podophyllin in preventing recurrence at 6–12 months. One small RCT found no significant difference in wart clearance or recurrence rates between laser and surgical excision.

*No placebo controlled RCTs found; categorisation based on consensus.

UNKNOWN EFFECTIVENESS

Imiquimod in people with HIV

One RCT in people with HIV found no significant difference in wart clearance over 16 weeks between imiquimod cream and placebo.

Interferon (intralesional)

We found no systematic review or RCTs that assessed interlesional interferon.

Laser surgery

We found no RCTs comparing laser surgery versus no treatment. One small RCT found no significant difference in wart clearance or recurrence rates between laser and surgical excision.

LIKELY TO BE INEFFECTIVE OR HARMFUL

Interferon, systemic

We found five RCTs comparing different formulations of systemic interferon versus placebo or no treatment. Two of the RCTs found that systemic interferon improved wart clearance compared with placebo or no treatment, whereas three of the RCTs found no significant difference between interferon and placebo in complete or partial wart clearance. Systemic interferon was associated with important adverse effects, including anaphylaxis, blood disorders, flu-like symptoms, headache, fatigue, myalgia, fever, and weight loss. One RCT found no significant difference in wart clearance at 6 months between electrosurgery and systemic interferon. One RCT found that systemic interferon was less effective than podophyllin in clearing warts at 3 months.

Genital warts

What are the effects of interventions to prevent transmission of external genital warts?

UNKNOWN EFFECTIVENESS

Condoms

Observational studies provided insufficient evidence to assess the effects of condom use on transmission of human papillomavirus. Penetrative intercourse is not required for spread because this can occur with external genital–genital or hand–genital touching. One case control and one cross-sectional study suggested that people who always used condoms were less likely to have genital warts than people who never or occasionally used them.

DEFINITION External genital warts are benign epidermal growths on the external perigenital and perianal regions. There are four morphological types: condylomatous, keratotic, papular, and flat warts. External genital warts are caused by the human papillomavirus (HPV). **Diagnosis** The majority of external genital warts are diagnosed by inspection. Some clinicians apply 5% acetic acid (white vinegar) to help visualise lesions because it produces so-called "acetowhite" change and, more importantly, defines vascular patterns characteristic for external genital warts. However, the "acetowhite" change also occurs with conditions other than external genital warts, so differential diagnoses should be considered. Some lesions, particularly those that are pigmented, should be biopsied to rule out severe dysplasia or melanoma.

INCIDENCE/ PREVALENCE In the USA in 2004, external genital warts accounted for more than 310 000 initial visits to private physicians' offices.[1] In the USA, 1% of sexually active men and women aged 18–49 years are estimated to have external genital warts.[2] It is believed that external and cervical lesions caused by HPV are the most prevalent sexually transmitted disease among persons 18–25 years of age. In the USA, 50–60% of women aged 18–25 years test positive for HPV DNA, but no more than 10–15% ever have genital warts.[3] By the age of 50 years, at least 80% of women will have acquired genital HPV infection. About 6.2 million Americans acquire a new genital HPV infection each year.[1,2]

AETIOLOGY/ RISK FACTORS External genital warts are caused by HPV and are sexually transmitted. They are more common in people with impaired immune function.[3] Although more than 100 types of HPV have been identified, most external genital warts in immunocompetent people are caused by HPV types 6 and 11.[4,5]

PROGNOSIS The ability to clear and remain free of external genital warts is a function of cellular immunity.[6] In immunocompetent people, the prognosis in terms of clearance and avoiding recurrence is good,[7] but people with impaired cellular immunity (e.g. people with HIV and AIDS) have great difficulty in achieving and maintaining wart clearance.[3] Without treatment, external genital warts may remain unchanged, may increase in size or number, or may resolve completely. Clinical trials found that recurrences may occur and may necessitate repeated treatment. External genital warts rarely, if ever, progress to cancer.[8] Juvenile laryngeal papillomatosis, a rare and sometimes life threatening condition, occurs in children of women with a history of genital warts. Its rarity makes it difficult to design studies that can evaluate whether treatment in pregnant women alters the risk.[9,10]

Please refer to clinicalevidence.com for full text and references.

Gonorrhoea

Search date July 2005

John Moran

What are the effects of treatments for uncomplicated infections in men and non-pregnant women?

BENEFICIAL

Single dose antibiotic regimens*

One systematic review of individual treatment arms of RCTs and observational studies found limited evidence that single dose regimens achieve cure rates of 95% or higher in urogenital or rectal infection. Cure rates were lower (about 80%) for pharyngeal infection. Resistance to penicillins, tetracyclines, and sulphonamides is now widespread, and resistance to fluoroquinolones has become common in some geographic areas.

*Based on results in individual arms of RCTs and observational studies.

What are the effects of treatments for uncomplicated infections in pregnant women?

BENEFICIAL

Single dose antibiotic regimens

One systematic review found that antibiotic treatment (amoxicillin plus probenecid, spectinomycin, ceftriaxone, cefixime) was effective for curing gonorrhoea in pregnant women. We found no reports of serious adverse effects.

What are the effects of treatments for disseminated gonococcal infection?

LIKELY TO BE BENEFICIAL

Multidose antibiotic regimens†

We found no RCTs assessing treatments for disseminated gonococcal infection, but there is consensus that multidose regimens using injectable cephalosporins or quinolones (except where quinolone resistant *N gonorrhoeae* have been reported) are the most effective treatments. We found no reports of treatment failures with these regimens.

†Based on non-RCT evidence and consensus.

What are the effects of dual treatment for gonorrhoea and chlamydia infection?

UNKNOWN EFFECTIVENESS

Dual antibiotic treatment

Dual treatment with an antimicrobial effective against gonorrhoea and chlamydia infections is based on theory and expert opinion rather than on evidence from RCTs. The balance between benefits and harms will vary with the prevalence of co-infection in each population.

Gonorrhoea

DEFINITION Gonorrhoea is caused by infection with *Neisseria gonorrhoeae*. In men, uncomplicated urethritis is the most common manifestation, with dysuria and urethral discharge. Less typically, signs and symptoms are mild and indistinguishable from those of chlamydial urethritis. In women, the most common site of infection is the uterine cervix where infection results in symptoms such as vaginal discharge, lower abdominal discomfort, and dyspareunia in only half of cases. Recent studies in the USA and UK found concurrent *Chlamydia trachomatis* in 7–14% of homosexual men with gonorrhea, in 20–30% of heterosexual men, and in 40–50% of women.[1-3] Overall, co-infection with *C trachomatis* is reported in 10–40% of people with gonorrhoea.[1-6]

INCIDENCE/ PREVALENCE Between 1975 and 1997, the reported incidence of gonorrhoea in the USA fell by 74%, reaching a nadir of 120 per 100 000 people. After a small increase in 1998, the rate of new gonorrhoeal infection has declined steadily since, with an incidence of 114 per 100 000 in 2004.[7] Rates are highest in younger people. In 2004, the incidence was highest in women aged 15–19 years (611 per 100 000) and men aged 20–24 years (431 per 100 000). In England, Wales and Northern Ireland diagnoses of gonorrhoea were 287 per 100 000 for 20–24 year old men and 208 per 100 000 for 16–19 year old women in 2002. In 2004, diagnoses of gonorrhoea had fallen to 240 per 100 000 for 20–24 year old men and 179 per 100 000 for 16–19 year old women.[8]

AETIOLOGY/ RISK FACTORS Most infections result from penile–vaginal, penile–rectal, or penile–pharyngeal contact. An important minority of infections are transmitted from mother to child during birth, which can cause a sight-threatening purulent conjunctivitis (ophthalmia neonatorum). Less common are ocular infections in older children and adults as a result of sexual exposure, poor hygiene, or the medicinal use of urine.

PROGNOSIS The natural history of untreated gonococcal infection is spontaneous resolution and microbiological clearance after weeks or months of unpleasant symptoms.[9] During this time, there is a substantial likelihood of transmission to others and of complications developing in the infected individual.[9] In many women, the lack of readily discernible signs or symptoms of cervicitis means that infections go unrecognised and untreated. An unknown proportion of untreated infections causes local complications, including lymphangitis, periurethral abscess, bartholinitis, and urethral stricture; epididymitis in men; and in women involvement of the uterus, fallopian tubes, or ovaries causing pelvic inflammatory disease (see pelvic inflammatory disease). One review found *N gonorrhoeae* was cultured from 8–32% of women with acute pelvic inflammatory disease in 11 European studies and from 27–80% of women in eight US studies.[10] The proportion of *N gonorrhoeae* infections in women that lead to pelvic inflammatory disease has not been well studied. However, one study of 26 women exposed to men with gonorrhoea found that 19 women were culture positive and, of these, five women had pelvic inflammatory disease and another four had uterine adnexal tenderness.[11] Pelvic inflammatory disease may lead to infertility (see pelvic inflammatory disease). In some people, localised gonococcal infection may disseminate. A US study estimated the risk of dissemination to be 0.6–1.1% among women, whereas a European study estimated it to be 2.3–3.0%.[12,13] The same European study found a lower risk in men, estimated to be 0.4–0.7%.[13] When gonococci disseminate, they cause petechial or pustular skin lesions; asymmetrical arthropathies, tenosynovitis, or septic arthritis; and rarely, meningitis or endocarditis.

Please refer to clinicalevidence.com for full text and references.

Partner notification

Search date April 2005

Catherine Mathews and Nicol Coetzee

What are the effects of different partner notification strategies in people with different sexually transmitted diseases?

LIKELY TO BE BENEFICIAL

Contract referral (as effective as provider referral in people with syphilis)

One systematic review of one large RCT comparing different partner notification strategies in people with syphilis found no significant difference in the proportion of partners notified between provider referral and contract referral, when people receiving the contract referral option were given 2 days to notify their partners.

Contract referral (*v* patient referral) in people with gonorrhoea

One systematic review found that, in people with gonorrhoea, contract referral increased the rate of partners presenting for treatment compared with patient referral.

Offering a choice between provider and patient referral (compared with offering only patient referral) in people with HIV

One systematic review of one RCT comparing different partner notification strategies found that, in people with HIV, offering a choice between provider referral (where the identity of the index patient was not revealed) and patient referral improved notification rates compared with offering patient referral alone.

Provider referral (*v* patient referral) in people with non-gonococcal urethritis (mainly chlamydia)

One RCT in people with non-gonococcal urethritis (mainly chlamydia) identified by the review found that provider referral increased the proportion of partners notified and of positive partners detected per patient compared with patient referral.

UNKNOWN EFFECTIVENESS

Contract referral in people with chlamydia

We found no RCTs assessing contract referral in people with chlamydia.

Contract referral in people with HIV

We found no RCTs assessing contract referral in people with HIV infection.

Outreach assistance in people with gonorrhoea or chlamydia

We found no RCTs assessing outreach assistance in people with gonorrhoea or chlamydia.

Outreach assistance in people with HIV

One RCT provided insufficient evidence to assess outreach assistance compared with patient referral in people with HIV infection.

Outreach assistance in people with syphilis

We found no RCTs assessing outreach assistance in people with syphilis.

Patient referral in people with syphilis

We found no RCTs assessing patient referral in people with syphilis.

►

Partner notification

Provider referral in people with gonorrhoea

We found no RCTs assessing provider referral in people with gonorrhoea.

What can be done to improve the effectiveness of patient referral?

UNKNOWN EFFECTIVENESS

Adding telephone reminders and contact cards to patient referral

One RCT identified by a systematic review provided insufficient evidence about the effects of adding telephone reminders and contact cards to patient referral in improving partner notification.

Educational videos

We found insufficient evidence about the effects of educational videos in improving partner notification.

Information pamphlets

One RCT identified by a systematic review provided insufficient evidence about the effects of information pamphlets in improving partner notification.

Patient referral by different types of healthcare professionals

One RCT identified by a systematic review provided insufficient evidence about the effects of patient referral by different types of healthcare professionals in improving partner notification.

DEFINITION Partner notification is a process whereby the sexual partners of people with a diagnosis of sexually transmitted infection are informed of their exposure to infection. The main methods are patient referral, provider referral, contract referral, and outreach assistance.

INCIDENCE/ PREVALENCE A large proportion of people with sexually transmitted infections will have neither symptoms nor signs of infection. For example, 22–68% of men with gonorrhoea who were identified through partner notification were asymptomatic.[1] Partner notification is one of the two strategies to reach such individuals, the other strategy being screening. Managing infection in people with more than one current sexual partner is likely to have the greatest impact on the spread of sexually transmitted infections.[2]

PROGNOSIS We found no studies showing that partner notification results in a health benefit, either to the partner or to future partners of infected people. Obtaining such evidence would be technically and ethically difficult. One RCT in asymptomatic women compared identifying, testing, and treating women at increased risk for cervical chlamydial infection versus usual care. It found these reduced the incidence of pelvic inflammatory disease (RR 0.44, 95% CI 0.20 to 0.90).[3] This evidence suggests that partner notification, which also aims to identify and treat people who are largely unaware of infection, would provide a direct health benefit to partners who are infected.

Please refer to clinicalevidence.com for full text and references.

Pelvic inflammatory disease

Search date May 2006

Jonathan Ross

What are the effects of empirical treatment compared with treatment delayed until the results of microbiological investigations are known?

UNKNOWN EFFECTIVENESS

Empirical antibiotic treatment versus treatment guided by test results

We found no systematic review or RCTs comparing empirical antibiotic treatment (before receiving results of microbiological tests) versus treatment that was guided by test result in women with suspected pelvic inflammatory disease (PID). However because there are no reliable clinical diagnostic criteria for PID, early empirical treatment is common. Observational evidence suggests that delaying treatment by 3 days or more may impair fertility.

How do different antimicrobial regimens compare?

LIKELY TO BE BENEFICIAL

Antibiotics (for symptoms and microbiological clearance in women with confirmed pelvic inflammatory disease)

There is consensus that antibiotic treatment is more effective than no treatment for women with confirmed pelvic inflammatory disease (PID). Two systematic reviews (the first combining observational studies and RCTs, the second only assessing RCTs) found that several different antibiotic regimens (including parenteral clindamycin plus parenteral aminoglycoside; parenteral cephalosporin with or without probenecid plus oral doxycycline; and oral ofloxacin) were similarly effective in relieving the symptoms of PID, and achieved high rates of clinical and microbiological cure.

Different durations of antibiotic treatment

We found no good evidence on the optimal duration of treatment.

Oral antibiotics (versus parenteral antibiotics)

Two RCTs found no significant difference between oral ofloxacin and parenteral cefoxitin plus doxycycline. Another RCT found no significant difference between outpatient treatment with intramuscular cefoxitin plus probenecid plus oral doxycycline and inpatient treatment with parenteral antibiotics in recurrence of pelvic inflammatory disease, chronic pelvic pain, infertility, or ectopic pregnancy rates at 84 months.

Outpatient (versus inpatient) antibiotic treatment

One RCT found no significant difference between outpatient treatment with intramuscular cefoxitin plus probenecid plus oral doxycycline and inpatient treatment with parenteral antibiotics in recurrence of pelvic inflammatory disease, chronic pelvic pain, infertility, or ectopic pregnancy rates at 84 months. ▶

Pelvic inflammatory disease

What are the effects of routine antibiotic prophylaxis to prevent pelvic inflammatory disease before intrauterine contraceptive device insertion?

UNKNOWN EFFECTIVENESS

Routine antibiotic prophylaxis before intrauterine device insertion in women at high risk

We found no good evidence about antibiotic prophylaxis before intrauterine device insertion in women at high risk of pelvic inflammatory disease.

UNLIKELY TO BE BENEFICIAL

Routine antibiotic prophylaxis before intrauterine device insertion in women at low risk

One systematic review found no significant difference in the incidence of pelvic inflammatory disease (PID) between routine prophylaxis with doxycycline and placebo before intrauterine contraceptive device insertion in women at low risk of PID.

DEFINITION Pelvic inflammatory disease (PID) is inflammation and infection of the upper genital tract in women, typically involving the fallopian tubes, ovaries, and surrounding structures.

INCIDENCE/PREVALENCE The exact incidence of PID is unknown because the disease cannot be diagnosed reliably from clinical symptoms and signs.[1-3] Direct visualisation of the fallopian tubes by laparoscopy is the best single diagnostic test, but it is invasive and not used routinely in clinical practice. PID is the most common gynaecological reason for admission to hospital in the USA, accounting for 18/10 000 recorded hospital discharges.[4] A diagnosis of PID is made in 1/62 (1.6%) women aged 16–45 years attending their primary care physician in England and Wales.[5] However, because most PID is asymptomatic, this figure underestimates the true prevalence.[1,6] A crude marker of PID in developing countries can be obtained from reported hospital admission rates, where it accounts for 17–40% of gynaecological admissions in sub-Saharan Africa, 15–37% in Southeast Asia, and 3–10% in India.[7]

AETIOLOGY/RISK FACTORS Factors associated with PID mirror those for sexually transmitted infections: young age, reduced socioeconomic circumstances, lower educational attainment, and recent new sexual partner.[2,8,9] Infection ascends from the cervix, and initial epithelial damage caused by bacteria (especially *Chlamydia trachomatis* and *Neisseria gonorrhoeae*) allows the opportunistic entry of other organisms. Many different microbes, including *Mycoplasma genitalium* and anaerobes, may be isolated from the upper genital tract.[10,11] The spread of infection to the upper genital tract may be increased by instrumentation of the cervix, but reduced by barrier methods of contraception, levonorgestrel implants, and oral contraceptives compared with other forms of contraception.[12-16]

PROGNOSIS PID has a high morbidity; about 20% of affected women become infertile, 30% develop chronic pelvic pain, and 1% of those who conceive have an ectopic pregnancy (see table 1) Ⓣ.[17,18] Uncontrolled observations suggest that clinical symptoms and signs resolve in a significant proportion of untreated women.[17] Repeated episodes of PID are associated with a four to six times increase in the risk of permanent tubal damage.[19] One case control study (76 cases and 367 controls) found that delaying treatment by even a few days is associated with impaired fertility (OR 2.6, 95% CI 1.2 to 5.9).[20]

Please refer to clinicalevidence.com for full text and references.

Acne vulgaris

Search date June 2005

Sarah Purdy

What are the effects of topical treatments in people with acne vulgaris?

BENEFICIAL

Benzoyl peroxide

One systematic review identified four RCTs, primarily in people with moderate acne, which found that topical benzoyl peroxide reduced either total lesion count or the number of inflammatory and non-inflammatory lesions at 4, 11, or 12 weeks compared with vehicle; these results were supported by more limited evidence from a fifth RCT with weak methods of analysis. None of the RCTs assessed patient perception of improvement. One of the RCTs found that benzoyl peroxide increased the proportion of people who had adverse effects, including dryness, scaling, burning, tingling, and redness, compared with vehicle. Another RCT found that more people using benzoyl peroxide had peeling compared with people using vehicle. A third RCT found similar rates of local adverse effects between benzoyl peroxide and vehicle.

Clindamycin (reduced the number of inflammatory lesions)

RCTs identified by a systematic review found that, in people with mild to severe acne, topical clindamycin 1% reduced the number of inflammatory lesions compared with placebo or vehicle. However, the RCTs found inconclusive evidence about the effects of clindamycin on non-inflammatory lesions. Three RCTs found that clindamycin increased the proportion of people who perceived that their acne was "markedly improved" or "improved". The RCTs gave little information on adverse effects.

Erythromycin (reduced the number of inflammatory lesions)

RCTs identified by a systematic review, in people with mild to severe acne, found that topical erythromycin reduced the number of inflammatory lesions at 12 weeks compared with vehicle. One RCT found that a similar proportion of people using erythromycin compared with vehicle perceived that their acne had improved from baseline at 12 weeks; the other RCTs did not assess patient perception of improvement. The RCTs found no significant difference in adverse effects between erythromycin and vehicle.

Tretinoin

Four large RCTs identified by a systematic review, primarily in people with mild to moderate acne, found that topical tretinoin reduced the number of inflammatory and non-inflammatory lesions at 8–12 weeks compared with vehicle. One RCT found tretinoin increased patient perception of acne improvement compared with vehicle; the other RCTs did not assess patient perception of improvement. The RCTs found that topical tretinoin was associated with erythema, peeling, burning, and pruritus. In the absence of data regarding the risk of birth defects, it is recommended that topical retinoids are not used in pregnancy or by women of childbearing age who are not taking adequate contraceptive precautions.

LIKELY TO BE BENEFICIAL

Adapalene

One large RCT in people with moderate acne, identified by a systematic review, found that topical adapalene reduced the number of non-inflammatory and inflammatory lesions at 12 weeks compared with vehicle. It found similar quality of life scores in people using adapalene or vehicle. It found that adapalene increased erythema, dryness, scaling, stinging/burning, and pruritus at 2 weeks compared with vehicle, but found no significant difference between groups in these outcomes at 12 weeks. In the absence of data regarding the risk of birth defects, it is recommended that topical retinoids are not used in pregnancy or by women of childbearing age who are not taking adequate contraceptive precautions.

Azelaic acid

Two RCTs, primarily in people with moderate acne, identified by two systematic reviews, found limited evidence that topical azelaic acid reduced the number of inflammatory and non-inflammatory lesions after 8–12 weeks compared with placebo. Neither of the RCTs assessed patient perception of improvement. The two RCTs, and a non-systematic review of controlled and uncontrolled studies, found that azelaic acid was associated with itching, stinging, burning, and erythema.

Erythromycin plus zinc

Two RCTs identified by a systematic review found that topical erythromycin plus zinc reduced acne severity compared with placebo. One of the RCTs found that topical erythromycin plus zinc reduced both inflammatory and non-inflammatory lesions; the other found that it reduced papules but not pustules. Neither RCT assessed patient perception of improvement. The RCTs give little information on adverse effects.

Isotretinoin

Two RCTs in people with mild to moderate acne identified by a systematic review found that topical isotretinoin reduced the number of inflammatory and non-inflammatory lesions compared with vehicle. These results were supported by more limited evidence from two other RCTs with weak methods of analysis. One of the RCTs found limited evidence from within group comparisons from baseline that a similar proportion of people using isotretinoin compared with vehicle perceived that their acne had improved from baseline at 12 weeks; the other RCTs did not assess patient perception of improvement. The RCTs found that topical isotretinoin was associated with severe erythema, dryness, soreness, and burning. In the absence of data regarding the risk of birth defects, it is recommended that topical retinoids are not used in pregnancy or by women of childbearing age who are not taking adequate contraceptive precautions.

Tetracycline

Three RCTs in people with moderate to severe acne identified by a systematic review found that topical tetracycline reduced acne severity at 12–16 weeks compared with placebo. This was supported by more limited evidence from a fourth RCT with weak methods of analysis. One of the RCTs found that a similar proportion of people taking topical tetracycline compared with placebo "considered that their condition was better than before treatment"; the other RCTs did not assess participant perception of improvement. Three of the RCTs found that topical tetracycline was associated with skin discolouration.

Acne vulgaris

UNKNOWN EFFECTIVENESS

Meclocycline

We found no RCTs comparing topical meclocycline versus placebo in people with acne vulgaris.

What are the effects of oral treatments in people with acne vulgaris?

LIKELY TO BE BENEFICIAL

Erythromycin

One systematic review identified no RCTs comparing oral erythromycin versus placebo in people with acne vulgaris. One RCT found that both oral erythromycin and oral doxycycline reduced the number of papules and pustules after 6 weeks, with no significant difference between groups. The RCT did not assess patient perception of improvement. Two RCTs in people with mild, moderate, or severe acne found that both erythromycin and oral tetracycline improved acne, but found no significant difference in the number of lesions or total inflammation scores between the drugs at 3–6 months. A third RCT did not compare oral erythromycin versus oral tetracycline directly, but found that fewer people within the group taking erythromycin had a "good" or "very good" response as assessed by their physician than people within the group taking tetracycline, although high proportions in both groups responded well. One of the RCTs found no significant difference between oral erythromycin and oral tetracycline in the proportion of people who perceived that their acne had improved; the other RCTs did not assess patient perception of improvement. Oral erythromycin may cause contraceptive failure during the initial weeks of treatment.

TRADE OFF BETWEEN BENEFITS AND HARMS

Doxycycline

One RCT identified by a systematic review provided insufficient evidence to compare oral doxycycline with placebo in people with acne vulgaris. A second RCT identified by another systematic review found that doxycycline reduced inflammatory lesions and comedones after 6 months compared with placebo. It found no significant difference in patient perception of improvement. One systematic review found no significant difference in inflammatory lesions, total lesion count, overall efficacy, or patient perception of improvement between oral doxycycline and oral minocycline. One RCT found that both oral doxycycline and oral erythromycin reduced the number of papules and pustules after 6 weeks, with no significant difference between groups. Another small RCT found no significant difference in mean lesion count at 8 weeks between oral doxycycline and oral oxytetracycline. The RCTs did not assess patient perception of improvement. Tetracyclines may harm bones and teeth and should not be taken by pregnant or breastfeeding women. They may cause contraceptive failure during the initial weeks of treatment.

Lymecycline

One systematic review identified no RCTs comparing oral lymecycline versus placebo in people with acne vulgaris. One RCT in people with moderate to severe acne identified by another systematic review found no significant difference between oral lymecycline and oral minocycline in inflammatory or non-inflammatory lesions or patient perception of improvement at 12 weeks.

Tetracyclines may harm bones and teeth, and should not be taken by pregnant or breastfeeding women. They may cause contraceptive failure during the initial weeks of treatment.

Minocycline

Two RCTs identified by a systematic review provided insufficient evidence to compare oral minocycline versus placebo or oral oxytetracycline. The review found no significant difference in inflammatory lesions, non-inflammatory lesions, total lesion count, overall efficacy, or patient perception of improvement between oral minocycline and oral doxycycline, lymecycline, or tetracycline. Two systematic reviews of one case control study and case reports suggested that oral minocycline was associated with an increased risk of developing the rare but serious condition systemic lupus erythematosus, and one review of case reports suggested that it may increase the risk of developing severe hepatic dysfunction. The evidence about adverse effects should be interpreted with caution because of wide variation between studies in numbers of reported adverse events. Tetracyclines may harm bones and teeth and should not be taken by pregnant or breastfeeding women. They may cause contraceptive failure during the initial weeks of treatment.

Oxytetracycline

One systematic review identified no RCTs comparing oral oxytetracycline versus placebo in people with acne vulgaris. One small RCT found no significant difference in mean lesion count at 8 weeks between oral doxycycline and oral oxytetracycline. The RCT did not assess patient perception of improvement. Another RCT identified by a systematic review provided insufficient evidence to compare oral oxytetracycline versus oral minocycline. Tetracyclines may harm bones and teeth and should not be taken by pregnant or breastfeeding women. They may cause contraceptive failure during the initial weeks of treatment.

Tetracycline

Four RCTs identified by a systematic review found that oral tetracycline reduced acne severity compared with placebo; these results were supported by more limited evidence from two further RCTs with weak methods of analysis. A seventh RCT identified by the review found no significant difference in the number of inflammatory lesions between oral tetracycline and placebo, but may have lacked power to detect a clinically important difference. One of the RCTs found that oral tetracycline increased the proportion of people who perceived that their acne was “markedly improved” or “improved” compared with placebo; this was supported by weaker evidence from within group comparisons from another RCT. RCTs identified by systematic reviews, in people with mild to severe acne, found that oral tetracycline and oral erythromycin or oral minocycline all reduced acne severity, with no significant difference between treatments. One of the RCTs found no significant difference between oral tetracycline and oral erythromycin in the proportion of people who perceived that their acne had improved; the other RCTs did not assess patient perception of improvement. The RCTs and controlled trials identified by the reviews found few adverse effects associated with oral tetracycline. Tetracyclines may harm bones and teeth, and should not be taken by pregnant or breastfeeding women. They may cause contraceptive failure during the initial weeks of treatment.

DEFINITION Acne vulgaris is a common inflammatory pilosebaceous disease characterised by comedones, papules, pustules, inflamed nodules, superficial pus filled cysts, and (in extreme cases) canalising and deep, inflamed, sometimes purulent sacs.[1] Lesions are most common on the face, but the neck, chest,

Acne vulgaris

upper back, and shoulders may also be affected. Acne can cause scarring and considerable psychological distress.[2] It is classified as mild, moderate, or severe.[1] Mild acne is defined as non-inflammatory lesions (comedones), a few inflammatory (papulopustular) lesions, or both. Moderate acne is defined as more inflammatory lesions, occasional nodules, or both, and mild scarring. Severe acne is defined as widespread inflammatory lesions, nodules, or both, and scarring; moderate acne that has not settled with 6 months of treatment; or acne of any "severity" with serious psychological upset. This chapter does not cover acne rosacea, acne secondary to industrial occupations, and treatment of acne in people under 13 years of age.

INCIDENCE/ PREVALENCE Acne is the most common skin disease of adolescence, affecting over 80% of teenagers (aged 13–18 years) at some point.[3] Estimates of prevalence vary depending on study populations and the method of assessment used. Prevalence of acne in a community sample of 14–16 year olds in the UK has been recorded as 50%.[4] In a sample of adolescents from schools in New Zealand, acne was present in 91% of males and 79% of females.[5] It has been estimated that up to 30% of teenagers have acne of sufficient severity to require medical treatment.[6] Acne was the presenting complaint in 3.1% of people aged 13–25 years attending primary care in a UK population.[7] Overall incidence is similar in both men and women, and peaks at 17 years of age.[6] The number of adults with acne, including people over 25 years, is increasing; the reasons for this increase are uncertain.[8]

AETIOLOGY/ RISK FACTORS The exact cause of acne is unknown. Four factors contribute to the development of acne: increased sebum secretion rate, abnormal follicular differentiation causing obstruction of the pilosebaceous duct, bacteriology of the pilosebaceous duct, and inflammation.[9] The anaerobic bacterium *Propionibacterium acnes* plays an important role in the pathogenesis of acne. Androgen secretion is the major trigger for adolescent acne.[10]

PROGNOSIS In the absence of treatment, acne persists in most sufferers for an average of 8–12 years.[11]

Please refer to clinicalevidence.com for full text and references.

Athlete's foot

Search date April 2006

Fay Crawford

What are the effects of topical treatments for athlete's foot?

BENEFICIAL

Topical allylamines (naftifine, terbinafine)

One systematic review and four subsequent RCTs found that allylamines were more effective than placebo for curing fungal skin infections. One small RCT identified by the review found no significant difference in cure rates between the naftifine and terbinafine. The review also found that topical allylamines increased cure rates at 3–12 weeks compared with topical azoles. However, three subsequent RCTs found no significant difference in cure rates between topical azoles and allylamines. We found no RCTs comparing topical allylamines versus topical ciclopirox olamine.

Topical azoles

One systematic review found that azole creams given for 4–6 weeks increased cure rates compared with placebo. One systematic review found insufficient evidence of a difference between individual azoles given for 3–7 weeks. The review also found that topical azoles were less effective than topical allylamines in increasing cure rates at 3–12 weeks. However, three subsequent RCTs found no significant difference in cure rates between topical azoles and allylamines. One systematic review of one RCT found no significant difference in cure rates between clotrimazole and ciclopirox olamine.

Topical ciclopirox olamine *New*

One systematic review and two subsequent RCTs found that topical ciclopirox olamine (0.77% or 1%) significantly increased cure rate compared with placebo. The review found no significant difference in cure rates between ciclopirox olamine and clotrimazole. We found no RCTs comparing ciclopirox olamine versus topical allylamines.

UNKNOWN EFFECTIVENESS

Improved foot hygiene, including socks, and hosiery

We found no systematic review or RCTs on the effects of foot hygiene and hosiery in the treatment of athlete's foot.

DEFINITION Athlete's foot is a cutaneous fungal infection caused by dermatophyte infection. It is characterised by itching, flaking, and fissuring of the skin. It may manifest in three ways: the skin between the toes may appear mascerated (white) and soggy; the soles of the feet may become dry and scaly; and the skin all over the foot may become red, and vesicular eruptions may appear.[1] It is conventional in dermatology to refer to fungal skin infections as superficial in order to distinguish them from systemic fungal infections.

INCIDENCE/ PREVALENCE Epidemiological studies have produced various estimates of the prevalence of athlete's foot. Studies are usually conducted in populations of people who attend dermatology clinics, sports centres, or swimming pools, or who are in the military. UK estimates suggest that athlete's foot is present in about 15% of the general population.[2] Studies conducted in dermatology clinics in Italy (722 people)[3] and China (1014 people)[4] found prevalences of 25% and 27%, respectively. A population based study conducted in 1148 children in Israel found the prevalence among children to be 30%.[5] ►

Athlete's foot

AETIOLOGY/ RISK FACTORS Swimming pool users and industrial workers may be at increased risk of fungal foot infection. However, one survey identified fungal foot infection in only 9% of swimmers, with the highest prevalence (20%) being in men aged 16 years and older.[2]

PROGNOSIS Fungal infections of the foot are not life threatening in people with normal immune status, but in some people they cause persistent itching and, ultimately, fissuring. Other people are apparently unaware of persistent infection. The infection can spread to other parts of the body and to other individuals.

Please refer to clinicalevidence.com for full text and references.

Atopic eczema

Search date February 2005

Fiona Bath-Hextall and Hywel Williams

What are the effects of self care treatments in adults and children with established atopic eczema?

LIKELY TO BE BENEFICIAL

Emollients* *New*

There is insufficient evidence to assess the effectiveness of emollients on atopic eczema; however, there is consensus that emollients are effective for treating the symptoms of atopic eczema. Five mixed quality RCTs provided insufficient evidence to compare different emollients and placebo. However, one RCT found that glycerin cream improved skin dryness and one RCT found that Kamillosan cream marginally improved pruritis, erythema, and desquamation compared with placebo and 0.5% hydrocortisone. In spite of this, emollients are widely used to improve the symptoms and appearance of associated dry skin, to prevent skin cracking, and to reduce dependence on topical corticosteroids. Two RCTs found different results with urea cream versus glycerin cream. One RCT found that urea cream reduced dryness compared with glycerin cream but another found no significant difference between the two treatments. Or benefits of emollients plus corticosteroids, see the section on corticosteroids. Transient burning has been reported with emollient use.

*Based on consensus.

What are the effects of topical medical treatments in adults and children with established atopic eczema?

BENEFICIAL

Corticosteroids *New*

One RCT found that flucinolone acetonide increased clearance compared with a peanut oil vehicle at 1 week. Two RCTs found that intermittent dosing with 0.005% fluticasone propionate in addition to regular emollient therapy decreased relapse rates compared with emollients alone at 16 weeks. Two RCTs comparing once daily versus twice daily fluticasone propionate versus a vehicle alone found different results. One RCT found that twice daily 0.005% fluticasone increased clearance compared with once daily application. However, another RCT found no significant difference in clearance between once daily and twice daily application of 0.05% or 0.005% fluticasone propionate. There was insufficient evidence to determine the superiority of one topical corticosteroid over another. One RCT found that a lipid mixture plus topical corticosteroids improved eczema compared with a lipid mixture alone. Two RCTs found that 0.05% fluticasone propionate cream decreased relapse rates at 16 weeks compared with emollients alone. Two RCTs found that topical corticosteroids were more effective at clearance compared with 1% pimecrolimus. Three RCTs found that 0.03% and 0.1% tacrolimus were more effective than mild topical corticosteroids but other RCTs found mixed results when compared with more potent corticosteroids. One systematic review found that studies that specifically gathered data on skin thinning and suppression of the pituitary–adrenal ▶

axis failed to find any evidence of harm. The most common adverse effect reported was burning, found in about 10% of people. Potent corticosteroids are generally used later in children compared with adults.

Pimecrolimus *New*

One systematic review and one subsequent RCT found that 1% pimecrolimus improved clearance between 3 weeks and 6 months compared with a vehicle. The systematic review found that 1% pimecrolimus reduced the proportion of people with acute flare at 6 months and 12 months compared with a vehicle. Two RCTs found that 1% pimecrolimus was less effective at achieving clearance compared with corticosteroids (0.1% betamethasone valerate and also 0.1% triamcinolone acetonide for trunk and limbs and 1% hydrocortisone acetate for the face). One RCT found no significant difference between 1% pimecrolimus and 0.03% tacrolimus in the proportion of children clear or almost clear at 6 weeks. One crossover RCT identified by the review found no significant difference in the proportion of people clear or almost clear between four times daily application versus twice daily application of 1% pimecrolimus cream at 3 weeks. The systematic review found no significant difference in the incidence of skin burning for 1% pimecrolimus and vehicle. However, the proportion of people with skin burning was significantly higher with 1% pimecrolimus compared with 0.1% betamethasone valerate or a combined regimen of 0.1% triamcinolone acetonide plus hydrocortisone acetate. The United States Food and Drug Administration has issued a public health advisory to inform healthcare professionals and the general public about a potential cancer risk from the use of pimecrolimus and tacrolimus, and recommends use as labelled and only where other treatments have failed. Pimecrolimus is used as a second line option for resistant cases in children over 2 years and in adults.

Tacrolimus *New*

Four RCTs identified by a systematic review found that 0.03% and 0.1% tacrolimus significantly increased clearance compared with a vehicle. Two RCTs identified by the review found that both 0.03% and 0.1% tacrolimus improved clearance compared with mild corticosteroids (1% hydrocortisone acetate or 0.1% aclometasone dipropionate) at 1 week and 3 weeks. One RCT found that 0.03% tacrolimus decreased clearance compared with a potent corticosteroid (0.1% hydrocortisone butyrate), however another RCT found no significant difference between 0.1% tacrolimus and a potent corticosteroid (0.12% betamethasone valerate). Three RCTs identified by the review found no significant difference in clearance between 0.03% tacrolimus versus 0.1% tacrolimus at 3 weeks. However, the other three RCTs in the review found that 0.1% tacrolimus significantly increased clearance at 12 weeks. Three similar RCTs, each examining a different population, found that 0.1% tacrolimus increased quality of life in adults, toddlers, and children compared with a vehicle. The systematic review found that 0.03% and 0.1% tacrolimus increased skin burning compared with vehicle. The United States Food and Drug Administration issued a public health advisory to inform healthcare professionals and the general public about a potential cancer risk from the use of pimecrolimus and tacrolimus, and recommend use as labelled and only where other treatments have failed. Tacrolimus is used as a second line option for resistant cases in children over 2 years and in adults.

What are the effects of dietary interventions in adults with established atopic eczema?

UNKNOWN EFFECTIVENESS

Vitamin E and multivitamins *New*

Three RCTs found insufficient evidence to assess vitamin E and multivitamins in atopic eczema. One RCT found no significant difference between selenium, selenium plus vitamin E, and placebo in severity of eczema at 12 weeks. One RCT found that vitamin E plus vitamin B2 reduced eczema severity compared with vitamin E or vitamin B2 alone at 4 weeks. One RCT found that vitamin E reduced eczema severity compared with placebo at 8 months.

What are the effects of dietary interventions in children with established atopic eczema?

UNKNOWN EFFECTIVENESS

Egg and cow's milk exclusion diet *New*

A systematic review and one subsequent RCT provided insufficient evidence to assess egg and milk free diets in people with atopic eczema. The RCT found that both extensively hydrolysed cow's milk formula and an amino acid based formula significantly improved eczema compared with baseline scores.

Elemental diet *New*

We found no RCTs of elemental diet in people with atopic eczema.

Few foods diet *New*

One RCT provided insufficient evidence to assess few foods diets in people with atopic eczema. It found that a few foods diet reduced eczema severity compared with a usual diet; however, there were a large number of withdrawals, mostly in the few foods diet group.

Probiotics *New*

One RCT provided insufficient evidence to assess probiotics in people with atopic eczema. The crossover RCT found that lactobacillus reduced total eczema severity compared with baseline measures; however, the change in severity was not statistically significant. It also found that lactobacillus increased perceived improvement in eczema compared with placebo. Another RCT found that heat inactivated, but not viable, lactobacillus increased episodes of diarrhoea in infants compared with placebo.

Pyridoxine (Vitamin B6) *New*

One RCT provided insufficient evidence to assess pyridoxine in people with atopic eczema. The RCT identified by a systematic review found no significant difference between pyridoxine and placebo in severity of eczema at 4 weeks.

Zinc supplementation *New*

One RCT provided insufficient evidence to assess zinc supplementation diets in people with atopic eczema. The RCT found no significant difference between zinc sulphate and placebo in severity of eczema at 8 weeks in children.

Atopic eczema

LIKELY TO BE INEFFECTIVE OR HARMFUL

Essential fatty acids (evening primrose oil, blackcurrant seed oil, fish oil) *New*

One systematic review and one subsequent RCT found no significant difference between essential fatty acids and placebo in severity of atopic eczema. The subsequent RCT found no significant difference between borage oil and placebo in the incidence of adverse effects.

What are the effects of primary preventive interventions in predisposed infants?

UNKNOWN EFFECTIVENESS

Prolonged breastfeeding by mother straight after birth *New*

We found no RCTs on the effect of breast feeding straight after birth on the development of atopic eczema in infants.

What are the effects of reducing allergens (maternal dietary restriction, control of house dust mite only)?

LIKELY TO BE BENEFICIAL

Early introduction of probiotics (in last trimester or shortly after birth) *New*

One RCT found that 1×10^{10} colony forming units of lactobacillus GG daily for 2–4 weeks before delivery decreased the proportion of infants who developed atopic eczema at 24 months by half and was maintained at 4 years.

UNKNOWN EFFECTIVENESS

Reduction of allergens (maternal dietary restriction, control of house dust mite only) *New*

One systematic review of methodologically poor RCTs found no significant difference between a maternal antigen avoidance diet during pregnancy and normal diet on the incidence of atopic eczema during the first 12–18 months of life. Subgroup analysis found limited evidence that a maternal antigen avoidance diet during lactation reduced the proportion of children developing atopic eczema during their first 12–18 months of life compared with normal diet. One RCT found no significant difference in the development of eczema between use of a mite impermeable mattress cover for the child's bed versus a simple educational package on allergen avoidance versus basic information about allergies at 24 months. One RCT identified by the review found that maternal antigen avoidance significantly decreased mean gestational weight gain by 1.8 kg for a 60 kg woman. Two RCTs identified by the review found that maternal antigen avoidance may be associated with a higher risk of preterm birth compared with no avoidance.

DEFINITION Atopic eczema (also known as atopic dermatitis) is a chronic, relapsing, and itchy inflammatory skin condition. In the acute stage, eczematous lesions are characterised by poorly defined erythema with surface change (oedema, vesicles, and weeping). In the chronic stage, lesions are marked by skin thickening (lichenification). Although lesions can occur anywhere on the body, babies often have eczematous lesions on their cheeks and outer limbs before developing the more typical flexural involvement behind the knees and in the folds of the elbow and neck later in childhood. Atopy, the tendency to produce specific immunoglobulin E responses to allergens, is associated with "atopic" eczema, but up to 60% of individuals with the disease phenotype may not be atopic.[1] This can cause confusion, for example around diagnosis, treatment, lifestyle recommendations, and genetic markers. The correct use of the term atopic eczema should therefore ideally only refer to those with a clinical picture of eczema who are also immunoglobulin E antibody high-responders. **Diagnosis:** There is no definitive "gold standard" for the diagnosis of atopic eczema, which is based on clinical features combined with a disease history. However, a UK working party developed a minimum list of reliable diagnostic criteria for atopic eczema using the Hanifin and Rajka list of clinical features as building blocks (see table 1 ⓣ).[2] In an independent validation study of children attending hospital dermatology outpatients, the criteria were shown to have a sensitivity of 85% and a specificity of 96% when compared with a dermatologist's diagnosis.[2] There are several severity scoring systems, used mainly in clinical trials, including the SCORing Atopic Dermatitis (SCORAD) and the six area, six sign atopic dermatitis severity score (SASSAD) indexes (see table 2 ⓣ). Quantitative scales used for measuring atopic eczema severity in clinical trials are too complex and difficult to interpret in clinical practice. The division of atopic eczema into mild, moderate, and severe mainly depends on the intensity of itching symptoms (e.g. resulting in sleep loss), the extent of involvement, and course of disease. **Population:** For the purposes of this review, we included all adults and children defined as having established atopic eczema. Where either adults or children are considered separately, this is highlighted in the text. We also included studies assessing primary prevention in those at risk of developing atopic eczema for specific interventions: prolonged breast feeding, maternal dietary restriction, house dust mite restriction, and early introduction of probiotics.

INCIDENCE/ PREVALENCE Atopic eczema affects 15–20% of school age children at some stage, and 2–10% of adults in the UK.[3] Prevalence data for the symptoms of atopic eczema were collected in the global International Study of Asthma and Allergies in Childhood (ISAAC). The results of the study suggest that atopic eczema is a worldwide problem affecting 5–20% of children.[4] One UK based population study showed that 2% of children under the age of 5 years have severe disease and 84% have mild disease.[5] Around 2% of adults have atopic eczema, and many of these have a more chronic and severe form.[6]

AETIOLOGY/ RISK FACTORS The causes of eczema are not well understood and are probably due to a combination of genetic and environmental factors.[7] In recent years, research has pointed to the possible role of environmental agents such as house dust mites,[8] pollution,[9] and prenatal or early exposure to infections.[10] The world allergy association's revised nomenclature for allergy also states that what is commonly called atopic eczema is not one specific disease but encompasses a spectrum of allergic mechanisms.[11]

PROGNOSIS Remission occurs by the age of 15 years in 60–70% of cases, although some relapse may occur later. Although no treatments are currently known to alter the natural history of atopic eczema, several interventions can help to control symptoms. Development and puberty may be delayed in the more severely affected child.[12]

Please refer to clinicalevidence.com for full text and references.

Cellulitis and erysipelas

Search date May 2005

Andrew D Morris

What are the effects of treatments for cellulitis and erysipelas?

LIKELY TO BE BENEFICIAL

Antibiotics

We found no RCTs or observational studies of sufficient quality comparing antibiotics versus placebo. RCTs comparing different antibiotic regimens found clinical cure in 50–100% of people.

UNKNOWN EFFECTIVENESS

Comparative effects of different antibiotic regimens

RCTs provided insufficient information on differences between regimens. However, most of the RCTs included only a small number of people with cellulitis or erysipelas, and were designed to test equivalence, rather than to detect a clinically important difference in cure rates between antibiotics.

Duration of antibiotics

We found one RCT comparing a 5 day course versus a 10 day course of antibiotics for uncomplicated cellulitis, which found no significant difference in the proportion of people with clinical cure at 14 days whose symptoms had not recurred by 28 days.

Oral versus intravenous antibiotics

We found no RCTs or observational studies of sufficient quality comparing oral antibiotics versus intravenous antibiotics.

Treatment of predisposing factors to prevent recurrence of cellulitis and erysipelas

We found no systematic review, RCTs, or observational studies of sufficient quality about the effects of treating predisposing factors to prevent recurrence of cellulitis or erysipelas.

DEFINITION **Cellulitis** is a spreading bacterial infection of the dermis and subcutaneous tissues. It causes local signs of inflammation such as warmth, erythema, pain, lymphangitis, and frequently systemic upset with fever and raised white blood cell count. **Erysipelas** is a form of cellulitis and is characterised by pronounced superficial inflammation. The lower limbs are by far the most common sites, but any area can be affected. The term erysipelas is commonly used when the face is affected.

INCIDENCE/ PREVALENCE We found no validated recent data on the incidence of cellulitis or erysipelas worldwide, but cellulitis is accepted to be a common problem. Cellulitis and abscess infections were responsible for 158 consultations per 10 000 people per year in the UK in 1991.[1] In 1985 in the UK, skin and subcutaneous tissue infections resulted in 29 820 hospital admissions and a mean occupancy of 664 hospital beds each day.[2] In 2002–2003 in England, the mean length of hospital stay for cellulitis was 9.3 days.[3]

AETIOLOGY/ RISK FACTORS The most common infective organisms for cellulitis and erysipelas in adults are streptococci (particularly *Streptococcus pyogenes*) and *Staphylococcus aureus*.[4] In children, *Haemophilus influenzae* was a frequent cause prior to the introduction of the *Haemophilus influenzae* type B vaccination. Several risk factors for cellulitis and erysipelas have been identified in a case control study (167 cases and 294 controls): lymphoedema (OR 71.2, 95% CI 5.6 to 908.0), leg ulcer (OR 62.5, 95% CI 7.0 to 556.0), toe web intertrigo (OR 13.9, 95% CI 7.2 to 27.0), and traumatic wounds (OR 10.7, 95% CI 4.8 to 23.8).[5]

PROGNOSIS Cellulitis can spread through the bloodstream and lymphatic system. A retrospective case study of people admitted to hospital with cellulitis found that systemic symptoms such as fever and raised white blood cell count were present in up to 42% of cases at presentation.[6] Lymphatic involvement can lead to obstruction and damage of the lymphatic system that predisposes to recurrent cellulitis.[7] Recurrence can occur rapidly, or after months or years. One prospective cohort study found that 29% of people with erysipelas had a recurrent episode within 3 years.[8] Local necrosis and abscess formation can also occur.[7] It is not known whether the prognosis of erysipelas differs from that of cellulitis. We found no evidence about factors that predict recurrence, or a better or worse outcome. We found no good evidence on the prognosis of untreated cellulitis.

Please refer to clinicalevidence.com for full text and references.

Fungal toenail infections

Search date June 2005

Fay Crawford and Jill Ferrari

What are the effects of treatments for fungal toenail infections?

BENEFICIAL

Oral itraconazole (more effective than placebo, but probably less effective than terbinafine)

One systematic review found that itraconazole increased cure rates of fungal toenail infection compared with placebo. It found that itraconazole had lower cure rates compared with terbinafine. It found no significant difference in cure rates between itraconazole and griseofulvin, or between pulsed and continuous itraconazole. We found no RCTs comparing itraconazole with ketoconazole or fluconazole.

Oral terbinafine

One systematic review found that terbinafine increased cure rates of fungal toenail infection compared with placebo, griseofulvin, and itraconazole. We found no RCTs comparing terbinafine with ketoconazole or fluconazole.

LIKELY TO BE BENEFICIAL

Oral fluconazole (although benefits are modest, even after long term treatment)

One systematic review found that fluconazole increased cure rates of fungal toenail infection compared with placebo, although benefits were modest. We found no RCTs comparing fluconazole with griseofulvin, terbinafine, itraconazole, or ketoconazole.

Topical ciclopirox (although benefits are modest, even after long term treatment)

One RCT found that 48 weeks of treatment with ciclopirox increased cure rates compared with placebo, although benefits were modest.

UNKNOWN EFFECTIVENESS

Oral griseofulvin

One systematic review found that griseofulvin produced lower cure rates compared with terbinafine. It found no significant difference in cure rates between griseofulvin, itraconazole, and ketoconazole. We found no RCTs comparing griseofulvin with placebo or fluconazole.

Oral ketoconazole

One systematic review found no significant difference in cure rates of fungal toenail infection between ketoconazole and griseofulvin. We found no RCTs comparing ketoconazole with placebo, terbinafine, itraconazole, or fluconazole.

Topical amorolfine

We found no RCTs on the effects of topical amorolfine in fungal toenail infection.

Topical butenafine

We found no RCTs on the effects of topical butenafine in fungal toenail infection. ▶

Topical fluconazole

We found no RCTs on the effects of topical fluconazole in fungal toenail infection.

Topical ketoconazole

We found no RCTs on the effects of topical ketoconazole in fungal toenail infection.

Topical terbinafine

We found no RCTs on the effects of topical terbinafine in fungal toenail infection.

Topical tioconazole

We found no RCTs on the effects of topical tioconazole in fungal toenail infection.

DEFINITION Fungal toenail infection (onychomycosis) is characterised as infection of part or all of the toenail unit, which includes the toenail plate, the toenail bed, and the toenail matrix.[1-3] Over time, the infection causes discolouration and distortion of part or all of the toenail unit.[4] The tissue under and around the toenail may also thicken. This chapter deals exclusively with dermatophyte toenail infections (see aetiology) and excludes candidal or yeast infections.

INCIDENCE/ PREVALENCE Fungal infections are reported to cause 23% of foot diseases and 50% of nail conditions in people seen by dermatologists but are less common in the general population, affecting 3–5% of people.[3] The prevalence varies among populations, which may be because of differences in screening techniques. In a large European project (13 695 people with a range of foot conditions), 35% had a fungal infection diagnosed by microscopy/culture.[5] However, a cross sectional study in Spanish people (10 007 adults aged ≥ 15 years) reported a prevalence of 2.6%,[6] while a survey in Scottish people (9332 adults aged ≥ 16 years) reported a prevalence of 2.1%.[7] The incidence of mycotic nail infections may have increased over the past few years, perhaps because of increasing use of systemic antibiotics, immunosuppressive treatment, more advanced surgical techniques, and the increasing incidence of HIV infection.[8] However, this was contradicted by a study in an outpatient department in Eastern Croatia, which compared the prevalence of fungal infections between two time periods (1986–1988, 47 832 people; 1997–2001, 75 691 people).[9] It found that the prevalence of fungal infection overall had increased greatly over the 10 years, but the percentage of fungal infections affecting the nail had decreased by 1% (fungal infections overall: 0.26% in 1986–1988 *v* 0.73% in 1997–2001; nail: 10.31% in 1986–1988 *v* 9.31% in 1997–2001).

AETIOLOGY/ RISK FACTORS Fungal nail infections are most commonly caused by anthropophilic fungi called dermatophytes. The genera *Trichophyton*, *Epidermophyton*, and *Microsporum* are typically involved,[1] specifically *T rubrum*, *T mentagrophytes* var. *interdigitale*, and *E floccosum*. Other fungi, moulds, or yeasts may be isolated, such as *Scopulariopsis brevicaulis*, *Aspergillus*, *Fusarium*, and *Candida albicans*.[3] *T rubrum* is now regarded as the most common cause of onychomycosis in the world.[10] Several factors that increase the risk of developing a fungal nail infection have been identified. One survey found that 26% of people with diabetes had onychomycosis and that diabetes increased the risk of infection, but the type and severity of diabetes was not correlated with infection (OR 2.77, 95% CI 2.15 to 3.57).[11] Another survey found that peripheral vascular disease and immunosuppression increased the risk of infection (OR 1.78, 95% CI 1.68 to 1.88 for peripheral vascular disease; OR 1.19, 95% CI 1.01 to 1.40 for immunosuppression). These factors may explain the general increase in prevalence of onychomycosis in the elderly population.[12] Environmental exposures such as occlusive footwear or warm, damp conditions have been cited as risk factors, as has trauma.[2,12] Fungal skin infection has been proposed as a risk

Fungal toenail infections

factor.[3,10,12] However, one large observational study, which included 5413 people with positive mycology, found that only a small proportion (21.3%) had both skin and toenail infections.[12]

PROGNOSIS Onychomycosis does not have serious consequences in otherwise healthy people. However, the Achilles project (846 people with fungal toenail infection) found that many people complain of discomfort in walking (51%), pain (33%), or limitation of their work or other activities (13%).[5] Gross distortion and dystrophy of the nail may cause trauma to the adjacent skin and may lead to secondary bacterial infection. In immunocompromised people, there is a risk that this infection will disseminate. Quality of life measures that are specific to onychomycosis have recently been developed. Studies using these indicators suggest that onychomycosis has negative physical and psychosocial effects.[13-15]

Please refer to clinicalevidence.com for full text and references.

Head lice

Search date October 2005

Ian Burgess

What are the effects of treatments for head lice?

LIKELY TO BE BENEFICIAL

Malathion

One RCT found that malathion lotion increased lice eradication rates compared with phenothrin lotion. One RCT found that malathion was more effective at eradicating live lice and lice eggs at 14 days than permethrin. One RCT identified by a systematic review found that malathion was more effective than wet combing with conditioner ("bug busting"). Another RCT found that pediculicide (malathion or permethrin) was less effective than "bug busting" for eradicating lice in a population with a high prevalence of insecticide resistance. We found no RCTs that compared malathion versus herbal treatments, pyrethrum, lindane, or co-trimoxazole.

Permethrin

One systematic review found that permethrin increased eradication rates compared with lindane. One RCT found that permethrin was less effective than malathion for eradication of lice and viable eggs at 14 days. Another RCT found that pediculicide (permethrin or malathion) was less effective than "bug busting" for eradicating lice in a population with a high prevalence of insecticide resistance. One RCT found that permethrin plus oral co-trimoxazole increased eradication rates compared with permethrin alone, but found high rates of adverse effects with co-trimoxazole. The RCT found no significant difference in eradication rates between permethrin alone and oral co-trimoxazole alone. We found no RCTs comparing permethrin versus phenothrin, pyrethrum, or herbal treatments.

TRADE OFF BETWEEN BENEFITS AND HARMS

Oral co-trimoxazole (trimethoprim plus sulfamethoxazole)

One RCT found no significant difference between oral co-trimoxazole alone and topical permethrin alone or oral co-trimoxazole plus topical permethrin in eradication of lice, nymphal stage, and eggs at 4 weeks. It found that co-trimoxazole plus permethrin increased eradication compared with permethrin alone. The RCT found that 25% of children taking co-trimoxazole developed intense pruritus after 3–4 days, but it disappeared after 1–3 hours. Potentially serious but rare adverse effects associated with co-trimoxazole include Stevens–Johnson syndrome, erythema multiforme, and blood disorders.

UNKNOWN EFFECTIVENESS

Combinations of insecticides

One RCT found no significant difference in eradication rates between a herbal product (coconut, anise, and ylang ylang) and a combination of insecticides (permethrin plus malathion, synergised with piperonyl butoxide). However, results may not generalise to different concentrations of these components or to different herbal preparations. We found no RCTs comparing combinations of insecticides versus single agents or co-trimoxazole.

Head lice

Dimeticone

We found one RCT that found no significant difference in eradication rates between 4% dimeticone lotion and 0.5% phenothrin liquid.

Herbal and essential oils

We found no RCTs that compared herbal products versus malathion, permethrin, phenothrin, pyrethrum, lindane, or co-trimoxazole. One RCT found no significant difference in eradication rates between a herbal product (coconut, anise, and ylang ylang) and a combination of insecticides (permethrin plus malathion, synergised with piperonyl butoxide). However, results may not generalise to different concentrations of these components or to different herbal preparations.

Lindane

One systematic review found that lindane was less effective at eliminating lice than permethrin. We found no RCTs comparing lindane versus other insecticides, mechanical removal of lice, herbal treatments, or co-trimoxazole. The possibility of central nervous system toxicity from lindane has led to its withdrawal in some countries.

Mechanical removal of lice or viable eggs by combing

One RCT identified by a systematic review found that wet combing with conditioner ("bug busting") was less effective than malathion at eradicating lice. Another RCT found that "bug busting" was more effective than pediculicide treatment (malathion or permethrin) in a population with a high prevalence of insecticide resistance. One methodologically weak RCT provided insufficient evidence to compare wet combing with conditioner versus phenothrin plus combing. One RCT found no difference in eradication rates using permethrin with adjuvant combing compared with permethrin alone. We found no RCTs comparing mechanical removal versus pyrethrum or lindane.

Phenothrin

We found no RCTs comparing phenothrin versus permethrin, pyrethrum, or lindane. One methodologically weak RCT provided insufficient evidence to compare phenothrin plus combing versus wet combing with conditioner. Another RCT found that malathion increased eradication rates compared with phenothrin. One RCT found no significant difference between 0.5% phenothrin liquid and 4% dimeticone lotion.

Pyrethrum

We found no RCTs comparing pyrethrum versus other insecticides, mechanical removal of lice, herbal treatments, or co-trimoxazole.

DEFINITION Head lice are obligate ectoparasites of socially active humans. They infest the scalp and attach their eggs to the hair shafts. Itching, resulting from multiple bites, is not diagnostic but may increase the index of suspicion. Eggs glued to hairs, whether hatched (nits) or unhatched, are not proof of active infection, because eggs may retain a viable appearance for weeks after death. A conclusive diagnosis can only be made by finding live lice. One observational study compared two groups of children with louse eggs but no lice at initial assessment.[1] Over 14 days, more children with five or more eggs within 6 mm of the scalp developed infestations compared with those with fewer than five eggs. Adequate follow up examinations using detection combing are more likely to be productive than nit removal to prevent reinfestation. Infestations are not self limiting.

INCIDENCE/ PREVALENCE We found no studies on the incidence and few recently published studies of prevalence in developed countries. Anecdotal reports suggest that prevalence has increased in the past few years in most communities in Europe, the Americas, and Australasia. A recent cross-sectional study from Belgium (6169 children, aged 2.5–12.0 years) found a prevalence of 8.9%.[2] An earlier pilot study (677 children, aged 3–11 years) showed that in individual schools the prevalence was as high as 19.5%.[3] One cross-sectional study from Belgium found that head lice were significantly more common in children from families with lower socioeconomic status (OR 1.25, 95% CI 1.04 to 1.47); in children with more siblings (OR 1.2, 95% CI 1.1 to 1.3); and in children with longer hair (OR 1.20, 95% CI 1.02 to 1.43), although hair length may influence ability to detect infestation. Socioeconomic status of the family was also a significant influence on the ability to treat infestations successfully; the lower the socioeconomic status the greater the risk of treatment failure (OR 1.70, 95% CI 1.05 to 2.70).[2]

AETIOLOGY/ RISK FACTORS Observational studies indicate that infestations occur most frequently in school children, although there is no evidence of a link with school attendance.[4,5] We found no evidence that lice prefer clean hair to dirty hair.

PROGNOSIS The infestation is almost harmless. Sensitisation reactions to louse saliva and faeces may result in localised irritation and erythema. Secondary infection of scratches may occur. Lice have been identified as primary mechanical vectors of scalp pyoderma caused by streptococci and staphylococci usually found on the skin.[6]

Please refer to clinicalevidence.com for full text and references.

Herpes labialis

Search date April 2006

Graham Worrall

What are the effects of antiviral treatments for the first attack of herpes labialis?

LIKELY TO BE BENEFICIAL

Oral antiviral agents (aciclovir)

One small RCT in children found that oral aciclovir reduced the mean duration of pain compared with placebo. Another small RCT in children found that oral aciclovir reduced the median time to healing compared with placebo.

UNKNOWN EFFECTIVENESS

Topical antiviral agents

We found no RCTs on the effects of topical antiviral agents.

What are the effects of interventions aimed at preventing recurrent attacks of herpes labialis?

LIKELY TO BE BENEFICIAL

Oral antiviral agents (aciclovir)

Six RCTs found limited evidence suggesting that prophylactic oral antiviral agents may reduce the frequency and severity of attacks compared with placebo, but the optimal timing and duration of treatment is uncertain.

Sunscreen

Two small crossover RCTs, one undertaken under laboratory conditions, found that ultraviolet sunscreen may reduce herpes recurrence compared with placebo.

UNKNOWN EFFECTIVENESS

Topical antiviral agents

We found no RCTs on the effects of topical antiviral agents used as prophylaxis.

What are the effects of treatments for recurrent attacks of herpes labialis?

LIKELY TO BE BENEFICIAL

Oral antiviral agents (aciclovir and valaciclovir)

Four RCTs found limited evidence that oral aciclovir and valaciclovir (if taken early in the attack) marginally reduced the duration of symptoms and pain compared with placebo. Two large RCTs found no significant difference between a 1 day and a 2 day course of valaciclovir and found that a higher proportion of people experienced headaches with valaciclovir compared with placebo.

UNKNOWN EFFECTIVENESS

Topical anaesthetic agents

One RCT found that topical tetracaine reduced the mean time to scab loss and increased the proportion of people who subjectively rated the treatment as effective compared with placebo. However, the clinical importance of these results is unclear as the absolute difference between groups was small.

Topical antiviral agents (slightly reduced healing time with aciclovir or penciclovir and limited effect on duration of pain)

Eight RCTs found that aciclovir or penciclovir slightly reduced healing time compared with placebo. Four RCTs found no significant difference in duration of pain between aciclovir and placebo but one RCT found that penciclovir reduced duration of pain compared with placebo.

Zinc oxide cream

One RCT found that zinc oxide cream reduced time to healing by 1.5 days compared with placebo, but found that it increased the risk of skin irritation.

DEFINITION Herpes labialis is a mild self limiting infection with herpes simplex virus type 1. It causes pain and blistering on the lips and perioral area (cold sores); fever and constitutional symptoms are rare. Most people have no warning of an attack, but some experience a recognisable prodrome.

INCIDENCE/ PREVALENCE Herpes labialis accounts for about 1% of primary care consultations in the UK each year; 20–40% of people have experienced cold sores at some time.[1]

AETIOLOGY/ RISK FACTORS Herpes labialis is caused by herpes simplex virus type 1. After the primary infection, which usually occurs in childhood, the virus is thought to remain latent in the trigeminal ganglion.[2] A variety of factors, including exposure to bright sunlight, fatigue, or psychological stress, can precipitate a recurrence.

PROGNOSIS In most people, herpes labialis is a mild, self limiting illness. Recurrences are usually shorter and less severe than the initial attack. Healing is usually complete in 7–10 days without scarring.[3] Rates of reactivation are unknown. Herpes labialis can cause serious illness in immunocompromised people.

Please refer to clinicalevidence.com for full text and references.

Malignant melanoma (non-metastatic)

Search date October 2005

Thomas Crosby and Philip Savage

What are the effects of interventions to prevent malignant melanoma?

UNKNOWN EFFECTIVENESS

Sunscreens

We found no RCTs examining the preventive effects of sunscreens on melanoma. Due to the nature of the intervention, it is unlikely that an RCT would be conducted. Systematic reviews of case control studies found inconclusive evidence about the effects of sunscreen use on reducing the incidence of malignant melanoma.

Is there an optimal surgical margin for the primary excision of melanoma?

LIKELY TO BE BENEFICIAL

Wider (3 cm) excision (reduced locoregional recurrence compared with narrower [1cm] excision in people with tumours of > 2 mm Breslow thickness)

We found one large RCT in people with thicker primary melanoma of > 2 mm Breslow depth, which found that a 1 cm excision margin increased locoregional recurrence compared with a 3 cm margin. It also found a non-statistically significant trend towards more deaths from melanoma with a 1 cm excision margin than with a 3 cm margin. We found no direct evidence comparing 2 cm and 3 cm excision margins in this group of people.

UNLIKELY TO BE BENEFICIAL

Wide excision (no better than narrower excision in people with tumours of < 2 mm Breslow thickness)

We found two systematic reviews and one subsequent RCT in people with primary cutaneous melanoma of < 2 mm Breslow depth. The reviews and the subsequent RCT found no significant difference in overall survival over 4–10 years between radical local surgery (4–5 cm excision margins) and less radical surgery (1–2 cm excision margins). The RCTs also found no significant difference in local recurrence rates between wider and narrower excision margins. One of the RCTs identified by the reviews found that wider excision increased the need for skin grafting and the duration of hospital stay compared with narrower excision; the other RCTs gave no information on adverse effects.

What are the effects of elective lymph node dissection in people with clinically uninvolved lymph nodes?

UNLIKELY TO BE BENEFICIAL

Elective lymph node dissection

One systematic review found no significant difference in survival at 5 years between elective lymph node dissection and delayed or no lymph node dissection in people with malignant melanoma without clinically detectable lymph node metastases.

What are the effects of sentinel lymph node biopsy in people with clinically uninvolved lymph nodes?

UNKNOWN EFFECTIVENESS

Sentinel lymph node biopsy

We found no systematic reviews or RCTs of sentinel lymph node biopsy that assessed survival in people with malignant melanoma.

What are the effects of adjuvant treatment?

UNKNOWN EFFECTIVENESS

Adjuvant vaccines in people with malignant melanoma

Four RCTs found no significant difference in survival between adjuvant vaccines and surgery alone or surgery plus placebo vaccine in people with malignant melanoma. One RCT found that ganglioside GM2 vaccine was less effective than high dose alfa interferon in improving relapse free and overall survival. A different vaccine preparation was used in each RCT, making it difficult to compare results from individual RCTs.

High dose adjuvant alfa interferon

One systematic review of three RCTs found that high dose alfa interferon reduced relapse rates compared with no adjuvant treatment. However, it found no significant difference between high dose alfa interferon and no adjuvant treatment in overall survival at 4–7 years. The review found evidence from two RCTs that higher doses of alfa interferon reduced relapse rate compared with low dose interferon, but found no significant difference in overall survival. One RCT found that high dose alfa interferon improved both relapse free and overall survival compared with ganglioside GM2 vaccine. Toxicity (myelosuppression, hepatotoxicity, and neurotoxicity) and withdrawal rates were high in people taking high dose alfa interferon; in one RCT, 76% of people had grade 3 or 4 toxicity.

Surveillance for early treatment of recurrence

We found no systematic reviews or RCTs examining the potential benefit of more or less intensive follow up or surveillance for early treatment of recurrent melanoma.

Malignant melanoma (non-metastatic)

UNLIKELY TO BE BENEFICIAL

Low dose adjuvant alfa interferon

One systematic review of seven RCTs found that low dose alfa interferon reduced relapse rates, but did not improve overall survival over 3–7 years, compared with no adjuvant treatment. Two subsequent RCTs found no significant difference in relapse free survival or overall survival at 5–8 years between low dose alfa interferon and no adjuvant treatment. The review found evidence from two RCTs that higher doses of alfa interferon reduced relapse rate compared with low dose interferon, but found no significant difference in overall survival. In one RCT, grade III or IV toxicity occurred in 10% of people taking low dose alfa interferon, and in another RCT, 15% of people withdrew owing to adverse effects.

DEFINITION Malignant melanoma is a tumour derived from melanocytes in the basal layer of the epidermis. After malignant transformation, the cancer cells become invasive by penetrating into and beyond the dermis. Metastatic spread can occur to the regional lymph nodes or to distant sites, particularly the lungs, liver, and central nervous system.

INCIDENCE/ PREVALENCE The incidence of melanoma varies widely in different populations (see table 1)Ⓣ and is about 10–20 fold higher in white than non-white populations. Estimates suggest that the number of cases of melanoma in the UK has increased approximately fourfold over the past 25 years.[1] Despite this rising incidence, death rates have changed more modestly and in some populations are now beginning to fall.[2,3] The increased early diagnosis of thin, good prognosis melanoma and melanoma in situ are the main reasons for the divergent findings on incidence and death rates.

AETIOLOGY/ RISK FACTORS The risk factors for the development of melanoma can be divided into genetic and environmental. Alongside the genetic risk factors of skin type and hair colour, the number of naevi a person has correlates closely with the risk of developing malignant melanoma.[4] Although the risk of developing malignant melanoma is higher in fair skinned populations living in areas of high sun exposure, the exact relationship between sun exposure, sunscreen use, skin type and risk is not clear. Both high total lifetime exposure to excessive sunlight and episodes of severe sunburn in childhood are associated with an increased risk of developing malignant melanoma in adult life. However, people do not necessarily develop malignancy at the sites of maximum exposure to the sun.

PROGNOSIS The prognosis of early stage malignant melanoma which is clinically limited to the primary skin site (stages I–II) (see table 2)Ⓣ is predominantly related to the depth of dermal invasion and the presence of ulceration. In stage III disease, where disease is present in the regional lymph nodes, the prognosis becomes worse with the increasing number of nodes involved.[5] For example, a person with a thin lesion (Breslow thickness < 1.0 mm) without lymph node involvement has a 95% chance of surviving 5 years. However, if the regional lymph nodes are macroscopically involved, the overall survival at 5 years is only 20–50%. In addition to tumour thickness and lymph node involvement, a number of studies have shown a better prognosis in women and in people with lesions on the limbs compared with those with lesions on the trunk.

Please refer to clinicalevidence.com for full text and references.

Psoriasis (chronic plaque)

Search date July 2005

Luigi Naldi and Berthold Rzany

What are the effects of non-drug treatments (other than ultraviolet light)?

UNKNOWN EFFECTIVENESS

Acupuncture

One RCT provided insufficient evidence on the effects of acupuncture for chronic plaque psoriasis.

Balneotherapy

One RCT provided insufficient evidence on the effects of balneotherapy in people with chronic plaque psoriasis.

Fish oil supplementation

RCTs provided insufficient evidence on the effects of fish oil supplementation for chronic plaque psoriasis.

Psychotherapy

We found no RCTs of sufficient quality of psychotherapy for chronic plaque psoriasis.

What are the effects of topical drug treatments?

BENEFICIAL

Tazarotene

RCTs found that tazarotene, a topical retinoid, improved mild to moderate chronic plaque psoriasis in the short term compared with placebo. One RCT found no significant difference between tazarotene and the topical corticosteroid fluocinonide in the reduction of lesion severity at 12 weeks. Three RCTs found that adding topical corticosteroids to tazarotene treatment improved response rate compared with tazarotene alone. A fourth RCT found that combined topical corticosteroid and tazarotene treatment increased the proportion of people with marked improvement compared with the vitamin D derivative calcipotriol. Tazarotene is contraindicated in women who are, or intend to become, pregnant because it is potentially teratogenic.

Vitamin D derivatives (topical)

One systematic review found that topical vitamin D derivatives improved plaque psoriasis compared with placebo. RCTs found that calcipotriol was more effective than other vitamin D derivatives. One systematic review found no significant difference in effectiveness between topical vitamin D derivatives and "potent" topical corticosteroids, but found that calcipotriol caused more perilesional and lesional irritation. One systematic review and one subsequent RCT found that topical vitamin D derivatives improved psoriasis at 4–12 weeks compared with dithranol, and caused fewer adverse effects. One systematic review found that calcipotriol improved psoriasis compared with coal tar, alone or in combination with allantoin and hydrocortisone. One RCT found that calcipotriol was less effective than combined topical corticosteroid and tazarotene treatment in increasing the proportion of people with marked improvement. RCTs found that ▶

Psoriasis (chronic plaque)

combination treatment with vitamin D derivatives plus "potent" topical corticosteroids improved psoriasis compared with either treatment alone or with placebo. In the short term, the combination of vitamin D derivatives plus topical corticosteroids decreased irritation compared with monotherapy. RCTs found that adding calcipotriol to oral fumaric acid or to dithranol improved psoriasis compared with fumaric acid or dithranol alone. RCTs provided insufficient evidence to compare vitamin D derivatives versus ultraviolet B or psoralen plus ultraviolet A or to assess other combination treatments containing topical vitamin D derivatives.

LIKELY TO BE BENEFICIAL

Dithranol

One systematic review of small RCTs found that dithranol improved chronic plaque psoriasis after 4–8 weeks compared with placebo. One systematic review of small RCTs found no significant difference between conventional and short contact dithranol treatment, but the RCTs may have lacked power to detect clinically relevant differences. One systematic review and one subsequent RCT found that dithranol was less effective than topical vitamin D derivatives and caused more adverse effects. One RCT found that adding calcipotriol, a vitamin D derivative, to dithranol improved psoriasis compared with dithranol alone. Small RCTs provided insufficient evidence to compare dithranol versus ultraviolet B or psoralen plus ultraviolet A in people with chronic plaque psoriasis. For information on the Ingram regimen, which contains dithranol, please see separate options.

Emollients*

We found no RCTs of emollients alone in people with chronic plaque psoriasis. However, there is consensus that they are effective and they are initial or adjunctive treatment for most people with chronic plaque psoriasis. One small RCT provided insufficient evidence on the effects of adding emollients to ultraviolet B radiation.

TRADE OFF BETWEEN BENEFITS AND HARMS

Corticosteroids (topical)

One systematic review found that topical corticosteroids, especially "potent" and "very potent" ones, improved psoriasis in the short term compared with placebo. Three small RCTs found limited evidence that occlusive polyethylene or hydrocolloid dressings enhanced the clinical activity of topical corticosteroids. The review found no significant difference in effectiveness between "potent" topical corticosteroids and vitamin D derivatives; another review found that calcipotriol caused more perilesional and lesional irritation than "potent" topical corticosteroids. One RCT found no significant difference between topical fluocinonide and the topical retinoid tazarotene in the reduction of lesion severity at 12 weeks. Three RCTs found that adding topical corticosteroids to tazarotene treatment improved response rate compared with tazarotene alone. A fourth RCT found that combined topical corticosteroid and tazarotene treatment increased the proportion of people with marked improvement compared with the vitamin D derivative calcipotriol. One systematic review found that a topical corticosteroid plus an oral retinoid was superior to the single treatments in improving psoriasis. RCTs found that combination treatment with "potent" topical corticosteroids plus vitamin D derivatives improved psoriasis compared with either treatment alone or with placebo. In the short term, the combination of topical corticosteroids plus vitamin D derivatives decreased irritation compared with monotherapy. Small RCTs provided insufficient evidence to compare topical corticosteroids versus ultraviolet B or psoralen plus ultraviolet A. Topical corticosteroids may cause striae and atrophy, which increase with potency and use of occlusive dressings. Continuous use may lead to adrenocortical suppression, and case reports suggest that severe flares of the disease may occur on withdrawal.

UNKNOWN EFFECTIVENESS

Salicylic acid

One small RCT provided insufficient evidence to assess topical salicylic acid compared with placebo in people with chronic plaque psoriasis. We found no RCTs of urea cream in people with chronic plaque psoriasis.

Tars

Small RCTs, some identified by a systematic review, provided insufficient evidence on the effects of coal tar compared with placebo, ultraviolet B, or psoralen plus ultraviolet A in people with chronic plaque psoriasis. Small RCTs found conflicting results on the effects of tars in combination with ultraviolet B exposure or dithranol. One small RCT provided insufficient evidence to compare coal tar plus fatty acids versus coal tar alone. One systematic review found that coal tar, alone or in combination with allantoin and hydrocortisone, was less effective than topical vitamin D derivatives (calcipotriol). For information on the Ingram regimen or Goeckerman treatment, which contain coal tar, please see separate options.

What are the effects of treatments with ultraviolet light?

LIKELY TO BE BENEFICIAL

Heliotherapy*

One RCT provided insufficient evidence on the effects of heliotherapy for chronic plaque psoriasis. Although we found limited evidence, there is consensus that heliotherapy is an effective option for most people with chronic plaque psoriasis.

Psoralen plus ultraviolet A (PUVA)*

One systematic review identified no RCTs that compared psoralen plus ultraviolet A versus no treatment. However, there is consensus that psoralen plus ultraviolet A is effective for clearance of psoriasis. One systematic review found that higher doses of psoralen improved psoriasis clearance more than lower doses of psoralen. One large RCT found that maintenance treatment with psoralen plus ultraviolet A reduced relapse compared with no maintenance treatment. One RCT found that psoralen plus ultraviolet A was more effective than the Ingram regimen in clearing psoriasis. RCTs provided insufficient evidence to compare psoralen plus ultraviolet A versus other treatments or to assess psoralen plus ultraviolet A combined with vitamin D derivatives or oral retinoids. Long term adverse effects of psoralen plus ultraviolet A treatment include photoaging and skin cancer (mainly squamous cell carcinoma).

Ultraviolet B*

We found no RCTs comparing ultraviolet B versus placebo or no treatment. However, there is consensus that ultraviolet B is effective in people with plaque psoriasis. RCTs provided insufficient evidence on the effects of ultraviolet B compared with other treatments, or on the effects of narrow band compared

Psoriasis (chronic plaque)

with broad band ultraviolet B for either clearance or maintenance treatment. One RCT found limited evidence that ultraviolet B given three times weekly cleared psoriasis faster than twice weekly treatment, with high clearance rates in both groups. RCTs provided insufficient evidence to assess combined treatment with ultraviolet B plus emollients, dithranol, vitamin D derivatives, or oral retinoids. For information on the Ingram regimen or Goeckerman treatment, which use ultraviolet B irradiation in combination with drug treatment, please see separate options.

UNKNOWN EFFECTIVENESS

Phototherapy plus balneotherapy

RCTs provided insufficient evidence on the effects of phototherapy plus balneotherapy in people with chronic plaque psoriasis.

Ultraviolet A

One RCT provided insufficient evidence on the effects of ultraviolet A sunbeds for chronic plaque psoriasis.

What are the effects of systemic drug treatments?

LIKELY TO BE BENEFICIAL

Alefacept

Three RCTs found that alefacept improved psoriasis and quality of life at 12 weeks compared with placebo. Alefacept is a relatively new drug for the treatment of psoriasis, and there is limited evidence regarding the possibility of long term or rare adverse effects.

Efalizumab

Three RCTs found that efalizumab improved psoriasis compared with placebo at 12 weeks. Two of the RCTs extended treatment to 24 weeks and found further improvements in people who had not initially had a complete response to treatment. Efalizumab is a relatively new drug for the treatment of psoriasis, and there is limited evidence regarding the possibility of long term or rare adverse effects.

Etanercept

Two RCTs found that etanercept increased the proportion of responders at 12–24 weeks compared with placebo. One of the RCTs found that quality of life improved more with etanercept than with placebo at 12 weeks. Etanercept is a relatively new drug for the treatment of psoriasis, and there is limited evidence regarding the possibility of long term or rare adverse events.

Infliximab

Two RCTs in people with severe psoriasis found that infliximab improved response rates at 10 weeks compared with placebo. Infliximab is a relatively new drug for the treatment of psoriasis, and there is limited evidence regarding the possibility of long term or rare adverse events.

TRADE OFF BETWEEN BENEFITS AND HARMS

Ciclosporin

One systematic review of people with severe psoriasis found that ciclosporin (cyclosporin) improved clearance compared with placebo and increased the proportion of people who remained in remission. One RCT found no significant difference between ciclosporin and methotrexate in complete or partial remission, duration of remission of psoriasis, or adverse effects. Two RCTs in people with severe psoriasis identified by a systematic review found that ciclosporin was more effective than etretinate for reducing psoriasis severity. RCTs provided insufficient evidence to assess adding calcipotriol to ciclosporin compared with ciclosporin alone in people with chronic plaque psoriasis. Two RCTs in people with severe psoriasis identified by the review found that a ciclosporin dose of 5.0 mg/kg daily increased response compared with a ciclosporin dose of 2.5 mg/kg daily. Any advantage of higher doses may be offset by an increase in dose related adverse effects, particularly increased renal toxicity and hypertension. The review found that a ciclosporin dose of 3.0 mg/kg daily was more effective than lower doses or than placebo for maintenance.

Fumaric acid derivatives

One systematic review of four small RCTs in people with severe psoriasis found limited evidence that oral fumaric acid esters reduced the severity of psoriasis after 16 weeks compared with placebo. However, acute adverse effects were common and included flushing and gastrointestinal symptoms. We found no RCTs on the effects of fumaric acid derivatives as maintenance treatment.

Methotrexate

One small RCT provided insufficient evidence about the effects of methotrexate compared with placebo. One RCT found no significant difference between methotrexate and ciclosporin (cyclosporin) in complete or partial remission, duration of remission of psoriasis, or adverse effects. Methotrexate can induce acute myelosuppression. Long term methotrexate carries the risk of hepatic fibrosis and cirrhosis, which is related to the dose regimen employed.

Retinoids (oral etretinate, acitretin)

One systematic review of people with severe psoriasis found limited evidence that oral retinoids improved clearance compared with placebo and was less effective than ciclosporin (cyclosporin) in improving clearance. RCTs provided insufficient evidence on the effects of oral retinoids as maintenance treatment. One systematic review found that an oral retinoid plus a topical corticosteroid was superior to the single treatments in improving psoriasis. One RCT provided insufficient evidence to assess adding calcipotriol to an oral retinoid compared with an oral retinoid alone. Adverse effects led to discontinuation of oral retinoid treatment in 10–20% of people. Teratogenicity renders oral retinoids less acceptable. Etretinate is no longer available in many countries.

UNKNOWN EFFECTIVENESS

Leflunomide

One RCT in people with psoriatic arthritis found limited evidence that leflunomide improved cutaneous psoriasis compared with placebo.

What are the effects of combined treatment with drugs plus ultraviolet light?

LIKELY TO BE BENEFICIAL

Ingram regimen*

One systematic review of weak RCTs provided insufficient evidence on the effects of the Ingram regimen. However, there is consensus that the Ingram regimen is likely to be beneficial for the clearance of psoriasis.

Psoriasis (chronic plaque)

TRADE OFF BETWEEN BENEFITS AND HARMS

Psoralen plus ultraviolet A (PUVA) plus oral retinoids

One systematic review found that adding oral retinoids to psoralen plus ultraviolet A significantly increased clearance rates compared with psoralen plus ultraviolet A alone. Teratogenicity renders oral retinoids less acceptable.

Ultraviolet B plus oral retinoids (combination better than either treatment alone)

RCTs found that combined treatment with ultraviolet B plus oral retinoids improved psoriasis compared with either treatment alone. Teratogenicity renders oral retinoids less acceptable.

UNKNOWN EFFECTIVENESS

Adding psoralen plus ultraviolet A (PUVA) or adding ultraviolet B to calcipotriol (topical)

We found inconclusive evidence about the effects of adding calcipotriol to psoralen plus ultraviolet A or to ultraviolet B in people with chronic plaque psoriasis. One systematic review found no significant difference between adding calcipotriol to either psoralen plus ultraviolet A or ultraviolet B and either treatment alone. However, one subsequent RCT found that fewer ultraviolet B treatments were required to achieve clearance with calcipotriol plus ultraviolet B compared with ultraviolet B alone.

Goeckerman treatment

Two small RCTs provided insufficient evidence to assess Goeckerman treatment in people with chronic plaque psoriasis.

Ultraviolet light plus emollients

One RCT found that ultraviolet B radiation plus an oil in water emollient temporarily improved psoriasis over 12 weeks compared with ultraviolet B radiation alone.

What are the effects of combined systemic plus topical drug treatment?

TRADE OFF BETWEEN BENEFITS AND HARMS

Retinoids (oral) plus topical corticosteroids (more effective than either treatment alone)

One systematic review found that a topical corticosteroid plus an oral retinoid was superior to the single treatments in improving psoriasis. Topical corticosteroids may cause striae and atrophy, which increase with potency and use of occlusive dressings. Continuous use may lead to adrenocortical suppression, and case reports suggest that severe flares of the disease may occur on withdrawal. Teratogenicity renders oral retinoids less acceptable.

UNKNOWN EFFECTIVENESS

Systemic drug treatment plus topical vitamin D derivatives

RCTs provide insufficient evidence to assess adding calcipotriol to an oral retinoid or to ciclosporin compared with drug alone in people with chronic plaque psoriasis.

*Based on consensus.

Psoriasis (chronic plaque)

DEFINITION Chronic plaque psoriasis, or psoriasis vulgaris, is a chronic inflammatory skin disease that is characterised by well demarcated erythematous scaly plaques on the extensor surfaces of the body and scalp. The lesions may occasionally itch or sting, and may bleed when injured. Dystrophic nail changes or nail pitting are found in more than a third of people with chronic plaque psoriasis, and psoriatic arthropathy occurs in 1% to more than 10%. The condition waxes and wanes, with wide variations in course and severity among individuals. Other varieties of psoriasis include guttate, inverse, pustular, and erythrodermic psoriasis. This review deals only with treatments for chronic plaque psoriasis and does not cover nail involvement or scalp psoriasis.

INCIDENCE/ PREVALENCE Psoriasis affects 1–3% of the general population. It is believed to be less frequent in people from Africa and Asia, but we found no reliable epidemiological data.[1]

AETIOLOGY/ RISK FACTORS About a third of people with psoriasis have a family history of the disease, but physical trauma, acute infection, and some medications (e.g. lithium salts and beta-blockers) are believed to trigger the condition. A few observational studies have linked the onset or relapse of psoriasis with stressful life events and personal habits, including cigarette smoking and, less consistently, alcohol consumption.[2] Others have found an association of psoriasis with body mass index and an inverse association with intake of fruit and vegetables.

PROGNOSIS We found no long term prognostic studies. With the exceptions of erythrodermic and acute generalised pustular psoriasis (severe conditions which affect < 1% of people with psoriasis and require intensive hospital care), psoriasis is not known to affect mortality. Psoriasis may substantially affect quality of life, by influencing a negative body image and self image, and limiting daily activities, social contacts, and work. One systematic review (search date 2000, 17 cohort studies) suggested that more severe psoriasis may be associated with lower levels of quality of life than milder psoriasis.[3] At present, there is no cure for psoriasis. However, in many people it can be well controlled with treatment, at least in the short term.

Please refer to clinicalevidence.com for full text and references.

Scabies

Search date March 2006

Paul Johnstone and Mark Strong

What are the effects of topical treatments for scabies?

BENEFICIAL

Crotamiton (as effective as lindane but less effective than permethrin)

One systematic review found that crotamiton was less successful at achieving clinical or parasitic cure after 28 days compared with permethrin. One systematic review identified one RCT that found no significant difference between crotamiton and lindane in clinical cure rates at 28 days.

Permethrin

One systematic review found that permethrin increased clinical and parasitic cure after 28 days compared with crotamiton. The systematic review found conflicting results with permethrin and lindane, but one subsequent RCT found that permethrin reduced failed clinical cure rates at 14 days compared with lindane. One subsequent RCT found evidence that permethrin increased clinical cure at 14 days compared with ivermectin.

TRADE OFF BETWEEN BENEFITS AND HARMS

Lindane

One systematic review identified one RCT that found no significant difference between lindane and crotamiton in clinical cure rates at 28 days. The systematic review found conflicting results between lindane and permethrin after 28 days but one subsequent RCT found lower clinical cure rates with lindane at 14 days than with permethrin. Another small RCT identified by the review found no significant difference between lindane and ivermectin in cure rates at 15 days. One subsequent RCT found no significant difference between lindane and ivermectin in failed clinical cure rates at 2 weeks, but found lower failed clinical cure rates at 4 weeks with ivermectin than with lindane. A second subsequent RCT found no significant difference between lindane and sulphur ointment in failed clinical or parasitic cure rates. We found reports of rare, serious adverse effects such as convulsions.

UNKNOWN EFFECTIVENESS

Benzyl benzoate

One systematic review identified one small RCT that found no significant difference between benzyl benzoate and ivermectin in clinical cure rates at 30 days. However, one subsequent RCT found that benzyl benzoate reduced clinical cure rates at 30 days compared with ivermectin. One systematic review identified one RCT that found no significant difference between benzyl benzoate and sulphur ointment in clinical cure rates at 8 or 14 days.

Malathion

One systematic review found no RCTs on the effects of malathion.

Sulphur compounds

One systematic review identified one RCT that found no significant difference between sulphur ointment and benzyl benzoate in clinical cure at 8 or 14 days. One subsequent RCT found no significant difference between sulphur ointment and lindane in failed clinical or parasitic cure rates.

What are the effects of systemic treatments for scabies?

LIKELY TO BE BENEFICIAL

Oral ivermectin

One systematic review identified one RCT that found that ivermectin increased clinical cure rates after 7 days compared with placebo. Another small RCT identified by the review found no significant difference between ivermectin and benzyl benzoate in clinical cure rates at 30 days. One subsequent RCT found that, compared with benzyl benzoate, ivermectin increased clinical cure rates at 30 days. One systematic review identified one small RCT that found no significant difference between ivermectin and lindane in clinical cure rates at 15 days. One subsequent RCT found no significant difference between ivermectin and lindane in failed clinical cure rates at 2 weeks, but it found that ivermectin decreased failed clinical cure rates at 4 weeks. One RCT found limited evidence that ivermectin reduced clinical cure rates at 14 days compared with permethrin.

DEFINITION Scabies is an infestation of the skin by the mite *Sarcoptes scabiei*.[1] Typical sites of infestation are skin folds and flexor surfaces. In adults, the most common sites are between the fingers and on the wrists, although infection may manifest in elderly people as a diffuse truncal eruption. In infants and children, the face, scalp, palms, and soles are also often affected. Infection with the scabies mite causes discomfort and intense itching of the skin, particularly at night, with irritating papular or vesicular eruptions. The discomfort and itching can be especially debilitating among immunocompromised people, such as those with HIV/AIDS.

INCIDENCE/ PREVALENCE Scabies is a common public health problem with an estimated prevalence of 300 million cases worldwide, mostly affecting people in developing countries, where prevalence can exceed 50%.[2] In industrialised countries it is most common in institutionalised communities. Case studies suggest that epidemic cycles occur every 7–15 years, and that these partly reflect the population's immune status.

AETIOLOGY/ RISK FACTORS Scabies is particularly common where there is social disruption, overcrowding with close body contact, and limited access to water.[3] Young children, immobilised elderly people, people with HIV/AIDS, and other medically and immunologically compromised people are predisposed to infestation and have particularly high mite counts.[4]

PROGNOSIS Scabies is not life threatening, but the severe, persistent itch and secondary infections may be debilitating. Occasionally, crusted scabies develops. This form of the disease is resistant to routine treatment and can be a source of continued reinfestation and spread to others.

Please refer to clinicalevidence.com for full text and references.

Seborrhoeic dermatitis

Search date February 2006

Juan Jorge Manriquez and Pablo Uribe

What are the effects of topical treatments for seborrhoeic dermatitis of the scalp in adults?

BENEFICIAL

Ketoconazole

Five RCTs found that ketoconazole 2% shampoo improved scalp symptoms (including scaling, itching, redness, and dandruff) compared with placebo over 4 weeks.

Selenium sulphide

One RCT found that selenium sulphide shampoo reduced dandruff compared with placebo.

LIKELY TO BE BENEFICIAL

Bifonazole

One small RCT found that bifonazole shampoo improved scalp symptoms compared with placebo.

Tar shampoo

One RCT found that tar shampoo was more effective at reducing scalp dandruff and redness than placebo.

Topical steroids (hydrocortisone, betamethasone valerate, clobetasone butyrate, mometasone furate, clobetasol propionate)*

We found no RCTs comparing topical steroids (hydrocortisone, betamethasone valerate, clobetasone butyrate, mometasone furate, or clobetasol propionate) versus placebo. There is consensus that topical steroids are effective in treating seborrhoeic dermatitis of the scalp in adults.

*Based on consensus opinion.

UNKNOWN EFFECTIVENESS

Terbinafine

We found no RCTs comparing terbinafine versus placebo in adults with seborrhoeic dermatitis of the scalp.

What are the effects of topical treatments for seborrhoeic dermatitis of the face and body in adults?

LIKELY TO BE BENEFICIAL

Bifonazole

One RCT found that bifonazole improved symptoms compared with placebo after 4 weeks.

◀ **Topical steroids (hydrocortisone, betamethasone valerate, clobetasone butyrate, mometasone furate, clobetasol propionate; short term episodic treatment in adults)***

We found no RCTs comparing topical steroids (hydrocortisone, betamethasone valerate, clobetasone butyrate, mometasone furate, or clobetasol propionate) versus placebo. There is consensus that short courses of topical steroids used episodically are effective in treating seborrhoeic dermatitis of the face and body in adults.

UNKNOWN EFFECTIVENESS

Emollients

We found no RCTs of sufficient quality comparing emollients versus no treatment in adults with seborrhoeic dermatitis of the face and body.

Ketoconazole

Two small RCTs found that ketoconazole 2% cream improved symptoms (erythema, scaling, papules, and pruritus) compared with placebo after 4 weeks, although the significance of the between group differences was not clear.

Lithium succinate

We found no RCTs of sufficient quality comparing lithium succinate versus placebo in adults with seborrhoeic dermatitis of the face and body.

Selenium sulphide

We found no RCTs of sufficient quality comparing selenium sulphide versus placebo in adults with seborrhoeic dermatitis of the face and body.

Terbinafine

We found no RCTs of sufficient quality comparing terbinafine versus placebo in adults with seborrhoeic dermatitis of the face and body.

DEFINITION Seborrhoeic dermatitis occurs in areas of the skin with a rich supply of sebaceous glands and manifests as red, sharply marginated lesions with greasy looking scales. On the face it mainly affects the medial aspect of the eyebrows, the area between the eyebrows, and the nasolabial folds. It also affects skin on the chest (commonly presternal) and the flexures. On the scalp it manifests as dry, flaking desquamation (dandruff) or yellow, greasy scaling with erythema. Dandruff is a lay term commonly used in the context of mild seborrhoeic dermatitis of the scalp. However, any scalp condition that produces scales could be labelled dandruff. Common differential diagnoses for seborrhoeic dermatitis of the scalp are psoriasis, eczema (see atopic eczema), and tinea capitis (see table 1)Ⓣ.

INCIDENCE/ PREVALENCE Seborrhoeic dermatitis is estimated to affect around 1–3% of the general population.[1] However, this is likely to be an underestimate because people do not tend to seek medical advice for mild dandruff.

AETIOLOGY/ RISK FACTORS *Malassezia* (*Pityrosporum*) *ovale* is considered to be the causative organism of seborrhoeic dermatitis and is responsible for producing an inflammatory reaction involving T cells and complement. Conditions that have been reported to predispose to seborrhoeic dermatitis include HIV,[2] neurological conditions such as Parkinson's disease, neuronal damage such as facial nerve palsy,[3] spinal injury,[4] ischaemic heart disease,[5] and alcoholic pancreatitis.[6] In this chapter we deal with treatment in immunocompetent adults who have no known predisposing conditions. ▶

Seborrhoeic dermatitis

PROGNOSIS Seborrhoeic dermatitis is a chronic condition that tends to flare and remit spontaneously, and is prone to recurrence after treatment.[1,7]

Please refer to clinicalevidence.com for full text and references.

Squamous cell carcinoma of the skin (non-metastatic)

Search date January 2006

Adèle Green and Robin Marks

Does the use of sunscreen help to prevent cutaneous squamous cell carcinoma?

LIKELY TO BE BENEFICIAL

Sunscreens in prevention of squamous cell carcinoma (daily compared with discretionary use)

One RCT in adults in a subtropical community in Queensland, Australia, about half of whom had previous solar keratoses, found that daily compared with discretionary use of sunscreen on the head, neck, arms, and hands reduced the incidence of squamous cell carcinoma tumours after 4.5 years.

Sunscreens to prevent development of new solar keratoses (compared with placebo or daily compared with discretionary use)

One RCT in people aged over 40 years living in Victoria, Australia, who had previous solar keratoses (a risk factor for squamous cell carcinoma) found that daily sunscreen reduced the incidence of new solar keratoses after 7 months compared with placebo. One RCT in adults in a subtropical community in Queensland, Australia, about half of whom had previous solar keratoses, found that daily compared with discretionary use of sunscreen reduced the increase of solar keratoses over the whole body after 2.5 years.

What is the optimal margin for primary excision of cutaneous squamous cell carcinoma?

UNKNOWN EFFECTIVENESS

Optimal primary excision margin

We found no RCTs or observational studies of sufficient quality relating size of primary excision margin to local recurrence rate.

Does micrographically controlled surgery result in lower rates of local recurrence than standard primary excision?

UNKNOWN EFFECTIVENESS

Micrographically controlled surgery versus primary excision

We found no RCTs or observational studies of sufficient quality comparing the effects of micrographically controlled (Mohs') surgery versus standard primary surgical excision on local recurrence rates.

BMJ Clin Evid Concise 2006;16:673–674.

Squamous cell carcinoma of the skin (non-metastatic)

Does radiotherapy after surgery affect local recurrence of cutaneous squamous cell carcinoma?

UNKNOWN EFFECTIVENESS

Radiotherapy after surgery (compared with surgery alone)

We found no RCTs or observational studies of sufficient quality comparing the effects of radiotherapy after surgery versus surgery alone on local recurrence rates.

DEFINITION Cutaneous squamous cell carcinoma is a malignant tumour of keratinocytes arising in the epidermis, showing histological evidence of dermal invasion.

INCIDENCE/ PREVALENCE Incidence rates are often derived from surveys because few cancer registries routinely collect notifications of squamous cell carcinoma of the skin. Incidence rates on exposed skin vary markedly around the world according to skin colour and latitude, and range from negligible rates in black populations and white populations living at high latit-udes to rates of about 1/100 in white residents of tropical Australia.[1]

AETIOLOGY/ RISK FACTORS People with fair skin colour who sunburn easily without tanning, people with xeroderma pigmentosum,[2-4] and those who are immunosuppressed[5] are susceptible to squamous cell carcinoma. The strongest environmental risk factor for squamous cell carcinoma is chronic sun exposure. Cohort and case control studies have found that the risk of squamous cell carcinoma is three times greater in people with fair skin colour, a propensity to burn on initial exposure to sunlight, or a history of multiple sunburns. Clinical signs of chronic skin damage, especially solar keratoses, are also risk factors for cutaneous squamous cell carcinoma.[3,4] In people with multiple solar keratoses (> 15), the risk of squamous cell carcinoma is 10–15 times greater than in people with no solar keratoses.[3,4]

PROGNOSIS Prognosis is related to the location and size of tumour, histological pattern, depth of invasion, perineural involvement, and immunosuppression.[6,7] A worldwide review of 95 case series, each consisting of at least 20 people, found that the overall metastasis rate for squamous cell carcinoma on the ear was 11% and on the lip 14%, compared with an average for all sites of 5%.[7] A review of 71 case series found that lesions less than 2 cm in diameter have less than half the local recurrence rate compared with lesions greater than 2 cm (7% *v* 15%), and less than a third of the rate of metastasis (9% *v* 30%).[7]

Please refer to clinicalevidence.com for full text and references.

Vitiligo

Search date March 2006

Rubeta Matin

What are the effects of medical treatments for vitiligo in adults?

BENEFICIAL

Corticosteroids (topical) *New*

One systematic review and one additional RCT found that potent topical corticosteroids improved repigmentation in localised vitiligo compared with placebo. The review found no significant difference in repigmentation of symmetrical localised patches of vitiligo between very potent topical corticosteroids and placebo. One RCT found that topical fluticasone propionate plus ultraviolet A improved repigmentation compared with topical fluticasone propionate alone. There were no RCTs comparing different strengths of topical corticosteroids versus each other or comparing the efficacy of topical corticosteroids on different parts of the body. Corticosteroid use is associated with skin atrophy, drug induced acne, and hypertrichosis. There is a consensus among clinicians that a limited course of potent and very potent topical corticosteroids in localised vitiligo is a useful first line treatment, particularly in newly formed lesions.

UNKNOWN EFFECTIVENESS

Immunomodulators (topical) *New*

We found no RCTs assessing the effect of topical immunomodulators (pimecrolimus, tacrolimus, imiquimod) in vitiligo in adults. We found one alert regarding a potential malignancy risk with topical tacrolimus and pimecrolimus.

Levamisole (oral) *New*

One RCT found no significant difference between oral levamisole plus topical mometasone furoate 0.1% and topical mometasone furoate 0.1% alone in the development of new lesions in adults and children with slowly spreading vitiligo at 6 months. The RCT was probably underpowered to show a significant difference owing to an unexpected lack of disease progression in the control group. Adverse effects were reported in the levamisole plus mometasone group; however, no direct comparison with the mometasone group was performed.

Vitamin D analogues (topical) *New*

We found insufficient evidence to assess topical vitamin D analogues (with or without psoralen plus ultraviolet A) in the management of vitiligo.

LIKELY TO BE INEFFECTIVE OR HARMFUL

Corticosteroids (oral)* *New*

We found no systematic reviews or RCTs investigating the effects of oral corticosteroids on vitiligo. There is consensus among clinicians that the adverse effects associated with oral corticosteroids far outweigh any benefit that may be achieved in people with vitiligo.

Vitiligo

What are the effects of ultraviolet light treatments for vitiligo in adults?

LIKELY TO BE BENEFICIAL

Ultraviolet A plus psoralen (oral)* *New*

One RCT found no significant difference between various psoralen derivatives (methoxsalen, trioxysalen, unsubstituted psoralen) plus ultraviolet A compared with ultraviolet A alone, whereas another RCT found a significant difference in repigmentation with unsubstituted psoralen plus sunlight compared with sunlight alone. One systematic review found no significant difference between oral and topical psoralens. One RCT found that methoxsalen plus trioxysalen plus ultraviolet A increased repigmentation of vitiliginous macules compared with oral unsubstituted psoralen plus ultraviolet A. The general consensus among clinicians is that ultraviolet A plus oral psoralen is effective for vitiligo.

Ultraviolet B (narrowband) *New*

One RCT found that narrowband ultraviolet B improved repigmentation in vitiligo compared with placebo. One RCT found that narrowband ultraviolet B improved repigmentation compared with topical psoralen plus ultraviolet A.

UNKNOWN EFFECTIVENESS

Ultraviolet B (broadband) *New*

One small RCT found limited evidence that more sessions of broadband ultraviolet B plus oral psoralen were required to produce repigmentation compared with ultraviolet A plus oral psoralen.

UNLIKELY TO BE BENEFICIAL

Ultraviolet A plus psoralen (topical) *New*

One RCT found no significant difference between topical psoralen plus ultraviolet A and no treatment at 18 months. One RCT found no significant difference between oral and topical psoralens. One RCT in a mixed population of adults and children found that topical psoralen plus ultraviolet A reduced repigmentation compared with narrowband ultraviolet B, although a significance assessment was not performed.

What are the effects of medical treatments for vitiligo in children?

BENEFICIAL

Corticosteroids (topical) *New*

One RCT found that clobetasol propionate 0.05% improved repigmentation compared with topical psoralen plus ultraviolet A at 6 months but another found that repigmentation was not significantly different from tacrolimus at 2 months. The most common adverse effect was mild atrophy.

LIKELY TO BE BENEFICIAL

Immunomodulators (topical) *New*

We found no RCTs comparing tacrolimus, pimecrolimus, or imiquimod versus placebo in children. One RCT compared 0.1% tacrolimus and 0.05% clobetasol propionate and found them to be equally effective in repigmentation.

UNKNOWN EFFECTIVENESS

Vitamin D analogues (topical) *New*

We found insufficient evidence to assess the effectiveness of topical calcipotriol in vitiligo in children.

LIKELY TO BE INEFFECTIVE OR HARMFUL

Corticosteroids (oral)* *New*

We found no systematic reviews or RCTs investigating the effects of oral corticosteroids on vitiligo in children. There is consensus among clinicians that the adverse effects associated with oral corticosteroids far outweigh any benefit that may be achieved in people with vitiligo.

What are the effects of ultraviolet light treatments for vitiligo in children?

LIKELY TO BE BENEFICIAL

Ultraviolet B (narrowband)* *New*

We found no systematic reviews or RCTs comparing narrowband ultraviolet B with placebo in children with vitiligo. One RCT in a mixed population of adults and children found narrowband ultraviolet B to be more effective compared with topical psoralen plus ultraviolet A, although a significance assessment was not performed. The general consensus is that narrowband ultraviolet B is safe and effective in children and may improve their quality of life.

LIKELY TO BE INEFFECTIVE OR HARMFUL

Ultraviolet A plus psoralen (oral or topical)* *New*

One RCT found that ultraviolet A (sunlight or sun lamp) plus oral trioxysalen improved vitiligo compared with ultraviolet A alone. One RCT in a mixed population of adults and children found that topical psoralen plus ultraviolet A reduced repigmentation compared with narrowband ultraviolet B, although a significance assessment was not performed. One RCT found that psoralen plus ultraviolet A reduced repigmentation at 6 months compared with clobetasol propionate 0.05%. The general consensus among clinicians is that ultraviolet A plus psoralen is not recommended in children under the age of 12 due to the risk of cataract formation and an increased risk of skin cancer.

*Categorisation based on consensus.

DEFINITION Vitiligo is an acquired skin disorder characterised by white (depigmented) patches in the skin, due to the loss of functioning melanocytes. The hair and rarely, the eyes may also lose colour too. Vitiligo patches can appear anywhere on the skin but common sites are usually around the orifices, the genitals, or sun exposed areas such as the face and hands. The disease is classified according to its extent and distribution, and can be subdivided into generalised or localised. In practice, there is considerable overlap between these types, and people often have vitiligo that cannot be categorised or will change during the course of their lifetime. Therefore, for the purposes of this review, we have included all people diagnosed with vitiligo of any type. Children were defined as people aged 15 years and below.

INCIDENCE/ PREVALENCE Vitiligo is estimated to affect 1% of the world population, regardless of age, gender, and skin colour.[1,2] Anyone of any age can develop vitiligo but it is very rarely reported to be present at birth. In a Dutch study, 50% of people reported that the disease appeared before the age of 20 years.[3,4]

AETIOLOGY/ RISK FACTORS The aetiology of vitiligo is uncertain, although genetic, immunological, and neurogenic factors seem to play a role.[1] In about a third of people affected with vitiligo, there is a family history of vitiligo, but there are very few epidemiological studies to confirm this.[5] Current research focuses on finding the genes responsible;[6,7] however, certain triggers (e.g. trauma to the skin, hormonal changes, and stress[8,9]) may be necessary for the disease to become apparent.[4] Autoimmune mechanisms are thought to be responsible in the pathogenesis of vitiligo (especially in generalised or focal non-dermatomal vitiligo).[10] This is supported by an increased incidence of antibodies found in people with vitiligo.[11] Furthermore, vitiligo is often associated with autoimmune diseases, such as thyroid diseases, pernicious anaemia, and diabetes mellitus. Another indication that vitiligo may be due to an autoimmune mechanism is the fact that melanocyte antibodies have been found in people with vitiligo; their incidence correlates with disease activity.[12,13] Involvement of cellular immunity has been considered because T lymphocytes and macrophages in perilesional skin have also been frequently reported.[14,15] Regarding segmental vitiligo, the neural hypothesis[10] suggests that it is due to an accumulation of a neurochemical substance, which decreases melanin production.

PROGNOSIS Vitiligo is not life threatening, and is mostly asymptomatic (although it does increase the risk of sunburn of the affected areas). The association of vitiligo and skin cancer remains an area of controversy. The occurrence of skin cancer in long lasting vitiligo is rare,[16] although studies have demonstrated increased psoralen plus ultraviolet A (PUVA) associated skin cancers. A Swedish study,[17] which followed up people treated with PUVA over 21 years, demonstrated an increased risk of squamous cell carcinomas. Furthermore, the risk of malignant melanoma increases among people treated with PUVA approximately 15 years after the first treatment.[18] The effects of vitiligo can be both cosmetically and psychologically devastating,[19] resulting in low self esteem[20] and poor body image.[21] The anxieties regarding the disease tend to occur in view of a lack of understanding of the aetiology and unpredictability of the course.[4] **Progression:** The course of generalised vitiligo is unpredictable; lesions may remain stable for years, or, more commonly, may progress with in between phases of stabilisation, or, less commonly, slowly progress for several years to cover the entire body surface.[22] In some instances, people may undergo rapid, complete depigmentation within 1 or 2 years.[23] In segmental vitiligo, lesions tend to spread rapidly at onset and show a more stable course thereafter.[24] **Predicting treatment responsiveness:** There are certain disease characteristics that help to predict the outcome of therapy. Besides age, duration of disease, localisation, and extent of depigmentation,[25,26] current disease activity should also be taken into consideration during clinical decision making. This is essential in people with vitiligo vulgaris, when the disease activity may fluctuate at a given time. Medical therapies and ultraviolet light treatments may be equally effective in active and stable disease,[27] but this may not be true for other treatments (e.g. surgery).[28] An associated skin manifestation is the phenomenon of "koebnerization",[29-32] which plays an important role in the appearance of new lesions in vitiligo. It occurs in most people with vitiligo.[3,33,34] This knowledge is important, because elimination of frictional trauma in the form of occlusive garments, wrist bands, and necklaces prevents occurrence of new lesions in the cosmetically important areas in a case of progressive vitiligo. Furthermore, it has been reported that the presence of positive experimentally induced Koebner phenomenon is associated with active disease but not necessarily more severe disease – that is, in terms of the extent of depigmentation.[35] The presence of Koebner phenomenon may be a valuable clinical factor to assess disease activity, and may predict responsiveness to certain treatments. A case series[35] reported that people who were Koebner phenomenon positive (induced experimentally) were significantly more responsive to topical fluticasone propionate combined with ultraviolet A therapy, but for narrowband ultraviolet B treatment, there was no difference in response, suggesting that people in active and stable stages of the disease may respond equally well to ultraviolet B.

Please refer to clinicalevidence.com for full text and references.

Warts

Search date August 2004

Michael Bigby and Sam Gibbs

What are the effects of treatments for warts?

BENEFICIAL

Salicylic acid (topical)

One systematic review found that simple topical salicylic acid increased complete wart clearance, successful treatment, or loss of one or more warts after 6–12 weeks compared with placebo. The review identified two RCTs comparing topical salicylic acid versus cryotherapy, which found no significant difference in the proportion of people with wart clearance at 3–6 months. One RCT provided insufficient evidence to compare topical salicylic acid versus cimetidine. The review gave no information on recurrence.

LIKELY TO BE BENEFICIAL

Contact immunotherapy (dinitrochlorobenzene)

One systematic review found that contact immunotherapy using dinitrochlorobenzene increased wart clearance compared with placebo. The review gave no information on recurrence.

Cryotherapy

One systematic review of two small RCTs found no significant difference between cryotherapy and placebo or no treatment in the proportion of people with wart clearance after 2–4 months. However, the RCTs may have been too small to detect a clinically important difference. The review found no significant difference between cryotherapy and salicylic acid in the proportion of people with wart clearance at 3–6 months. One RCT identified by the review found that cryotherapy was less effective than photodynamic treatment in reducing the number of warts at 4–6 weeks. Another RCT found that fewer people having cryotherapy than occlusive treatment with duct tape had complete clearance of warts at 2 months. A third RCT provided insufficient evidence to compare cryotherapy versus cimetidine. The systematic review found weak evidence that aggressive cryotherapy increased the proportion of people with wart clearance after 1–3 months compared with gentle cryotherapy. We found no information on recurrence.

Duct tape occlusion

One RCT found that more people having occlusive treatment with duct tape than cryotherapy had complete clearance of warts at 2 months. The RCT did not assess recurrence.

UNKNOWN EFFECTIVENESS

Bleomycin (intralesional)

RCTs found conflicting evidence on the effects of intralesional bleomycin. Two RCTs found that intralesional bleomycin increased the number of warts cured after 6 weeks compared with placebo. One RCT found no significant difference between bleomycin and placebo in the proportion of people with wart clearance after 30 days, and another RCT found weak evidence that bleomycin cured fewer warts than placebo after 3 months. None of these RCTs assessed recurrence. A fifth RCT found no significant difference between different concentrations of bleomycin in the proportion of warts that were cured and did not recur over 3 months.

Carbon dioxide laser

One systematic review identified no RCTs on the effects of carbon dioxide laser in people with non-genital warts.

Cimetidine

Three small RCTs provided insufficient evidence to compare cimetidine versus placebo, and one small RCT provided insufficient evidence to compare cimetidine versus topical treatments (cryotherapy or topical salicylic acid). One small RCT found that cimetidine plus levamisole increased wart clearance at 12 weeks compared with cimetidine alone. None of the RCTs assessed recurrence.

Distant healing

One RCT provided insufficient evidence to assess distant healing in people with non-genital warts.

Hypnotic suggestion

We found no RCTs on the effects of hypnotic suggestion in the clearance of warts.

Inosine pranobex

One RCT provided insufficient evidence about the effects of inosine pranobex on wart clearance.

Interferon alfa (systemic)

We found no systematic review and no RCTs of sufficient quality on the effects of systemic interferon alfa in people with non-genital warts.

Levamisole

Two RCTs and one CCT provided insufficient evidence on the effects of levamisole compared with placebo on the clearance of warts. One RCT found that levamisole plus cimetidine increased wart clearance at 12 weeks compared with cimetidine alone. None of the RCTs assessed recurrence.

Photodynamic treatment

RCTs with heterogeneous methods of analysis that assessed a variety of types of photodynamic treatment provided insufficient evidence to draw conclusions on wart clearance or recurrence.

Pulsed dye laser

One RCT provided insufficient evidence on the effects of pulsed dye laser in people with non-genital warts.

Surgical procedures

One systematic review identified no RCTs on the effects of surgical procedures on wart clearance.

Zinc sulphate (oral)

One weak RCT found that oral zinc sulphate increased the proportion of people with complete resolution of warts at 2 months compared with placebo. The RCT followed up responders every 2 weeks for 2–6 months and found no recurrences.

Warts

UNLIKELY TO BE BENEFICIAL

Homeopathy

Two RCTs found no significant difference between homeopathy and placebo in the proportion of people with wart clearance after 8–18 weeks. The RCTs did not assess recurrence.

DEFINITION Non-genital warts (verrucas) are an extremely common, benign, and usually self limiting skin disease. Infection of epidermal cells with the human papillomavirus [HPV] results in cell proliferation and a thickened, warty papule on the skin. There are over 100 different types of HPV. The appearance of warts is determined by the type of virus and the location of the infection. Any area of skin can be infected, but the most common sites involved are the hands and feet. Genital warts are not covered in this review (see chapter on genital warts). Common warts are most often seen on the hands and present as skin coloured papules with a rough "verrucous" surface. Flat warts are most often seen on the backs of the hands and on the legs. They appear as slightly elevated, small plaques that are skin coloured or light brown. Plantar warts occur on the soles of the feet and look like very thick callouses.

INCIDENCE/ PREVALENCE There are few reliable, population based data on the incidence and prevalence of non-genital warts. Prevalence probably varies widely between different age groups, populations, and periods of time. Two large population based studies found prevalence rates of 0.84% in the USA[1] and 12.9% in Russia.[2] Prevalence is highest in children and young adults, and two studies in school populations have shown prevalence rates of 12% in 4–6 year olds in the UK[3] and 24% in 16–18 year olds in Australia.[4]

AETIOLOGY/ RISK FACTORS Warts are caused by HPV, of which there are over 100 different types. They are most common at sites of trauma, such as the hands and feet, and probably result from inoculation of virus into minimally damaged areas of epithelium. Warts on the feet can be acquired from walking barefoot in communal areas where other people walk barefoot. One observational study (146 adolescents) found that the prevalence of warts on the feet was 27% in those that used a communal shower room and 1.3% in those that used the locker (changing) room.[5] Warts on the hand are also an occupational risk for butchers and meat handlers. One cross-sectional survey (1086 people) found that the prevalence of warts on the hand was 33% in abattoir workers, 34% in retail butchers, 20% in engineering fitters, and 15% in office workers.[6] Immunosuppression is another important risk factor. One observational study in immunosuppressed renal transplant recipients found that at 5 years or longer after transplantation 90% had warts.[7]

PROGNOSIS Non-genital warts in immunocompetent people are harmless and usually resolve spontaneously as a result of natural immunity within months or years. The rate of resolution is highly variable and probably depends on several factors, including host immunity, age, HPV type, and site of infection. One cohort study (1000 children in long stay accommodation) found that two thirds of warts resolved without treatment within a 2 year period.[8] One systematic review (search date 2000, 17 RCTs) comparing local treatments versus placebo found that about 30% of people using placebo (range 0–73%) had no warts after about 10 weeks (range 4–24 weeks).[9]

Please refer to clinicalevidence.com for full text and references.

Wrinkles

Search date December 2004

Miny Samuel, Rebecca Brooke, and Christopher Griffiths

What are the effects of interventions to prevent skin wrinkles?

UNKNOWN EFFECTIVENESS

Sunscreens

We found no RCTs on the effects of sunscreens in preventing wrinkles.

Vitamin C or E (topical)

We found no RCTs on the effects of topical vitamins C or E on wrinkles.

What are the effects of treatments for skin wrinkles?

BENEFICIAL

Tazarotene (improved fine wrinkles)

Two RCTs in people with moderately photodamaged skin found that tazarotene cream improved fine wrinkling compared with placebo at 24 weeks. One RCT found no significant difference between tazarotene cream and tretinoin cream in fine wrinkling at 24 weeks. However, another RCT found that tazarotene improved fine and coarse wrinkling compared with tretinoin, although tazarotene increased burning sensation on the skin in the first week of treatment.

Tretinoin (improved fine wrinkles)

RCTs in people with mild to moderate photodamage found that topical tretinoin applied for up to 12 months improved fine wrinkles compared with vehicle cream but the effect on coarse wrinkles differed among studies. Four RCTs in people with moderate to severe photodamage found that topical tretinoin applied for 6 months improved fine and coarse wrinkles on the face compared with vehicle cream. All of the RCTs that examined higher strength creams (tretinoin 0.1%, 0.05%, and 0.02%) found that tretinoin improved fine wrinkles compared with vehicle cream in people with mild, moderate, or severe photodamage. Common short term adverse effects with tretinoin included itching, burning, and erythema. Skin peeling was the most common persistent adverse effect, which was most frequent and severe at 12–16 weeks. One RCT found no significant difference between tretinoin and tazarotene cream in fine wrinkling at 24 weeks. However, another RCT found that tazarotene improved fine and coarse wrinkling compared with tretinoin, although tretinoin was associated with less burning sensation on the skin in the first week of treatment.

TRADE OFF BETWEEN BENEFITS AND HARMS

Isotretinoin

In people with mild to severe photodamage, two RCTs found that isotretinoin cream improved fine and coarse wrinkles after 36 weeks compared with vehicle cream. Severe facial irritation occurred in 5–10% of people using isotretinoin.

UNKNOWN EFFECTIVENESS

Carbon dioxide laser

We found no RCTs comparing carbon dioxide laser versus placebo or no treatment in people with wrinkles. Two small RCTs in women with perioral wrinkles found no significant difference between carbon dioxide laser and ▶

Wrinkles

dermabrasion in improvement in wrinkles at 4–6 months. A third RCT found that laser was slightly more effective than dermabrasion in improving wrinkles. Adverse effects were commonly reported. Erythema was reported in all three RCTs, two of which found that erythema was more common with laser than with dermabrasion. Small RCTs provided insufficient evidence about carbon dioxide laser compared with chemical peel, or other laser treatments.

Chemical peel

Small RCTs provided insufficient evidence about chemical peel compared with carbon dioxide laser.

Dermabrasion

We found no RCTs comparing dermabrasion versus placebo or no treatment in people with wrinkles. Two small RCTs in women with perioral wrinkles found no significant difference between dermabrasion and carbon dioxide laser in improvement in wrinkles at 4–6 months, but a third RCT found that dermabrasion was slightly less effective than laser in improving wrinkles. Adverse effects were commonly reported. Erythema was reported in all three RCTs, two of which found that erythema was more common with laser than with dermabrasion.

Facelift

We found no RCTs on the effects of facelifts in people with wrinkles.

Oral natural cartilage polysaccharides

One RCT found no significant difference between an oral preparation of cartilage polysaccharide and placebo in wrinkle appearance at 3 months. Smaller RCTs found that oral cartilage polysaccharide reduced fine, moderate, or severe wrinkles compared with placebo. However, these studies were small and of limited reliability. We found limited evidence that some preparations may be more effective than others.

Retinyl esters

We found no RCTs of retinyl esters that evaluated clinical outcomes in people with wrinkles.

Topical natural cartilage polysaccharides

One small RCT found that a topical preparation of cartilage polysaccharide reduced fine and coarse wrinkles at 120 days compared with placebo. However, we were unable to draw reliable conclusions from this study.

Variable pulse erbium: YAG laser

Small RCTs provided insufficient evidence about variable pulse erbium: YAG laser compared with carbon dioxide laser.

Vitamin C or E (topical)

One poor quality RCT found limited evidence that an ascorbic acid formulation applied daily to the face for 3 months improved fine and coarse wrinkling compared with a vehicle cream. Stinging and erythema were common but were not quantified according to treatment. We were unable to draw reliable conclusions from this study because of deficiencies in its methodology.

DEFINITION Wrinkles, also known as rhytides, are visible creases or folds in the skin. Wrinkles less than 1 mm in width and depth are defined as fine wrinkles and those greater than 1 mm as coarse wrinkles. Most RCTs have studied wrinkles on the face, forearms, and hands.

INCIDENCE/ PREVALENCE We found no information on the incidence of wrinkles alone, only on the incidence of skin photodamage, which includes a spectrum of features such as wrinkles, hyperpigmentation, tactile roughness, and telangiectasia. The incidence of skin disorders associated with ultraviolet light increases with age and develops over several decades. One Australian study (1539 people, aged 20–55 years living in Queensland) found moderate to severe photodamage in 72% of men and 47% of women under 30 years of age.[1] Severity of photodamage was significantly greater with increasing age, and was independently associated with solar keratoses ($P < 0.01$) and skin cancer ($P < 0.05$). Wrinkling was more common in people with white skin, especially skin phototypes I and II. One study reported that the incidence of photodamage in European and North American populations with Fitzpatrick skin types I, II, and III is about 80–90%.[2] We found few reports of photodamage in black skin (phototypes V and VI).

AETIOLOGY/ RISK FACTORS Wrinkles may be caused by intrinsic factors (e.g. aging, hormonal status, and intercurrent diseases) and by extrinsic factors (e.g. exposure to ultraviolet radiation and cigarette smoke). These factors contribute to epidermal thinning, loss of elasticity, skin fragility, and creases and lines in the skin. The severity of photodamage varies with skin type, which includes skin colour and the capacity to tan.[3] One review of five observational studies found that facial wrinkles in men and women were more common in smokers than in non-smokers.[4] It also found that the risk of moderate to severe wrinkles in lifelong smokers was more than twice that in current smokers (RR 2.57, 95% CI 1.83 to 3.06). Oestrogen deficiency may contribute to wrinkles in postmenopausal women.[5]

PROGNOSIS Although wrinkles cannot be considered to be a medical illness requiring intervention, concerns about aging may affect quality of life. Such concerns are likely to be influenced by geographical differences, culture, and personal values. In some cases concerns about physical appearance can lead to difficulties with interpersonal interactions, occupational functioning, and self esteem.[6] In societies in which the aging population is growing and a high value is placed on the maintenance of a youthful appearance, there is a growing preference for interventions that ameliorate the visible signs of aging.

Please refer to clinicalevidence.com for full text and references.

Insomnia in the elderly

Search date August 2005

Danielle Dunne and Paul Montgomery

What are the effects of non-drug treatments for insomnia in elderly people?

UNKNOWN EFFECTIVENESS

Cognitive behavioural therapy

One small RCT found that individual or group cognitive behavioural therapy improved sleep quality at the end of treatment and at 3 months compared with no treatment, although mean sleep quality scores were consistent with continuing insomnia with or without cognitive behavioural therapy.

Exercise programmes

One small RCT found that sleep quality improved after a 16 week programme of regular, moderate intensity exercise four times a week compared with no treatment. However, mean sleep quality scores were consistent with persisting insomnia both with and without exercise.

Timed exposure to bright light

We found no RCTs comparing the effects of timed bright light exposure with other treatments or no treatment in elderly people.

What are the effects of drug treatments for insomnia in elderly people?

LIKELY TO BE BENEFICIAL

Zaleplon *New*

Two large RCTs measuring subjective sleep outcomes found that zaleplon improved sleep latency, but not sleep duration, number of awakenings, or sleep quality compared with placebo at 7 and 14 days. One small RCT measuring subjective and objective outcomes found that 5 and 10 mg doses of zaleplon improved sleep latency and slightly increased total time asleep compared with placebo at 2 days. The two large RCTs found increased rates of rebound insomnia with zaleplon 10 mg compared with placebo after discontinuation of treatment.

Zolpidem *New*

RCTs found that zolpidem improved sleep latency, reduced the number of awakenings during the night, and increased sleep duration and quality compared with placebo at 1–28 days. Three RCTs suggested broad equivalence between zolpidem and triazolam. Two RCTs found no significant difference in outcomes between 10 and 20 mg doses of zolpidem, and one RCT found no significant difference between 5 and 10 mg.

TRADE OFF BETWEEN BENEFITS AND HARMS

Benzodiazepines (quazepam, flurazepam, brotizolam, nitrazepam, and triazolam) *New*

Three small RCTs provided limited evidence of modest improvements in sleep outcomes with benzodiazepines compared with placebo, but increased impairment of memory, cognitive, and psychomotor function, and rebound insomnia ▶

compared with placebo. Three RCTs provided limited evidence suggesting a broad equivalence between triazolam and zolpidem. One small RCT provided limited evidence of no significant difference in sleep outcomes between nitrazepam and zopiclone at 7 days.

UNKNOWN EFFECTIVENESS

Diphenhydramine *New*

We found no RCTs looking at the effects of diphenhydramine on insomnia in elderly people.

Zopiclone *New*

We found no RCTs comparing the effects of zopiclone on insomnia in elderly people.

DEFINITION Insomnia is defined by the US National Institutes of Health as experience of poor quality sleep, with difficulty in initiating or maintaining sleep, waking too early in the morning, or failing to feel refreshed.[1] Chronic insomnia is defined as insomnia occurring for at least three nights a week for 1 month or more.[2] Primary insomnia is defined as chronic insomnia without specific underlying medical, psychiatric, or other sleep disorders such as sleep apnoea, depression, dementia, periodic limb movement disorder, or circadian rhythm sleep disorder. This topic only covers primary insomnia in people aged 60 years and over.

INCIDENCE/ PREVALENCE Across all adult age groups, up to 40% of people have insomnia.[3] However, prevalence increases with age, with estimates ranging from 31–38% in people aged 18–64 years to 45% in people aged 65–79 years.[4]

AETIOLOGY/ RISK FACTORS The cause of insomnia is uncertain. The risk of primary insomnia increases with age and may be related to changes in circadian rhythms associated with age. Psychological factors and lifestyle changes may exacerbate perceived effects of changes in sleep patterns associated with age, leading to reduced satisfaction with sleep.[5] Other possible risk factors in all age groups include hyperarousal, chronic stress, and daytime napping.[2,6]

PROGNOSIS We found few reliable data on long term morbidity and mortality in people with primary insomnia. Primary insomnia is a chronic and relapsing condition.[7] Likely consequences include reduced quality of life and increased risk of accidents owing to daytime sleepiness. People with primary insomnia may be at greater risk of dependence on hypnotic medication, depression, dementia, and falls, and may be more likely to require residential care.[8]

Please refer to clinicalevidence.com for full text and references.

Jet lag

Search date November 2005

Andrew Herxheimer

What are the effects of interventions to prevent or minimise jet lag?

LIKELY TO BE BENEFICIAL

Melatonin*

One systematic review found that melatonin reduced mean jet lag scores on eastward and westward flights compared with placebo. The review found case reports of possible adverse effects, and suggested that people with epilepsy or taking warfarin (or other oral anticoagulants) should not use melatonin without medical supervision. It concluded that the pharmacology and toxicology of melatonin needs systematic study, and routine pharmaceutical quality control of melatonin products is necessary.

*The adverse effects of melatonin have not yet been adequately investigated.

TRADE OFF BETWEEN BENEFITS AND HARMS

Hypnotics

Three small RCTs found limited evidence that hypnotics (zopiclone, zolpidem) improved sleep duration or sleep quality or jet lag compared with placebo. Adverse effects reported with hypnotics include headache, dizziness, nausea, confusion, and amnesia. Short term benefits of hypnotics must be considered in the light of potential adverse effects.

UNKNOWN EFFECTIVENESS

Lifestyle and environmental adaptations (eating, avoiding alcohol or caffeine, sleeping, daylight exposure, arousal)

We found no RCTs on the effects of eating, avoiding alcohol or caffeine, sleeping, daylight exposure, or arousal. Such RCTs are unlikely to be carried out.

DEFINITION Jet lag is a syndrome associated with rapid long haul flights across several time zones, characterised by sleep disturbances, daytime fatigue, reduced performance, gastrointestinal problems, and generalised malaise.[1] As with most syndromes, not all of the components must be present in any one case. It is due to the "body clock" continuing to function in the day–night rhythm of the place of departure. The rhythm adapts gradually under the influence of light and dark, mediated by melatonin secreted by the pineal gland: darkness switches on melatonin secretion, exposure to strong light switches it off.

INCIDENCE/ PREVALENCE Jet lag affects most air travellers crossing five or more time zones. The incidence and severity of jet lag increases with the number of time zones crossed.

AETIOLOGY/ RISK FACTORS Someone who has previously experienced jet lag is liable to do so again. Jet lag is worse the more time zones crossed in one flight, or series of flights, within a few days. Westward travel generally causes less disruption than eastward travel as it is easier to lengthen, rather than to shorten, the natural circadian cycle.[2]

PROGNOSIS Jet lag is worst immediately after travel and gradually resolves over 4–6 days as the person adjusts to the new local time.[2] The more time zones that are crossed, the longer it takes to wear off.

Please refer to clinicalevidence.com for full text and references.

Sleep apnoea

Search date May 2005

Michael Hensley and Cheryl Ray

What are the effects of treatment of severe obstructive sleep apnoea-hypopnoea syndrome?

BENEFICIAL

Nasal continuous positive airway pressure

One systematic review found that nasal continuous positive airway pressure reduced daytime sleepiness compared with placebo, no treatment, or conservative treatment in people with severe obstructive sleep apnoea-hypopnoea syndrome.

LIKELY TO BE BENEFICIAL

Oral appliances

Two small RCTs found that oral appliances that produced anterior advancement of the mandible improved sleep disordered breathing and daytime sleepiness in people with severe obstructive sleep apnoea-hypopnoea syndrome compared with appliances that did not advance the mandible.

UNKNOWN EFFECTIVENESS

Measures aimed at improving compliance with nasal continuous positive airway pressure *New*

One systematic review found no significant difference in measures of compliance between standard continuous positive airway pressure (CPAP) and automatically titrated CPAP, bi-level positive airway pressure, patient-titrated CPAP, or CPAP plus humidification. The review and one subsequent RCT provided limited evidence that some educational or psychological interventions may improve compliance with CPAP.

Weight loss

One systematic review found no RCTs on the effects of weight loss in people with severe obstructive sleep apnoea-hypopnoea syndrome.

What are the effects of treatment for non-severe obstructive sleep apnoea-hypopnoea syndrome?

LIKELY TO BE BENEFICIAL

Nasal continuous positive airway pressure

Two systematic reviews found no significant difference in daytime sleepiness between nasal continuous positive airway pressure (CPAP) and conservative treatment, placebo pill, or sham/subtherapeutic nasal CPAP in people with non-severe obstructive sleep apnoea-hypopnoea syndrome, but found that CPAP improved some measures of cognitive performance, functional outcomes, symptoms, energy and vitality, and depression. One subsequent crossover RCT in people with non-severe obstructive sleep apnoea-hypopnoea syndrome found that nasal CPAP improved sleep outcomes, vigilance, executive cognitive function, and quality of life compared with placebo pill at 3 months. One systematic review and two subsequent RCTs found that nasal CPAP improved apnoea/hypopnoea index compared with an oral appliance.

◀ **Oral appliances (more effective than no treatment, control appliance or placebo but less effective than nasal CPAP)**

Three RCTs found that an oral appliance that produced mandibular advancement reduced daytime sleepiness and sleep disordered breathing compared with no treatment, a control appliance, or placebo pills. One systematic review and two subsequent RCTs found that oral appliances were less effective than nasal continuous positive airway pressure at improving apnoea/hypopnoea index.

UNKNOWN EFFECTIVENESS

Measures aimed at improving compliance with nasal continuous positive airway pressure

One systematic review found no RCTs comparing standard continuous positive airway pressure (CPAP) versus automatically titrated CPAP, bi-level positive airway pressure, patient titrated CPAP, or CPAP plus humidification solely in people with non-severe obstructive sleep apnoea-hypopnoea syndrome. One RCT found that an educational video improved attendance for the next appointment compared with no video, but found no evidence of a difference between groups in sleepiness or quality of life.

Weight loss

One systematic review found no RCTs on the effect of weight loss in people with non-severe obstructive sleep apnoea-hypopnoea syndrome.

DEFINITION Sleep apnoea is the popular term for obstructive sleep apnoea-hypopnoea syndrome (OSAHS). OSAHS is abnormal breathing during sleep that causes recurrent arousals, sleep fragmentation, and nocturnal hypoxaemia. The syndrome includes daytime sleepiness, impaired vigilance and cognitive functioning, and reduced quality of life.[1,2] Apnoea is the absence of airflow at the nose and mouth for at least 10 seconds, and hypopnoea is a major reduction (> 50%) in airflow also for at least 10 seconds. Apnoeas may be "central", in which there is cessation of inspiratory effort, or "obstructive", in which inspiratory efforts continue but are ineffective because of upper airway obstruction. The diagnosis of OSAHS is made when a person with daytime symptoms has significant sleep disordered breathing revealed by polysomnography (study of sleep state, breathing, and oxygenation) or by more limited studies. Criteria for the diagnosis of significant sleep disordered breathing have not been rigorously assessed, but they have been set by consensus and convention.[3,4] Diagnostic criteria have variable sensitivity and specificity. For example, an apnoea/hypopnoea index (AHI) of less than five episodes of apnoea or hypopnoea per hour of sleep is considered normal;[5] however, people with upper airway resistance syndrome have an index below five episodes per hour,[6] and many healthy elderly people have an index greater than five episodes per hour.[7] In an effort to achieve international consensus, new criteria have been proposed and are becoming more widely used.[8] The severity of OSAHS can be classified by the severity of two factors: daytime sleepiness (see table 1)Ⓣ and AHI (see table 2)Ⓣ. Severe OSAHS is defined as severe sleep disordered breathing (AHI > 35 episodes per hour) plus symptoms of excessive daytime sleepiness (such as Epworth Sleepiness Scale > 10 or Multiple Sleep Latency Test < 5 minutes – see table 3Ⓣ). Central sleep apnoea and sleep associated hypoventilation syndromes are not covered in this chapter.

INCIDENCE/ PREVALENCE The Wisconsin Sleep Cohort Study of over 1000 people (mean age 47 years) in North America found prevalence rates for AHI more than five episodes per hour of 24% in men and 9% in women, and for OSAHS with an index greater than five episodes per hour plus excessive sleepiness of 4% in men and 2% ▶

Sleep apnoea

in women.[22] There are international differences in the occurrence of OSAHS, of which obesity is considered to be an important determinant.[23] Ethnic differences in prevalence have also been found after adjustment for other risk factors.[7,23] Little is known about the burden of illness in developing countries.

AETIOLOGY/ RISK FACTORS The site of upper airway obstruction in the OSAHS is around the level of the tongue, soft palate, or epiglottis. Disorders that predispose to either narrowing of the upper airway or reduction in its stability (e.g. obesity, certain craniofacial abnormalities, vocal cord abnormalities, and enlarged tonsils) have been associated with an increased risk of OSAHS. It has been estimated that a 1 kg/m^2 increase in body mass index (3.2 kg for a person 1.8 m tall) leads to a 30% increase (95% CI 13% to 50%) in the relative risk of developing abnormal sleep disordered breathing (AHI ≥ 5 episodes/hour) over a period of 4 years.[23] Other strong associations include increasing age and sex (male to female ratio is 2 : 1). Weaker associations include menopause, family history, smoking, and night time nasal congestion.[23]

PROGNOSIS The long term prognosis of people with untreated severe OSAHS is poor with respect to quality of life, likelihood of motor vehicle accidents, hypertension, and possibly cardiovascular disease and premature mortality.[24] Unfortunately, the prognosis of both treated and untreated OSAHS is unclear.[7] The limitations in the evidence include bias in the selection of participants, short duration of follow up, and variation in the measurement of confounders (e.g. smoking, alcohol use, and other cardiovascular risk factors). Treatment is widespread, making it difficult to find evidence on prognosis for untreated OSAHS. Observational studies support a causal association between OSAHS and systemic hypertension, which increases with the severity of OSAHS (OR 1.21 for non-severe OSAHS to 3.07 for severe OSAHS).[24] OSAHS increases the risk of motor vehicle accidents threefold to sevenfold.[24,25] It is associated with increased risk of premature mortality, cardiovascular disease, and impaired neurocognitive functioning.[24]

Please refer to clinicalevidence.com for full text and references.

Breast cancer (metastatic)

Search date June 2005

Justin Stebbing, Jeremy Crane, and Andrew Gaya

What are the effects of first line hormonal treatment?

BENEFICIAL

Hormonal treatment with antioestrogens (tamoxifen) or progestins (no significant difference in survival compared with non-taxane combination chemotherapy so may be preferable in women with oestrogen receptor positive disease)

One systematic review found no significant difference in survival at 12 or 24 months between first line hormonal treatment with tamoxifen or progestins and non-taxane combination chemotherapy. The review suggested that hormonal treatment may be preferable to chemotherapy as first line treatment in women with oestrogen receptor positive disease unless disease is rapidly progressing. It found that response rates were lower with hormonal treatment than with chemotherapy, but hormonal treatment was associated with less nausea, vomiting, and alopecia.

Selective aromatase inhibitors in postmenopausal women (at least as effective as tamoxifen in delaying disease progression)

Two RCTs found that the aromatase inhibitor anastrozole as first line treatment in metastatic postmenopausal breast cancer was at least as effective as tamoxifen in delaying disease progression and may cause fewer thromboembolic adverse events and vaginal bleeding. One RCT found that the aromatase inhibitor letrozole increased time to disease progression compared with tamoxifen.

Tamoxifen in oestrogen receptor positive women

RCTs have found that antioestrogens (primarily tamoxifen) resulted in tumour responses in a substantial proportion of women with metastatic breast cancer. The likelihood of benefit with antioestrogen treatment was greatest in postmenopausal women with oestrogen receptor positive tumours. RCTs found no significant difference in response rates, remission rates, or overall survival between tamoxifen and progestins or ovarian ablation, but tamoxifen was associated with fewer adverse effects. One RCT found that medroxyprogesterone increased overall response and weight gain compared with tamoxifen, but found no significant difference in survival between treatments. Two RCTs in women with metastatic postmenopausal breast cancer found that tamoxifen and the aromatase inhibitor anastrozole were similarly effective in delaying disease progression but that tamoxifen may cause more thromboembolic adverse effects and vaginal bleeding. One RCT found that tamoxifen was less effective than the aromatase inhibitor letrozole in delaying disease progression.

LIKELY TO BE BENEFICIAL

Combined gonadorelin analogues plus tamoxifen in premenopausal women

RCTs in premenopausal women with oestrogen receptor positive metastatic breast cancer found that first line treatment with gonadorelin analogues plus tamoxifen improved response rates, overall survival, and progression free survival compared with gonadorelin analogues alone.

TRADE OFF BETWEEN BENEFITS AND HARMS

Ovarian ablation in premenopausal women (no significant difference in response rates or survival compared with tamoxifen but associated with substantial adverse effects)

One systematic review and one subsequent RCT in premenopausal women found no significant difference in response rate, duration of response, or survival between ovarian ablation (surgery or irradiation) and tamoxifen as first line treatment. Ovarian ablation is associated with substantial adverse effects such as hot flushes and "tumour flare".

Progestins (beneficial in women with bone metastases or anorexia compared with tamoxifen; higher doses associated with adverse effects)

One systematic review found no significant difference in response rates, remission rates, or survival between medroxyprogesterone and tamoxifen as first line treatment. One subsequent RCT found that medroxyprogesterone increased overall response and weight gain compared with tamoxifen, but found no significant difference in survival between treatments. Observational evidence suggested that progestins may increase appetite, weight gain, and wellbeing, and reduce pain from bone metastases. One non-systematic review found that higher doses of medroxyprogesterone increased nausea, vaginal bleeding, and exacerbations of hypertension. One systematic review found no significant difference in survival at 12 or 24 months between first line hormonal treatment (with progestins or tamoxifen) and non-taxane combination chemotherapy. The review suggested that hormonal treatment may be preferable to chemotherapy as first line treatment in women with oestrogen receptor positive disease unless disease is rapidly progressing. It found that response rates were lower with hormonal treatment than with chemotherapy but it was associated with less nausea, vomiting, and alopecia.

What are the effects of second line hormonal treatment in women who have not responded to tamoxifen?

BENEFICIAL

Selective aromatase inhibitors in postmenopausal women (prolonged survival compared with progestins, no significant difference in time to progression compared with antioestrogens)

RCTs found that, in postmenopausal women with metastatic breast cancer who had relapsed on adjuvant tamoxifen or progressed during first line treatment with tamoxifen, the selective aromatase inhibitors letrozole, and exemestane prolonged survival compared with progestins (megestrol) or non-selective aromatase inhibitors (aminoglutethimide), and had fewer adverse effects. One RCT found no significant difference between anastrozole and progestins (megestrol) in objective response, but it did not assess survival. Two RCTs found no significant difference between anastrozole and fulvestrant in time to progression. The evidence suggests that selective aromatase inhibitors are most effective in oestrogen receptor positive women.

LIKELY TO BE INEFFECTIVE OR HARMFUL

Progestins (less effective in prolonging survival than selective aromatase inhibitors and have more adverse effects)

RCTs found that, in postmenopausal women with metastatic breast cancer who had relapsed on adjuvant tamoxifen or progressed during first line treatment with tamoxifen, progestins were less effective in prolonging survival as second line treatment than selective aromatase inhibitors and were associated with more adverse effects.

What are the effects of first line chemotherapy?

BENEFICIAL

Anthracycline based non-taxane combination chemotherapy regimens (CAF) containing doxorubicin (delayed progression, increased response rates and survival compared with non-anthracycline based regimens)

RCTs found that combination chemotherapy regimens containing an anthracycline, such as doxorubicin (CAF) as first line treatment increased response rates, time to progression, and survival compared with other regimens.

Classical non-taxane combination chemotherapy (CMF) (increases response rates and survival compared with modified CMF)

One systematic review found that classical CMF as first line treatment increased response rate and survival compared with modified CMF regimens. One RCT found that doxorubicin plus cyclophosphamide delayed both treatment failure and disease progression compared with epirubicin plus cyclophosphamide. It found no significant difference in overall response or survival between treatments.

TRADE OFF BETWEEN BENEFITS AND HARMS

Taxane based combination chemotherapy (may increase response rates compared with non-taxane combination chemotherapy but with increased adverse effects)

One systematic review found that taxane based chemotherapy as first or second line treatment increased overall survival, time to progression, and overall response compared with non-taxane chemotherapy. If the analysis was restricted to RCTs of first line chemotherapy it found that the increase in overall response with taxane based chemotherapy remained significant, but there was no significant difference in overall survival or time to progression. A second systematic review of a subset of the RCTs included in the first review found no significant difference between first line treatment with taxanes plus anthracycline and standard anthracycline based combination regimens in time to progression or overall survival. Both reviews found that taxane based chemotherapy increased adverse events such as neurotoxicity, neutropenia, and alopecia. One RCT found no significant difference between first line treatment with sequential and concomitant treatment with epirubicin plus paclitaxel in progression free survival time and overall survival time but found that sequential treatment increased grade 3–4 neutropenia and grade 2–4 neuropathy. One RCT found no significant difference between paclitaxel plus epirubicin and paclitaxel plus carboplatin as first line treatment in overall survival or adverse effects between treatments. It found that paclitaxel plus carboplatin increased time to treatment failure.

LIKELY TO BE INEFFECTIVE OR HARMFUL

High dose chemotherapy (no significant difference in overall survival compared with standard chemotherapy and increased adverse effects)

One systematic review and one subsequent RCT found no significant difference in overall survival over 1–5 years between high dose chemotherapy (requiring

Breast cancer (metastatic)

haematopoietic transplant) and standard dose chemotherapy. The review and the RCT found that high dose chemotherapy increased treatment related morbidity and mortality compared with standard chemotherapy.

What are the effects of first line chemotherapy in combination with a monoclonal antibody?

BENEFICIAL

Chemotherapy plus monoclonal antibody (trastuzumab) in women with overexpressed *HER2/neu* oncogene

One RCT found that, in women whose tumours overexpress the *HER2/neu* oncogene, standard chemotherapy plus the monoclonal antibody trastuzumab as first line treatment increased the time to disease progression, objective response, and overall survival compared with standard chemotherapy alone. The most serious adverse effect observed was cardiac dysfunction in women who received an anthracycline plus trastuzumab.

What are the effects of second line chemotherapy?

LIKELY TO BE BENEFICIAL

Taxane based combination chemotherapy (increases response rate in women with anthracycline resistant disease compared with non-taxane combination chemotherapy)

One systematic review found that taxane based chemotherapy as first or second line treatment increased overall survival, time to progression, and overall response compared with non-taxane based chemotherapy. If the analysis was limited to women who had previously received anthracyclines, the improvement with taxane based chemotherapy remained significant for time to progression and overall response, but not for overall survival.

UNKNOWN EFFECTIVENESS

Capecitabine for anthracycline resistant disease

One RCT found similar response rates and time to disease progression between capecitabine and paclitaxel after anthracycline failure.

Semisynthetic vinca alkaloids for anthracycline resistant disease

One RCT found no significant difference in progression or overall survival between fluorouracil plus vinorelbine and docetaxel given as second line chemotherapy. Another RCT found that second line vinorelbine improved survival and reduced progression compared with melphalan. A third RCT found no significant difference in survival or quality of life between vinorelbine plus doxorubicin and doxorubicin alone.

What are the effects of treatments for bone metastases?

BENEFICIAL

Radiotherapy plus appropriate analgesia*

We found no RCTs. We found limited evidence from non-randomised studies that persistent and localised bone pain can be treated successfully in over 80% of women with radiotherapy plus concomitant appropriate analgesia (from non-steroidal anti-inflammatory drugs to morphine and its derivatives) and that cranial nerve compression can be treated successfully with radiotherapy in 50–80% of people. RCTs found no evidence that short courses were less effective for pain relief than long courses of radiotherapy. One RCT found that different fractionation schedules can be used to treat neuropathic bone pain effectively.

LIKELY TO BE BENEFICIAL

Bisphosphonates

RCTs in women receiving standard chemotherapy or hormonal treatment for bone metastases secondary to metastatic breast cancer found that bisphosphonates reduced and delayed skeletal complications compared with placebo. They found no significant difference in survival.

What are the effects of treatments for spinal cord metastases?

BENEFICIAL

Radiotherapy*

We found no RCTs. Spinal cord compression is an emergency. Retrospective studies suggested that early radiotherapy improved outcomes. However, fewer than 10% of people walked again if severe deterioration of motor function occurred before radiotherapy.

Radiotherapy plus high dose corticosteroids in women with spinal cord compression

One small RCT in women with spinal cord compression found that adding high dose corticosteroids to radiotherapy improved the chance of walking 6 months after treatment compared with radiotherapy alone.

What are the effects of treatments for cerebral metastases?

LIKELY TO BE BENEFICIAL

Radiotherapy*

We found no RCTs. Retrospective studies suggested that whole brain irradiation improved neurological function in some women with brain metastases secondary to breast cancer.

UNKNOWN EFFECTIVENESS

Intrathecal chemotherapy

We found no RCTs or observational studies of intrathecal chemotherapy in people with cerebral metastases.

Radiation sensitisers

We found no RCTs of radiation sensitisers. One open label case control study provided limited evidence that adding intravenous RSR13, a radiation sensitiser, during whole brain radiotherapy may prolong survival.

Surgical resection

We found no RCTs. One retrospective cohort study provided insufficient evidence to assess surgical resection in people with cerebral metastases.

Breast cancer (metastatic)

What are the effects of treatments for choroidal metastases?

LIKELY TO BE BENEFICIAL

Radiotherapy*

We found no RCTs. Retrospective studies suggested that radiotherapy benefited some women with choroidal metastases.

*Not based on RCT evidence.

DEFINITION Metastatic or advanced breast cancer is the presence of disease at distant sites such as the bone, liver, or lung. It is not treatable by primary surgery and is currently considered incurable. However, young people with good performance status may survive for 15–20 years.[1] Symptoms may include pain from bone metastases, breathlessness from spread to the lungs, and nausea or abdominal discomfort from liver involvement.

INCIDENCE/ PREVALENCE Breast cancer is the second most frequent cancer in the world and is by far the most common malignant disease in women (22% of all new cancer cases). Worldwide, the ratio of mortality to incidence is about 36%. It ranks fifth as a cause of death from cancer overall (although it is the leading cause of cancer mortality in women — the 370 000 annual deaths represent 13.9% of cancer deaths in women). In the USA, metastatic breast cancer causes 46 000 deaths annually, and in the UK causes 15 000 deaths annually.[2] It is the most prevalent cancer in the world today and there are an estimated 3.9 million women alive who have had breast cancer diagnosed in the past 5 years (compared, for example, with lung cancer, where there are 1.4 million alive). The true prevalence of metastatic disease is high because some women live with the disease for many years. Since 1990, there has been an overall increase in incidence rates of about 1.5% annually.[3]

AETIOLOGY/ RISK FACTORS The risk of metastatic disease relates to known adverse prognostic factors in the original primary tumour. These factors include oestrogen receptor negative disease, primary tumours 3 cm or more in diameter, and axillary node involvement — recurrence occurred within 10 years of adjuvant chemotherapy for early breast cancer in 60–70% of node positive women and 25–30% of node negative women in one large systematic review.[4]

PROGNOSIS Prognosis depends on age, extent of disease, and oestrogen receptor status. There is also evidence that overexpression of the product of the *HER2/neu* oncogene, which occurs in about a third of women with metastatic breast cancer, is associated with a worse prognosis.[5] A short disease free interval (e.g. < 1 year) between surgery for early breast cancer and developing metastases suggests that the recurrent disease is likely to be resistant to adjuvant treatment.[6] In women who receive no treatment for metastatic disease, the median survival from diagnosis of metastases is 12 months.[7] The choice of first line treatment (hormonal or chemotherapy) is based on a variety of clinical factors (see table 1)Ⓣ.[8-11] In many countries, such as the USA, Canada, and some countries in Europe, there is evidence of a decrease in death rates in recent years. This probably reflects improvements in treatment (and therefore improved survival) as well as earlier diagnosis.[2,12]

Please refer to clinicalevidence.com for full text and references.

Breast cancer (non-metastatic)

Search date February 2006

Alan Rodger, Justin Stebbing and Alastair M Thompson

What are the effects of interventions after breast conserving surgery for ductal carcinoma in situ?

LIKELY TO BE BENEFICIAL

Radiotherapy (reduced recurrence)

Two RCTs identified by a systematic review found that radiotherapy after breast conserving surgery for ductal carcinoma *in situ* reduced local recurrence and invasive carcinoma compared with no radiotherapy after 4 and 8 years. However, they found no evidence of an effect on survival. One RCT in women having local excision found no significant difference between tamoxifen plus radiotherapy and radiotherapy alone in total invasive or ductal carcinoma *in situ* events after a median follow up of 1 year. One RCT found that radiotherapy plus placebo was less effective at reducing breast cancer events in women who had undergone wide excision, after a median follow up of 6 years, compared with adjuvant tamoxifen, although subgroup analysis suggested that the benefit of adding tamoxifen may be limited to oestrogen receptor positive tumours. The RCT found no evidence of an effect on survival.

Tamoxifen plus radiotherapy (reduced recurrence in women with oestrogen receptor positive tumours)

One RCT found that adjuvant tamoxifen reduced breast cancer events in women who had undergone wide excision and radiotherapy after a median follow up of 6 years compared with adjuvant placebo, although subgroup analysis suggested that benefit may be limited to women with oestrogen receptor positive tumours. It found no evidence of an effect on survival. One RCT in women having local excision found no significant difference between tamoxifen plus radiotherapy and radiotherapy alone in invasive or ductal carcinoma *in situ* events after a median follow up of 1 year.

What are the effects of treatments for primary operable breast cancer?

BENEFICIAL

Adjuvant aromatase inhibitors

One RCT found that, compared with placebo, letrozole reduced breast cancer events and improved disease free survival in postmenopausal women who had completed 5 years of postoperative tamoxifen therapy. The RCT found no significant difference in overall survival. Two RCTs found that adjuvant aromatase inhibitors (anastrozole and exemestane) reduced breast cancer events and significantly increased disease free survival compared with tamoxifen in postmenopausal women with early breast cancer. Adjuvant aromatase inhibitors (letrozole, anastrozole, and exemestane) are associated with a higher incidence of arthralgia and fractures compared with placebo or tamoxifen, but reduced thromboembolic and endometrial events compared with tamoxifen.

Adjuvant combination chemotherapy (better than no chemotherapy)

One systematic review found that adjuvant combination chemotherapy reduced recurrence and improved survival at 10 years compared with no chemotherapy. ▶

Breast cancer (non-metastatic)

The benefit seemed to be independent of nodal or menopausal status, although the absolute improvements were greater in women with node positive disease, and probably greater in younger women. Adverse effects of chemotherapy include fatigue, nausea and vomiting, hair loss, bone marrow suppression, neuropathy, and gastrointestinal disturbance. Chemotherapy may impair fertility and ovarian function.

Adjuvant tamoxifen (in women with oestrogen receptor positive tumours)

One systematic review found that adjuvant tamoxifen taken for up to 5 years reduced the risk of recurrence and death in women with oestrogen receptor positive tumours, irrespective of age, menopausal status, nodal involvement, or the addition of chemotherapy. Treatment for 5 years was more effective than were shorter durations, but available evidence did not find benefit associated with prolongation of treatment beyond 5 years. Tamoxifen slightly increased the risk of endometrial cancer and thrombotic complications, but we found no evidence of an overall adverse effect on non-breast cancer mortality.

Anthracycline regimens as adjuvant chemotherapy (better than standard CMF [cyclophosphamide, methotrexate, and fluorouracil] regimens)

One systematic review found that adjuvant regimens containing an anthracycline reduced recurrence and improved survival compared with a standard multidrug chemotherapy regimen (cyclophosphamide, methotrexate, and fluorouracil) at 5 years. Adverse effects of chemotherapy include nausea and vomiting, hair loss, bone marrow suppression, fatigue, and gastrointestinal disturbance. Chemotherapy may impair fertility and ovarian function.

Chemotherapy plus monoclonal antibody (trastuzumab) in women with overexpressed *HER2/neu* oncogene New

Three RCTs found that trastuzumab, started after or during chemotherapy, increased disease-free survival compared with observation after 2 years in HER2 positive women. These results compelled the interim data safety monitoring boards to stop the trials after the first interim analyses.

Combined chemotherapy plus tamoxifen

One RCT found that adding chemotherapy to tamoxifen improved survival at 5 years in women with lymph node negative, oestrogen receptor positive early breast cancer. It found that adding combined chemotherapy to tamoxifen was associated with increased adverse effects such as nausea, neutropenia, alopecia, thromboembolism, and phlebitis.

Less extensive mastectomy (similar survival to more extensive surgery, and better cosmetic outcome)

Two systematic reviews and long term follow up of included RCTs found that more extensive (radical) mastectomy did not improve outcomes compared with less extensive (simple) mastectomy in women with early invasive breast cancer, providing that all local disease was excised. Cosmetic appearance is worse with more extensive surgery.

Ovarian ablation in premenopausal women

One systematic review found that in premenopausal women with early breast cancer, ovarian ablation improved survival compared with no ablation after 15 years' follow up.

Radiotherapy after breast conserving surgery (reduced local recurrence and breast cancer mortality compared with breast conserving surgery alone)

One systematic review found that adding radiotherapy to breast conserving surgery reduced the risk of local recurrence, breast cancer mortality, and overall mortality compared with breast conserving surgery alone. One systematic review and one additional RCT found no significant difference in survival and local recurrence with breast conserving surgery plus radiotherapy compared with mastectomy. Radiotherapy may be associated with late adverse effects, which are rare, including pneumonitis, pericarditis, arm oedema, brachial plexopathy, and radionecrotic rib fracture.

Radiotherapy after mastectomy in women at high risk of local recurrence

One systematic review found that radiotherapy after mastectomy (alone or with axillary clearance or sampling) reduced the 5 year risk of isolated local recurrence compared with no radiotherapy in people with node positive and node negative disease. In people with node positive disease, the review found that radiotherapy after mastectomy with axillary clearance reduced breast cancer mortality compared with no radiotherapy. In people with node negative disease, the review found that radiotherapy after mastectomy with axillary clearance increased breast cancer mortality compared with no radiotherapy. The review found no significant difference in breast cancer mortality between radiotherapy after mastectomy (alone or with axillary sampling) and no radiotherapy in people with node positive and node negative disease. Women at high risk of recurrence include those with more axillary node involvement, larger tumours, higher histological grade, lymphovascular invasion, and involvement of tumour margins. Radiotherapy may be associated with late adverse effects, which are rare, including pneumonitis, pericarditis, arm oedema, brachial plexopathy, and radionecrotic rib fracture.

LIKELY TO BE BENEFICIAL

Primary chemotherapy (reduced mastectomy rates and had similar survival rates to adjuvant chemotherapy)

Five RCTs found no significant difference in survival with primary chemotherapy compared with adjuvant chemotherapy. Three RCTs found that primary chemotherapy reduced mastectomy rates compared with adjuvant chemotherapy. Adverse effects of chemotherapy include fatigue, nausea and vomiting, hair loss, bone marrow suppression, neuropathy, and gastrointestinal disturbance. Chemotherapy may impair fertility and ovarian function.

Radiotherapy plus tamoxifen after breast conserving surgery (reduced local recurrence rates)

One RCT in women aged over 50 years found that radiotherapy (with or without tamoxifen) reduced ipsilateral breast cancer recurrence compared with tamoxifen alone after median follow up of 87 months. It found no significant difference in survival. One RCT in women aged over 50 years found that postoperative radiotherapy plus tamoxifen reduced relapse rates in the ipsilateral breast and improved disease free survival compared with postoperative tamoxifen alone after 5 years. Subgroup analysis found greater benefit in women with receptor positive tumours. Another RCT in women aged over 70 years found that radiotherapy plus tamoxifen reduced local or regional recurrence rates compared with tamoxifen alone in women who had undergone lumpectomy for receptor positive tumours after 5 years. The RCT found no difference in time to distant metastasis or overall survival. Radiotherapy may be associated with late adverse effects, which are rare, including pneumonitis, pericarditis, arm oedema, brachial plexopathy, and radionecrotic rib fracture.

Total nodal radiotherapy

One systematic review found that postmastectomy radiotherapy, including total nodal irradiation, reduced locoregional recurrence. However, it found conflicting evidence on breast cancer mortality.

TRADE OFF BETWEEN BENEFITS AND HARMS

Axillary clearance

There is consensus that axillary clearance reduces regional recurrence compared with no axillary management. RCTs found no significant difference in survival at 5–10 years between axillary clearance and axillary sampling (followed by axillary radiotherapy in women found to be node positive) or axillary radiotherapy (regardless of axillary nodal status). One systematic review found that axillary radiotherapy reduced isolated local recurrence compared with axillary clearance, but this difference was not significant. One systematic review of mainly poor quality RCTs found that the risk of arm lymphoedema was highest with axillary clearance plus radiotherapy, lower with axillary sampling plus radiotherapy, and lowest with sampling alone.

Axillary radiotherapy

One systematic review found that axillary radiotherapy reduced isolated local recurrence compared with axillary clearance, but this difference was not significant. The review found no significant difference in survival at 10 years between axillary radiotherapy and axillary clearance. One systematic review of mainly poor quality RCTs found that the risk of arm lymphoedema was highest with axillary clearance plus radiotherapy, lower with axillary sampling plus radiotherapy, and lowest with sampling alone.

Axillary sampling

One RCT found no significant difference in survival at 5 years between axillary clearance and axillary sampling (followed by axillary radiotherapy in women found to be node positive). One systematic review of mainly poor quality RCTs found that the risk of arm lymphoedema was highest with axillary clearance plus radiotherapy, lower with axillary sampling plus radiotherapy, and lowest with sampling alone.

Radiotherapy after mastectomy in women not at high risk of local recurrence

One systematic review found that radiotherapy after mastectomy (alone or with axillary clearance or sampling) reduced the 5 year risk of isolated local recurrence compared with no radiotherapy in people with node positive and node negative disease. In people with node positive disease, the review found that radiotherapy after mastectomy with axillary clearance reduced breast cancer mortality compared with no radiotherapy. In people with node negative disease, the review found that radiotherapy after mastectomy with axillary clearance increased breast cancer mortality compared with no radiotherapy. The review found no significant difference in breast cancer mortality between radiotherapy after mastectomy (alone or with axillary sampling) and no radiotherapy in people with node positive and node negative disease. Women at high risk of recurrence include those with more axillary node involvement, larger tumours, higher histological grade, lymphovascular invasion, and involvement of tumour margins. Radiotherapy may be associated with late adverse effects, which are rare, including pneumonitis, pericarditis, arm oedema, brachial plexopathy, and radionecrotic rib fracture. There is, therefore, a trade off between absolute benefits and harms in women not at high risk of local recurrence.

UNKNOWN EFFECTIVENESS

Different primary chemotherapy regimens (insufficient evidence regarding which regimen is most effective)

We found insufficient evidence of any difference between the common primary chemotherapy regimens in survival, recurrence, or quality of life.

Less than whole breast radiotherapy plus breast conserving surgery *New*

We found insufficient evidence on less than whole breast radiotherapy after breast conserving surgery.

Radiotherapy to the internal mammary chain

One RCT found no significant difference in relapse or survival at 2–3 years between radiotherapy and no radiotherapy to the internal mammary chain. Treatment may increase radiation induced cardiac morbidity.

Radiotherapy to the ipsilateral supraclavicular fossa

We found insufficient evidence about the effects of irradiation of the ipsilateral supraclavicular fossa on survival. RCTs have found that radiotherapy to the chest wall and lymph nodes is associated with reduced risk of locoregional recurrence, including supraclavicular fossa nodal recurrence. Morbidity associated with irradiation of the supraclavicular fossa is rare and, where it occurs, is mild and temporary.

Sentinel node biopsy (versus axillary dissection plus sentinel node dissection)

One RCT found that sentinel node biopsy reduced postoperative pain, and physical and psychological morbidity compared with axillary dissection, although there was no significant difference in survival between treatments. Follow up may have been too short to detect a significant difference in survival between treatments. A second RCT found that sentinel node biopsy reduced arm swelling and loss of sensation compared with axillary node dissection.

UNLIKELY TO BE BENEFICIAL

Enhanced dose regimens of adjuvant combination chemotherapy

RCTs did not find additional survival advantage from enhanced dose regimens of adjuvant combination chemotherapy. Adverse effects of chemotherapy include nausea and vomiting, hair loss, bone marrow suppression, fatigue, and gastrointestinal disturbance. Chemotherapy may impair fertility and ovarian function.

Prolonged adjuvant combination chemotherapy (8–12 months *v* 4–6 months)

One systematic review found no additional survival benefit from prolonging adjuvant chemotherapy from 4–6 to 8–12 months. Adverse effects of chemotherapy include nausea and vomiting, hair loss, bone marrow suppression, fatigue, and gastrointestinal disturbance. Chemotherapy may impair fertility and ovarian function.

Breast cancer (non-metastatic)

LIKELY TO BE INEFFECTIVE OR HARMFUL

High dose chemotherapy plus autologous stem cell transplantation

One systematic review found no significant difference between high dose chemotherapy plus autologous stem cell transplantation and conventional chemotherapy in 5 year survival for women with early, poor prognosis breast cancer. The review found that high dose chemotherapy plus autologous stem cell transplantation increased treatment related and non-cancer related deaths compared with conventional chemotherapy.

What are the effects of interventions in locally advanced breast cancer (stage III B)?

LIKELY TO BE BENEFICIAL

Adding hormonal treatment to radiotherapy (improves survival compared with radiotherapy alone)

One RCT found that hormonal treatment (tamoxifen or ovarian ablation) plus radiotherapy delayed locoregional recurrence and improved survival at 8 years in locally advanced breast cancer compared with radiotherapy alone.

Postoperative radiotherapy (in women also receiving postoperative systemic treatment)

Two RCTs found that postoperative radiotherapy increased overall and disease free survival at 5 and 10 years in women who also received systemic treatment (chemotherapy or hormone therapy) following mastectomy. One small RCT found no reliable evidence that postoperative radiotherapy improved outcomes in women who had systemic therapy after surgery. One RCT found no evidence that postmastectomy radiotherapy improved relapse rates or survival compared with no radiotherapy in women who were not receiving further systemic treatment after surgery.

Radiotherapy (similar effectiveness to surgery)

Two small RCTs that included women with locally advanced disease (stage III B) found that radiotherapy or surgery as a sole local treatment had a similar effect on response rates, duration of response, and overall survival for locally advanced breast cancer that was rendered operable by prior chemotherapy.

Surgery (similar effectiveness to radiotherapy)

Two small RCTs that included women with locally advanced disease (stage III B) found that radiotherapy or surgery as a sole local treatment had a similar effect on response rates, duration of response, and overall survival for locally advanced breast cancer that was rendered operable by prior chemotherapy.

UNKNOWN EFFECTIVENESS

Adding chemotherapy (cyclophosphamide/methotrexate/fluorouracil or anthracycline based regimens) to radiotherapy

Three RCTs found insufficient evidence that radiotherapy plus cytotoxic chemotherapy using cyclophosphamide plus methotrexate plus fluorouracil, or an anthracycline based multidrug regimen, improved survival, disease free survival, or long term locoregional control compared with radiotherapy alone in locally advanced breast cancer. One RCT found no difference between adjuvant chemotherapy and primary plus adjuvant chemotherapy in women also receiving radiotherapy.

Radiotherapy (low dose versus tamoxifen)

One small RCT found no difference in response or survival between low dose radiotherapy (40 Gy in 15 fractions) and tamoxifen in women with locally advanced breast cancer.

UNLIKELY TO BE BENEFICIAL

Hormonal treatment versus multimodal treatment

One RCT found that tamoxifen followed by salvage treatments upon tumour progression did not improve remission rates after 6 months compared with multimodal treatment (primary chemotherapy, surgery, radiotherapy, and tamoxifen).

DEFINITION This chapter examines the effects of treatment for non-metastatic, primary breast cancer. **Ductal carcinoma in situ** is a non-invasive tumour characterised by the presence of malignant cells in the breast ducts but with no evidence that they breach the basement membrane and invade into periductal connective tissues. **Invasive breast cancer** occurs when cancer cells spread beyond the basement membrane, which covers the underlying connective tissue in the breast. This tissue is rich in blood vessels and lymphatic channels that are capable of carrying cancer cells beyond the breast. Invasive breast cancer can be separated into three main groups: early invasive breast cancer, locally advanced breast cancer, and metastatic breast cancer (see breast cancer (metastatic)). **Operable breast cancer** is apparently restricted to the breast and to local lymph nodes and can be removed surgically. Although women do not have overt metastases at the time of staging, they remain at risk of local recurrence and of metastatic spread. They can be divided into those with tumours greater than 4 cm or with multifocal cancers that are usually treated by mastectomy, and those with tumours less than 4 cm or with unifocal cancers that can be treated by breast conserving surgery. **Locally advanced breast cancer** is defined according to the TNM staging system of the UICC[1] as stage III B (includes T4 a–d; N2 disease, but absence of metastases [see table 3]Ⓣ). It is a disease presentation with clinical or histopathological evidence of skin and/or chest wall involvement and/or axillary nodes matted together by tumour extension. **Metastatic breast cancer** is presented in a separate chapter (see breast cancer (metastatic)).

INCIDENCE/ PREVALENCE Breast cancer affects 1/10–1/11 women in the UK and causes about 21 000 deaths a year. Prevalence is about five times higher, with over 100 000 women in the UK living with breast cancer at any one time. Of the 36 000 new cases of breast cancer a year in England and Wales, most will present with primary operable disease.[2]

AETIOLOGY/ RISK FACTORS The risk of breast cancer increases with age, doubling every 10 years up to the menopause. Risk factors include an early age at menarche, older age at menopause, older age at birth of first child, family history, atypical hyperplasia, excess alcohol intake, radiation exposure to developing breast tissue, oral contraceptive use, postmenopausal hormone replacement therapy, and obesity. Risk in different countries varies five-fold. The cause of breast cancer in most women is unknown. About 5% of breast cancers can be attributed to mutations in the genes *BRCA1* and *BRCA2*,[3] but the contribution to inherited breast cancer of other genes, including *Chk2*, *ATM*, *p53*, and *PTEN*, is currently less well established.

PROGNOSIS **Non-metastatic carcinoma** of the breast is potentially curable. The risk of relapse depends on various clinicopathological features, of which axillary node involvement, tumour grade, tumour size, and oestrogen receptor status are the most prognostically important. Of women with operable disease, 80% are alive

Breast cancer (non-metastatic)

5 years after diagnosis and treatment (adjuvant treatment is given to most women after surgery). Risk of recurrence is highest during the first 5 years, but the risk remains even 15–20 years after surgery. Those with node positive disease have a 50–60% chance of recurrence within 5 years, compared with 30–35% for node negative disease. Recurrence at 10 years, according to one large systematic review,[4] is 60–70% in node positive women and 25–30% in node negative women. The prognosis for disease free survival at 5 years is worse for stage III B (33%) than that for stage III A (71%). Overall survival at 5 years is 44% for stage III B and 84% for stage III A.[5] Poor survival and high rates of local recurrence characterise locally advanced breast cancer.

Please refer to clinicalevidence.com for full text and references.

Breast pain

Search date January 2005

Nigel Bundred

What are the effects of treatments for breast pain?

LIKELY TO BE BENEFICIAL

Topical non-steroidal anti-inflammatory drugs

One RCT found that topical diclofenac reduced breast pain compared with placebo at 6 months. There is widespread consensus that topical non-steroidal anti-inflammatory drugs are effective and well tolerated in relieving breast pain, and they are easily available over the counter.

TRADE OFF BETWEEN BENEFITS AND HARMS

Danazol

One RCT found that danazol reduced cyclical breast pain after 12 months compared with placebo, but it increased adverse effects (weight gain, deepening of the voice, menorrhagia, and muscle cramps). It found no significant difference in pain relief between danazol and tamoxifen.

Gestrinone

One RCT found that gestrinone reduced breast pain after 3 months compared with placebo, but increased adverse effects (greasy skin, hirsutism, acne, reduction in breast size, headache, and depression).

Gonadorelin analogues (luteinising hormone releasing hormone analogues)

One RCT found that goserelin injection reduced breast pain compared with placebo, but increased adverse effects (vaginal dryness, hot flushes, decreased libido, oily skin/hair, decreased breast size, irritability).

Tamoxifen

Three RCTs found limited evidence that tamoxifen was more effective than placebo at reducing breast pain. The two RCTs that reported on adverse effects found more hot flushes and vaginal discharge with tamoxifen compared with placebo, although differences between groups did not reach significance. One RCT found similar efficacy but fewer adverse effects with a lower dose of 10 mg compared with 20 mg. One RCT found no significant difference in pain relief between tamoxifen and danazol. One meta-analysis of four large breast cancer prevention trials found that tamoxifen used long term was associated with an increased risk of venous thromboembolism. Tamoxifen is not licensed for mastalgia in the UK or USA.

UNKNOWN EFFECTIVENESS

Antibiotics

We found no systematic review or RCTs of sufficient quality on the effects of antibiotics in women with breast pain.

Diet (low fat, high carbohydrate)

One small RCT found limited evidence that advice to follow a low fat, high carbohydrate diet reduced self reported premenstrual breast swelling and breast tenderness at 6 months compared with general dietary advice. However, it found no significant difference between groups in the combined outcome of breast swelling, tenderness, and nodularity on physical examination at 6 months.

Diuretics

We found no systematic review or RCTs of sufficient quality on the effects of diuretics in women with breast pain.

Lisuride

One RCT with weak methods found limited evidence that lisuride maleate (a dopamine agonist) reduced breast pain over 2 months compared with placebo.

Pyridoxine

We found no systematic review or RCTs of sufficient quality on the effects of pyridoxine in women with breast pain.

Tibolone

One RCT found no significant difference between tibolone and placebo in breast pain and tenderness at 12 months.

Vitamin E

We found no systematic review or RCTs of sufficient quality on the effects of vitamin E in women with breast pain.

UNLIKELY TO BE BENEFICIAL

Bromocriptine

One RCT with high withdrawal rates and one small crossover RCT reporting results after crossover found limited evidence that bromocriptine (a dopamine agonist) reduced breast pain compared with placebo. However, both RCTs found a higher incidence of adverse effects with bromocriptine than with placebo. Adverse events included nausea, dizziness, postural hypotension, and constipation. One of the RCTs found that withdrawals related to adverse effects were more frequent with bromocriptine compared with placebo, although differences between groups did not reach significance. Bromocriptine is now used rarely because of frequent and intolerable adverse effects, and the US Food and Drug Administration has withdrawn its licence for this indication.

Hormone replacement therapy (oestrogen)

We found no placebo controlled RCTs of hormone replacement therapy for breast pain. Hormone replacement therapy is associated with an increased risk of breast cancer, venous thromboembolism, and gall bladder disease.

Progestogens

Two small crossover RCTs found no significant difference between either progesterone cream or medroxyprogesterone acetate tablets and placebo in breast pain.

LIKELY TO BE INEFFECTIVE OR HARMFUL

Evening primrose oil

One RCT found no significant difference between evening primrose oil and placebo in frequency of pain at 6 months. In the UK, the Committee for Safety of Medicines has withdrawn the prescription licence from evening primrose oil because of lack of efficacy, but it is still available to purchase without prescription.

Breast pain

DEFINITION Breast pain can be differentiated into cyclical mastalgia (worse before a menstrual period) or non-cyclical mastalgia (unrelated to the menstrual cycle).[1,2] Cyclical pain is often bilateral, usually most severe in the upper outer quadrants of the breast, and may be referred to the medial aspect of the upper arm.[1-3] Non-cyclical pain may be caused by true breast pain or chest wall pain located over the costal cartilages.[1,2,4] Specific breast pathology and referred pain unrelated to the breasts are not included in this chapter.

INCIDENCE/ PREVALENCE Up to 70% of women develop breast pain in their lifetime.[1,2] Of 1171 US women attending a gynaecology clinic, 69% suffered regular discomfort, which was judged as severe in 11% of women, and 36% had consulted a doctor about breast pain.[2]

AETIOLOGY/ RISK FACTORS Breast pain is most common in women aged 30–50 years.[1,2]

PROGNOSIS Cyclical breast pain resolves spontaneously within 3 months of onset in 20–30% of women.[5] The pain tends to relapse and remit, and up to 60% of women develop recurrent symptoms 2 years after treatment.[1] Non-cyclical pain responds poorly to treatment but may resolve spontaneously in about 50% of women.[1]

Please refer to clinicalevidence.com for full text and references.

Candidiasis (vulvovaginal)

Search date October 2005

Des Spence

What are the effects of drug treatments for acute vulvovaginal candidiasis in non-pregnant symptomatic women?

BENEFICIAL

Intravaginal imidazoles

Three RCTs found that intravaginal imidazoles (butoconazole, clotrimazole, or miconazole) reduced persistent symptoms of vulvovaginal candidiasis after 4–5 weeks compared with placebo. RCTs found no significant difference in efficacy among the various intravaginal imidazoles. They also found no clear evidence of any difference in persistent symptoms between single dose and multiple doses, or different durations of multiple dose regimens, but may have been too small to detect clinically significant effects. RCTs found no significant difference in persistent symptoms at 1–12 weeks between intravaginal imidazoles and oral fluconazole or itraconazole. RCTs found that intravaginal imidazoles were associated with less nausea, headache, and abdominal pain but more vulval irritation and vaginal discharge than oral fluconazole. One small RCT found that intravaginal miconazole (with or without oral nystatin) was more effective at reducing symptoms at 6 months than intravaginal nystatin but found no significant differences for comparisons against other intravaginal imidazoles or intravaginal nystatin plus oral nystatin. A second RCT provided insufficient evidence to compare intravaginal imidazoles versus intravaginal nystatin.

Oral fluconazole

We found no RCTs comparing oral fluconazole versus placebo, no treatment, or intravaginal nystatin. One systematic review found no significant difference in persistent symptoms of vulvovaginal candidiasis over 1–12 weeks between oral fluconazole or oral itraconazole and intravaginal imidazoles. It found that oral fluconazole was associated with more nausea, headache, and abdominal pain but less vulval irritation and vaginal discharge compared with intravaginal imidazoles. One methodologically weak RCT provided insufficient evidence to compare oral fluconazole versus oral itraconazole.

Oral itraconazole

One RCT found that oral itraconazole reduced persistent symptoms of vulvovaginal candidiasis at 1 week after treatment compared with placebo. One systematic review found no significant difference in persistent symptoms over 1–12 weeks between oral itraconazole or oral fluconazole and intravaginal imidazoles. One methodologically weak RCT provided insufficient evidence to compare oral itraconazole versus oral fluconazole.

LIKELY TO BE BENEFICIAL

Intravaginal nystatin

One RCT found that intravaginal nystatin reduced the proportion of women with a poor symptomatic response after 14 days' treatment compared with placebo. Two RCTs provided insufficient evidence to compare intravaginal nystatin versus intravaginal imidazoles. One RCT found that intravaginal nystatin was less effective than boric acid in increasing clinical cure rates at 4 weeks. It gave no ▶

information on the adverse effects of intravaginal nystatin compared with intravaginal boric acid. We found no RCTs comparing intravaginal nystatin versus oral fluconazole or itraconazole.

What are the effects of alternative or complementary treatments for acute vulvovaginal candidiasis in non-pregnant symptomatic women?

UNKNOWN EFFECTIVENESS

Douching

Two systematic reviews identified no RCTs of douching in women with acute vulvovaginal candidiasis. Douching was associated with serious sequelae, including pelvic inflammatory disease, endometritis, ectopic pregnancy, gonorrhoea, and chlamydia.

Garlic

One systematic review identified no RCTs of garlic in women with acute vulvovaginal candidiasis.

Intravaginal boric acid

One RCT identified by a systematic review found that intravaginal boric acid increased clinical cure rates at 4 weeks compared with intravaginal nystatin. It gave no information on the adverse effects of intravaginal boric acid compared with intravaginal nystatin. Intravaginal boric acid can cause skin irritation.

Intravaginal tea tree oil

One systematic review identified no RCTs of intravaginal tea tree oil in women with acute vulvovaginal candidiasis.

Yoghurt containing *Lactobacillus acidophilus* (oral or vaginal)

One systematic review identified no RCTs of treatment with lactobacillus yoghurt (oral or vaginal) in women with acute vulvovaginal candidiasis.

What are the effects of treating a male sexual partner to resolve symptoms and prevent recurrence in non-pregnant women with symptomatic acute vulvovaginal candidiasis?

UNLIKELY TO BE BENEFICIAL

Treating a male sexual partner to resolve symptoms and prevent symptomatic recurrence in women with symptomatic acute vulvovaginal candidiasis

RCTs found no significant difference between treating and not treating a woman's male sexual partner in the resolution of the woman's symptoms of acute vulvovaginal candidiasis over 1–4 weeks or in the rate of symptomatic recurrence at 4–5 weeks after treatment.

Candidiasis (vulvovaginal)

What are the effects of drug treatments for recurrent vulvovaginal candidiasis in non-pregnant symptomatic women?

LIKELY TO BE BENEFICIAL

Oral fluconazole

One RCT found that fluconazole reduced symptomatic recurrence compared with placebo after 6 months of treatment and increased clinical cure rate 6 months after treatment was discontinued.

Oral itraconazole

One RCT found that monthly prophylaxis with oral itraconazole reduced symptomatic recurrence of vulvovaginal candidiasis over 6 months compared with placebo. One methodologically weak, open label RCT provided insufficient evidence to compare twice weekly prophylaxis with oral itraconazole versus intravaginal clotrimazole.

UNKNOWN EFFECTIVENESS

Intravaginal imidazoles

Two RCTs provided insufficient evidence about the effects of regular prophylaxis with intravaginal clotrimazole compared with placebo in preventing symptomatic recurrence of vulvovaginal candidiasis. One RCT found no significant difference in the number of episodes of symptomatic vaginitis over 6 months between monthly prophylaxis with intravaginal clotrimazole and treatment as required, although women who took monthly prophylaxis had fewer episodes and the RCT may have been underpowered to detect a clinically important difference. More women preferred treatment as required. One RCT found insufficient evidence about the effects of regular prophylaxis with intravaginal clotrimazole compared with oral itraconazole.

What are the effects of alternative or complementary treatments for symptomatic recurrent vulvovaginal candidiasis in non-pregnant women?

UNKNOWN EFFECTIVENESS

Douching

Two systematic reviews identified no RCTs of douching in women with recurrent vulvovaginal candidiasis. Douching is associated with serious sequelae, including pelvic inflammatory disease, endometritis, ectopic pregnancy, gonorrhoea, and chlamydia. One RCT found no significant difference in risk of pelvic inflammatory disease at 1 year between douche and cloth towel.

Garlic

One systematic review identified no RCTs of garlic in women with recurrent vulvovaginal candidiasis.

Intravaginal boric acid

We found no RCTs of intravaginal boric acid in women with recurrent vulvovaginal candidiasis.

Intravaginal tea tree oil

One systematic review identified no RCTs of intravaginal tea tree oil in women with recurrent vulvovaginal candidiasis.

Yoghurt containing *Lactobacillus acidophilus* (oral or vaginal)

Two poor quality crossover RCTs identified by a systematic review provided insufficient evidence about the effects of a diet containing oral lactobacillus yoghurt in women with recurrent vulvovaginal candidiasis. Oral yoghurt may cause gastrointestinal disturbance in people with lactose intolerance. The review identified no RCTs of vaginal lactobacillus yoghurt.

What are the effects of treating a male sexual partner in non-pregnant women with symptomatic recurrent vulvovaginal candidiasis?

UNKNOWN EFFECTIVENESS

Treating a male sexual partner to resolve symptoms and prevent recurrence in women with symptomatic recurrent vulvovaginal candidiasis

We found no RCTs on treating a male sexual partner to resolve symptoms and prevent recurrence in previously symptomatic women.

What are the effects of treating asymptomatic non-pregnant women with a positive swab for candidiasis?

UNKNOWN EFFECTIVENESS

Alternative or complementary treatments

We found no systematic reviews or RCTs on the effects of yoghurt containing *Lactobacillus acidophilus*, douching, garlic, tea-tree oil, or intravaginal boric acid in asymptomatic non-pregnant women with a positive swab for candidiasis.

Drug treatments

We found no systematic reviews or RCTs on the effects of intravaginal imidazoles (butoconazole, clotrimazole, miconazole, fenticonazole, terconazole, tioconazole, econazole), oral fluconazole, oral itraconazole, or intravaginal nystatin in asymptomatic non-pregnant women with a positive swab for candidiasis.

DEFINITION **Vulvovaginal candidiasis** is defined as symptomatic vaginitis (inflammation of the vagina), which often involves the vulva, caused by infection with a *Candida* yeast. Predominant symptoms are vulval itching and abnormal vaginal discharge (which may be minimal, a "cheese-like" material, or a watery secretion).[1] Differentiation from other forms of vaginitis requires the presence of yeast on microscopy of vaginal fluid. **Recurrent vulvovaginal candidiasis** is commonly defined as four or more symptomatic episodes a year.[2]

INCIDENCE/ PREVALENCE Vulvovaginal candidiasis is estimated to be the second most common cause of vaginitis after bacterial vaginosis. Estimates of its incidence are limited and often derived from women who attend hospital clinics. Asymptomatic prevalence has been reported in 10% of women[3] and self reported history of at least one episode of vulvovaginal candidiasis has been as high as 72%.[4] Recurrent symptoms are common but are caused by candidiasis in only a third of cases.[5]

AETIOLOGY/ RISK FACTORS *Candida albicans* accounts for 85–90% of cases of vulvovaginal candidiasis.[6,7] Development of symptomatic vulvovaginal candidiasis probably represents increased growth of yeast that previously colonised the vagina without causing symptoms. Risk factors for vulvovaginal candidiasis include pregnancy, diabetes mellitus, and systemic antibiotics. The evidence that different types of contraceptives are associated with risk factors is contradictory. The incidence of vulvovaginal candidiasis rises with initiation of sexual activity, but we found no direct evidence that vulvovaginal candidiasis is sexually transmitted.[8-10]

PROGNOSIS We found few descriptions of the natural history of untreated vulvovaginal candidiasis. Discomfort is the main complication and can include pain while passing urine or during sexual intercourse. Balanitis in male partners of women with vulvovaginal candidiasis can occur, but it is rare.

Please refer to clinicalevidence.com for full text and references.

Cervical cancer

Search date June 2005

Sudha Sundar, Amanda Horne, and Sean Kehoe

What are the effects of interventions to manage early stage cervical cancer?

LIKELY TO BE BENEFICIAL

Conisation of the cervix for microinvasive carcinoma (stage Ia1)*

We found no systematic review or RCTs comparing conisation of the cervix versus simple hysterectomy for microinvasive carcinoma (stage Ia1). However, there is consensus that conisation of the cervix is effective for microinvasive carcinoma (stage Ia1) provided that excision margins are clear of cancer or intraepithelial neoplasia. Conisation of the cervix can, unlike hysterectomy, preserve fertility.

Radiotherapy or surgery*

One RCT found no significant difference in overall survival or disease free survival between radiotherapy and radical hysterectomy plus lymphadenectomy (with or without adjuvant radiotherapy) for early stage cervical cancer. It found that surgery significantly increased the risk of severe adverse effects compared with radiotherapy. Consensus regards both surgery and radiotherapy as likely to be beneficial.

*Based on consensus.

UNKNOWN EFFECTIVENESS

Radical trachelectomy plus lymphadenectomy (preserved fertility compared with hysterectomy)

We found no systematic review or RCTs comparing radical trachelectomy plus lymphadenectomy versus radical hysterectomy in women with early stage cervical cancer. Radical trachelectomy plus lymphadenectomy can, unlike hysterectomy, preserve fertility.

What are the effects of interventions to manage bulky early stage cervical cancer?

BENEFICIAL

Chemoradiotherapy (increased survival compared with radiotherapy alone)

Two RCTs found that chemoradiotherapy improved overall survival and progression free survival compared with radiotherapy, when used either before or after hysterectomy. Combined chemoradiotherapy was associated with more haematological and gastrointestinal toxicity than radiotherapy alone.

UNKNOWN EFFECTIVENESS

Neoadjuvant chemotherapy

Two RCTs found that neoadjuvant chemotherapy before surgery, radiotherapy, or surgery plus radiotherapy increased overall survival compared with these treatments without neoadjuvant chemotherapy. However, another RCT found no significant difference in overall survival between neoadjuvant chemotherapy before surgery, and radiotherapy alone.

BMJ Clin Evid Concise 2006;16:715–716.

Cervical cancer

DEFINITION Cervical cancer is a malignant neoplasm arising from the uterine cervix. About 80% of cervical cancers are of the squamous type; the remainder are adenocarcinomas, adenosquamous carcinomas, and other rare types.[1] Staging of cervical cancer is based on clinical evaluation (FIGO classification; see table 1 Ⓣ). Management is determined by tumour bulk and stage. **Population:** This topic deals with treatments for early stage cancer (defined as FIGO stage Ia1, Ia2, Ib1, and small IIa tumours) and bulky early stage disease (defined as FIGO stage Ib2 and larger IIa tumours).

INCIDENCE/ PREVALENCE Cervical cancer is the second most common cancer in women, with about 450 000 new cases diagnosed worldwide each year.[2] Most (80%) cases occur in less developed countries without an effective screening programme. The incidence of cervical cancer in the UK and Europe has significantly reduced since the introduction of a screening programme for detecting precancerous cervical intraepithelial neoplasia. Cervical cancer incidence fell by 42% between 1988 and 1997 (England and Wales). This fall has been reported to be related to the cervical screening programme.[3] In England and Wales, cervical cancer has an annual incidence of 3200 women, and causes about 1000 deaths each year.[4]

AETIOLOGY/ RISK FACTORS Risk factors for cervical cancer include sexual intercourse at an early age, multiple sexual partners, tobacco smoking, long term oral contraceptive use, low socioeconomic status, immunosuppressive therapy, and micronutrient deficiency. Persistent infection by oncogenic, high risk strains of human papilloma virus (HPV) is strongly associated with the development of cervical cancer.[5-7] HPV is acquired mainly by sexual intercourse and has a peak prevalence of 20–30% in women aged 20–30 years,[8] although in 80% of cases the infection is transient and resolves within 12–18 months.

PROGNOSIS Overall, 5 year disease free survival is 50–70% for stages Ib2 and IIb, 30–50% for stage III, and 5–15% for stage IV.[1] In women who receive treatment, 5 year survival in stage Ia approaches 100%, falling to 70–85% for stage Ib1 and smaller IIa tumours. Survival in women with more locally advanced tumours is influenced by tumour bulk, the person's age, and coexistent medical conditions. Untreated mortality in locally advanced disease is high.

Please refer to clinicalevidence.com for full text and references.

Dysmenorrhoea

Search date July 2005

Michelle L Proctor and Cynthia M Farquhar

What are the effects of treatments for dysmenorrhoea?

BENEFICIAL

Non-steroidal anti-inflammatory drugs (other than aspirin)

One systematic review and four subsequent RCTs found that non-steroidal anti-inflammatory drugs (NSAIDs, including cyclo-oxygenase-2 [COX-2] inhibitors, but excluding niflumic acid) reduced moderate to severe pain compared with placebo in women with primary dysmenorrhoea. The review also found that NSAIDs (excluding COX-2 inhibitors) reduced restriction of daily activities, absence from work or school, and the need for additional analgesia compared with placebo. It remains unclear from direct comparisons which of the NSAIDs have better efficacy or safety. One small RCT identified by the review found no significant difference in pain relief between an NSAID (naproxen) and paracetamol. The review found that naproxen was associated with fewer adverse effects than co-proxamol. It also found that mefenamic acid reduced symptoms more than co-proxamol. One small RCT identified by another systematic review found no significant difference in pain relief between ibuprofen alone and ibuprofen plus vitamin E. The harms of NSAIDs, including the COX-2 inhibitor class, are considered in detail elsewhere in *Clinical Evidence* (see non-steroidal anti-inflammatory drugs topic) and include gastrointestinal ulceration and haemorrhage for traditional NSAIDs and, for at least some of the COX-2 inhibitors, increased cardiovascular risk. Co-proxamol has been withdrawn in some countries due to evidence that fatal toxicity may occur with a small multiple of the normal therapeutic dose and, therefore, a proportion of fatalities are caused by inadvertent overdose. Rofecoxib and valdecoxib, NSAIDs of the COX-2 inhibitor class, have been withdrawn worldwide because of cardiovascular adverse effects.

LIKELY TO BE BENEFICIAL

Aspirin, paracetamol, and compound analgesics

One systematic review found that aspirin was more effective than placebo for pain relief in women with primary dysmenorrhoea. Two systematic reviews found no significant difference in pain relief between paracetamol and placebo, aspirin, or naproxen, although some of the RCTs may have been too small to detect clinically important differences. The first review found limited evidence that co-proxamol reduced pain compared with placebo. One small RCT identified by a systematic review found no significant difference in pain relief between paracetamol and a non-steroidal anti-inflammatory drug (naproxen). One systematic review found that naproxen was associated with fewer adverse effects than co-proxamol. It also found that mefenamic acid reduced symptoms to a greater extent than co-proxamol. Co-proxamol has been withdrawn in some countries due to evidence that fatal toxicity may occur with a small multiple of the normal therapeutic dose and, therefore, a proportion of fatalities are caused by inadvertent overdose.

Thiamine

One large RCT identified by a systematic review found that thiamine reduced pain after 60 days compared with placebo in women with primary dysmenorrhoea.

BMJ Clin Evid Concise 2006;16:717–720.

Dysmenorrhoea

Toki-shakuyaku-san (herbal remedy)

One systematic review found limited evidence that toki-shakuyaku-san reduced pain after 6 months and reduced the need for additional medication, compared with placebo in women with primary dysmenorrhoea.

Topical heat (about 39 °C)

One RCT found that topical heat treatment was more effective than placebo in reducing pain in women with primary dysmenorrhoea and that it may be as effective as ibuprofen. Another RCT found that topical heat was more effective in reducing pain than was paracetamol.

Transcutaneous electrical nerve stimulation (high frequency stimulation only; effects of low frequency stimulation remain unclear)

One systematic review found limited evidence from small RCTs that high frequency transcutaneous electrical nerve stimulation reduced pain compared with sham transcutaneous electrical nerve stimulation but was less effective in achieving pain relief compared with ibuprofen in women with primary dysmenorrhoea. Small RCTs provided insufficient evidence to assess the effects of low frequency transcutaneous electrical nerve stimulation compared with either placebo tablets, or high frequency or placebo transcutaneous electrical nerve stimulation.

Vitamin E

One systematic review and one subsequent RCT found that vitamin E reduced pain compared with placebo in women with primary dysmenorrhoea. A second systematic review identified one RCT, which found no significant difference in pain relief between vitamin E plus ibuprofen and ibuprofen alone.

UNKNOWN EFFECTIVENESS

Acupuncture

One systematic review of one small RCT provided insufficient evidence to assess the clinical effects of acupuncture versus placebo or no treatment in women with primary dysmenorrhoea.

Behavioural interventions

Two poor quality RCTs assessing relaxation and aerobic exercise provided insufficient evidence about the effects of behavioural interventions in women with primary dysmenorrhoea.

Combined oral contraceptives

One systematic review and one subsequent RCT provided insufficient evidence about effects of combined oral contraceptives on pain relief compared with placebo in women with primary dysmenorrhoea.

Fish oil

One small crossover RCT identified by a systematic review and one additional RCT provided limited evidence that fish oil (with or without vitamin B_{12}) reduced pain and symptoms after 1–3 months compared with placebo in women with primary dysmenorrhoea.

Herbal remedies (other than toki-shakuyaku-san)

We found no RCTs of herbal remedies other than toki-shakuyaku-san in women with primary dysmenorrhoea.

Magnesium

One systematic review found limited evidence from two out of three small RCTs that magnesium reduced pain after 5–6 months compared with placebo in women with primary dysmenorrhoea. The third RCT found no significant difference between treatments.

Surgical interruption of pelvic nerve pathways

One systematic review of three small RCTs provided insufficient evidence to assess surgical nerve interruption in women with primary dysmenorrhoea.

Vitamin B_{12}

We found no RCTs comparing vitamin B_{12} versus placebo in women with primary dysmenorrhoea. One small RCT provided insufficient evidence for vitamin B_{12} compared with a low fat vegetarian diet. One RCT provided limited evidence that vitamin B_{12} plus fish oil reduced pain and symptoms after 1–3 months compared with placebo.

UNLIKELY TO BE BENEFICIAL

Spinal manipulation

One systematic review identified one good quality RCT, which found no significant difference between spinal manipulation and placebo manipulation in pain after 1 month in women with primary dysmenorrhoea. The review also found two small poorer quality RCTs, which found inconclusive results regarding the effectiveness of spinal manipulation versus placebo or no treatment.

DEFINITION Dysmenorrhoea is painful menstrual cramps of uterine origin. It is commonly divided into primary dysmenorrhoea (pain without organic pathology) and secondary dysmenorrhoea (pelvic pain associated with an identifiable pathological condition, such as endometriosis [see Endometriosis topic] or ovarian cysts). The initial onset of primary dysmenorrhoea is usually shortly after menarche (6–12 months), when ovulatory cycles are established. Pain duration is commonly 8–72 hours and is usually associated with the onset of menstrual flow. Secondary dysmenorrhoea can also occur at any time after menarche, but may arise as a new symptom during a woman's fourth and fifth decades, after the onset of an underlying causative condition.[1] This chapter deals with both primary and secondary dysmenorrhoea; however, it should be noted that most RCTs are in women with primary dysmenorrhoea. Endometriosis, which can cause secondary dysmenorrhoea, is covered in a separate chapter [see Endometriosis topic].

INCIDENCE/ PREVALENCE Variations in the definition of dysmenorrhoea make it difficult to determine prevalence precisely. Studies tend to report on prevalence in adolescent girls, and the type of dysmenorrhoea is not always specified. Adolescent girls tend to have a higher prevalence of primary dysmenorrhoea than older women, as primary dysmenorrhoea can improve with age (see Prognosis). Secondary dysmenorrhoea rates may be lower in adolescents, as onset of causative conditions may not yet have occurred. Therefore, the results from prevalence studies of adolescents may not always be extrapolated to older women, or be accurate estimates of the prevalence of secondary dysmenorrhoea. However, various types of studies have found a consistently high prevalence in women of different ages and nationalities. One systematic review (search date 1996) of the prevalence of chronic pelvic pain, summarising both community and hospital surveys from developed countries, estimated prevalence to be 45–95%.[2] A second systematic review of studies in developing countries (search date 2002) found that 25–50% of adult women and about 75% of adolescents experience pain with menstruation, with 5–20% reporting severe

Dysmenorrhoea

dysmenorrhoea or pain that prevents them from participating in their usual activities.[3] Additional studies of prevalence are summarised in Table 1 (see table 1)Ⓣ.

AETIOLOGY/ RISK FACTORS A longitudinal study of a representative sample of women born in 1962, residing in G teborg, Sweden, found that the severity of dysmenorrhoea was significantly associated with the duration of menstrual flow (average duration of menstrual flow was 5.0 days for women with no dysmenorrhoea and 5.8 days for women with severe dysmenorrhoea, where severe dysmenorrhoea was defined as pain that did not respond well to analgesics and clearly inhibited daily activity; $P < 0.001$; WMD –0.80, 95% CI –1.36 to –0.24); younger age at menarche (13.1 years in women without dysmenorrhoea *v* 12.6 years in women with severe dysmenorrhoea; $P < 0.01$; WMD 0.50, 95% CI 0.09 to 0.91); and cigarette smoking (41% of smokers and 26% of non-smokers experienced moderate or severe dysmenorrhoea).[4] There is also some evidence of a dose–response relationship between exposure to environmental tobacco smoke and increased incidence of dysmenorrhoea.[5]

PROGNOSIS Primary dysmenorrhoea is a chronic recurring condition that affects most young women. Studies of the natural history of this condition are sparse. One longitudinal study in Scandinavia found that primary dysmenorrhoea often improves in the third decade of a woman's reproductive life, and is also reduced after childbirth.[4] We found no studies that reliably examined the relationship between the prognosis of secondary dysmenorrhoea and the severity of the underlying pathology, such as endometriosis.

Please refer to clinicalevidence.com for full text and references.

Endometriosis

Search date March 2005

Neil Johnson and Cynthia Farquhar

What are the effects of hormonal treatments given at diagnosis?

BENEFICIAL

Combined oral contraceptives or medroxyprogesterone

RCTs found that hormonal treatments at diagnosis (combined oral contraceptives, danazol, gestrinone, gonadorelin analogues, or medroxyprogesterone acetate) reduced pain attributed to endometriosis over 3–6 months of treatment, and were all similarly effective. Two RCTs found that gonadorelin analogues reduced dysmenorrhoea, pelvic pain, and dyspareunia compared with combined oral contraceptives, but one RCT found no significant difference in pain between combined oral contraceptives and combined oral contraceptives plus gonadorelin analogues. Adverse effects of hormonal treatments are common. Two RCTs found that combined oral contraceptives reduced bone mineral density loss, hot flushes, insomnia, and vaginal dryness compared with gonadorelin analogues.

TRADE OFF BETWEEN BENEFITS AND HARMS

Danazol, gestrinone, or gonadorelin analogues

RCTs found that hormonal treatments at diagnosis (combined oral contraceptives, danazol, gestrinone, gonadorelin analogues, or medroxyprogesterone acetate) reduced pain attributed to endometriosis over 3–6 months of treatment compared with placebo, and were all similarly effective. Two RCTs found that gonadorelin analogues reduced dysmenorrhoea, pelvic pain, and dyspareunia compared with combined oral contraceptives, but one RCT found no significant difference in pain between combined oral contraceptives and combined oral contraceptives plus gonadorelin analogues. Adverse effects of hormonal treatments are common, and include hot flushes and bone loss with gonadorelin analogues or gestrinone and androgenic adverse effects with danazol. Two RCTs found that combined oral contraceptives reduced bone mineral density loss, hot flushes, insomnia, and vaginal dryness compared with gonadorelin analogues. One RCT found that danazol increased withdrawal because of adverse effects compared with gonadorelin analogues. One RCT identified by a systematic review found that gonadorelin analogues plus add-back oestrogen or oestrogen/progestogen reduced short term loss in bone mineral density compared with gonadorelin analogues alone.

UNKNOWN EFFECTIVENESS

Dydrogesterone

One small RCT provided insufficient evidence to compare dydrogesterone versus placebo.

BMJ Clin Evid Concise 2006;16:721–724.

What are the effects of hormonal treatments before surgery?

UNKNOWN EFFECTIVENESS

Hormonal treatment before surgery

Four RCTs provided insufficient evidence on the effects of hormonal treatment before surgery in women with pain attributed to endometriosis.

What are the effects of surgical treatments?

LIKELY TO BE BENEFICIAL

Combined laparoscopic removal of endometriotic deposits and uterine nerve ablation

One RCT found limited evidence that laparoscopic removal of deposits plus laparoscopic uterine nerve ablation reduced pain compared with diagnostic laparoscopy at 6 months, and that pain reduction persisted for up to 5 years in more than half of the women. Two small RCTs identified by a systematic review and two subsequent RCTs found no significant difference between laparoscopic removal of endometriotic deposits plus laparoscopic uterine nerve ablation and laparoscopic removal alone in rates of recurrent dysmenorrhoea at 6 months to 3 years. One of the subsequent RCTs found no significant difference between treatments in overall treatment satisfaction at 1 year. However, the RCTs may have been too small to detect clinically important differences.

UNKNOWN EFFECTIVENESS

Laparoscopic removal of endometriotic deposits alone

One RCT found limited evidence that laparoscopic removal of endometriotic deposits alone improved pain symptoms and quality of life compared with diagnostic laparoscopy at 6 months. Two small RCTs identified by a systematic review and two subsequent RCTs found no significant difference between laparoscopic removal of endometriotic deposits plus laparoscopic uterine nerve ablation and laparoscopic removal alone in rates of recurrent dysmenorrhoea at 6 months to 3 years. One of the subsequent RCTs found no significant difference between treatments in overall treatment satisfaction at 1 year. However, the RCTs may have been too small to detect clinically important differences. We found no RCTs comparing laser versus electrosurgical removal of endometriosis, and no RCTs comparing excisional versus ablative surgical removal of endometriosis, other than in people with ovarian endometrioma. Two RCTs found that laparoscopic cystectomy reduced recurrence of pelvic pain symptoms compared with laparoscopic drainage and cyst wall electrosurgical ablation. Complication rates were similar.

Laparoscopic uterine nerve ablation alone

We found no systematic review or RCTs evaluating laparoscopic uterine nerve ablation alone in women with pain attributed to endometriosis. One RCT found limited evidence that laparoscopic uterine nerve ablation plus laparoscopic removal of deposits reduced pain at 6 months compared with diagnostic laparoscopy, and that pain reduction persisted for up to 5 years in more than half of the women. Two small RCTs identified by a systematic review and two subsequent RCTs found no significant difference between laparoscopic uterine nerve ablation plus laparoscopic removal of endometrial deposits and laparoscopic removal alone in rates of recurrent dysmenorrhoea at 6 months to 3 years. One of the subsequent RCTs found no significant difference between treatments in overall treatment satisfaction at 1 year. However, the RCTs may have been too small to detect clinically important differences.

What are the effects of hormonal treatment after conservative surgery?

LIKELY TO BE BENEFICIAL

Hormonal treatment after conservative surgery

One systematic review found that hormonal treatment after conservative surgery improved American Fertility Society scores compared with placebo or expectant management, but found no significant difference in pain between groups at 12 and 24 months. RCTs found that, compared with placebo or expectant management, 6 months of hormonal treatment with danazol or gonadorelin analogues after surgery reduced pain and delayed the recurrence of pain at 12 and 24 months. Treatment for 3 months with danazol or gonadorelin analogues or treatment with combined oral contraceptives for 6 months did not seem to be effective. One RCT found that cyproterone acetate and combined oral contraceptives were similarly effective in women with modest and severe pain. One small RCT found that a levonorgestrel releasing intrauterine device inserted after surgery reduced dysmenorrhoea compared with surgery alone at 1 year. One RCT found no significant difference in pain control or American Fertility Score between danazol and triptorelin, although danazol increased breakthrough bleeding. Adverse effects of hormonal treatment are common and include hot flushes and bone loss with gonadorelin analogues and androgenic adverse effects with danazol. Two RCTs found insufficient evidence comparing hormonal treatment after surgery versus hormonal treatment before surgery and hormonal treatment before and after surgery.

What are the effects of hormonal treatment after oophorectomy (with or without hysterectomy)?

UNKNOWN EFFECTIVENESS

Hormonal treatment after oophorectomy

One RCT in women who previously had an oophorectomy found insufficient evidence on the effects of hormone replacement therapy on recurrence of endometriosis compared with no treatment.

What are the effects of treatments for ovarian endometrioma?

LIKELY TO BE BENEFICIAL

Laparoscopic cystectomy for ovarian endometrioma (reduces pain compared with drainage and cyst wall electrosurgical ablation)

Two RCTs found that laparoscopic cystectomy reduced recurrence of pelvic pain symptoms compared with laparoscopic drainage and cyst wall electrosurgical ablation. Complication rates were similar.

DEFINITION Endometriosis is characterised by ectopic endometrial tissue, which can cause dysmenorrhoea, dyspareunia, non-cyclical pelvic pain, and subfertility. Diagnosis is made by laparoscopy. Most endometrial deposits are found in the pelvis (ovaries, peritoneum, uterosacral ligaments, pouch of Douglas, and

Endometriosis

rectovaginal septum). Extrapelvic deposits, including those in the umbilicus and diaphragm, are rare. Severity of endometriosis is defined by the American Fertility Society: this review uses the terms mild (stage I and II), moderate (stage III), and severe (stage IV).[1] Endometriomas are cysts of endometriosis within the ovary. This review assesses dysmenorrhoea, dyspareunia, and non-cyclical pelvic pain associated with endometriosis. For subfertility associated with endometriosis see infertility and subfertility [web only].

INCIDENCE/ PREVALENCE In asymptomatic women, the prevalence of endometriosis is 2–22%.[2-5] Variations in estimates of prevalence are thought to be mostly because of differences in diagnostic thresholds and criteria between studies, and in variations in childbearing age between populations, rather than underlying genetic differences. In women with dysmenorrhoea, the incidence of endometriosis is 40–60%, and in women with subfertility is 20–30%.[3,6,7] The severity of symptoms and the probability of diagnosis increase with age.[8] Incidence peaks at about 40 years of age.[9] Symptoms and laparoscopic appearance do not always correlate.[10]

AETIOLOGY/ RISK FACTORS The cause of endometriosis is unknown. Risk factors include early menarche and late menopause. Embryonic cells may give rise to deposits in the umbilicus, whereas retrograde menstruation may deposit endometrial cells in the diaphragm.[11,12] Use of oral contraceptives reduces the risk of endometriosis, and this protective effect persists for up to 1 year after their discontinuation.[9]

PROGNOSIS We found two RCTs in which laparoscopy was repeated after treatment in women given placebo.[13,14] Over 6–12 months, endometrial deposits resolved spontaneously in up to a third of women, deteriorated in nearly half, and were unchanged in the remainder.

Please refer to clinicalevidence.com for full text and references.

Female infertility

Search date April 2004

Hesham Al-Inany

What are the effects of treatments for infertility caused by ovulation disorders?

LIKELY TO BE BENEFICIAL

Clomifene

One systematic review found that clomifene (clomiphene) increased pregnancy rates compared with placebo in women who ovulate infrequently. Two RCTs in anovulatory women found no significant difference between clomifene and tamoxifen in pregnancy or ovulation rates. One small crossover trial in anovulatory women found that clomifene plus tamoxifen improved ovulation rate per cycle compared with clomifene alone. One systematic review found that clomifene plus metformin increased pregnancy and ovulation rates over 6 months compared with clomifene alone in women with polycystic ovary syndrome.

In vitro fertilisation*

We found no RCTs comparing in vitro fertilisation versus no treatment in women with ovulation disorders; however, RCTs are unlikely to be conducted. One RCT found that immediate compared with delayed in vitro fertilisation increased pregnancy and live birth rates in women with any cause of infertility. One RCT identified by a systematic review found no significant difference between in vitro fertilisation and intracytoplasmic sperm injection in pregnancy rate in women with various causes of infertility.

Metformin

One systematic review found that metformin increased ovulation rates compared with placebo. However, it found no significant difference in pregnancy or live birth rates between metformin and placebo, but is likely to have been underpowered to detect a clinically important difference. The systematic review also found that metformin plus clomifene (clomiphene) increased pregnancy and ovulation rates over 6 months compared with clomifene alone. One RCT, in women with clomifene resistant polycystic ovary syndrome, found no significant difference in pregnancy or ovulation rates between metformin and laparoscopic ovarian drilling.

TRADE OFF BETWEEN BENEFITS AND HARMS

Gonadotrophins

We found no RCTs comparing gonadotrophins versus placebo or clomifene (clomiphene). One systematic review found no significant difference in pregnancy or ovulation rates between human menopausal gonadotrophin and urinary follicle stimulating hormone (urofollitropin) in women with polycystic ovary syndrome. One systematic review found no significant difference between human menopausal gonadotrophin and recombinant follicle stimulating hormone (follitropin) in ongoing pregnancy or live birth rates in women having in vitro fertility treatment. One systematic review found no significant difference between follitropin and urofollitropin in ovulation or pregnancy rates. One systematic review and two subsequent RCTs found no significant difference in pregnancy rates between gonadotrophins and laparoscopic ovarian drilling after 6–12 months' follow up. One case control study provided limited evidence that ▶

BMJ Clin Evid Concise 2006;16:725–729.

Female infertility

gonadotrophins may be associated with an increased risk of epithelial ovarian cancer. Systematic reviews found that gonadotrophins were associated with ovarian hyperstimulation syndrome and multiple pregnancies.

UNKNOWN EFFECTIVENESS

Cyclofenil

One RCT provided insufficient evidence about the effects of cyclofenil in women with ovulatory disorders.

Gonadotrophin priming of oocytes before in vitro maturation

Three small RCTs provided insufficient evidence to assess gonadotrophin priming of oocytes using recombinant follicle stimulating hormone (follitropin) or human chorionic gonadotrophin, or follitropin plus human chorionic gonadotrophin in women with ovulation disorders.

Gonadotrophin releasing hormone agonists plus gonadotrophins

We found no systematic review or RCTs comparing gonadotrophin releasing hormone agonists plus gonadotrophins versus gonadotrophins alone, in women with ovulation disorders. One systematic review in women with various causes of infertility having in vitro fertilisation, found that gonadotrophin releasing hormone agonists plus gonadotrophins increased clinical pregnancy rate per cycle compared with gonadotrophins alone. Gonadotrophin agonists plus gonadotrophin combination treatments are associated with an increased risk of ovarian hyperstimulation.

Gonadotrophin releasing hormone antagonists

We found no RCTs comparing gonadotrophin releasing hormone antagonists versus gonadotrophin releasing hormone agonists in women with infertility caused by ovulation disorders. One systematic review in couples being treated for infertility (including infertility owing to male factor infertility, but excluding women with polycystic ovary syndrome) found that gonadotrophin releasing hormone antagonists reduced clinical pregnancy rates compared with gonadotrophin releasing hormone agonists (long protocol).

Intrauterine insemination plus controlled ovarian stimulation

We found no RCTs assessing intrauterine insemination plus controlled ovarian stimulation treatment in women with ovulation disorders. Consensus regards this combination as likely to be beneficial for the treatment of women with unexplained infertility or infertility owing to cervical hostility.

Laparoscopic ovarian drilling

We found no RCTs comparing laparoscopic ovarian drilling versus no treatment. One systematic review and two subsequent RCTs found no significant difference in pregnancy rates between laparoscopic ovarian drilling and gonadotrophins after 6–12 months follow up. One RCT in women with clomifene (clomiphene) resistant polycystic ovary syndrome found no significant difference in pregnancy or ovulation rates between laparoscopic ovarian drilling and metformin.

Ovarian wedge biopsy

We found no RCTs assessing ovarian wedge biopsy or resection in women with infertility caused by ovulation disorders. However, this procedure is no longer routinely performed. Laparoscopic ovarian drilling, which reduces the risk of adhesion formation, is performed in preference.

Pulsatile gonadotrophin releasing hormone

One systematic review of small, weak RCTs provided insufficient evidence to assess pulsatile gonadotrophin releasing hormone treatment.

Tamoxifen

We found no systematic review or RCTs comparing the effects of tamoxifen versus placebo. Two RCTs in anovulatory women found no significant difference between clomifene (clomiphene) and tamoxifen in pregnancy or ovulation rates.

What are the effects of treatments for tubal infertility?

BENEFICIAL

In vitro fertilisation*

We found no RCTs comparing in vitro fertilisation versus no treatment in women with tubal infertility. RCTs are unlikely to be conducted. One RCT found that immediate compared with delayed in vitro fertilisation increased pregnancy and live birth rates in women with any cause of infertility. One RCT identified by a systematic review found no significant difference in pregnancy rates between in vitro fertilisation and intracytoplasmic sperm injection in women with various causes of infertility including tubal infertility.

LIKELY TO BE BENEFICIAL

Tubal flushing with oil soluble media

We found no systematic review or RCTs solely in women with tubal infertility. One systematic review in women with various causes of infertility found that tubal flushing with oil soluble media increased pregnancy rates compared with no intervention. It found no significant difference in pregnancy rate between tubal flushing with oil and water soluble medium, however tubal flushing with oil soluble media increased live birth rate compared with flushing with water soluble media.

Tubal surgery before in vitro fertilisation

One systematic review in women with hydrosalpinges having in vitro fertilisation found that tubal surgery increased pregnancy and live birth rates compared with no treatment or medical treatment. One systematic review found no significant difference in pregnancy rates between different types of tubal surgery. One systematic review found no significant difference in pregnancy rates between tubal surgery plus additional treatments to prevent adhesion formation (steroids, dextran, noxytioline) and tubal surgery alone. Another systematic review provided insufficient evidence to assess postoperative hydrotubation or second look laparoscopy after tubal surgery.

UNKNOWN EFFECTIVENESS

Selective salpingography plus tubal catheterisation

We found no RCTs on the effects of selective salpingography plus tubal catheterisation in women with tubal infertility.

Tubal flushing with water soluble media

We found no systematic review or RCTs solely in women with tubal infertility. One systematic review in women with various causes of infertility identified no RCTs comparing tubal flushing with water soluble media versus no intervention. It found no significant difference in pregnancy rate between tubal flushing with

Female infertility

water and oil soluble medium, however tubal flushing with water soluble media decreased live birth rate compared with flushing with oil soluble media.

What are the effects of treatments for infertility associated with endometriosis?

LIKELY TO BE BENEFICIAL

Intrauterine insemination plus gonadotrophins

One RCT found that intrauterine insemination plus gonadotrophins (follicle stimulating hormone) increased live birth rates compared with no treatment. One RCT found that intrauterine insemination plus gonadotrophins (human menopausal gonadotrophin) increased pregnancy rate after the first treatment cycle compared with intrauterine insemination alone.

In vitro fertilisation*

We found no RCTs comparing in vitro fertilisation versus no treatment in women with infertility associated with endometriosis. RCTs are unlikely to be conducted. One RCT found that immediate compared with delayed in vitro fertilisation increased pregnancy and live birth rates in women with any cause of infertility. One RCT identified by a systematic review found no significant difference in pregnancy rate between in vitro fertilisation and intracytoplasmic sperm injection in women with various causes of infertility.

Laparoscopic ablation of endometrial deposits

We found no RCTs comparing laparoscopic surgery versus no treatment or versus ovarian suppression. One systematic review found that laparoscopic ablation or resection of endometrial deposits increased live birth rates and ongoing pregnancy rates compared with diagnostic laparoscopy.

LIKELY TO BE INEFFECTIVE OR HARMFUL

Drug induced ovarian suppression

One systematic review found no significant difference in pregnancy rates between drugs that induce ovarian suppression and placebo. The review also found no significant difference in pregnancy rates between ovulation suppression agents and danazol.

*No RCTs, but strong observational evidence that in vitro fertilisation increases live birth rates.

DEFINITION This chapter focuses on infertility related to factors associated with the woman rather than the man. Normal fertility has been defined as achieving a pregnancy within 2 years by regular unprotected sexual intercourse.[1] However, many define infertility as the failure to conceive after 1 year of unprotected intercourse. Infertility can be primary, in women who have never conceived, or secondary, in women who have previously conceived. This chapter will deal with infertility owing to endometriosis, ovulation disorders, and tubal infertility. Endometriosis is a progressive disease which occurs when the endometrial tissue lining the uterus grows outside the uterus and attaches to the ovaries, fallopian tubes, or other organs in the abdominal cavity (See endometriosis). Ovulation disorders are defined by the failure of an ovum to be expelled because of a malfunction in the ovary, and are a major cause of infertility. Tubal infertility is the inability to conceive owing to a blockage in one or both fallopian tubes, and is a common cause of infertility.

Female infertility

INCIDENCE/ PREVALENCE Although there is no evidence of a major change in the prevalence of female infertility, many more couples are seeking help than previously. Currently, about 1/6 (17%) couples in industrialised countries will seek medical advice for infertility.[2] Rates of primary infertility vary widely between countries, ranging from < 6% in China, Malawi, Tanzania, and Zambia; 9% in the Philippines; > 10% in Finland, Sweden, and Canada; and 18% in Switzerland.[3,4] Reported rates of secondary infertility are less reliable.

AETIOLOGY/ RISK FACTORS In the UK, about 10–20% of infertility cases are unexplained.[5] The rest are caused by ovulatory failure (27%), tubal damage (14%), endometriosis (5%), low sperm count or quality (19%), and other causes (5%).[6]

PROGNOSIS In developed countries, 80–90% of couples attempting to conceive are successful after 1 year and 95% after 2 years.[7] The chances of becoming pregnant vary with the cause and duration of infertility, the woman's age, the woman's previous pregnancy history, and the availability of different treatment options.[8,9] For the first 2–3 years of unexplained infertility, cumulative conception rates remain high (27–46%) but decrease with increasing age of the woman and duration of infertility.[9] The background rates of spontaneous pregnancy in infertile couples can be calculated from longitudinal studies of infertile couples who have been observed without treatment.[9]

Please refer to clinicalevidence.com for full text and references.

Fibroids (uterine myomatosis, leiomyomas)

Search date November 2005

Anne Lethaby and Beverley Vollenhoven

What are the effects of medical treatment alone in women with fibroids?

LIKELY TO BE BENEFICIAL

Gonadorelin analogues (GnRHa) plus progestogen (no significant difference in heavy bleeding compared with GnRHa alone, but adding progestogen reduces vasomotor symptoms and hot flushes associated with GnRHa)

One small RCT found no significant difference between leuprorelin (leuprolide) acetate plus progestogen and leuprorelin acetate alone in the proportion of women who had heavy bleeding at 12 months. One small RCT found that goserelin acetate plus medroxyprogesterone acetate reduced vasomotor symptoms over 12 months compared with goserelin acetate alone. One small RCT found that leuprorelin acetate plus progestogen reduced the proportion of women with hot flushes over 24 weeks compared with leuprorelin acetate alone.

Gonadorelin analogues (GnRHa) plus raloxifene (reduces fibroid size and bone mineral density loss, no significant difference in fibroid-related symptoms, cognitive measures, mood, quality of life, and hot flushes)

One RCT found that adding raloxifene to leuprolide acetate reduced fibroid size and bone mineral density loss compared with leuprolide acetate alone. It found no significant difference in fibroid related symptoms, cognition, mood, quality of life, or hot flushes.

Gonadorelin analogues (GnRHa) plus tibolone (no significant difference in fibroid symptoms compared with GnRHa alone, but adding tibolone reduces hot flushes and prevents loss in bone mineral density associated with GnRHa)

Two small RCTs found no significant difference between gonadorelin analogues alone and gonadorelin analogues plus tibolone in fibroid related symptoms or uterine and fibroid size. They found that adding tibolone reduced hot flushes, vaginal dryness, and night sweats and prevented loss in bone mineral density.

TRADE OFF BETWEEN BENEFITS AND HARMS

Gonadorelin analogues alone

RCTs found that gonadorelin analogues increased the proportion of women with amenorrhoea compared with placebo after about 3 months, but were associated with menopausal symptoms and bone loss, which may make them unsuitable for long term use. Two RCTs found that nafarelin reduced bone density from baseline after 16 weeks' treatment compared with placebo, but that bone density returned to pretreatment levels 6 months after treatment was stopped. Two RCTs found that hot flushes were more common with nafarelin than with placebo or buserelin. One RCT found that hot flushes and sweating were more common with goserelin than with placebo. We found no systematic review or RCTs comparing gonadorelin analogues alone versus surgical treatment.

UNKNOWN EFFECTIVENESS

Gonadorelin analogues (GnRHa) plus combined oestrogen–progestogen (insufficient evidence on effects compared with GnRHa plus progestogen)

One small RCT provided insufficient evidence to compare leuprorelin plus combined oestrogen–progestogen hormone replacement therapy versus leuprorelin plus progestogen only hormone replacement therapy.

Gonadorelin analogues (GnRHa) plus tibolone (similar reductions in bone mineral density compared with hysterectomy plus oophorectomy)

One RCT found that, in those women who became menopausal 12 months after treatment with gonadorelin analogues plus tibolone, there were no differences in the reduction in measures of bone mineral density or bone turnover markers from baseline when compared with women treated by hysterectomy plus bilateral oophorectomy (whereby surgical menopause is induced).

Levonorgestrel intrauterine system

We found no RCTs of the levonorgestrel intrauterine system in women with fibroids.

Non-steroidal anti-inflammatory drugs

We found no systematic review or RCTs of non-steroidal anti-inflammatory drugs in women with fibroids.

In women scheduled for fibroid surgery, what are the effects of preoperative medical treatments?

LIKELY TO BE BENEFICIAL

Gonadorelin analogues

One systematic review found that gonadorelin analogues for at least 3 months before fibroid surgery improved preoperative haemoglobin concentration and haematocrit, and reduced uterine and pelvic symptoms compared with placebo or no pretreatment. Preoperative gonadorelin also reduced the rate of vertical incisions during laparotomy. Women having hysterectomy were more likely to have a vaginal rather than an abdominal procedure after gonadorelin analogue pretreatment compared with placebo or no pretreatment. Preoperative goserelin reduced intraoperative blood loss, although the difference was small and the clinical importance is uncertain. One subsequent RCT found no significant difference between preoperative triptorelin and immediate surgery in intraoperative blood loss. One small RCT found that gonadorelin analogue combined with endometrial resection reduced the need for further treatment (either medical or surgical) over 1 year compared with gonadorelin analogue alone. However, preoperative gonadorelin analogue was associated with adverse hypo-oestrogenic effects, such as hot flushes, vaginal symptoms, and sweating, and women receiving gonadorelin analogue were more likely to withdraw from treatment because of adverse effects.

Fibroids (uterine myomatosis, leiomyomas)

What are the effects of surgical treatments in women with fibroids?

BENEFICIAL

Laparoscopic myomectomy (maintains fertility compared with hysterectomy; reduces recovery time and postoperative pain compared with abdominal myomectomy)

RCTs found that laparoscopic myomectomy reduced recovery time or stay in hospital, postoperative pain and fever, and blood loss compared with abdominal myomectomy. One RCT found no significant difference in recurrence rates of fibroids, and another RCT found no significant difference in pregnancy rates between laparoscopic and abdominal myomectomy. We found no RCTs comparing laparoscopic myomectomy versus total abdominal, vaginal, or laparoscopic hysterectomy, but the main benefit of myomectomy compared with hysterectomy is that it maintains fertility. We found no systematic review or RCTs comparing total laparoscopic myomectomy versus medical treatments.

LIKELY TO BE BENEFICIAL

Laparoscopically assisted vaginal hysterectomy (reduces recovery time and postoperative pain compared with total abdominal hysterectomy, but increases operating time and blood loss compared with total vaginal hysterectomy)

Two RCTs found that women having laparoscopically assisted vaginal hysterectomy had shorter recovery times and less postoperative pain compared with women having total abdominal hysterectomy. One RCT found that women having laparoscopically assisted vaginal hysterectomy had longer operating time and more blood loss than women having total vaginal hysterectomy. We found no systematic review or RCTs comparing total laparoscopically assisted vaginal hysterectomy versus laparoscopic or total abdominal myomectomy or versus medical treatments. The main benefit of myomectomy compared with hysterectomy is that it maintains fertility.

Total abdominal hysterectomy (reduces fibroid related symptoms compared with no treatment)*

We found no RCTs comparing total abdominal hysterectomy versus no treatment or sham surgery. An RCT is unlikely to be conducted. There is consensus that total abdominal hysterectomy is superior to no treatment in reducing fibroid related symptoms. RCTs found that women having total abdominal hysterectomy had longer surgery; more blood loss, pain, and fever; longer hospital stay; later return to work; and less satisfaction than women having total vaginal hysterectomy. Two RCTs found that women having total abdominal hysterectomy had longer recovery times and more postoperative pain but shorter operating times and less blood loss than women having laparoscopically assisted vaginal hysterectomy. One RCT found that women having total abdominal hysterectomy had more postoperative fever, and longer hospital stay and recovery times than women having total laparoscopic hysterectomy. Two RCTs found that total abdominal hysterectomy increased length of hospital stay and recovery time compared with uterine embolisation. It found no significant difference in intraprocedural complications, postprocedural complications, emergency department visits, and readmission to hospital. We found no systematic review or RCTs comparing total abdominal hysterectomy versus laparoscopic or total abdominal myomectomy or versus medical treatments. The main benefit of myomectomy compared with hysterectomy is that it maintains fertility.

Total abdominal myomectomy (maintains fertility compared with hysterectomy but increases recovery time and postoperative pain compared with laparoscopic myomectomy)

Three RCTs found that abdominal myomectomy had increased recovery time or stay in hospital compared with laparoscopic myomectomy. Two RCTs found that abdominal myomectomy had increased pain and blood loss compared with laparoscopic myomectomy. One RCT found a reduction in fever but no significant difference in recurrence rates of fibroids, and another RCT found no significant difference in pregnancy rates or other obstetrical outcomes between laparoscopic and abdominal myomectomy. We found no RCTs comparing abdominal myomectomy versus total abdominal, vaginal, or laparoscopic hysterectomy, but the main benefit of myomectomy compared with hysterectomy is that it maintains fertility. We also found no systematic review or RCTs comparing myomectomy versus medical interventions.

Total laparoscopic hysterectomy (reduces postoperative fever, hospital stay, and recovery time compared with total abdominal hysterectomy)

One RCT found that women having total laparoscopic hysterectomy had less postoperative fever, shorter hospital stay, and shorter recovery times compared with women having total abdominal hysterectomy. We found no systematic review or RCTs comparing total laparoscopic hysterectomy versus laparoscopic or total abdominal myomectomy or versus medical treatments. The main benefit of myomectomy compared with hysterectomy is that it maintains fertility.

Total vaginal hysterectomy (reduces operation time, blood loss, pain, fever, and hospital stay compared with total abdominal hysterectomy and increases satisfaction with operation)

Two RCTs found that women having total vaginal hysterectomy had shorter operation time; less blood loss, pain, and fever; shorter hospital stay; earlier return to work; and greater satisfaction than women having total abdominal hysterectomy. One RCT found that women having total vaginal hysterectomy had shorter operation times and less blood loss than women having laparoscopically assisted vaginal hysterectomy. We found no systematic review or RCTs comparing total vaginal hysterectomy versus laparoscopic or total abdominal myomectomy or versus medical treatments. The main benefit of myomectomy compared with hysterectomy is that it maintains fertility.

UNKNOWN EFFECTIVENESS

Hysteroscopic resection

We found no RCTs of hysteroscopic resection in women with fibroids.

Magnetic resonance guided focused ultrasound (magnetic resonance imaging guided focused ultrasound surgery)

We found no systematic reviews or RCTs of magnetic resonance imaging guided focused ultrasound surgery in women with fibroids.

Rollerball endometrial ablation

We found no RCTs comparing rollerball endometrial ablation versus medical treatment or hysterectomy. One RCT compared rollerball endometrial ablation versus thermal balloon ablation in women with fibroids smaller than the average size of a 12 week pregnancy, all of whom had been pretreated with gonadorelin analogues. It found no significant difference between rollerball and thermal balloon ablation in amenorrhoea rates, pictorial bleeding assessment chart score, haemoglobin, or hysterectomy rates at 12 months. It found that rollerball ablation increased operation time and intraoperative complication rate compared with thermal balloon ablation. About a third of women reported being "not very satisfied" with either operation.

Thermal balloon ablation

We found no RCTs comparing thermal balloon ablation versus non-surgical treatment or hysterectomy. One RCT compared thermal balloon ablation versus rollerball endometrial ablation in women with fibroids smaller than the average size of a 12 week pregnancy, all of whom had been pretreated with gonadorelin analogues. It found no significant difference between thermal balloon and rollerball ablation in amenorrhoea rates, pictorial bleeding assessment chart score, haemoglobin, or hysterectomy rates at 12 months. It found that thermal balloon ablation reduced operation time and intraoperative complication rate compared with rollerball ablation. About a third of women reported being "not very satisfied" with either operation. We found no systematic review or RCTs comparing thermal balloon ablation versus medical treatments.

Thermal myolysis with laser

We found no RCTs of thermal myolysis with laser in women with fibroids.

Uterine embolisation

Two RCTs found that uterine embolisation reduced length of hospital stay and recovery time compared with total abdominal hysterectomy. One RCT found that uterine embolisation increased the rate of minor complications (mainly vaginal discharge, expulsion of fibroid, and urinary tract infection) and readmission to hospital, but this was not confirmed by the other RCT, which did not carry out intention to treat analysis of adverse effects. We found no systematic review or RCTs comparing uterine embolisation versus medical treatments.

*Based on consensus, RCTs unlikely to be conducted.

DEFINITION Fibroids (uterine leiomyomas) are benign tumours of the smooth muscle cells of the uterus. Women with fibroids can be asymptomatic or may present with menorrhagia (30%), pelvic pain with or without dysmenorrhoea or pressure symptoms (34%), infertility (27%), and recurrent pregnancy loss (3%).[1] Much of the data describing the relationship between the presence of fibroids and symptoms are based on uncontrolled studies that have assessed the effect of myomectomy on the presenting symptoms.[2] One observational study (142 women) undertaken in the USA suggested that the prevalence of fibroids in infertile women can be as high as 13%, but no direct causal relationship between fibroids and infertility has been established.[3]

INCIDENCE/ PREVALENCE The reported incidence of fibroids varies from 5.4–77.0%, depending on the method of diagnosis used (the gold standard is histological evidence). It is not possible to state the actual incidence of fibroids because some women with fibroids will not have symptoms and will therefore not be tested for fibroids. Observational evidence suggests that, in premenopausal women, the incidence of fibroids increases with age, reducing during menopause.[4,5] Based on postmortem examination, 50% of women were found to have these tumours.[6] Gross serial sectioning at 2 mm intervals of 100 consecutive hysterectomy specimens revealed the presence of fibroids in 50/68 (73%) premenopausal women and 27/32 (84%) postmenopausal women. These women were having hysterectomies for reasons other than fibroids.[7] The incidence of fibroids in black women is three times greater than that in white women, based on ultrasound or hysterectomy diagnosis.[8] Submucosal fibroids have been diagnosed in 6–34% of women having a hysteroscopy for abnormal bleeding, and in 2–7% of women having infertility investigations.[9]

Fibroids (uterine myomatosis, leiomyomas)

AETIOLOGY/ RISK FACTORS The cause of fibroids is unknown. Each fibroid is of monoclonal origin and arises independently.[10,11] Factors thought to be involved include the sex steroid hormones oestrogen and progesterone, as well as the insulin-like growth factors, epidermal growth factor, and transforming growth factor. Risk factors for fibroid growth include nulliparity and obesity. Risk also reduces consistently with increasing number of term pregnancies; women with five term pregnancies have a quarter of the risk of nulliparous women ($P < 0.001$).[5] Obesity increases the risk of fibroid development by 21% with each 10 kg weight gain ($P = 0.008$).[5] The combined oral contraceptive pill also reduces the risk of fibroids with increasing duration of use (women who have taken oral contraceptives for 4–6 years compared with women who have never taken oral contraceptives: OR 0.8, 95% CI 0.5 to 1.2; women who have taken oral contraceptives for ≥ 7 years compared with women who have never taken oral contraceptives: OR 0.5, 95% CI 0.3 to 0.9).[12] Women who have had injections containing 150 mg depot medroxyprogesterone acetate also have a reduced incidence compared with women who have never had injections of this drug (OR 0.44, 95% CI 0.36 to 0.55).[13]

PROGNOSIS There are few data on the long term untreated prognosis of these tumours, particularly in women who are asymptomatic at diagnosis. One small case control study reported that in a group of 106 women treated with observation alone over 1 year, there was no significant change in symptoms and quality of life over that time.[14] Fibroids tend to shrink or fibrose after the menopause.[5]

Please refer to clinicalevidence.com for full text and references.

Genital prolapse in women

Search date August 2005

Joseph Loze Onwude

What are the effects of non-surgical treatments in women with genital prolapse?

LIKELY TO BE BENEFICIAL

Vaginal pessaries*

We found no RCTs or observational studies of sufficient quality examining effects of vaginal pessaries on the symptoms of genital prolapse. However, consensus opinion suggests that they are effective for short term relief of genital prolapse before surgery, or in the long term if surgery is contraindicated.

UNKNOWN EFFECTIVENESS

Pelvic floor muscle exercises

We found no RCTs or observational studies of sufficient quality examining the effects of pelvic floor muscle exercises on the symptoms of genital prolapse.

Vaginal oestrogen

We found no systematic review, RCTs, or observational studies of sufficient quality on the effects of vaginal oestrogen in women with genital prolapse.

What are the effects of surgical treatments in women with genital prolapse?

BENEFICIAL

Abdominal sacral colpopexy versus sacrospinous colpopexy (vaginal sacral colpopexy) for upper vaginal wall vault prolapse

One systematic review in women with upper vaginal wall vault prolapse found that abdominal sacral colpopexy was more effective than sacrospinous colpopexy (vaginal sacral colpopexy) in reducing recurrent vault prolapse, preventing postoperative dyspareunia and stress incontinence, and reducing reoperation rates. It was associated with a longer operating time and a longer time to return to normal activities.

Anterior colporrhaphy with mesh reinforcement versus traditional anterior colporrhaphy in women with anterior vaginal wall prolapse

One systematic review found that anterior colporrhaphy with mesh reinforcement was more effective than anterior colporrhaphy alone in reducing recurrent cystocoele rates, with similar postoperative complication rates.

Posterior colporrhaphy versus transanal repair in women with posterior vaginal wall prolapse

One systematic review found that posterior colporrhaphy was better than transanal repair of rectocoele or enterocoele in reducing the proportion of women with recurrent posterior vaginal wall prolapse.

Traditional anterior colporrhaphy versus abdominal Burch colposuspension in women with anterior vaginal wall prolapse

One RCT identified by a systematic review found that anterior vaginal wall repair reduced recurrent cystocoele rates compared with Burch colposuspension, with similar postoperative complication rates.

LIKELY TO BE BENEFICIAL

Abdominal sacrohysteropexy versus vaginal hysterectomy and repair for upper vaginal wall prolapse

One systematic review in women with uterine prolapse found that abdominal sacrohysteropexy (with uterine preservation) reduced recurrence of prolapse compared with vaginal hysterectomy and repair but was less effective in reducing the proportion of women with symptoms. Abdominal sacrohysteropexy also increased the need for reoperation.

Posterior colporrhaphy with mesh versus posterior colporrhaphy without mesh reinforcement in women with posterior vaginal wall prolapse

One RCT identified by a systematic review found no significant difference in rates of recurrent rectocoeles between adding mesh reinforcement to posterior colporrhaphy and posterior colporrhaphy alone. However, it may have lacked power to detect a clinically important difference between groups.

Posterior intravaginal slingplasty (infracoccygeal sacropexy) versus vaginal sacrospinous colpopexy for upper vaginal wall prolapse

One systematic review in women with upper vaginal wall vault prolapse found that posterior intravaginal slingplasty was similar to vaginal sacrospinous colpopexy in reducing recurrent vault prolapses at 17–19 months' follow up.

Ultralateral anterior colporrhaphy versus traditional anterior colporrhaphy

One systematic review found that ultralateral anterior colporrhaphy was similar to traditional anterior colporrhaphy in reducing the incidence of recurrent cystocoeles.

UNKNOWN EFFECTIVENESS

Surgical versus non-surgical treatment in women with anterior vaginal wall prolapse

We found no systematic review or RCTs comparing surgical versus non-surgical treatment in women with upper vaginal wall prolapse.

Surgical versus non-surgical treatment in women with posterior vaginal wall prolapse

We found no systematic review or RCTs comparing surgical versus non-surgical treatment in women with posterior vaginal wall prolapse.

Surgical versus non-surgical treatment in women with upper vaginal wall prolapse

We found no systematic review or RCTs comparing surgical versus non-surgical treatment in women with upper vaginal wall prolapse.

*Consensus regards vaginal pessaries as effective.

DEFINITION Genital prolapse (also known as pelvic organ prolapse) refers to uterine, uterovaginal, or vaginal prolapse. Genital prolapse has several causes but occurs primarily from loss of muscle support in the pelvic region. In this chapter we have attempted to use the most common and descriptive

Genital prolapse in women

terminology, for ease of understanding. In uterine prolapse the uterus descends into the vaginal canal with the cervix at its leading edge; this may in turn pull down the vagina, in which case it may be referred to as uterovaginal prolapse. In the case of vaginal prolapse one or more regions of the vaginal wall protrude into the vaginal canal. Vaginal prolapse is classified according to the region of the vaginal wall that is affected: a cystocoele involves the upper anterior vaginal wall, urethrocoele the lower anterior vaginal wall, rectocoele the lower posterior vaginal wall, and enterocoele the upper posterior vaginal wall. After hysterectomy, the apex of the vagina may prolapse as a vault prolapse. This usually pulls down the anterior and posterior vaginal walls as well. The two main systems for grading the severity of genital prolapse, the Baden–Walker halfway system[1] and the Pelvic Organ Prolapse Quantification (POPQ) system,[2] are summarised in Table 1 Ⓣ. Mild genital prolapse may be asymptomatic. Symptoms of genital prolapse are mainly non-specific. Common symptoms include pelvic heaviness, genital bulge, and difficulties during sexual intercourse, such as pain or loss of vaginal sensation. Symptoms that may be more commonly associated with specific forms of prolapse include urinary incontinence, which is associated with cystocoele; incomplete urinary emptying, which is associated with cystocoele or uterine prolapse, or both; and need to apply digital pressure to the perineum or posterior vaginal wall for defaecation, which is associated with rectocoele.[3]

INCIDENCE/ PREVALENCE Prevalence estimates vary widely, depending on the population and the way in which women were recruited into studies. One study conducted in the USA (497 women aged 18–82 years attending a routine general gynaecology clinic) found that 93.6% had some degree of genital prolapse (43.3% POPQ stage 1, 47.7% POPQ stage 2, 2.6% POPQ stage 3, and 0% POPQ stage 4).[4] In that study the incidence of clinically relevant prolapse (≥ POPQ stage 2) was found to increase with advancing parity: non-parous, 14.6%; one to three births, 48.0%; and more than three births, 71.2%. One Swedish study (487 women) found that 30.8% of women between the ages of 20 and 59 years had some degree of genital prolapse on clinical assessment.[5] The prevalence of genital prolapse increased with age, from 6.6% in women aged 20–29 years to 55.6% in women aged 50–59 years. A cross-sectional study (241 perimenopausal women aged 45–55 years seeking to enter a trial of hormone replacement therapy) found that 23% had POPQ stage 1 genital prolapse, 4% had POPQ stage 2 prolapse, and no women had POPQ stage 3 or 4 prolapse.[6] One cross-sectional study conducted in the UK (285 perimenopausal and postmenopausal women attending a menopause clinic with climacteric symptoms) found that 20% had some degree of uterovaginal or vault prolapse, 51% some degree of anterior wall vaginal prolapse, and 27% some degree of posterior wall vaginal prolapse.[7] Severe prolapse (equivalent to POPQ stage 3 or 4) was found in 6% of women. One prospective study (412 postmenopausal women aged 50–79 years) found that the baseline prevalence of cystocoele was 24.6% (prevalence for grade 1 was 14.4%, 2 was 9.5%, and 3 was 0.7%), the baseline prevalence of rectocoele was 12.9% (prevalence for grade 1 was 7.8% and 2 was 5.1%), and the baseline prevalence of uterine prolapse was 3.8% (prevalence for grade 1 was 3.3% and 2 was 0.6%).[8] Among women who entered the study, the annual incidence of cystocoele was 9%, rectocoele was 6%, and uterine prolapse was 2%.

AETIOLOGY/ RISK FACTORS The strongest risk factor for pelvic organ prolapse is parity[9] because childbirth can cause damage to the pudendal nerves,[10] fascia, and supporting structures, as well as muscle.[11] A Swedish population based study found that the prevalence of genital prolapse was higher in parous women (44%) than in non-parous women (5.8%). In addition, it found an association with pelvic floor muscle-tone and genital prolapse.[5] One case control study found that other strong risk factors for severe (POPQ stages 3 or 4) genital prolapse are increasing age (OR 1.12 for each additional year, 95% CI 1.09 to 1.15), increasing weight of largest baby delivered vaginally (OR 1.24 for each additional 1 lb (450 g; 2.00, 95% CI 1.06 to 1.44), previous hysterectomy (OR 2.37, 95% CI 1.16 to 4.86), and previous surgery for genital prolapse (OR 5.09, 95% CI 1.49 to 17.26).[12] The study did not find a significant association between severe genital prolapse and chronic medical conditions such as obesity, hypertension, or chronic obstructive pulmonary disease.

PROGNOSIS We found no reliable information about the natural history of untreated mild genital prolapse (POPQ stages 1 and 2, Baden–Walker grades 1 and 2). We found one prospective study on the progression of genital prolapse in women who were treated or untreated with hormone replacement therapy (oestrogen plus progesterone).[8] However, the results were not reported separately by treatment group and therefore they may not apply to untreated women. In addition, the investigators used an examination technique whose reliability, reproducibility, and ability to discriminate between absence of prolapse and mild prolapse was not known. It found that, over 1 year, cystocoeles progressed from grade 1 to grades 2–3 in 9% of cases, regressed from grades 2–3 to grade 0 in 9%, and regressed from grade 1 to grade 0 in 23%. Rectocoeles progressed from grade 1 to grades 2–3 in 1%, but regressed from grades 2–3 to grade 0 in 3%, and from grade 1 to grade 0 in 2%. Uterine prolapse regressed from grade 1 to grade 0 in 48%. The incidence of morbidity associated with genital prolapse is also difficult to estimate. The annual incidence of hospital admission for prolapse in the UK has been estimated at 2.04 per 1000 women under the age of 60 years.[13] Genital prolapse is also a major cause of gynaecological surgery.

Please refer to clinicalevidence.com for full text and references.

Intimate partner violence towards women

Search date December 2005

Joanne Klevens and Laura Sadowski

What are the effects of interventions in female victims of intimate partner violence?

LIKELY TO BE BENEFICIAL

Advocacy

One RCT and one non-randomised controlled trial found that advocacy reduced reabuse compared with no treatment. The RCT also found an improvement in women's quality of life with advocacy compared with no treatment. One controlled trial found no significant difference in rates of reabuse between combined counselling plus mentoring (similar to advocacy) and a resource card, but found that counselling plus mentoring slightly reduced rates of reabuse compared with unlimited counselling alone.

Cognitive trauma therapy

One RCT found limited evidence that cognitive trauma therapy reduced post-traumatic stress disorder and depression compared with no treatment at 6 weeks.

Peer support groups

One RCT showed improvements in perceived social support, psychological distress, and utilisation of healthcare services for women in a domestic violence shelter participating in a support group.

Safety planning

One RCT and two non-randomised controlled trials of good quality found consistent positive effects of helping women develop a safety plan on health, reabuse, or both.

UNKNOWN EFFECTIVENESS

Different types of counselling (relative benefits unclear)

One controlled trial found that grief resolution oriented counselling improved self esteem and self efficacy from baseline, whereas feminist oriented counselling did not. However, the study did not compare effects of interventions directly. Similarly, one controlled trial found that cognitive behaviour oriented therapy improved women's assertiveness and reduced exposure to abuse from baseline, whereas non-specific support did not. One controlled trial did not find any difference in reduction of physical violence or reabuse and improvement in psychological wellbeing between group and individual couple counselling, whereas another non-randomised controlled trial found that group couple counselling reduced reabuse after 6 months compared with no counselling while individual couple counselling did not. One RCT and one non-randomised controlled trial reported that gender specific or group couple therapy reduced subsequent exposure to violence among couples from baseline, but found no significant differences between these two types of counselling.

Shelters

We found no reliable controlled trials. One cohort study of limited quality found a reduced incidence of violence in the weeks after shelter stay for women ▶

choosing to use the shelter compared with women not choosing to stay at the shelter. However, the benefits were limited to women who were also seeking additional help elsewhere.

UNLIKELY TO BE BENEFICIAL

Counselling (type not reported)

Two controlled trials and one comparative cohort study found no effect of counselling (type not reported) compared with no treatment on medical care utilisation rates, reported exposure to violence and threats of violence, or depression, state anxiety, and self esteem.

DEFINITION Intimate partner violence (IPV) is actual or threatened physical or sexual violence, or emotional or psychological abuse (including coercive tactics) by a current or former spouse or dating partner (including same sex partners).[1] Other terms commonly used to describe IPV include domestic violence, domestic abuse, spouse abuse, marital violence, and battering.

INCIDENCE/ PREVALENCE Between 10% and 69% of women participating in population based surveys in 48 countries from around the world reported being physically assaulted by a partner during their lifetime.[2] Rates of reported assault by a partner are 4.3 times higher among women than men.[3] Nearly 25% of surveyed women in the USA reported being physically, sexually, or both physically and sexually assaulted by a current or former partner at some time during their lives, and 1.5% were victimised during the previous 12 months.[3] Rates of violence against pregnant women range from 0.9% to 20%.[4] Between 11.7% and 24.5% of women in prenatal clinics[5-8] and 5.5% and 17.0% of women in primary or ambulatory care reported being abused by a partner in the past year.[9-12]

AETIOLOGY/ RISK FACTORS A systematic review found that physical IPV toward women is associated with lower levels of education and unemployment, low family income, marital discord, and with the partner's lower level of occupation, childhood experiences of abuse, witnessing interparental violence, higher levels of anger, depression, heavy or problem drinking, drug use, jealousy, and lack of assertiveness with spouse.[13] A similar review of research on psychological aggression found that the few demographic and psychological variables assessed were either inconsistently associated with psychological IPV or were found to be associated with psychological IPV in studies with serious methodological limitations.[14]

PROGNOSIS There are few prospective studies documenting the course of IPV and its outcomes. Cross-sectional surveys suggest that IPV persists for at least two thirds of women.[15,16] Among black and Hispanic people, persistence of IPV seems to be dependent on initial severity.[17] For all ethnic groups, half of those reporting moderate IPV did not report occurrences of IPV at the 5 year follow up, but for people of black or Hispanic origin reporting severe IPV only a third did not report occurrences of domestic violence at the 5 year follow up. A case control study conducted in middle class working women found that, compared with non-abused women, women abused by their partners during the previous 9 years were significantly more likely to have or report headaches (48% *v* 35%), back pain (40% *v* 25%), sexually transmitted diseases (6% *v* 2%), vaginal bleeding (17% *v* 6%), vaginal infections (30% *v* 21%), pelvic pain (17% *v* 9%), painful intercourse (13% *v* 7%), urinary tract infections (22% *v* 12%), appetite loss (9% *v* 3%), digestive problems (35% *v* 19%), abdominal pain (22% *v* 11%), and facial injuries (8% *v* 1%).[18] After adjusting for age, race, insurance status, and cigarette smoking, a cross-sectional survey found that women experiencing psychological abuse are also more likely to report poor physical and mental health, disability preventing work, arthritis, chronic pain, migraine and other frequent headaches, sexually transmitted infections, chronic pelvic pain, stomach ulcers, spastic colon, frequent indigestion, diarrhoea, or constipation (see table 1)Ⓣ.[19]

Please refer to clinicalevidence.com for full text and references.

Menopausal symptoms

Search date December 2005

Edward Morris and Janice Rymer

What are the effects of medical treatments for menopausal symptoms?

BENEFICIAL

Progestogens alone

Five RCTs found that progestogens alone reduced vasomotor symptoms compared with placebo and one RCT found no significant difference in vasomotor symptoms between progestogens and placebo. One RCT found no significant difference in vasomotor symptoms between progesterone alone and oestrogen alone. We found no RCTs examining effects of progestogens alone on urogenital symptoms. One RCT found no significant difference in psychological symptoms or quality of life between progesterone and placebo.

Tibolone

Two RCTs found that tibolone improved vasomotor symptoms compared with placebo. One RCT found that tibolone improved sexual function compared with placebo. Two RCTs provided limited evidence that tibolone was not as effective for reducing vasomotor symptoms as oestrogen plus progestogen. Two RCTs found that tibolone improved sexual function compared with oestrogen plus progestogen. We found no RCTs assessing psychological symptoms or quality of life.

TRADE OFF BETWEEN BENEFITS AND HARMS

Oestrogens alone (improved menopausal symptoms but increased risk of breast cancer, endometrial cancer, stroke, and venous thromboembolism after long term use)

Systematic reviews and subsequent RCTs found that oestrogen improved vasomotor symptoms, urogenital symptoms, psychological symptoms, and quality of life in the short term (3–6 months) compared with placebo. However, important adverse effects of oestrogen include increased risk of breast cancer, endometrial cancer, stroke, and venous thromboembolic disease. Adding progestogen reduces the risk of endometrial hyperplasia.

Oestrogens plus progestogens (improved menopausal symptoms but increased risk of breast cancer, endometrial cancer, stroke, and venous thromboembolism after long term use)

One systematic review and subsequent RCTs found that oestrogen plus progestogens improved vasomotor symptoms, urogenital symptoms, and psychological symptoms in the short term compared with placebo. However, important adverse effects include increased risk of breast cancer, stroke, stress incontinence, and venous thromboembolic disease. Two RCTs provided limited evidence that oestrogen plus progestogen reduced vasomotor symptoms compared with tibolone, but that tibolone improved sexual function compared with oestrogen plus progestogen.

UNKNOWN EFFECTIVENESS

Antidepressants

We found no systematic review or RCTs on the effects of antidepressants on menopausal symptoms.

Menopausal symptoms

Clonidine

One small RCT found that transdermal clonidine reduced the number and intensity of hot flushes after 8 weeks compared with placebo. However, we were unable to draw reliable conclusions from this study. We found no RCTs that assessed the effects of clonidine on sexual function, psychological symptoms, or quality of life.

Phyto-oestrogens

Nine RCTs provided no consistent evidence that phyto-oestrogens reduced vasomotor or other menopausal symptoms compared with placebo. We found no RCTs that assessed quality of life. One RCT found that isoflavone increased the proportion of women with simple endometrial hyperplasia at 5 years compared with placebo.

Testosterone

Small RCTs provided no consistent evidence about the effects of testosterone plus oestrogens on vasomotor symptoms or sexual function compared with oestrogen alone or placebo. We found no RCTs that assessed psychological symptoms or quality of life.

DEFINITION Menopause is defined as the end of the last menstrual period. A woman is deemed to be postmenopausal 1 year after her last period. For practical purposes, most women are diagnosed as menopausal after 1 year of amenorrhoea. Menopausal symptoms often begin in the perimenopausal years. The complex of menopausal symptomatology includes vasomotor symptoms (hot flushes), sleeplessness, mood changes, reduction in energy levels, loss of libido, vaginal dryness, and urinary symptoms.

INCIDENCE/ PREVALENCE In the UK, the mean age for the start of the menopause is 50 years and 9 months. The median onset of the perimenopause is 45.5–47.5 years. One Scottish survey (6096 women aged 45–54 years) found that 84% of women had experienced at least one of the classic menopausal symptoms, with 45% finding one or more symptoms to be a problem.[1]

AETIOLOGY/ RISK FACTORS Urogenital symptoms of menopause are caused by decreased oestrogen concentrations, but the cause of vasomotor symptoms and psychological effects is complex and remains unclear.

PROGNOSIS Menopause is a physiological event. Timing of the natural menopause in healthy women may be determined genetically. Although endocrine changes are permanent, menopausal symptoms such as hot flushes, which are experienced by about 70% of women, usually resolve with time.[2] Some symptoms, however, such as genital atrophy, may remain the same or worsen.

Please refer to clinicalevidence.com for full text and references.

Menorrhagia

Search date September 2004

Kirsten Duckitt and Keri McCully

What are the effects of medical treatments?

BENEFICIAL

Non-steroidal anti-inflammatory drugs

One systematic review found that non-steroidal anti-inflammatory drugs (NSAIDs) reduced menstrual blood loss compared with placebo. Systematic reviews found no significant difference in menstrual blood loss between mefenamic acid and naproxen, or between NSAIDs and oral progestogens given in the luteal phase, but the comparisons may have lacked power to exclude clinically important differences between treatments. Systematic reviews found that mefenamic acid was less effective than tranexamic acid or danazol in reducing menstrual blood loss, but caused fewer adverse effects than danazol. RCTs identified by several systematic reviews provided insufficient evidence to compare NSAIDs versus etamsylate (ethamsylate), combined oral contraceptives, or intrauterine progestogens. We found no RCTs comparing NSAIDs versus gonadorelin analogues. One RCT identified by a systematic review found that medical treatment, including NSAIDs, was less effective than endometrial resection in reducing menstrual blood loss at 4 months and 2 years, and increased the proportion of women who had adverse effects over 4 months.

Tranexamic acid

Systematic reviews found that tranexamic acid reduced menstrual blood loss compared with placebo, mefenamic acid, flurbiprofen, diclofenac, etamsylate (ethamsylate), or oral progestogens. We found no RCTs comparing tranexamic acid versus danazol, combined oral contraceptives, or gonadorelin analogues. RCTs identified by several systematic reviews provided insufficient evidence to compare tranexamic acid versus intrauterine progestogens. One RCT identified by a systematic review found that medical treatment, including tranexamic acid, was less effective than endometrial resection in reducing menstrual blood loss at 4 months and 2 years, and increased the proportion of women who had adverse effects over 4 months. Adverse effects of tranexamic acid include leg cramps and nausea, which occur in about a third of women using this drug. One long term population based observational study found no evidence that tranexamic acid increased the risk of thromboembolism.

TRADE OFF BETWEEN BENEFITS AND HARMS

Danazol

Systematic reviews found that danazol reduced blood loss compared with placebo, mefenamic acid, naproxen, or luteal phase oral progestogens but found that danazol increased adverse effects compared with either non-steroidal anti-inflammatory drugs or oral progestogens. RCTs identified by several systematic reviews provided insufficient evidence to compare danazol versus combined oral contraceptives or intrauterine progestogens. We found no RCTs comparing danazol versus tranexamic acid or gonadorelin analogues. One RCT identified by a systematic review found that medical treatment, including danazol, was less effective than endometrial resection in reducing menstrual blood loss at 4 months and 2 years, and increased the proportion of women who had adverse effects over 4 months.

Menorrhagia

UNKNOWN EFFECTIVENESS

Combined oral contraceptives

One RCT identified by three systematic reviews provided insufficient evidence to compare oral contraceptives versus other drugs. Another RCT identified by a systematic review found that medical treatment, including oral contraceptives, was less effective than endometrial resection in reducing menstrual blood loss at 4 months and 2 years, and increased the proportion of women who had adverse effects over 4 months.

Etamsylate

One systematic review provided insufficient evidence to compare etamsylate (ethamsylate) versus placebo or mefenamic acid. Two systematic reviews found that etamsylate was less effective than tranexamic acid in reducing menstrual blood loss. We found no RCTs comparing etamsylate versus danazol, combined oral contraceptives, oral progestogens, intrauterine progestogens, or gonadorelin analogues.

Gonadorelin analogues

We found no RCTs of gonadorelin analogues in women with menorrhagia.

Intrauterine progestogens

We found no RCTs comparing intrauterine progestogens versus placebo. RCTs identified by several systematic reviews provided insufficient evidence to compare intrauterine progestogens versus other drugs. RCTs identified by two systematic reviews provided insufficient evidence to compare intrauterine versus oral progestogens. One systematic review found that intrauterine progestogens were less effective than hysterectomy or endometrial destruction in reducing menstrual blood loss over 1 year, but caused fewer serious adverse effects than hysterectomy.

UNLIKELY TO BE BENEFICIAL

Oral progestogens (longer cycle)

We found no RCTs comparing oral progestogens versus placebo. One RCT identified by a systematic review found no significant difference in menstrual blood loss between a longer treatment cycle of oral progestogen and a levonorgestrel releasing intrauterine device.

LIKELY TO BE INEFFECTIVE OR HARMFUL

Oral progestogens in luteal phase only

We found no RCTs comparing oral progestogens versus placebo. One systematic review found no significant difference in menstrual blood loss between oral progestogens given in the luteal phase and non-steroidal anti-inflammatory drugs, but the comparison may have lacked power to exclude clinically important differences between treatments. One systematic review found that luteal phase oral progestogens were less effective in reducing mean menstrual blood loss than tranexamic acid or danazol. RCTs identified by two systematic reviews provided insufficient evidence to compare oral versus intrauterine progestogens. One RCT identified by a systematic review found that medical treatment, including oral progestogens, was less effective than endometrial resection in reducing menstrual blood loss at 4 months and 2 years, and increased the proportion of women who had adverse effects over 4 months.

What are the effects of surgical treatments?

BENEFICIAL

Hysterectomy (reduces menstrual blood loss compared with intrauterine progestogens or endometrial destruction; also reduces need for further surgery compared with endometrial destruction)

One systematic review found that surgery (hysterectomy or endometrial destruction) reduced menstrual blood loss over 1 year compared with intrauterine progestogens but that hysterectomy was associated with more serious adverse effects than progestogens. Two systematic reviews found that hysterectomy reduced menstrual blood loss and the number of women requiring further operations, and increased participant satisfaction compared with endometrial destruction. Five small RCTs found no evidence of a difference in effectiveness between different types of hysterectomy, although operating and recovery times differed. One large cohort study reported major or minor complications in about a third of women having hysterectomy.

LIKELY TO BE BENEFICIAL

Endometrial destruction (reduces menstrual blood loss compared with medical treatment)

One systematic review found that surgery (hysterectomy or endometrial destruction) reduced menstrual blood loss over 1 year compared with intrauterine progestogens. One RCT identified by a systematic review found that endometrial resection reduced blood loss at 4 months and 2 years compared with medical treatment, and reduced the proportion of women who had adverse effects over 4 months. Two systematic reviews found that endometrial destruction increased menstrual blood loss and the need for further operations and reduced participant satisfaction compared with hysterectomy. RCTs found that complications, such as infection, haemorrhage, and uterine perforation, occurred in up to 15% of women having endometrial destruction.

Hysteroscopic endometrial destruction (increases amenorrhoea compared with non-hysteroscopic destruction)

One systematic review found that hysteroscopic methods of endometrial destruction increased amenorrhoea at 12 months compared with non-hysteroscopic methods. We found no consistent evidence of a difference in amenorrhoea or satisfaction rates among different types of hysteroscopic procedure. RCTs found that complications, such as infection, haemorrhage, and uterine perforation, occurred in up to 15% of women having endometrial destruction.

UNKNOWN EFFECTIVENESS

Dilatation and curettage

We found no RCTs on the effects of dilatation and curettage.

Myomectomy

We found no RCTs on the effects of myomectomy.

Menorrhagia

What are the effects of endometrial thinning before endometrial destruction?

BENEFICIAL

Gonadorelin analogues

One systematic review found that preoperative gonadorelin analogues reduced postoperative moderate or heavy menstrual blood loss at 6–12 months after surgery and increased amenorrhoea at 24 months after surgery compared with placebo or no preoperative treatment. It found no significant difference between gonadorelin analogues and danazol in postoperative amenorrhoea at 12 months.

UNKNOWN EFFECTIVENESS

Danazol

Two small RCTs identified by a systematic review and one subsequent RCT provided insufficient evidence to compare preoperative danazol versus placebo or no preoperative treatment. One systematic review found no significant difference between danazol and gonadorelin analogues in postoperative amenorrhoea at 12 months. Two RCTs identified by a systematic review provided insufficient evidence to compare danazol versus other medical treatments.

Oral progestogens

Three RCTs identified by a systematic review provided insufficient evidence about the effects of oral progestogens compared with placebo, no preoperative treatment, or other medical treatments.

DEFINITION Menorrhagia is defined as heavy but regular menstrual bleeding. Idiopathic ovulatory menorrhagia is regular heavy bleeding in the absence of recognisable pelvic pathology or a general bleeding disorder. Objective menorrhagia is taken to be a total menstrual blood loss of 80 mL or more in each menstruation.[1] Subjectively, menorrhagia may be defined as a complaint of regular excessive menstrual blood loss occurring over several consecutive cycles in a woman of reproductive years.

INCIDENCE/ PREVALENCE In the UK, 5% of women (aged 30–49 years) consult their general practitioner each year with menorrhagia.[2] In New Zealand, 2–4% of primary care consultations by premenopausal women are for menstrual problems.[3]

AETIOLOGY/ RISK FACTORS Idiopathic ovulatory menorrhagia is thought to be caused by disordered prostaglandin production within the endometrium.[4] Prostaglandins may also be implicated in menorrhagia associated with uterine fibroids, adenomyosis, or the presence of an intrauterine device. Fibroids have been reported in 10% of women with menorrhagia (80–100 mL/cycle) and 40% of those with severe menorrhagia (≥ 200 mL/cycle).[5]

PROGNOSIS Menorrhagia limits normal activities and causes iron deficiency anaemia in two thirds of women proved to have objective menorrhagia.[1,6,7] One in five of all women in the UK and one in three women in the USA have a hysterectomy before the age of 60 years; menorrhagia is the main presenting problem in at least 50% of these women.[8-10] About 50% of the women who have a hysterectomy for menorrhagia are found to have a normal uterus.[11]

Please refer to clinicalevidence.com for full text and references.

Ovarian cancer (advanced)

Search date June 2005

Aarti Sharma, Usha Menon and Jonathan Ledermann

What are the effects of surgical treatments for ovarian cancer that is advanced at first presentation?

UNKNOWN EFFECTIVENESS

Primary surgery plus chemotherapy versus chemotherapy alone *New*

We found no systematic review or RCTs comparing primary surgery plus chemotherapy versus chemotherapy alone.

Primary surgery plus chemotherapy versus surgery alone *New*

We found no systematic review or RCTs comparing primary surgery plus chemotherapy versus surgery alone.

Primary surgery versus no surgery *New*

One systematic review found no RCTs comparing surgery versus no surgery. It found limited evidence from case series that maximal surgical cytoreduction is a strong determinant of survival in advanced ovarian cancer. It concluded that more studies are required in the area.

UNLIKELY TO BE BENEFICIAL

Interval debulking in women who have residual tumours after primary surgery *New*

One RCT showed that debulking surgery improved survival in women with greater than 1 cm of residual disease after primary surgery, but only if less than 1 cm of residual tumour remained after debulking. Two other RCTs failed to show any benefit from interval debulking surgery.

Second look surgery compared with watchful waiting *New*

One RCT found no evidence that second look surgery improved overall survival compared with watchful waiting in women having chemotherapy after primary surgery for advanced ovarian cancer.

What are the effects of platinum based chemotherapy for ovarian cancer that is advanced at first presentation?

LIKELY TO BE BENEFICIAL

Carboplatin plus taxane versus cisplatin plus taxane *New*

Three RCTs showed no difference in overall or progression free survival from regimens based on carboplatin or cisplatin. Carboplatin based regimens are associated with less gastrointestinal toxicity but more haematological adverse effects compared with cisplatin based regimens.

UNLIKELY TO BE BENEFICIAL

Combination platinum based chemotherapy versus single agent platinum (cisplatin or carboplatin alone may be as effective as platinum and non-taxane combination regimens) *New*

One systematic review and three additional RCTs that compared single agent platinum based chemotherapy versus platinum plus non-platinum combination ▶

regimens found no difference between regimens in the outcomes of death, progression free survival, or overall survival at up to 10 years' follow up. Leucopenia, nausea and vomiting, and alopecia were more common with combination treatment than with platinum alone.

What are the effects of taxane based chemotherapy for ovarian cancer that is advanced at first presentation?

UNLIKELY TO BE BENEFICIAL

Adding a taxane to a platinum based compound *New*

Two RCTs showed a longer median progression free and overall survival from a taxane plus platinum regimen compared with a platinum plus cyclophosphamide regimen over 25–37 months' follow up. Two RCTs showed no difference in progression free or overall survival from the addition of a taxane to platinum based monotherapy, after up to 51 months follow up, although the crossover rate between treatment groups in one of these trials was high. Overall taxanes are associated with increased haematological and neurological toxicity. Amifostine has not been shown to reduce neurotoxicity but increases gastrointestinal and haematological toxicity associated with paclitaxel plus carboplatin.

Paclitaxel versus docetaxel *New*

One RCT found no evidence of a difference in progression free or overall survival between paclitaxel and docetaxel when both were combined with carboplatin.

DEFINITION Ovarian tumours are classified according to the assumed cell type of origin (surface epithelium, stroma, or germ cells). Epithelial tumours account for over 90% of all ovarian cancers.[1] These can be further grouped into histological types (serous, mucinous, endometroid, and clear cell). Epithelial ovarian cancer is staged using the FIGO classification (see table 1 T).[2] This review is limited to first line treatment in women with advanced (FIGO stage 2–4) invasive epithelial ovarian cancer at first presentation.

INCIDENCE/ PREVALENCE The worldwide incidence of ovarian cancer according to the GLOBOCAN database was 204 499 cases in 2002. There is a worldwide variation with highest rates in Lithuania, Denmark, and Estonia and lowest in Egypt, Malawi, and Mali. This may be because of variation in reproductive practice, use of the oral contraceptive pill, breastfeeding habits, and age at menarche and menopause. The incidence of ovarian cancer rises steadily with increasing age and peaks in the seventh and eighth decades of life. In the UK, it is the fourth most common cause of cancer deaths with about 6900 new cases diagnosed annually and 4600 deaths from the disease each year.[3] The incidence of ovarian cancer seems to be stabilising in some other countries, and in some affluent countries (Finland, Denmark, New Zealand, and the US) rates are declining.

AETIOLOGY/ RISK FACTORS Risk factors include family history of ovarian cancer, increasing age, and low parity.[4-6] . More controversial are subfertility and use of fertility drugs[7,8] . Use of the oral contraceptive pill for more than 5 years reduces the risk by 30–40%.[4,9-11] Other factors associated with risk reduction are tubal ligation, hysterectomy, breast feeding, increasing age at menarche, decreasing age at menopause, and use of non-steroidal anti-inflammatory drugs.[12-16]

PROGNOSIS Survival rates vary according to the age of the woman, stage of the disease, and residual tumour after surgery. The most important determinant of survival appears to be the stage of disease at diagnosis. Diagnosis at an early stage has a five-year survival rate of greater than 70% but for those diagnosed with advanced stage disease it is approximately 15%.[17] Younger women survive longer than older women, even after adjustments for general life expectancy. In the UK, the five-year relative survival rate at diagnosis for women aged 15–39 is nearly 70%. In comparison, it is only 12% for women diagnosed over 80 years of age.[17]

Please refer to clinicalevidence.com for full text and references.

Polycystic ovary syndrome

Search date October 2005

Hesham Al-Inany

What are the effects of treatments?

LIKELY TO BE BENEFICIAL

Finasteride (may be similarly effective in reducing hirsutism compared with spironolactone, and cyproterone acetate–ethinylestradiol)

Two RCTs found that finasteride reduced hirsutism after 6 months of treatment compared with placebo. Small RCTs, which included women with idiopathic hirsutism, found differing results for the comparison of finasteride versus flutamide. Of the three RCTs that directly compared these treatments, two found no significant difference in hirsutism among treatments, and the third found that finasteride was less effective than flutamide in reducing hirsutism at 12 months. One RCT found that spironolactone 100 mg daily reduced symptoms of hirsutism compared with finasteride 5 mg daily after 12 months of treatment. Another RCT found no significant difference in hirsutism between spironolactone 100 mg daily and finasteride 5 mg daily at 6 months. One RCT found no significant difference between finasteride and cyproterone acetate–ethinylestradiol in improvement in hirsutism after 9 months of treatment. Another RCT found that adding finasteride to cyproterone acetate–ethinylestradiol reduced hirsutism at 6 months compared with cyproterone acetate–ethinylestradiol alone. One RCT found limited evidence that adding finasteride to spironolactone reduced hirsutism compared with spironolactone alone. We found no RCTs that assessed effects on oligomenorrhoea.

Flutamide (may be similarly effective in reducing hirsutism compared with finasteride and spironolactone)

One small RCT found that flutamide improved hirsutism compared with placebo at 6 months. Small RCTs, which included women with idiopathic hirsutism, provided limited evidence on the relative effectiveness of flutamide, finasteride, and spironolactone. Of the three RCTs that directly compared treatments, two found no significant difference in hirsutism among treatments, and the third found that flutamide was more effective than finasteride in reducing hirsutism at 12 months. One RCT found no significant difference between flutamide alone and flutamide plus cyproterone acetate–ethinylestradiol in reducing hirsutism at 6 months, but found that combined treatment reduced the number of women with oligomenorrhoea from baseline.

Metformin (improved menstrual pattern compared with placebo; reduced hirsutism compared with cyproterone acetate–ethinylestradiol)

One RCT found limited evidence that metformin improved menstrual pattern over 3 months compared with placebo. Another RCT found that adding metformin to a low calorie diet reduced oligomenorrhoea at 6 months compared with placebo, and found limited evidence that it also reduced hirsutism. A third RCT found that metformin was more effective in reducing hirsutism at 12 months than cyproterone acetate–ethinylestradiol.

Spironolactone (may be similarly effective for reducing hirsutism as flutamide and finasteride)

One systematic review of two RCTs found that spironolactone reduced hirsutism at 6 months compared with placebo in women with idiopathic hirsutism or hirsutism attributed to polycystic ovary syndrome. One RCT found that spironolactone 100 mg daily reduced symptoms of hirsutism compared with finasteride 5 mg daily after 12 months of treatment. Another RCT, which included women with idiopathic hirsutism, found no significant difference in hirsutism between spironolactone 100 mg daily, finasteride 5 mg daily, and flutamide 250 mg daily at 6 months. One small RCT found limited evidence that spironolactone was less effective in reducing hirsutism at 6 months than ketoconazole. One RCT provided limited evidence that adding finasteride to spironolactone reduced hirsutism compared with spironolactone alone. One RCT provided insufficient evidence to compare spironolactone versus cyproterone acetate–ethinylestradiol. We found no RCTs that assessed the effects of spironolactone on oligomenorrhoea.

TRADE OFF BETWEEN BENEFITS AND HARMS

Cyproterone acetate–ethinylestradiol (co-cyprindiol; reduced hirsutism but increased risk of venous thromboembolism)

One small RCT found limited evidence that cyproterone acetate–ethinylestradiol reduced hair growth compared with placebo at 12 months. One small RCT found limited evidence that although cyproterone acetate–ethinylestradiol reduced symptoms of hirsutism at 6 months from baseline, it was not as effective as ketoconazole. RCTs provided insufficient evidence to compare cyproterone acetate–ethinylestradiol versus desogestrel–ethinylestradiol, gonadotrophin releasing hormone agonists, or spironolactone. One RCT found that cyproterone acetate–ethinylestradiol was less effective than metformin for reducing hirsutism at 12 months. One RCT found that adding finasteride to cyproterone acetate–ethinylestradiol reduced hirsutism more than did cyproterone acetate–ethinylestradiol alone. One RCT found no significant difference between cyproterone acetate–ethinylestradiol and finasteride in improvement in hirsutism at 9 months. RCTs provided insufficient evidence about the effects of cyproterone acetate–ethinylestradiol on oligomenorrhoea. Cyproterone acetate–ethinylestradiol is associated with an increased risk of venous thromboembolism.

UNKNOWN EFFECTIVENESS

Interventions to achieve weight loss

We found no systematic review or RCTs assessing the effects of weight loss on clinical outcomes in women with polycystic ovary syndrome. One RCT found limited evidence by assessing changes within groups from baseline that a high or a low protein diet aimed at achieving weight loss may improve menstrual pattern over 16 weeks.

Ketoconazole

One small RCT found limited evidence that ketoconazole reduced hirsutism at 6 months compared with low dose cyproterone acetate–ethinylestradiol, cyproterone acetate–ethinylestradiol plus sequential cyproterone acetate, or spironolactone. We found no RCTs that assessed effects on oligomenorrhoea.

Mechanical hair removal

One RCT found that high intensity laser treatment reduced the self reported severity of hirsutism compared with control (low intensity laser treatment).

Polycystic ovary syndrome

DEFINITION Polycystic ovary syndrome (PCOS; Stein–Leventhal syndrome, sclerocystic ovarian disease) is defined as an accumulation of many incompletely developed follicles in the ovaries owing to chronic anovulation with an increase in ovarian androgen production.

INCIDENCE/ PREVALENCE PCOS is diagnosed in 4–10% of women attending gynaecology clinics in developed countries,[1,2] but this figure may not reflect the true prevalence because there have been no specific population based studies and the criteria used for diagnosis are varied. Most women present in their thirties.[2]

AETIOLOGY/ RISK FACTORS The aetiology is unknown. Genetic factors may play a part, but the exact mechanisms are unclear. Two studies found some evidence of familial aggregation of hyperandrogenaemia (with or without oligomenorrhoea) in first degree relatives of women with PCOS.[2,3] In the first study, 22% of sisters of women with PCOS fulfilled diagnostic criteria for PCOS.[2] In the second study, of the 78 mothers and 50 sisters evaluated clinically, 19 (24%) mothers and 16 (32%) sisters had PCOS.[3]

DIAGNOSIS The diagnosis excludes secondary causes such as androgen producing neoplasm, hyperprolactinaemia, and adult onset congenital adrenal hyperplasia.[1] It is characterised by irregular menstrual cycles, scanty or absent menses, multiple small cysts on the ovaries (polycystic ovaries), mild hirsutism, and infertility. Many women also have insulin resistance, acne, and weight gain.[1] Until recently, there was no overall consensus on the criteria for diagnosing PCOS. In some studies, it has been diagnosed based on the ultrasound findings of polycystic ovaries, rather than on clinical criteria. An international consensus definition of PCOS has now been published, which defines PCOS as at least two of the following criteria: reduced or no ovulation; clinical and/or biochemical signs of excessive secretion of androgens; and/or polycystic ovaries (the presence of at least 12 follicles measuring 2–9 mm in diameter, an ovarian volume in excess of 10 mL, or both).[4] Other aetiologies should also be excluded (congenital adrenal hyperplasias, androgen secreting tumours, Cushing's syndrome).

PROGNOSIS There is some evidence that women with PCOS are at increased risk of developing type 2 diabetes and cardiovascular disorders secondary to hyperlipidaemia compared with women who do not have PCOS.[5] Oligomenorrhoeic and amenorrhoeic women are at increased risk of developing endometrial hyperplasia and, later, endometrial carcinoma.[6]

Please refer to clinicalevidence.com for full text and references.

Premenstrual syndrome

Search date November 2005

Irene Kwan and Joseph Loze Onwude

What are the effects of drug treatments in women with premenstrual syndrome?

BENEFICIAL

Spironolactone

RCTs found that luteal phase spironolactone improved psychological and physical symptoms of premenstrual syndrome over 2–6 months compared with placebo.

LIKELY TO BE BENEFICIAL

Alprazolam

RCTs found that luteal phase alprazolam improved most physical and psychological symptoms of premenstrual syndrome after 3–6 months' treatment compared with placebo, including severe symptoms in women with premenstrual dysphoric disorder. Mild adverse effects were common. Benzodiazepines are associated with dependence.

Buspirone

One RCT found that buspirone (luteal or continuous) was more effective than placebo in improving self rated global improvement at 4 months in women with premenstrual dysphoric disorder. Results for individual psychological and physical symptoms were inconclusive. Mild adverse effects were common.

Gonadorelin analogues for < 6 months

One systematic review found that gonadorelin analogues reduced overall symptoms of premenstrual syndrome over 3–6 months compared with placebo. Women taking gonadorelin analogues were three times more likely to have adverse effects, including hot flushes, aches, night sweats, nausea, and headaches, than women taking placebo. The addition of hormonal addback therapy to reduce long term adverse effects did not reduce efficacy. However, treatment with gonadorelin analogues without hormonal addback for more than 6 months carries a serious risk of osteoporosis, limiting their usefulness for long term treatment.

Metolazone

One RCT found that luteal phase metolazone reduced premenstrual swelling and weight gain and improved mood symptoms compared with placebo.

Non-steroidal anti-inflammatory drugs

RCTs found that luteal phase mefenamic acid or naproxen sodium improved physical and psychological premenstrual symptoms over 3–6 months compared with placebo. The RCTs provided little information on adverse effects.

TRADE OFF BETWEEN BENEFITS AND HARMS

Clomipramine

RCTs found that clomipramine (luteal or continuous) improved psychological symptoms of premenstrual syndrome over three treatment cycles, but not physical symptoms. A proportion of women stopped treatment because of adverse effects such as drowsiness, nausea, vertigo, and headache.

BMJ Clin Evid Concise 2006;16:755–759.

Premenstrual syndrome

Danazol

RCTs found that danazol reduced overall premenstrual symptoms after 3 months' treatment compared with placebo, but had important adverse effects associated with masculinisation when used continuously in the long term.

Selective serotonin reuptake inhibitors (SSRIs)

One systematic review and subsequent RCTs found that selective serotonin reuptake inhibitors improved premenstrual symptoms over two to six cycles compared with placebo, but caused frequent adverse effects. Current evidence indicates no clear relationship between selective serotonin reuptake inhibitors and increased risk for suicide, but there is concern that selective serotonin reuptake inhibitors may increase the risk of self harm and suicidal ideation. Regulatory authorities in Europe, the UK, and the USA have issued warnings about the use of selective serotonin reuptake inhibitors in children and adolescents.

What are the effects of hormonal treatments?

TRADE OFF BETWEEN BENEFITS AND HARMS

Progesterone

One systematic review found an improvement in overall premenstrual symptoms in women taking luteal phase progesterone for 2–6 months compared with placebo. Although the review found a wide range of adverse effects associated with progesterone (including excessive bleeding, dysmenorrhoea, abdominal pain, nausea, and headache), it found no significant difference in the frequency of withdrawals owing to adverse effects.

Progestogens

One systematic review found that progestogens reduced premenstrual symptoms over three or four cycles compared with placebo. It found no significant difference between progestogens and placebo in the proportion of women who withdrew owing to adverse effects. The most common adverse effects associated with progestogens are nausea, breast discomfort, headache, and menstrual irregularity. Progestogen may induce premenstrual syndrome symptoms in some women.

UNKNOWN EFFECTIVENESS

Oestrogens

Limited evidence from one RCT suggested that continuous estradiol may improve symptoms of premenstrual syndrome after 3 months' treatment compared with placebo. However the magnitude of any effect is unclear. Important adverse effects of oestrogen include increased risk of breast cancer, endometrial cancer, stroke, and venous thromboembolic disease.

Oral contraceptives

One RCT found that oral contraceptives improved certain premenstrual symptoms (appetite, acne, and food cravings) compared with placebo, but did not improve mood related symptoms.

Tibolone

One small RCT found limited evidence that continuous tibolone improved premenstrual symptom score over 6 months compared with placebo (multivitamins).

What are the effects of psychological interventions in women with premenstrual syndrome?

UNKNOWN EFFECTIVENESS

Cognitive behavioural therapy

Weak RCTs provided insufficient evidence to assess cognitive behavioural therapy in women with premenstrual syndrome.

What are the effects of physical therapy in women with premenstrual syndrome?

UNKNOWN EFFECTIVENESS

Bright light therapy

One systematic review found no significant difference between bright light therapy and placebo in reducing depressive symptoms related to premenstrual dysphoric disorder.

Chiropractic manipulation

One weak crossover trial provided insufficient evidence to assess chiropractic manipulation in women with premenstrual syndrome.

Exercise

We found no systematic review or RCTs of exercise in women with premenstrual syndrome.

Reflexology

One RCT found limited evidence that reflexology was better than sham reflexology in reducing premenstrual symptoms at 8 weeks.

Relaxation

One RCT found limited evidence that relaxation treatment was better than reading leisure material or charting symptoms in reducing premenstrual symptoms over 5 months. Two further weak RCTs provided insufficient evidence to assess relaxation.

What are the effects of dietary supplements in women with premenstrual syndrome?

BENEFICIAL

Pyridoxine

One systematic review found that luteal phase or continuous pyridoxine (vitamin B_6) was better than placebo in relieving overall symptoms of premenstrual syndrome over 2–6 months.

LIKELY TO BE BENEFICIAL

Calcium supplements

Two RCTs identified by a systematic review found that calcium supplements improved symptoms compared with placebo.

Premenstrual syndrome

UNKNOWN EFFECTIVENESS

Evening primrose oil

Weak RCTs provided insufficient evidence to assess the effects of evening primrose oil in women with premenstrual symptoms.

Magnesium supplements

Weak RCTs provided insufficient evidence to assess the effects of magnesium supplements in women with premenstrual syndrome.

What are the effects of surgical treatments in women with premenstrual syndrome?

LIKELY TO BE BENEFICIAL

Hysterectomy with bilateral oophorectomy*

We found no systematic review or RCTs of hysterectomy alone or hysterectomy with bilateral oophorectomy in women with premenstrual syndrome. Cohort studies have found almost complete eradication of the symptoms of premenstrual syndrome after hysterectomy plus bilateral oophorectomy and continuous oestrogen placement and there is consensus that it is effective. Surgery is rarely used but may be indicated if there are coexisting gynaecological problems.

Laparoscopic bilateral oophorectomy*

We found no systematic review or RCTs of laparoscopic bilateral oophorectomy in women with premenstrual syndrome; an RCT is unlikely to be performed. Cohort studies have found almost complete eradication of the symptoms of premenstrual syndrome after hysterectomy plus bilateral oophorectomy and continuous oestrogen placement and there is consensus that it is effective. Surgery is rarely used but may be indicated if there are coexisting gynaecological problems.

*No RCTs but consensus that effective and an RCT unlikely to be performed.

UNKNOWN EFFECTIVENESS

Endometrial ablation

We found no systematic review or RCTs of endometrial ablation in women with premenstrual syndrome.

DEFINITION A woman has premenstrual syndrome if she complains of recurrent psychological or physical symptoms (or both) occurring specifically during the luteal phase of the menstrual cycle, and often resolving by the end of menstruation.[1] The symptoms can also persist during the bleeding phase. (For details of psychological, behavioural, and physical symptoms commonly reported in women with premenstrual syndrome see web table A.) **Severe premenstrual syndrome:** The definition of severe premenstrual syndrome varies among RCTs, but in recent studies standardised criteria have been used to diagnose one variant of severe premenstrual syndrome (termed the premenstrual dysphoric disorder), based on at least five symptoms, including one of four core psychological symptoms (from a list of 17 physical and psychological symptoms), being severe premenstrually and mild or absent postmenstrually.[2,3] The 17 symptoms are depression, feeling hopeless or guilty, anxiety/tension, mood swings, irritability/persistent anger, decreased interest, poor concentration, fatigue, food craving or increased appetite, sleep disturbance, feeling out of control or overwhelmed, poor coordination, headache, aches, swelling/bloating/weight gain, cramps, and breast tenderness.

INCIDENCE/ PREVALENCE Premenstrual symptoms occur in 95% of all women of reproductive age; severe, debilitating symptoms (premenstrual syndrome) occur in about 5% of those women.[1]

AETIOLOGY/ RISK FACTORS The aetiology is unknown, but hormonal and other (possibly neuroendocrine) factors probably contribute.[4,5]

PROGNOSIS Except after oophorectomy, symptoms of premenstrual syndrome usually recur when treatment is stopped.

Please refer to clinicalevidence.com for full text and references.

Pyelonephritis (acute) in non-pregnant women

Search date February 2006

Ignacio Neumann, M Fernanda Rojas, and Philippa Moore

What are the effects of antibiotic treatments for acute pyelonephritis?

LIKELY TO BE BENEFICIAL

Intravenous antibiotics in women admitted to hospital with uncomplicated infection*

We found no systematic review or RCTs comparing intravenous antibiotics versus no antibiotics. Consensus holds that intravenous antibiotics are effective, and it is unlikely that a placebo controlled RCT would now be performed.

Oral antibiotics for women with uncomplicated infection*

We found no systematic review or RCTs comparing oral antibiotics versus no antibiotics. However, consensus holds that these drugs are effective, and it is unlikely that such an RCT would now be performed.

*Categorisation is not based on placebo controlled RCTs. Such studies are likely to be considered unethical.

UNKNOWN EFFECTIVENESS

Intravenous antibiotics plus oral antibiotics versus oral antibiotics alone

One RCT found no significant difference in rates of clinical success between intravenous antibiotics plus oral ciprofloxacin and oral ciprofloxacin alone.

Relative effectiveness of different intravenous antibiotic regimens

One RCT found limited evidence of no significant difference between intravenous ampicillin plus intravenous gentamicin and intravenous co-trimoxazole plus intravenous gentamicin for relief of symptoms and recurrence of bacteriuria at 28 days. We found insufficient evidence to compare clinical effects of different intravenous regimens. We found no RCTs comparing different lengths of treatment with the same intravenous antibiotic.

Relative effectiveness of different oral antibiotic regimens

One systematic review and two subsequent RCTs in women with uncomplicated pyelonephritis (some of whom were admitted to hospital) found no consistent differences between different antibiotics in bacteriological or clinical cure rates. However, observational data suggest that broader spectrum antibiotics, such as quinolones, may be more effective than narrow spectrum antibiotics such as amoxicillin (amoxycillin) and trimethoprim–sulfamethoxazole in areas with a high prevalence of resistance to these drugs. We found no RCTs comparing different lengths of treatment with the same oral antibiotic.

Relative effectiveness of inpatient versus outpatient management

We found no systematic review or RCTs comparing inpatient versus outpatient management of women with acute uncomplicated pyelonephritis.

Relative effectiveness of oral versus intravenous antibiotics

We found no RCTs comparing oral versus intravenous antibiotics in women with acute pyelonephritis.

What are the effects of analgesia for acute pyelonephritis?

UNKNOWN EFFECTIVENESS

Non-steroidal anti-inflammatory drugs

We found no systematic review or RCTs comparing non-steroidal anti-inflammatory drugs (NSAIDs) versus placebo or versus simple systemic analgesics (non-opiates) in the management of women with acute uncomplicated pyelonephritis. Recognised adverse effects of non-steroidal anti-inflammatory drugs include impairment of renal function, suggesting that they should be used with caution in uncomplicated acute pyelonephritis.

Simple systemic analgesics (non-opiates)

We found no systematic review or RCTs comparing simple analgesics (excluding urinary tract analgesics and opiates) versus placebo or versus non-steroidal anti-inflammatory drugs in the management of women with acute uncomplicated pyelonephritis. to be considered unethical.

DEFINITION Acute pyelonephritis, or upper urinary tract infection, is an infection of the kidney characterised by pain when passing urine, fever, chills, flank pain, nausea, and vomiting. White blood cells are almost always present in the urine. White blood cell casts are occasionally seen on urine microscopy. There is no consensus on the definitions for grades of severity. However, people with acute pyelonephritis may be divided into those able to take oral antibiotics and without signs of sepsis, who may be managed at home, and those requiring intravenous antibiotics in hospital. Pyelonephritis is considered uncomplicated if it is caused by a typical pathogen in an immunocompetent person who has normal renal anatomy and renal function.[1] There is little difference in the treatment of men and non-pregnant women.

INCIDENCE/ PREVALENCE The estimated annual incidence per 10 000 people is 27.6 cases in the USA[2] and 35.7 cases in South Korea.[3] Worldwide prevalence and incidence are unknown.

AETIOLOGY/ RISK FACTORS Pyelonephritis is most commonly caused when bacteria in the bladder ascend the ureters and invade the kidneys. In some cases, this may result in bacteria entering and multiplying in the bloodstream. The most frequently isolated organism is *Escherichia coli* (56–85%); others include *Enterococcus faecalis*, *Klebsiella pneumoniae*, and *Proteus mirabilis*.[2,4,5] People with structural or functional urinary tract abnormalities are more prone to pyelonephritis that is refractory to oral therapy or complicated by bacteraemia. Risk factors associated with pyelonephritis in healthy women are sexual intercourse, use of spermicide, urinary tract infection in the previous 12 months, a mother with a history of urinary tract infection, diabetes, and urinary incontinence.[2] The incidence of drug resistant microorganisms varies in different geographical areas. Recent hospitalisation, recent use of antibiotics, immunosuppression, recurrent pyelonephritis, and nephrolithiasis increase the risk of drug resistance.[4]

PROGNOSIS Prognosis is good if uncomplicated pyelonephritis is treated appropriately. Complications include renal abscess, septic shock, and renal impairment, including acute renal failure. Short term independent risk factors for mortality include age above 65 years, septic shock, being bedridden, and immunosuppression.[4] Conditions such as underlying renal disease, diabetes mellitus, and immunosuppression may worsen prognosis, but we found no good long term evidence about rates of sepsis or death among people with such conditions.

Please refer to clinicalevidence.com for full text and references.

Recurrent cystitis in non-pregnant women

Search date May 2005

Ayan Sen

Which interventions prevent further recurrence of cystitis in women experiencing at least two infections per year?

BENEFICIAL

Continuous antibiotic prophylaxis (trimethoprim, co-trimoxazole, nitrofurantoin, cefaclor, or a quinolone)

One systematic review found that continuous antibiotic prophylaxis lasting 6–12 months with cefalexin, co-trimoxazole, nitrofurantoin, norfloxacin, or a quinolone reduced rates of recurrent cystitis during prophylaxis compared with placebo, and found no consistent difference in recurrence rates among different continuous regimens. However, two RCTs identified by the review found no significant difference in recurrence rates at 6 months after completing prophylaxis compared with placebo. RCTs comparing continuous daily antibiotic prophylaxis versus postcoital antibiotic prophylaxis found no significant difference in recurrence rates. RCTs provided insufficient evidence to compare continuous antibiotic prophylaxis versus continuous prophylaxis with methenamine hippurate. There is no clear consensus about when to start continuous antibiotic prophylaxis and how long it should continue.

Postcoital antibiotic prophylaxis (co-trimoxazole, nitrofurantoin, or a quinolone)

One RCT identified by a systematic review found that co-trimoxazole up to 2 hours after sexual intercourse reduced clinical recurrence rates compared with placebo. Another RCT comparing continuous daily antibiotic prophylaxis versus postcoital antibiotic prophylaxis found no significant difference in rates of microbiological recurrence.

LIKELY TO BE BENEFICIAL

Cranberry juice and cranberry products

One systematic review found that cranberry products (juice or capsules) reduced symptomatic recurrence of cystitis over 12 months compared with placebo.

UNKNOWN EFFECTIVENESS

Continuous prophylaxis with methenamine hippurate

RCTs provided insufficient evidence to assess continuous prophylaxis with methenamine hippurate (hexamine hippurate) compared with placebo or continuous antibiotic prophylaxis in women with recurrent cystitis.

Passing urine after intercourse

We found no systematic review or RCTs of passing urine after intercourse in women with recurrent cystitis.

Single dose self administered co-trimoxazole

One small RCT found that single dose, self administered co-trimoxazole started at the onset of cystitis symptoms was less effective in reducing recurrence rates over 1 year than continuous co-trimoxazole prophylaxis. However, evidence was too limited to draw firm conclusions, as the higher rate of cystitis in women using ▶

single dose prophylaxis is to be expected because treatment was only administered after the onset of symptoms. We found no RCTs of other single dose antibiotics.

DEFINITION In most cases, cystitis is a bacterial infection of the lower urinary tract which causes pain when passing urine and causes frequency, urgency, haematuria, and suprapubic pain not associated with passing urine. White blood cells and bacteria are almost always present in the urine. A recurrent urinary tract infection is a symptomatic urinary tract infection that follows clinical resolution of an earlier infection generally, but not necessarily, after treatment.[1] Recurrent cystitis is usually defined in the literature as three episodes of urinary tract infection in the past 12 months or two episodes in the past 6 months. Recurrent urinary tract infections cause serious discomfort to women and have a high impact on ambulatory health care costs as a result of outpatient visits, diagnostic tests, and prescriptions.

INCIDENCE/ PREVALENCE Recurrent cystitis is common among young healthy women, even though they generally have anatomically and physiologically normal urinary tracts. One study found that nearly half of the women whose uncomplicated urinary tract infections resolved spontaneously developed a recurrent urinary tract infection within the first year.[2] In a study of college women with their first urinary tract infection, 27% experienced at least one culture confirmed recurrence within the 6 months following initial infection and 2.7% had a second recurrence over this time period.[3] In a Finnish study of women aged 17–82 years who had *Escherichia Coli* cystitis, 44% had a recurrence within 1 year, 53% in women older than 55 years, 36% in younger women.[4] No large population based studies have been performed yet to determine what proportion of women with urinary tract infection develops a pattern of high frequency recurrence. Occasionally, recurrences are due to a persistent focus of infection, but the vast majority is thought to represent reinfection.[1] A recurrence is defined clinically as a relapse if it is caused by the same species as that causing the original urinary tract infection and if it occurs within 2 weeks after treatment. It is considered reinfection if it occurs more than 2 weeks after treatment of the original infection.[1] Most women are able to diagnose their own episodes of recurrent cystitis from symptoms (positive predictive value in one RCT 92%).[5]

AETIOLOGY/ RISK FACTORS Cystitis is caused by uropathogenic bacteria in the faecal flora that colonise the vaginal and periurethral openings, and ascend the urethra into the bladder. Sexual intercourse, diaphragm–spermicide use, and a history of recurrent urinary tract infection have been shown to be strong and independent risk factors for cystitis.[6] Spermicide coated condom use may also increase the risk of urinary tract infection.[7,8] Antimicrobial use has been shown to adversely affect the vaginal flora in animals and humans,[9] and recent use of antibiotics is strongly associated with risk of cystitis.[10] however, risk factors specific to women with recurrent cystitis have received little study. In a large, case controlled study of women, comprising 229 cases and 253 controls, with and without a history of recurrent urinary tract infection, the strongest risk factor for recurrence in a multivariate analysis was the frequency of sexual intercourse.[11] Other risk factors included spermicide use in the past year, new sex partner during the past year, having a first urinary tract infection at or before 15 years of age, and having a mother with history of urinary tract infections. Urine voiding disorders such as those associated with prolapse, multiple sclerosis, bladder cancer, or bladder stones are also associated with increased risk.[11] An association has been found between pre- and postcoital voiding, frequency of urination, delayed voiding habits, douching, and body mass index. A possible association between smoking (which is strongly associated with bladder cancer) and recurrent cystitis has not been assessed. These behavioural patterns have never been evaluated in prospective, randomised trials. Data suggest that pelvic anatomical differences may have a role in predisposing some young

Recurrent cystitis in non-pregnant women

women to recurrent urinary tract infection, especially those who do not have other risk factors.[12] In postmenopausal women, reduced oestrogen levels appear to contribute to recurrent cystitis in healthy women. The vagina, bladder, and urethra respond to oestrogen, and when the hormonal level in the body is reduced, the tissues of these organs become thinner, weaker, and dry. The changes in the tissues of the bladder and urethra and the associated loss of protection against infection-causing germs may cause an increased risk of urinary tract infection in postmenopausal women. Cystitis is also more common during pregnancy because of changes in the urinary tract. As the uterus grows, its increased weight can block the drainage of urine from the bladder, causing an infection. Women are at increased risk for recurrent cystitis from weeks 6–24 of pregnancy.

PROGNOSIS We found little evidence on the long term effects of untreated cystitis.[2] One study found that progression to pyelonephritis was infrequent, and that most cases of cystitis regressed spontaneously, although symptoms sometimes persisted for several months. However, bacteriuria in pregnant women carries a much greater risk of progressing to pyelonephritis than in non-pregnant women (28% *v* 1%) and is associated with serious risks.[2]

Please refer to clinicalevidence.com for full text and references.

Stress incontinence

Search date December 2005

Joseph L Onwude

What are the effects of non-surgical treatments for women with stress incontinence?

BENEFICIAL

Serotonin reuptake inhibitors (duloxetine)

One systematic review found that duloxetine at doses of 80 mg or above daily improved the frequency of incontinence episodes, the proportion of people who had improved at end of treatment, rates of subjective cure or improvement, and quality of life outcomes compared with placebo. The review found that lower doses of 20–40 mg daily also increased the proportion of people who improved at the end of treatment but for other outcomes found no significant difference between these doses and placebo. Duloxetine was associated with more adverse effects, including nausea, diarrhoea, headache, dizziness, fatigue, and dry mouth, compared with placebo. One RCT included in the systematic review found that duloxetine 80 mg daily plus imitation pelvic floor muscle exercises reduced the frequency of incontinence compared with pelvic floor muscle exercises plus placebo, but found no significant difference between groups in quality of life scores.

LIKELY TO BE BENEFICIAL

Pelvic floor electrical stimulation

RCTs found that pelvic floor electrical stimulation was more effective than no treatment or sham pelvic floor electrical stimulation at increasing subjective improvement in symptoms at between 4 to 8 weeks. One systematic review found no significant difference in cure or improvement rates at 12 months between pelvic muscle electrical stimulation and pelvic floor muscle exercises. It found that pelvic floor electrical stimulation was associated with a small number of cases of vaginal irritation and difficulties in maintaining motivation for treatment. Another systematic review found no significant difference between pelvic floor electrical stimulation and vaginal cones in self reported cure or improvement rates, or in urinary leakage over 4 weeks to 12 months, but it may have lacked power to detect a clinically important difference. A third systematic review found no significant difference in cure or improvement rates between pelvic floor electrical stimulation and oestrogen supplements, but it may have lacked the power to detect a clinically important difference.

Pelvic floor muscle exercises

One systematic review found that pelvic floor muscle exercises increased cure or improvement rates and reduced the number of daily leakages over 3–6 months compared with no treatment or placebo. One subsequent RCT found that pelvic floor muscle exercises plus placebo reduced pad use at 12 weeks compared with placebo, but found no significant difference between groups in incontinence episode frequency, Incontinence Quality of Life (I-QOL) scores, or Patient Global Impression of Improvement (PGI-I) scores. The review found no significant difference in cure or improvement rates at 12 months between pelvic floor muscle exercises and pelvic floor electrical stimulation. It found that pelvic floor muscle exercises reduced the number of daily leakage episodes at 6 months compared with vaginal cones, but there was no significant difference between treatments in cure or improvement rates at 12 months. One systematic review ▶

found that pelvic floor muscle exercises increased cure or improvement rates compared with oestrogen supplements at 9 months. One RCT found that pelvic floor muscle exercises plus placebo was less effective at reducing frequency of incontinence compared with duloxetine 80 mg daily plus imitation pelvic floor muscle exercises, but found no significant difference in quality of life scores between groups.

Vaginal cones

One systematic review found that vaginal cones improved self reported cure or improvement rates compared with no treatment or advice to use a continence guard over 6–12 months. It found no significant difference in daily leakage episodes. RCTs found no significant difference between vaginal cones and pelvic floor muscle exercises in self reported cure or improvement rates over 12 months. It found that vaginal cones were less effective than pelvic floor muscle exercises in reducing the number of leakage episodes over 6 months. RCTs also found no significant difference between vaginal cones and pelvic floor electrical stimulation in self reported cure or improvement rates, or urinary leakage over 4 weeks to 12 months, but they may have lacked power to detect a clinically important difference. One RCT also found no significant difference between vaginal cones and combined pelvic floor electrical stimulation and biofeedback in subjective and objective improvement rates after 6 weeks. The most common adverse effect associated with vaginal cones was difficulty maintaining motivation for use, but a small number of more serious events such as vaginitis and abdominal pain were reported.

TRADE OFF BETWEEN BENEFITS AND HARMS

Oestrogen supplements

One systematic review found that short term treatment with oestrogen supplements improved cure or improvement rates compared with placebo. The review found lower rates of cure or improvement with oestrogen supplements compared with pelvic floor muscle exercises at 9 months. It found no significant difference in rates of cure or improvement between short term treatment with oestrogen supplements and pelvic floor electrical stimulation, but it may have lacked the power to detect a clinically important difference. It found no significant difference in rates of cure or improvement between pelvic floor electrical stimulation and short term treatment with oestrogen supplements, but it may have lacked the power to detect a clinically important difference. One RCT found no significant difference in subjective cure or improvement rates between vaginal oestrogen (estriol) and an adrenergic agonist (phenylpropanolamine). There are concerns about the safety of long term oestrogen use. One RCT found that oral oestrogen supplements increased the risk of strokes in postmenopausal women without a uterus at 6 years. There is limited evidence that unopposed oestrogen is associated with an increased risk of endometrial cancer in women with a uterus.

UNKNOWN EFFECTIVENESS

Adrenergic agonists

Pooled results from two small RCTs suggested that phenylpropanolamine increased subjective cure or improvement rates compared with placebo, although this difference was not significant. Two RCTs found that midodrine or clenbuterol increased subjective cure or improvement rates compared with placebo. One RCT found that phenylpropanolamine increased subjective cure or improvement rates compared with pelvic floor muscle exercises. A second RCT found no significant difference between clenbuterol and pelvic floor muscle exercises. One RCT identified by the review found no significant difference in subjective cure or improvement rates between phenylpropanolamine and vaginal oestrogen (estriol). Phenylpropanolamine has been withdrawn from the US market because of an increased risk of haemorrhagic stroke.

What are the effects of surgical treatments for women with stress incontinence?

BENEFICIAL

Laparoscopic colposuspension (similar cure rates to open retropubic colposuspension and tension free vaginal tape)

We found no RCTs comparing laparoscopic colposuspension versus no treatment, non-surgical treatment, anterior vaginal repair, suburethral slings, or needle suspension. One systematic review found that open retropubic colposuspension improved objective cure rates at 1 year compared with laparoscopic colposuspension. One systematic review found that laparoscopic colposuspension was less effective than open retropubic colposuspension at improving objective cure rates at 1 year. However, it found no significant difference in objective cure rates at 5 years, or in subjective cure rates at 1 or 5 years. One RCT identified by a review found a higher cure rate with tension free vaginal tape than with laparoscopic colposuspension at 6 months to 2 years, while two subsequent RCTs found no significant difference in cure rate between treatments at 6 weeks to 1 year.

Open retropubic colposuspension (higher cure rates than non-surgical treatment, anterior vaginal repair, or needle suspension, but more adverse effects than non-surgical treatment)

We found no RCTs comparing open retropubic colposuspension versus no treatment or sham treatment. One systematic review found that open retropubic colposuspension increased cure rates at 1–5 years compared with non-surgical treatment, anterior vaginal repair, or needle suspension. Open retropubic colposuspension was associated with more adverse effects than non-surgical treatment, but fewer surgical complications than needle suspension. It found that open retropubic colposuspension improved objective cure rates at 1 year compared with laparoscopic colposuspension. However, it found no significant difference in objective cure rates at 5 years, or in subjective cure rates at 1 or 5 years. It also found no significant difference in cure rates at 1 year between open retropubic colposuspension and suburethral slings. One systematic review found no significant difference in cure rate between tension free vaginal tape and open retropubic colposuspension at up to 2 years. However, the included trials may have lacked power to exclude a clinically important difference in cure rates. RCTs included in the review found that open retropubic colposuspension was associated with a lower incidence of bladder perforation than tension free vaginal tape, but a higher incidence of postoperative fever.

LIKELY TO BE BENEFICIAL

Suburethral slings other than tension free vaginal tape (similar cure rates to open retropubic colposuspension and needle suspension, but more perioperative complications than needle suspension)

We found no RCTs comparing suburethral slings versus no treatment, sham treatment, non-surgical treatment, anterior vaginal repair, or laparoscopic colposuspension. Five RCTs identified by a systematic review found no significant difference in cure rates at up to 6 years between suburethral slings and open retropubic colposuspension, although the studies may have lacked power to detect a clinically important difference. One small RCT identified by the review found no significant difference in cure rates at 1 year between suburethral slings and needle suspension, but it may have lacked power to detect a clinically important difference. The RCT found that suburethral slings increased perioperative complications compared with needle suspension. Two RCTs found no significant difference in subjective cure rates between suburethral slings and tension free vaginal tape at 6–12 months.

TRADE OFF BETWEEN BENEFITS AND HARMS

Tension free vaginal tape

We found no RCTs comparing tension free vaginal tape versus no treatment, sham treatment, non-surgical treatment, anterior vaginal repair, or needle suspension. Two RCTs found no significant difference in cure rates between tension free vaginal tape and other types of suburethral slings at 6–12 months. One systematic review found no significant difference in cure rates between tension free vaginal tape and open retropubic colposuspension at up to 2 years. RCTs included in the review found that tension free vaginal tape was associated with a higher incidence of bladder perforation than open retropubic colposuspension, but a lower incidence of postoperative fever. Five RCTs found no significant difference in cure rate between tension free vaginal tape and laparoscopic colposuspension at 6 weeks to 2 years.

UNKNOWN EFFECTIVENESS

Transobturator foramen procedures (limited evidence similar cure rates to tension free vaginal tape) *New*

One RCT found no significant difference in cure rates between transobturator foramen procedures and tension free vaginal tape at 15 months. We found no RCTs comparing transobturator foramen procedures versus no treatment, sham treatment, non-surgical treatment, anterior vaginal repair, non-tension free vaginal tape, suburethral slings, open retropubic colposuspension, laparoscopic colposuspension, and needle suspension.

UNLIKELY TO BE BENEFICIAL

Anterior vaginal repair (lower cure rates than open retropubic colposuspension)

We found no RCTs comparing anterior vaginal repair versus no treatment, suburethral slings, laparoscopic colposuspension, or tension free vaginal tape. One RCT provided insufficient evidence to compare anterior vaginal repair versus non-surgical treatment. One systematic review found that anterior vaginal repair was less effective than open retropubic colposuspension at increasing cure rates at 12 months or 5 years, and found no significant difference in overall operative complications between the two procedures. It found no significant difference in cure rates at 12 months between anterior vaginal repair and needle suspension.

Needle suspension (lower cure rates and more surgical complications than open retropubic colposuspension)

We found no RCTs comparing needle suspension versus no treatment, non-surgical treatment, tension free vaginal tape, or laparoscopic colposuspension. One systematic review found no significant difference in cure rates between needle suspension and anterior vaginal repair or suburethral slings, but found that needle suspension was associated with fewer perioperative complications than suburethral slings. Another systematic review found that open retropubic colposuspension improved cure rates and was associated with fewer surgical complications than needle suspension at 5 years.

DEFINITION Stress incontinence is involuntary leakage of urine on effort or exertion, or on sneezing or coughing.[1] Stress incontinence predominantly affects women, and can cause social and hygiene problems. Typically, there is no anticipatory feeling of needing to pass urine. Under urodynamic testing, urodynamic stress incontinence is confirmed by demonstrating loss of urine when intravesical pressure exceeds maximum urethral pressure, in the absence of a detrusor contraction. A confirmed diagnosis of urodynamic stress incontinence is particularly important before surgical treatment,[2] given that the symptoms of stress incontinence can occur in people with detrusor overactivity, which is confirmed by the demonstration of uninhibited bladder contractions. This topic deals with stress incontinence in general.

INCIDENCE/ PREVALENCE Stress incontinence is a common problem. Prevalence has been estimated at 17–45% of adult women in the setting of a high income country.[3] One cross-sectional study (15 308 women in Norway < 65 years) found that the prevalence of stress incontinence was 4.7% in women who have not borne a child, 6.9% in women who had caesarean deliveries only, and 12.2% in women who had vaginal deliveries only.[4]

AETIOLOGY/ RISK FACTORS Aetiological factors include pregnancy, vaginal or caesarean delivery, cigarette smoking, and obesity.[4-7] One cross-sectional study (15 308 women in Norway) found that when compared with women who have not borne a child, the risk of stress incontinence was increased in women who have delivered by caesarean section (age adjusted OR 1.4, 95% CI 1.0 to 2.0) or by vaginal delivery (age adjusted OR 3.0, 95% CI 2.5 to 3.5).[4] The risk of stress incontinence was also increased in women who had a vaginal delivery compared with women who had a caesarean section (adjusted OR 2.4, 95% CI 1.7 to 3.2). One case control study (606 women) found that the risk of "genuine", now called "urodynamic", stress incontinence was increased in former smokers (adjusted OR 2.20, 95% CI 1.18 to 4.11) and in current smokers (adjusted OR 2.48, 95% CI 1.60 to 3.84).[7] We found no reliable data measuring the risks associated with obesity.

PROGNOSIS We found no reliable data about the natural history of stress incontinence. Untreated stress incontinence is believed to be a persistent, lifelong condition.

Please refer to clinicalevidence.com for full text and references.

Bites (mammalian)

Search date August 2005

David Jerrard

What are the effects of interventions to prevent mammalian bites?

LIKELY TO BE BENEFICIAL

Education

We found no RCTs of the effect of education programmes on the incidence of mammalian bites. One RCT in school children found that an educational programme increased precautionary behaviour around dogs compared with no education.

UNKNOWN EFFECTIVENESS

Education in specific occupational groups

We found no RCTs of education to prevent bites in specific occupational groups.

What are the effects of measures to prevent complications from mammalian bites?

LIKELY TO BE BENEFICIAL

Antibiotic prophylaxis for human bites on the hand

Meta-analysis in one systematic review according to the site of the wound found that antibiotics reduced infections of the hand only. One small RCT in the review found that in people with human bites on the hand, antibiotics reduced the rate of infection compared with placebo. One subsequent RCT found no significant difference in infection rate between antibiotics and placebo in people with low risk human bites.

Debridement, irrigation, and decontamination*

We found no reliable studies assessing debridement, irrigation, decontamination measures, or infiltration of serum into the wound. However, there is consensus that such measures are likely to be beneficial.

Primary wound closure

One poor quality RCT comparing primary wound closure with no closure in people with dog bites found no significant difference in the incidence of infection, but the RCT was too small to exclude clinically important effects. There is consensus that primary closure of most bite wounds is likely to be beneficial and does not increase the risk of subsequent infection.

Tetanus immunisation after mammalian bites*

We found no evidence on the effects of tetanus toxoid or tetanus immunoglobulin in preventing tetanus after human or animal bites. There is clinical consensus that tetanus immunisation should be given routinely as part of wound care for mammalian bites. An RCT comparing tetanus immunisation versus no immunisation would be considered unethical.

UNKNOWN EFFECTIVENESS

Antibiotic prophylaxis for non-human mammalian bites

The effects of antibiotic prophylaxis in preventing complications of mammalian bites remain unclear. Limited evidence from one systematic review found that, when all causes and sites of mammalian bite were combined, there was no evidence of a difference in infection rate between antibiotics and placebo.

What are the effects of treatments for infected mammalian bites?

LIKELY TO BE BENEFICIAL

Antibiotics*

We found no RCTs of antibiotics compared with placebo for infected mammalian bites. However, there is consensus that antibiotics are likely to be beneficial.

UNKNOWN EFFECTIVENESS

Comparative effectiveness of different antibiotics

One RCT in people with infected and uninfected animal and human bites found no significant difference in failure rate (which was undefined) with penicillin, with or without dicloxacillin, compared with amoxicillin (amoxycillin)/clavulanic acid.

*No RCT evidence, but there is consensus that treatment is likely to be beneficial.

DEFINITION Bite wounds are mainly caused by humans, dogs, or cats. They include superficial abrasions (30–43%), lacerations (31–45%), and puncture wounds (13–34%).[1]

INCIDENCE/ PREVALENCE Bite wounds account for about 1–2% of all emergency department visits annually in the USA, costing over US $100 million annually.[2,3] In the USA, an estimated 3.5–4.7 million dog bites occur each year.[4] About one in five people bitten by a dog seek medical attention, and 1% of those require admission to hospital.[5,6] Between a third and half of all mammalian bites occur in children.[7] Human bites are the most prevalent mammalian bites after those of dogs and cats, accounting for up to 2–3% of mammalian bites.[2,8]

AETIOLOGY/ RISK FACTORS In over 70% of cases, people are bitten by their own pets or by an animal known to them. Males are more likely to be bitten than females, and are more likely to be bitten by dogs, whereas females are more likely to be bitten by cats.[4] One study found that children under 5 years old were significantly more likely than older children to provoke animals before being bitten.[9] One study of infected dog and cat bites found that the most commonly isolated bacteria was *Pasteurella*, followed by *Streptococci*, *Staphylococci*, *Moraxella*, *Corynebacterium*, and *Neisseria*.[10] Mixed aerobic and anaerobic infection was more common than anaerobic infection alone. Human bites commonly occur in children as a result of fighting or playing. In adults, bites commonly occur during physical or sexual abuse.[8] Tooth abrasions to the knuckles (or "clenched fist injuries") can occur during fist fighting.[2]

PROGNOSIS In the USA, dog bites cause about 20 deaths a year.[11] In children, dog bites frequently involve the face, potentially resulting in severe lacerations and scarring.[12] Rabies, a life threatening viral encephalitis, may be contracted as a consequence of being bitten or scratched by a rabid animal. More than 99% of human rabies occurs in developing countries where canine rabies is endemic.[13] Transmission of rabies from domestic animals such as dogs and cats to humans is extremely rare in the USA, Europe, and Canada. The incidence of rabies

Bites (mammalian)

transmission in dog bites sustained in Africa, Southeast Asia, and India is significantly higher.[14] Human bites, particularly those to the hand, are often complicated by infection. One study reported infection in 48% of untreated bites to the hand.[8]

Please refer to clinicalevidence.com for full text and references.

Burns (minor thermal)

Search date January 2006

Jason Wasiak and Heather Cleland

What are the effects of treatments for minor thermal burns?

UNKNOWN EFFECTIVENESS

Alginate dressing *New*

We found no systematic reviews or RCTs examining the effects or harms of alginate dressing for minor thermal burns.

Antibiotics

We found no systematic reviews or RCTs comparing routine prophylactic use of topical or oral antibiotics versus placebo or no treatment for minor burns.

Chlorhexidine impregnated paraffin gauze dressing

We found no systematic reviews or RCTs comparing chlorhexidine impregnated paraffin gauze dressing versus placebo or no treatment for minor thermal burns. Two RCTs comparing chlorhexidine impregnated paraffin gauze versus hydrocolloid dressing found no significant difference in time to wound healing but, subjectively, both investigators and participants in one of the RCTs rated the hydrocolloid dressing more favourably. One RCT found that chlorhexidine impregnated paraffin gauze dressing decreased healing time slightly compared with hydrocolloid dressing plus silver sulfadiazine cream, but the significance of this difference was not assessed. One RCT found that chlorhexidine impregnated paraffin gauze dressing increased time to wound healing and was perceived as more painful compared with polyurethane film. One RCT found no significant difference between chlorhexidine impregnated tulle gras wide meshed gauze dressing and povidone iodine ointment impregnated rayon dressing in mean pain score. However, it found that a larger proportion of people required oral analgesia with chlorhexidine dressing compared with povidone iodine dressing. It found no significant difference between dressings in adherence to or bleeding from the wound.

Foam dressing *New*

We found no systematic reviews or RCTs examining the effects of foam dressing for minor thermal burns.

Hydrocolloid dressing

We found no systematic reviews or RCTs comparing hydrocolloid dressing versus placebo or no treatment for minor thermal burns. Two RCTs comparing hydrocolloid dressing versus chlorhexidine impregnated paraffin gauze dressing found no significant difference between treatments in time to wound healing but, subjectively, both investigators and participants in one of the RCTs rated the hydrocolloid dressing more favourably. One RCT found no significant difference in time to wound healing, pain, or interference with activities of daily living between hydrocolloid dressing and chlorhexidine impregnated paraffin gauze dressing plus silver sulfadiazine cream. One RCT found that hydrocolloid dressing reduced time to healing, pain, and limitation of activity compared with silver sulfadiazine cream. One RCT found that healing time was shorter with hydrocolloid dressing alone compared with hydrocolloid dressing plus silver sulfadiazine cream.

▶

Burns (minor thermal)

Hydrogel dressing *New*

We found no systematic reviews or RCTs examining the effects of hydrogel dressing for minor thermal burns.

Paraffin gauze dressing

We found no systematic reviews or RCTs comparing paraffin gauze dressing versus placebo or no treatment for minor thermal burns. One RCT comparing paraffin gauze versus polyurethane film found no significant difference in pain or time to wound healing.

Polyurethane film

We found no systematic reviews or RCTs comparing polyurethane film versus placebo or no treatment for minor thermal burns. One RCT, which compared polyurethane film versus paraffin gauze, found no significant difference in pain or time to wound healing. One RCT found that polyurethane film reduced time to wound healing and was perceived as less painful compared with chlorhexidine impregnated paraffin gauze.

Silicone coated nylon dressing

We found no systematic reviews or RCTs comparing silicone dressing coated nylon versus placebo or no treatment for minor thermal burns. Two RCTs in children found that silicone coated nylon dressing reduced time to wound healing compared with silver sulfadiazine cream covered by gauze dressing. One of the RCTs also found that silicone mesh dressing reduced pain compared with silver sulfadiazine cream in the first 5 days after burn injury.

LIKELY TO BE INEFFECTIVE OR HARMFUL

Silver sulfadiazine cream

We found no systematic reviews or RCTs comparing silver sulfadiazine cream versus placebo or no treatment for minor thermal burns. One RCT found that silver sulfadiazine cream increased time to healing, pain, and limitation of activity compared with hydrocolloid dressing. One RCT found that healing time was longer with hydrocolloid dressing plus silver sulfadiazine cream compared with hydrocolloid dressing alone. Two RCTs in children found that silver sulfadiazine cream covered by gauze dressing increased time to wound healing compared with silicone coated nylon dressing. One of the RCTs also found that silver sulfadiazine cream increased pain compared with silicone mesh dressing in the first 5 days after burn injury. One RCT comparing a combination of chlorhexidine impregnated paraffin gauze dressing plus silver sulfadiazine cream versus hydrocolloid dressing found no significant difference in time to wound healing, pain levels, or interference with activities of daily living.

DEFINITION Burn depth is classified as erythema (first degree) involving the epidermis only, superficial partial thickness (second degree) involving the epidermis and upper dermis, deep partial thickness (second degree) involving the epidermis and dermis, and full thickness burns (third degree) involving the epidermis, dermis, and damage to appendages. This chapter deals with minor thermal burns – that is, superficial partial thickness burns that do not involve the hands or face. Superficial partial thickness burns are caused by exposure to heat sufficient to cause damage to the epidermis and papillary dermis of the skin. They are characterised by pain and hypersensitivity. The skin seems moist and pink or red, and is perfused, as demonstrated by blanching on pressure. This type of injury will blister within hours and heal within 2–3 weeks with minimal scarring if no infection is present. The severity of a superficial partial thickness burn is usually judged by the percentage of total body surface area involved: less than 15% total body surface area for adults and 10% total body surface area for children.

INCIDENCE/ PREVALENCE The incidence of minor thermal burns is difficult to estimate. Generally, less than 5% of all burn injuries requiring treatment will necessitate admission to hospital.[1] Worldwide estimates surrounding all thermal burn injuries suggest that about two million people are burned, up to 80 000 are hospitalised, and 6500 die of burn wounds every year.[1]

AETIOLOGY/ RISK FACTORS The pattern of injury varies among different age groups. Males aged 18–25 years seem more susceptible to injury owing to a variety of causes — mainly flame, electrical, and, to a lesser extent, chemicals.[2] Many burn injuries in this age group are due to the inappropriate use of flammable agents such as petrol. However, most burns occur in the home. Thermal burns, in particular scalds, are common among the young as well as the elderly. The kitchen is reported to be the most common place of injury for children, as is the bathroom for the elderly. Those with concomitant conditions or complicating factors such as motor or neurological impairment are at greater risk.

PROGNOSIS Superficial partial thickness burns will heal spontaneously with minimal hypertrophic scarring within 2–3 weeks if the wound remains free of infection.[3] The capacity to heal is also dependent on the health and age of the individual, with the elderly and those with concomitant medical conditions prone to delayed healing. Cooling the burn, as part of the initial emergency treatment, significantly reduces pain and wound oedema if started within 3 hours of injury.[2] The optimal time to cool a wound may vary from 20–30 minutes using tap water (at a temperature of 5–25 °C).[4] Use of iced water or prolonged periods of cooling can deepen tissue injury, induce hypothermia, and are best avoided.[3] Cleaning solutions and dressings aim to prevent wound infection. The ideal dressing will establish an optimum microenvironment for wound healing. It will maintain the wound temperature and moisture level, permit respiration, allow epithelial migration,[5] and exclude environmental bacteria.

Please refer to clinicalevidence.com for full text and references.

Pressure ulcers

Search date February 2006

Nicky Cullum and Emily Petherick

What are the effects of preventive interventions in people at risk of developing pressure ulcers?

BENEFICIAL

Foam alternatives (compared with standard foam mattresses)

One systematic review found that foam alternatives to the standard hospital foam mattress reduced the incidence of pressure ulcers over 10–14 days in people at high risk. A subsequent RCT found that 4 hourly repositioning on a viscoelastic foam mattress reduced the incidence of pressure ulcers compared with standard care. It found no significant difference between 2 or 3 hourly repositioning on a standard hospital mattress or 6 hourly repositioning on a viscoelastic foam mattress and standard care. We found no clear evidence of a "best" foam alternative.

Pressure relieving overlays on operating tables (compared with standard tables)

Three RCTs identified by a systematic review found that pressure relieving overlays on operating tables reduced the incidence of pressure ulcers compared with standard tables. However, a fourth RCT identified by the review found that more people developed ulcers when a foam overlay was used on an operating table compared with standard care.

LIKELY TO BE BENEFICIAL

Low air loss beds in intensive care (more effective than standard beds; effects relative to alternating pressure mattresses unclear)

One RCT in people in intensive care found that low air loss beds reduced the risk of new pressure ulcers compared with standard intensive care beds. One small RCT found no significant difference in the risk of pressure ulcer development using low air loss beds compared with an alternating pressure mattress.

Medical sheepskin overlays (compared with standard care)

Two RCTs found that medical sheepskin overlays reduced the incidence of pressure ulcers compared with standard treatment in people in hospital aged over 18 years at risk of pressure ulcers.

UNKNOWN EFFECTIVENESS

Alternating pressure surfaces (compared with standard foam mattress or constant low pressure supports)

Two small RCTs found that alternating pressure mattresses reduced pressure ulcers compared with a standard foam mattress. However, one of these RCTs had flawed methods. One systematic review found no significant difference between alternating pressure devices and constant low pressure mattresses in the incidence of pressure ulcers. However, the meta-analysis performed by the review may have been underpowered to detect a clinically important difference. One subsequent RCT also found no significant difference in pressure ulcer ▶

incidence between alternating pressure overlays and viscoelastic foam mattresses. Three small RCTs identified by the systematic review comparing alternating pressure surfaces versus each other found no significant difference between them. However, all were underpowered to detect clinically important differences.

Different seat cushions

Three underpowered RCTs identified by a systematic review provided insufficient evidence about the effects of different seat cushions in preventing pressure ulcers.

Electric profiling beds

One RCT identified by a systematic review provided insufficient evidence about the effects of electric profiling beds in preventing pressure ulcers.

Hydrocellular heel supports (compared with orthopaedic wool padding)

One RCT found that hydrocellular heel supports reduced the development of pressure ulcers compared with orthopaedic wool padding.

Low tech constant low pressure supports

Weak RCTs identified by a systematic review provided insufficient evidence about the effects of low tech constant low pressure supports in preventing pressure ulcers.

Nutritional supplements (New)

One systematic review found insufficient evidence from RCTs with flawed methods about the effects of nutritional supplements for preventing pressure ulcers.

Repositioning (regular "turning")

One systematic review provided insufficient evidence about the effects of repositioning (regular "turning") in preventing pressure ulcers. A subsequent RCT found that 4 hourly repositioning on a viscoelastic foam mattress reduced the incidence of pressure ulcers compared with 2 or 3 hourly repositioning on a standard hospital mattress or 6 hourly repositioning on a viscoelastic foam mattress, or standard care. It found no significant difference between standard care and 2 or 3 hourly repositioning on a standard hospital mattress or 6 hourly repositioning on a viscoelastic foam mattress.

Topical lotions and dressings

One systematic review provided insufficient evidence about the effects topical lotions or dressings in preventing pressure ulcers. One subsequent double blind RCT found that a compound of eight different fatty acids applied topically twice daily to pressure areas reduced pressure ulcer incidence compared with a topical placebo preparation in people at medium to very high risk of pressure ulcers.

LIKELY TO BE INEFFECTIVE OR HARMFUL

Air filled vinyl boots

One small RCT identified by a systematic review found that air filled vinyl boots with foot cradles were associated with more rapid development of pressure ulcers compared with hospital pillows.

Pressure ulcers

Low air loss hydrotherapy beds (compared with other pressure relieving surfaces)

One small RCT found a non-significant trend towards an increased the risk of developing a pressure ulcer with low air loss hydrotherapy beds compared with a range of support surfaces in people with incontinence. The RCT was likely to have been underpowered to detect a clinically significant difference between groups.

What are the effects of treatments in people with pressure ulcers?

LIKELY TO BE BENEFICIAL

Air fluidised supports (compared with standard care)

Two RCTs found that air fluidised supports reduced pressure ulcers after 15 days compared with standard care. One RCT with weak methods found no significant difference between air fluidised supports and standard care.

Hydrocolloid dressings (compared with standard dressings)

One systematic review and two other RCTs provided limited evidence that hydrocolloid dressings improved ulcer healing at up to 12 weeks compared with standard dressings (gauze soaked in saline, hypochlorite, or povidone iodine). One additional RCT found no significant difference between hydrocolloid dressings and standard dressings in ulcer healing. Systematic reviews and RCTs provided insufficient evidence to compare hydrocolloid dressings versus dressings other than standard dressings or topical phenytoin.

UNKNOWN EFFECTIVENESS

Alternating pressure surfaces

RCTs identified by a systematic review provided insufficient evidence on the effects of alternating pressure surfaces in healing pressure ulcers.

Debridement

RCTs provided insufficient evidence to compare effects of different debriding agents on healing of pressure ulcers.

Dressings other than hydrocolloid

Small, methodologically weak RCTs provided insufficient evidence about the effects of dressings other than hydrocolloid in people with pressure ulcers.

Electrotherapy

Three RCTs found limited evidence that electrotherapy increased healing compared with sham treatment, however, one RCT found no significant difference in healing between electrotherapy and sham treatment. However, the RCTs were small and of limited quality, and their results may therefore be unreliable.

Low air loss beds

Small RCTs identified by a systematic review provided insufficient evidence on the effects of low air loss beds in healing pressure ulcers.

Low level laser therapy

Five RCTs provided insufficient evidence about the effects of low level laser therapy on healing of pressure ulcers.

Low tech constant low pressure supports

One RCT identified by a systematic review provided insufficient evidence on the effects of low tech constant low pressure supports in healing pressure ulcers.

Nutritional supplements

Four RCTs identified by a systematic review found no significant difference in healing between nutritional supplements and control interventions (low dose or no supplements). However, studies were small and may have lacked power to detect clinically important differences between treatments. A subsequent small RCT found improved wound healing scores when a standard hospital diet was supplemented by calories, protein, vitamin C, zinc, and arginine compared with an alternative supplement, or a standard hospital diet alone.

Seat cushions

Two RCTs provided insufficient evidence to assess the effects of seat cushions in healing pressure ulcers.

Surgery

We found no systematic review or RCTs of surgical treatments for pressure ulcers.

Therapeutic ultrasound

One systematic review of two RCTs found no significant difference in healing between ultrasound and sham ultrasound.

Topical negative pressure

Two systematic reviews provided insufficient evidence about the effects of topical negative pressure on healing of pressure ulcers.

Topical phenytoin

Two small RCTs provided insufficient evidence about the effects of topical phenytoin on healing of pressure ulcers.

DEFINITION Pressure ulcers (also known as pressure sores, bed sores, and decubitus ulcers) may present as persistently hyperaemic, blistered, broken, or necrotic skin and may extend to underlying structures, including muscle and bone. Pressure ulcers are usually graded on a scale of 1 to 4, with a higher grade indicating greater ulcer severity.[1]

INCIDENCE/ PREVALENCE Reported prevalence rates range between 4.7% and 32.1% for hospital populations, between 4.4% and 33.0% for community care populations, and between 4.6% and 20.7% for nursing home populations.[2]

AETIOLOGY/ RISK FACTORS Pressure ulcers are caused by unrelieved pressure, shear, or friction. They are most common below the waist and at bony prominences, such as the sacrum, heels, and hips. They occur in all healthcare settings. Increased age, reduced mobility, impaired nutrition, vascular disease, faecal incontinence, and skin condition at baseline consistently emerge as risk factors.[3,4] However, the relative importance of these and other factors is uncertain.

PROGNOSIS There are little data on untreated prognosis of pressure ulcers. The presence of pressure ulcers has been associated with a twofold to fourfold increased risk of death in elderly people and people in intensive care.[5,6] However, pressure ulcers are a marker for underlying disease severity and other comorbidities rather than an independent predictor of mortality.[5]

Please refer to clinicalevidence.com for full text and references.

Venous leg ulcers

Search date July 2005

E Andrea Nelson, Nicky Cullum, and June Jones

What are the effects of treatments?

BENEFICIAL

Compression bandages and stockings

One systematic review and one additional RCT found that compression bandages or stockings healed more venous leg ulcers than no compression. One systematic review and one subsequent RCT found insufficient evidence to suggest a difference between multilayer elastomeric and non-elastomeric high compression bandages. One systematic review and five subsequent RCTs found no significant difference in healing rates between multilayer elastomeric high compression bandages and short stretch bandages or Unna's boot. One systematic review found that multilayer compression increased ulcer healing compared with single layer bandages. One systematic review and three subsequent RCTs found no significant difference in the proportion of people healed with four layer elastomeric bandages compared with other high compression multilayer bandages. One RCT found no significant difference in healing rates between a non-elastic legging and Unna's boot. One RCT found no significant difference in healing between a short stretch bandage and a stocking system (see comment). We found insufficient evidence from one small RCT about the effects of compression bandages compared with intermittent pneumatic compression.

Oral pentoxifylline

One systematic review and two subsequent RCTs found that oral pentoxifylline increased the proportion of ulcers healed over 6–12 months compared with placebo.

LIKELY TO BE BENEFICIAL

Cultured allogenic bilayer skin replacement

Two RCTs found that cultured allogenic bilayer skin replacement increased the proportion of ulcers healed after 6 months compared with a non-adherent dressing.

Oral flavonoids

Two RCTs found that adding flavonoids to compression increased the proportion of ulcers healed after 2–6 months compared with compression alone.

Oral sulodexide

Three RCTs found that sulodexide plus compression increased the proportion of ulcers healed after 2–3 months' treatment compared with compression alone.

Peri-ulcer injection of granulocyte-macrophage colony stimulating factor

One RCT found that peri-ulcer injection of granulocyte-macrophage colony stimulating factor increased the proportion of ulcers healed after 13 weeks' treatment compared with placebo.

Systemic mesoglycan

One RCT found that systemic mesoglycan plus compression increased the proportion of ulcers healed after 24 weeks' treatment compared with compression alone.

UNKNOWN EFFECTIVENESS

Cultured allogenic single layer dermal replacement

One RCT compared 12, four, or one piece of human dermal replacement plus compression versus compression alone. It found no difference between treatments in the number of ulcers healed at 12 weeks. However this RCT may have been too small to detect anything but a very large difference in effectiveness.

Debriding agents

One systematic review of small RCTs provided insufficient evidence about the effects of debriding agents on ulcer healing.

Foam, film, hyaluronic acid-derived dressings, or alginate (semi-occlusive) dressings

One systematic review provided insufficient evidence to compare the effects of semi-occlusive dressings (foam, film, hyaluronic acid-derived, or alginate) versus simple low adherent dressings, in the presence of compression. One systematic review and four subsequent RCTs found no significant difference in healing rates between semi-occlusive and occlusive dressings.

Intermittent pneumatic compression

One small RCT found insufficient evidence to compare intermittent pneumatic compression with compression bandages or stockings. One RCT found that intermittent pneumatic compression plus compression stockings improved ulcer healing at 3 months compared with compression stockings alone. Two other RCTs found no significant difference in healing at 6 months between intermittent pneumatic compression plus elastic stockings and Unna's boot, and between intermittent pneumatic compression plus Unna's boot and Unna's boot alone.

Laser treatment (low level)

RCTs provided insufficient evidence about the effects of low level laser on ulcer healing.

Oral aspirin

One RCT provided insufficient evidence about the effects of oral aspirin on ulcer healing.

Oral rutosides

RCTs provided insufficient evidence about the effects of oral rutosides on ulcer healing.

Oral thromboxane alpha$_2$ antagonists

One RCT provided insufficient evidence about the effects of oral thromboxane alpha$_2$ antagonists on ulcer healing.

Oral zinc

RCTs provided no evidence that oral zinc improved ulcer healing.

Platelet derived growth factor

Two RCTs provided insufficient evidence to compare the effects of recombinant human derived platelet derived growth factor versus placebo for ulcer healing.

Skin grafting

RCTs provided insufficient evidence about the effects of skin grafting on ulcer healing.

Venous leg ulcers

Superficial vein surgery

Three RCTs found no evidence of a benefit associated with superficial vein surgery for ulcer healing. One systematic review identified one RCT which compared two forms of surgery. It found no difference between open surgery and endoscopic surgery in healing rates, but it found that higher rates of infection were associated with open surgery.

Therapeutic ultrasound

RCTs provided limited evidence of benefit about the effects of therapeutic ultrasound on ulcer healing.

Topical antimicrobial agents

RCTs provided insufficient evidence about the effects of topical antimicrobial agents on ulcer healing.

Topical calcitonin gene related peptide plus vasoactive intestinal polypeptide

One RCT provided insufficient evidence about the effects of topical calcitonin gene related peptide plus vasoactive intestinal polypeptide on ulcer healing.

Topical mesoglycan

One RCT provided insufficient evidence about the effects of topical mesoglycan on ulcer healing.

Topical negative pressure

One systematic review provided insufficient evidence about the effects of topical negative pressure on ulcer healing.

Topical recombinant keratinocyte growth factor 2

One RCT provided insufficient evidence about the effects of topical recombinant keratinocyte growth factor 2 on ulcer healing.

UNLIKELY TO BE BENEFICIAL

Freeze dried keratinocyte lysate

One RCT found no significant difference in the proportion of people with healed ulcers after 24 weeks of compared with vehicle or standard care.

Hydrocolloid (occlusive) dressings in the presence of compression

One systematic review found that, in the presence of compression, hydrocolloid dressings did not heal more venous leg ulcers than simple, low adherent dressings. One systematic review and four subsequent RCTs found no significant difference in healing rates between occlusive and semi-occlusive dressings.

Topically applied autologous platelet lysate

One RCT found no significant difference in the proportion of people with healed ulcers after 9 months between topically applied autologous platelet lysate compared with placebo.

What are the effects of interventions to prevent recurrence?

BENEFICIAL

Compression stockings

One RCT found that compression stockings reduced recurrence at 6 months compared with no compression, and that non-compliance with compression is a risk factor for recurrence.

LIKELY TO BE BENEFICIAL

Superficial vein surgery

Three RCTs provided evidence that superficial vein surgery with or without compression reduced recurrence compared with compression alone. One RCT compared open versus endoscopic surgery and found fewer recurrences in the endoscopic surgery group and higher infection rates with open surgery. Vein surgery has the usual risks of surgery and anaesthesia.

UNKNOWN EFFECTIVENESS

Oral rutoside

One RCT identified by a systematic review provided insufficient evidence on the effects of oral rutoside compared with placebo on ulcer recurrence.

Oral stanozolol

One RCT identified by a systematic review provided insufficient evidence on the effects of oral stanozolol compared with placebo on ulcer recurrence.

DEFINITION Definitions of leg ulcers vary, but the following is widely used: loss of skin on the leg or foot that takes more than 6 weeks to heal. Some definitions exclude ulcers confined to the foot, whereas others include ulcers on the whole of the lower limb. This review deals with ulcers of venous origin in people without concurrent diabetes mellitus, arterial insufficiency, or rheumatoid arthritis.

INCIDENCE/ PREVALENCE Between 1.5 and 3.0/1000 people have active leg ulcers. Prevalence increases with age to about 20/1000 in people aged over 80 years.[1]

AETIOLOGY/ RISK FACTORS Leg ulceration is strongly associated with venous disease. However, about a fifth of people with leg ulceration have arterial disease, either alone or in combination with venous problems, which may require specialist referral.[1] Venous ulcers (also known as varicose or stasis ulcers) are caused by venous reflux or obstruction, both of which lead to poor venous return and venous hypertension.

PROGNOSIS People with leg ulcers have a poorer quality of life than age matched controls because of pain, odour, and reduced mobility.[2] In the UK, audits have found wide variation in the types of care (hospital inpatient care, hospital clinics, outpatient clinics, home visits), in the treatments used (topical agents, dressings, bandages, stockings), in healing rates and recurrence rates (26–69% in 1 year).[3,4]

Please refer to clinicalevidence.com for full text and references.

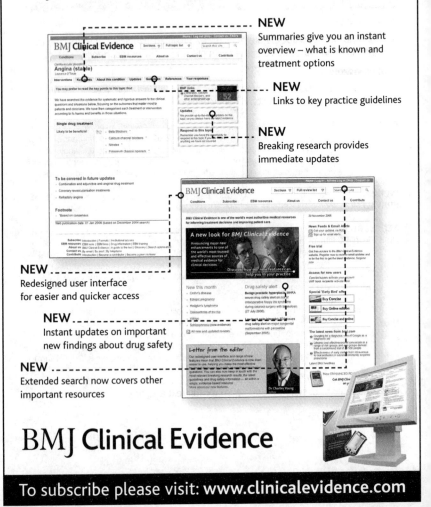

Note

When looking up a class of drug, the reader is advised to also look up specific examples of that class of drug where additional entries may be found. The reverse situation also applies.

Index

Subject index

Subject index

Subject index

Subject index

Subject index

Subject index

Subject index

Subject index

Subject index

Subject index

Subject index

Subject index

Subject index

BMJ Clinical evidence concise comments

BMJ Clinical Evidence Concise is an evolving resource and we welcome any feedback on the content of this issue and suggestions for future issues.

Please photocopy and complete this form, then return it to us.

For UK and rest of world - Fax: + 44 (0) 20 7383 6242, mail: BMJ Clinical Evidence Concise, BMJ Publishing Group, BMA House, Tavistock Square, London WC1H 9JR, UK

For North and South America - Fax: 1-240-646-7005, mail: BMJ Clinical Evidence Concise, PO Box 512, Annapolis Jct, MD20701-0512, USA

Alternatively, email us at CEfeedback@bmjgroup.com

Name: ....

Address: ....

....

....Email: ....

Position

- ☐ GP/Primary Care Physician
- ☐ Hospital Doctor/ Specialist Physician
- ☐ Pharmacist
- ☐ Resident/Registrar
- ☐ Nurse
- ☐ PAM
- ☐ Manager
- ☐ Press
- ☐ Researcher
- ☐ Administrator
- ☐ Librarian
- ☐ Medical Student
- ☐ Member of Public/ Patient Support Group
- ☐ Other..................

1. Comments concerning the selection of studies

Section..

Topic ....

Reference ....

Comment..

....

....

2. Suggestions for future issues

....

....

....

3. Other comments/questions

....

....

....

Approaches to primary prevention

Written by Stacey Sheridan, Assistant Professor of Medicine, University of North Carolina, USA.

Coronary heart disease (CHD) is a major cause of mortality throughout the world; it is responsible for 13% of deaths worldwide.[1] It is also a leading cause of disability and is responsible for a growing proportion of health care costs. Most of the burden of heart disease can be attributed to several risk factors, including increasing age, male sex, increasing blood pressure, increasing serum cholesterol, smoking, diabetes, and left ventricular hypertrophy.[2] Importantly, if an individual's exposure to these risk factors can be reduced, the risk of subsequent CHD deaths can also be reduced.

In the past, guidelines focused on assessment and treatment of individual risk factors. More recently, it has become apparent that it is better to assess and base treatment decisions on estimates of an individual's overall (or global) risk of CHD events. Global CHD risk assesses the combined effect of exposure to all relevant risk factors.[3] Using global CHD risk, as opposed to an individual risk factor based approach, has several advantages: it mitigates against clinicians' and patients' tendency to watch rather than treat small elevations in one or more risk factors;[4,5] it helps physicians and patients balance the intensity of treatment with the safety, cost, and time commitment necessary for treatment;[6] and it has been shown to be more cost effective in guiding CHD intervention decisions than a risk factor based approach.[7]

Global CHD risk can be calculated from multivariate statistical equations that have been derived from large prospective cohort studies or randomised trials.[8–14] These equations estimate a person's risk of having a CHD event over 5–10 years after input of relevant risk factor information. One popular and well validated risk equation has been derived from the Framingham Heart Study.[14] It has been used in several clinical risk tools (e.g. the Framingham risk tables, the New Zealand risk tables, the modified Sheffield tables, the Joint British Societies risk prediction charts, the Joint European Societies risk prediction charts, the Canadian risk nomogram, the BMJ Cardio Risk Manager, the National Cholesterol Education Program risk calculator, and the American Heart Association's risk calculator). These tools predict the degree of risk well in white and African-American men and women aged 30-65 years in the US, the UK, Northern Europe, Australia and Israel. They predict risk less well in men and women aged younger than 30 years or older than 65 years, diabetic persons, other ethnic populations in the US (e.g. Japanese men, Hispanic men, and Native American Women),[15–17] and Southern European populations.[11,18] As such, Framingham risk tools should be used with caution in these groups. In southern European populations, clinicians should consider risk tools derived from the Seven Countries Study, the Italian Rural Areas Study, or the Rome Occupational Group.[11,12,18,19] However, these tools also have limitations. For example, they include relatively few risk factors, are derived from truncated middle aged or male only populations, and have been prospectively validated in limited populations.

Most tools provide information on the combined risk of stable and unstable angina, myocardial infarction, and CHD death. However, some tools report only the risk of myocardial infarction and CHD death; these tools will produce smaller numeric estimates of risk than tools that also include angina. A few tools also predict risk of stroke. When using CHD risk tools for clinical decision making, the user must remember that these tools do not account for the non-cardiovascular benefits of treatment. As such, they cannot be used as the sole basis for decision making about whether or not to recommend smoking cessation, exercise, diet or hypertension treatment, because these treatments have multiple potential benefits apart from their effect on cardiovascular disease.

In choosing which risk tool to use, providers should choose tools that are readily available and easy for them to use. Providers may also wish to consider their practice environment and who will be performing the risk assessments. Providers who have access to a computer with an available spreadsheet program or dedicated internet access should consider spreadsheet and web based programs for risk calculation.[19,20] These tools allow calculation of fine gradations of risk and frequently provide comparisons to individuals with low risk. Some providers may find that a combination of products is most useful, particularly if the outcome of interest varies according to patient concerns.

Providers may also wish to choose tools that provide risk information in a format that can be used with current guidelines for risk reduction.[20] For instance, to allow risk based decision making about lipid lowering treatment in the US, providers need a tool that allows stratification of risk into less than 10%, 10–20%, and greater than 20%.[21] To adhere to evidence based guidelines on aspirin use, providers need a tool with finer gradations of risk because the risk : benefit ratio for aspirin use transitions from helpful to harmful at a 10 year risk of CHD events between 3–5% and 10%.[22]

At present it is unclear how providers should address risk calculation in people with diabetes. The National Cholesterol Education Program and the American Heart Association currently recommend that physicians treat people with diabetes as though they have a risk for subsequent CHD events that is equivalent to that in people with known CHD.[21,23] In accordance with this, they have recommended that their Framingham risk calculators be used only in people without diabetes. However, many persons with diabetes, particularly young women, will have a risk much lower than 20% over 10 years. Whether treating all diabetic people as having high risk is superior, equal, or inferior to individualised assessment has not been studied.

In addition to choosing which type of risk tool to use, providers must assure that they have sufficient information to complete the risk assessment. Some information, such as age, smoking status, and presence or absence of diabetes can be obtained by interview at the time the risk calculation is performed. Other information, such as blood pressure, cholesterol levels, and presence or absence of left ventricular hypertrophy on electrocardiogram must be obtained before risk calculation.

Table 1 provides links to Framingham calculators that may be useful in clinical practice. No easy to use paper based or web based calculators derived from the Seven Countries Study, the Italian Rural Areas Study, or the Rome Occupational Group were identified.

TABLE 1 Predicted outcomes in a selected sample of available Framingham risk calculators

Calculators that predict total† CHD events:
Framingham Risk Tables[14,24]
Modified Sheffield Tables[25]
Stat Cardiac Risk[26]
Heart-to-Heart[27]
Calculators that predict hard* events:
Joint British Societies Risk Prediction Charts[28]
National Cholesterol Education Program[29]
American Heart Association[30]

†Total events = stable and unstable angina, myocardial infarction and death; *hard events = myocardial infarction and death

REFERENCES

1. The World Health Report, 2000. Health Systems-Improving Performance. WHO.
2. Greenland P, Knoll MD, Stamler J, et al. Major risk factors as antecedents of fatal and nonfatal coronary heart disease events. *JAMA* 2003;290:891–897.
3. Jackson R, Lawes C, Bennett D, et al. Treatment with drugs to lower blood pressure and blood cholesterol based on an individual's absolute cardiovascular risk. *Lancet* 2005;365:434–441.
4. Phillips LS, Branch WT, Cook CB, et al. Clinical inertia. *Ann Intern Med* 2001; 135:825–834.
5. Oliveria SA, Lapuerta P, McCarthy BD, et al. Physician-related barriers to the effective management of uncontrolled hypertension. *Arch Intern Med* 2002; 162:413–420.
6. Pearson 2003. New tools for coronary risk assessment: what are their advantages and limitations? *Circulation* 2002;105:886–892.
7. Murray CJ, Lauer JA, Hutubessy RC, et al. Effectiveness and costs of interventions to lower systolic blood pressure and cholesterol: a global and regional analysis on reduction of cardiovascular-disease risk. *Lancet* 2003;361: 717–725.
8. Assmann G, Cullen P, Schulte H. Simple scoring scheme for calculating the risk of acute coronary events based on the 10-year follow-up of the prospective cardiovascular Munster (PROCAM) study. *Circulation* 2002;105:310–315. [Erratum in: *Circulation* 2002;105:900].
9. Tunstall-Pedoe H. The Dundee coronary risk-disk for management of change in risk factors. *BMJ* 1991;303:744–747.
10. ERICA Research Group. Prediction of coronary heart disease in Europe. The 2nd report of the WHO-ERICA Project. *Eur Heart J* 1991;12:291–297.
11. Menotti A, Lanti M, Puddu PE, et al. Coronary heart disease incidence in Northern and Southern European populations: a reanalysis of the seven countries study for a European coronary risk chart. *Heart* 2000;84:238–244.
12. Menotti A, Spagnolo A, Dima F, et al. The prediction of coronary heart disease in different population samples. *Eur J Epidemiol* 1992;8:516–521.
13. Simons LA, Simons J, Friedlander Y, et al. Risk functions for prediction of cardiovascular disease in the elderly Australians: the Dubbo Study. *Med J Aust* 2003;178:113–116.
14. Wilson PW, D'Agostino RB, Levy D, et al. Prediction of coronary heart disease using risk factor categories. *Circulation* 1998;97:1837–1847.
15. Liao Y, McGee DL, Cooper RS, et al. How generalizable are coronary risk prediction models? Comparison of Framingham and two national cohorts. *Am Heart J* 1999;137:837–845.
16. Grundy SM, D'Agostino RB Sr, Mosca L, et al. Cardiovascular risk assessment based on US cohort studies: findings from a National Heart, Lung, and Blood institute workshop. *Circulation* 2001;104:491–496.
17. D'Agostino RB Sr, Grundy S, Sullivan LM, et al. Validation of the Framingham coronary heart disease prediction scores: results of a multiple ethnic groups investigation. *JAMA* 2001;286:180–187.
18. Menotti A, Puddu PE, Lanti M. Comparison of the Framingham risk function-based coronary chart with risk function from an Italian population study. *Eur Heart J* 2000;21:365–370.
19. Menotti A, Puddu PE, Lanti M. The estimate of cardiovascular risk. Theory, tools and problems. *Ann Ital Med Int* 2002:17:81–94.

20. Sheridan S, Pignone M, Mulrow C. Framingham-based tools to measure global risk of coronary heart disease: a systematic review of tools for clinicians. *J Gen Intern Med* 2003;18:1039–1052.

21. Expert Panel on Detection, Evaluation, and Treatment of High Blood Cholesterol in Adults. Executive summary of the third report of the National Cholesterol Education Program (NCEP) Expert Panel on Detection, Evaluation, and Treatment of High Blood Cholesterol in Adults (Adult Treatment Panel III). *JAMA* 2001;285:2486–2497.

22. Hayden M, Pignone M, Phillips C, et al. Aspirin for the primary prevention of cardiovascular events: a summary of the evidence for the U.S. Preventive Services Task Force. *Ann Intern Med* 2002;136:161–172.

23. Grundy SM, Pasternak R, Greenland P, et al. Assessment of cardiovascular risk by use of multiple-risk-factor assessment equations: a statement for healthcare professionals from the American Heart Association and the American College of Cardiology. *Circulation* 1999;100:1481–1492.

24. www.nhlbi.nih.gov/about/framingham/risktmen.pdf (last accessed 5 July 2005).

25. Wallis EJ, Ramsay LE, Ul Haq I, et al. Coronary and cardiovascular risk estimation for primary prevention: validation of a new Sheffield table in the 1995 Scottish health survey population. *BMJ* 2000;320:671–676. [Erratum in: BMJ 2000;320:1034].

26. www.statcoder.com (last accessed 5 July 2005).

27. www.med-decision.com (last accessed 5 July 2005).

28. www.hyp.ac.uk/bhs/riskview/resources_prediction_chart.htm (last accessed 5 July 2005).

29. www.nhlbi.nih.gov/guidelines/cholesterol/index.htm (last accessed 5 July 2005).

30. www.americanheart.org (last accessed 5 July 2005).

Estimating cardiovascular risk and treatment benefit

Adapted from the New Zealand guidelines on management of dyslipidaemia[1] and raised blood pressure[2] by Rod Jackson

How to use these colour charts

The charts help the estimation of a person's absolute risk of a cardiovascular event and the likely benefit of drug treatment to lower cholesterol or blood pressure. For these charts, cardiovascular events include: myocardial infarction, new angina, ischaemic stroke, transient ischaemic attack, peripheral vascular disease, congestive heart failure, and cardiovascular-related death.

There is a group of patients in whom risk can be assumed to be high (>20% in 5 years) without using the charts. They include those with symptomatic cardiovascular disease (angina, myocardial infarction, congestive heart failure, stroke, TIA, and peripheral vascular disease), or left ventricular hypertrophy on ECG.

To estimate a person's absolute 5 year risk:

- Find the table relating to their sex, diabetic status (on insulin, oral hypoglycaemics, or fasting blood glucose over 8 mmol/L), smoking status, and age. The age shown in the charts is the mean for that category, i.e. age 60 = 55 to 65 years.
- Within the table find the cell nearest to the person's blood pressure and total cholesterol : HDL ratio. For risk assessment it is enough to use a mean blood pressure based on two readings on each of two occasions, and cholesterol measurements based on one laboratory or two non-fasting Reflotron measurements. More readings are needed to establish the pre-treatment baseline. When the systolic and diastolic values fall in different risk levels, the higher category applies.
- The colour of the box indicates the person's 5 year cardiovascular disease risk (see below).

RISK LEVEL
5 year CVD risk
(non-fatal and fatal)

Very High	>30%
	25–30%
	20–25%
High	15–20%
Moderate	10–15%
Mild	5–10%
	2.5–5%
	<2.5%

Notes: (1) People with a strong history of CVD (first degree male relatives with CVD before 55 years, female relatives before 65 years) or obesity (body mass index above 30 kg/m^2) are likely to be at greater risk than the tables indicate. The magnitude of the independent predictive value of these risk factors remains unclear — their presence should influence treatment decisions for patients at borderline treatment levels. (2) If total cholesterol or total cholesterol : HDL ratio is greater than 8 then the risk is at least 15%. (3) Nearly all people aged 75 years or over also have an absolute cardiovascular risk over 15%.

Charts reproduced with permission from The National Heart Foundation of New Zealand. Also available on http://www.nzgg.org.nz/guidelines/0035/CVD_Risk_Full.pdf

REFERENCES

1. Dyslipidaemia Advisory Group. 1996 National Heart Foundation clinical guidelines for the assessment and management of dyslipidaemia. *NZ Med J* 1996;109:224–232.
2. National Health Committee. Guidelines for the management of mildly raised blood pressure in New Zealand: Ministry of Health National Health Committee Report, Wellington, 1995.

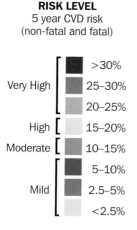

Estimating cardiovascular risk and treatment benefit

RISK LEVEL: MEN

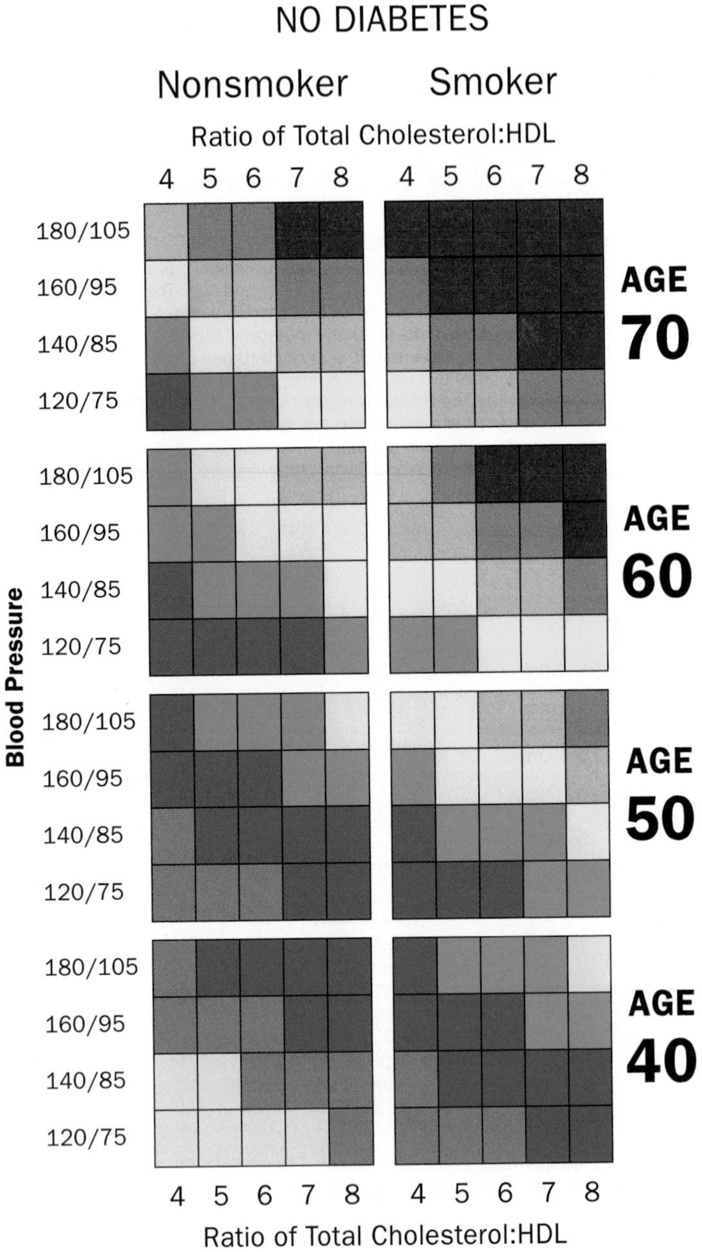

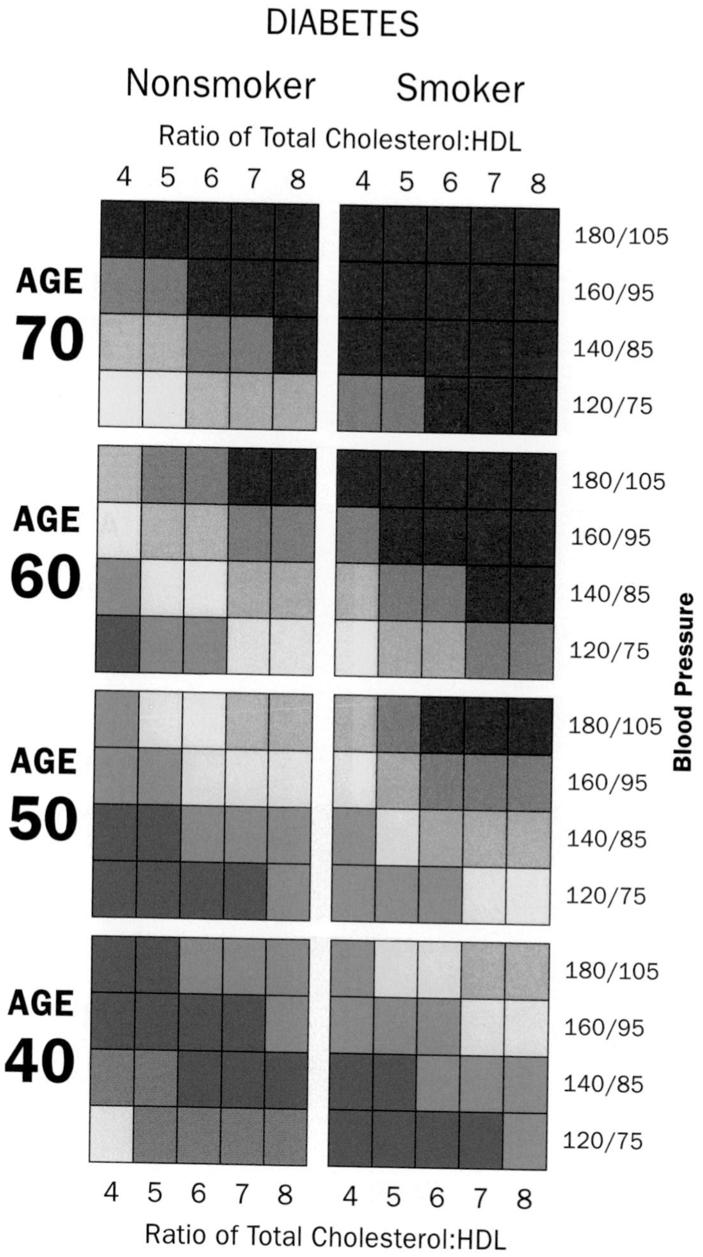
DIABETES
Nonsmoker
Smoker
Ratio of Total Cholesterol:HDL
4 5 6 7 8 4 5 6 7 8
AGE 70
AGE 60
AGE 50
AGE 40
180/105
160/95
140/85
120/75
Blood Pressure
4 5 6 7 8 4 5 6 7 8
Ratio of Total Cholesterol:HDL

Estimating cardiovascular risk and treatment benefit

RISK LEVEL: WOMEN

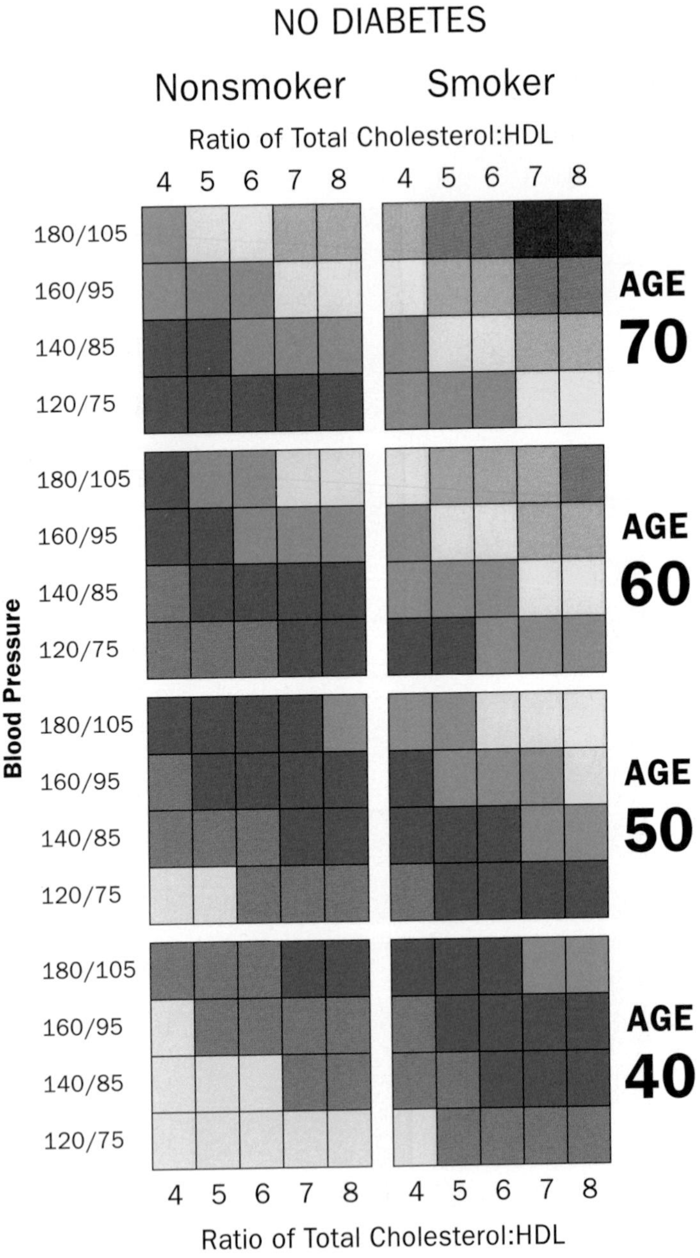

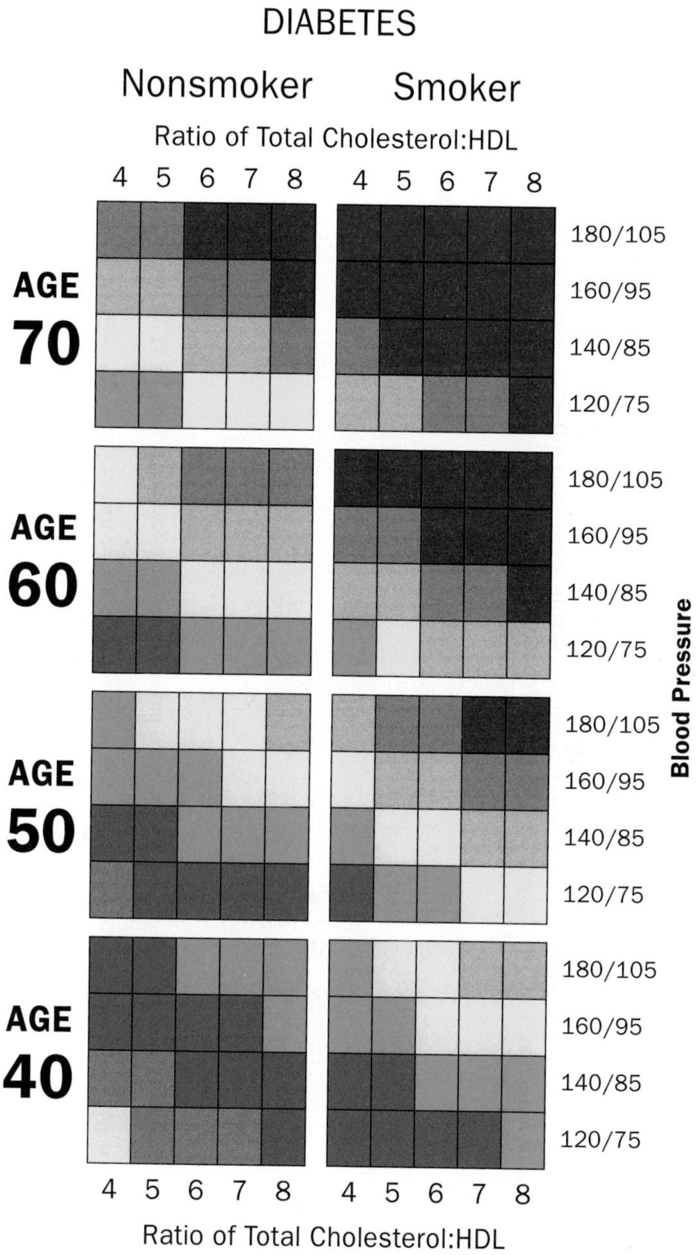
DIABETES
Nonsmoker
Smoker
Ratio of Total Cholesterol:HDL
4 5 6 7 8
4 5 6 7 8
AGE 70
AGE 60
AGE 50
AGE 40
180/105
160/95
140/85
120/75
Blood Pressure
Ratio of Total Cholesterol:HDL

Appendix 2

Estimating cardiovascular risk and treatment benefit

Mid-range value	Benefit CVD events prevented per 100 treated over 5 years			Benefit NNT to prevent one event over 5 years		
	One intervention Estimated absolute risk reduction (ARR) 25%	Two interventions Estimated absolute risk reduction (ARR) 45%	Three interventions Estimated absolute risk reduction (ARR) 55%	One intervention 1/ARR	Two interventions 1/ARR	Three interventions 1/ARR
>30%	>8	>14	>17	<13	<7	<6
27.5	7	12	15	15	8	7
22.5	6	10	12	18	10	8
17.5	4	8	10	23	13	10
12.5	3	6	7	32	18	15
7.5	2	3	4	53	30	24
2.75	0.7	1.2	1.5	145	81	66
<2.5	<0.6	<1.1	<1.4	>160	>89	>73

Assumptions:

- A conservative estimate that each intervention: aspirin, blood pressure treatment (lowering systolic BP by 10 mm Hg) or lipid modification (lowering LDL-C by 20%) reduces cardiovascular risk by about 25% over 5 years;
- The relative risk of a CVD event over 5 years after one intervention compared to no treatment is 0.75, after two is 0.75 x 0.75, and after three is 0.75 x 0.75 x 0.75 (i.e. the risk is multiplicative).

The number needed to treat: adjusting for baseline risk

Adapted with permission from Chatellier et al, 1996[1]

BACKGROUND

The number needed to treat (NNT) to avoid a single additional adverse outcome is a meaningful way of expressing the benefit of an active treatment over a control. It can be used both to summarise the results of a therapeutic trial or series of trials and to help medical decision making about an individual patient.

If the absolute risk of adverse outcomes in a therapeutic trial is ARC in the control group and ART in the treatment group, then the absolute risk reduction (ARR) is defined as (ARC – ART). The NNT is defined as the inverse of the ARR:

$$NNT = 1/(ARC - ART)$$

Since the Relative Risk Reduction (RRR) is defined as (ARC – ART)/ARC, it follows that NNT, RRR, and ARC are related by their definitions in the following way:

$$NNT \times RRR \times ARC = 1$$

This relationship can be used to estimate the likely benefits of a treatment in populations with different levels of baseline risk (that is different levels of ARC). This allows extrapolation of the results of a trial or meta-analysis to people with different baseline risks. Ideally, there should be experimental evidence of the RRR in each population. However, in many trials, subgroup analyses show that the RRR is approximately constant in groups of patients with different characteristics. Cook and Sackett therefore proposed that decisions about individual patients could be made by using the NNT calculated from the RRR measured in trials and the baseline risk in the absence of treatment estimated for the individual patient.[2]

The method may not apply to periods of time different to that studied in the original trials.

USING THE NOMOGRAM

The nomogram shown on the next page allows the NNT to be found directly without any calculation: a straight line should be drawn from the point corresponding to the estimated absolute risk for the patient on the left hand scale to the point corresponding to the relative risk reduction stated in a trial or meta-analysis on the central scale. The intercept of this line with the right hand scale gives the NNT. By taking the upper and lower limits of the confidence interval of the RRR, the upper and lower limits of the NNT can be estimated.

REFERENCES

1. Chatellier G, Zapletal E, Lemaitre D, *et al*. The number needed to treat: a clinically useful nomogram in its proper context. *BMJ* 1996;321:426–429.
2. Cook RJ, Sackett DL. The number needed to treat: a clinically useful measure of treatment effect. *BMJ* 1995;310:452–454.

Number needed to treat

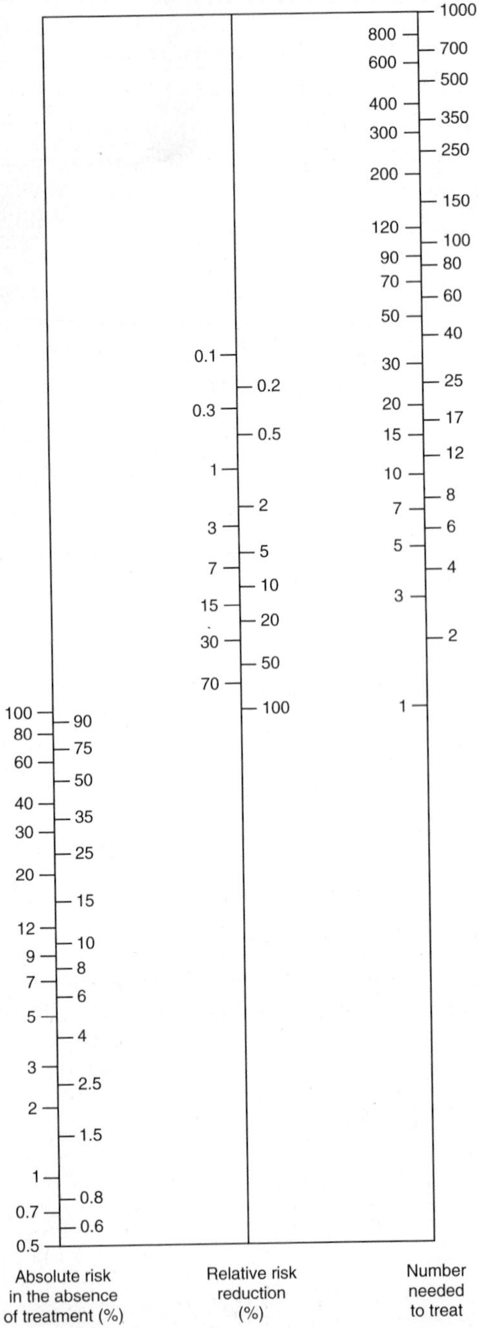

FIGURE **Nomogram for calculating the number needed to treat. Published with permission.[1]**